Pediatric Rheumatology

Pediatric Rheumatology

Edited by Leslie Schwartz

hayle medical

New York

Hayle Medical,
750 Third Avenue, 9th Floor,
New York, NY 10017, USA

Visit us on the World Wide Web at:
www.haylemedical.com

ISBN: 978-1-63241-733-6

Cataloging-in-Publication Data

Pediatric rheumatology / edited by Leslie Schwartz.
p. cm.
Includes bibliographical references and index.
ISBN 978-1-63241-733-6
1. Pediatric rheumatology. 2. Rheumatism in children. 3. Rheumatology. 4. Pediatrics.
I. Schwartz, Leslie.
RJ482.R48 P43 2019
618.920 723--dc23

Table of Contents

Preface

The autoimmune and inflammatory conditions affecting the infants, children and adolescents are called pediatric rheumatic diseases. The field of medicine dealing with such diseases is known as pediatric rheumatology. It is an important subfield of pediatrics. A specialist in this field is called a pediatric rheumatologist. Some of the common types of pediatric rheumatic diseases include juvenile rheumatoid arthritis, juvenile dermatomyositis, juvenile lupus, mixed connective tissue disease, Kawasaki disease and fibromyalgia. Juvenile rheumatoid arthritis is a type of arthritis affecting children below the age of sixteen. Juvenile dermatomyositis is a type of inflammatory condition that causes muscle weakness and skin rash. This book includes some of the vital pieces of work being conducted across the world, on various topics related to pediatric rheumatology. It strives to provide a fair idea about this discipline and to help develop a better understanding of the latest advances within this field. This book is a vital tool for all researching and studying this discipline.

Significant researches are present in this book. Intensive efforts have been employed by authors to make this book an outstanding discourse. This book contains the enlightening chapters which have been written on the basis of significant researches done by the experts.

Finally, I would also like to thank all the members involved in this book for being a team and meeting all the deadlines for the submission of their respective works. I would also like to thank my friends and family for being supportive in my efforts.

Editor

1

Outcomes of non-infectious Paediatric uveitis in the era of biologic therapy

Megan Cann[1], Athimalaipet V. Ramanan[1,2*†], Andrew Crawford[3,4], Andrew D. Dick[1,2,5,6], Sarah L. N. Clarke[1,4], Fatima Rashed[2] and Catherine M. Guly[1†]

Abstract

Background: There is a paucity of data on the ocular outcomes in paediatric non-infectious uveitis since the introduction of the biologic agents. The purpose of this study was to outline the clinical characteristics of children with non-infectious uveitis and determine the visual outcomes and ocular complication rates in the modern era.

Methods: Children with non-infectious uveitis from January 2011 to December 2015 were identified. Data was collected at baseline, 1, 3, 5, and 10 years post diagnosis. The incidence rates of visual impairment, structural ocular complications and surgical intervention were calculated. Using logistic regression the association between various baseline characteristics and later visual impairment was investigated.

Results: Of the 166 children, 60.2% ($n = 100$) had a systemic disease association. 72.9% ($n = 121$) children received methotrexate, 58 children progressed to a biologic. The incidence rates of visual acuity loss to > 0.3 LogMAR (6/12) and to ≥1.0 LogMAR (6/60) were 0.05/Eye Year (EY) and 0.01/EY, respectively. Visual outcomes in the Juvenile Idiopathic Arthritis associated Uveitis (JIA-U) and Idiopathic Uveitis cohorts were not statistically significant. Of the 293 affected eyes, posterior synechiae was the predominant complication on presentation, while cataract had the highest incidence rate (0.05/EY). On direct comparison, children with JIA-U were statistically significantly more likely to develop glaucoma while children with Idiopathic Uveitis were statistically significantly more likely to develop macular oedema.

Conclusion: One third of children received a biological therapy, reflecting increasing utilisation and importance of biological agents in the management of inflammatory conditions. Rates of visual impairment and ocular complications are an improvement on previously published data.

Keywords: Uveitis, Biologics, Paediatrics, Visual outcomes

Background

Uveitis is rare in the paediatric population, with an estimated incidence of 4.3 per 100,000 and a prevalence of 27.9 per 100,000 [1, 2] but there is a high rate of chronic disease [3]. Non-infectious uveitis accounts for between 69 and 95% of childhood uveitis [4–7]. Juvenile Idiopathic Arthritis associated Uveitis (JIA-U) makes up 41–47% of cases but equally in 28–51% of children no cause is found [7–9]. Ocular complications including cataract, glaucoma and macular oedema are reported in up to 76% of all cases of paediatric uveitis [4]. Visual impairment is common but reporting is variable making comparisons difficult. Using incidence rates of visual impairment, visual loss in children with JIA-U has been reported at 0.10/EY [10]. Other studies have reported overall rates of visual impairment in at least one affected eye between 17 and 37% and 5 year rates of 36.36 and 15.1% for visual acuity worse then 20/50 and 20/200 respectively [3, 4, 8].

Topical corticosteroids carry a risk of cataract and glaucoma [11] and increasingly early use of immunosuppressive agents is advocated in chronic non-infectious uveitis to reduce the risk of visual loss [12, 13]. Methotrexate is the most commonly prescribed immunosuppressive therapy in

* Correspondence: avramanan@hotmail.com
†Athimalaipet V. Ramanan and Catherine M. Guly contributed equally to this work.
[1]University Hospitals Bristol NHS Foundation Trust, Bristol, UK
[2]Translational Health Sciences, Bristol Medical School, Faculty of Health sciences, Bristol, UK
Full list of author information is available at the end of the article

paediatric uveitis [13], but 27–48% children do not achieve control of inflammation and 20% experience adverse events [14–16]. Use of infliximab in the management of refractory paediatric uveitis was first reported in 2005 [17]. The following year a small case series of adalimumab for paediatric uveitis was published [18]. Adalimumab was licenced for adult and paediatric non-infectious uveitis in 2016 and 2017 respectively following successful outcome of randomised controlled trials (RCTs) [19, 20].

There is a paucity of data on longer term outcomes of paediatric uveitis (including JIA-U) in the era of biologic treatment. The aim of this retrospective study is to determine the visual outcomes and ocular complications of children attending a tertiary service covering the South-West of England and the South of Wales (approximate population of 5.5 million).

Methods

Patient identification

Bristol Eye Hospital Databases were reviewed to identify all patients with uveitis. Children were included if they had been diagnosed with non-infectious uveitis prior to the age of 16 years and been managed at the Bristol Eye Hospital between January 2011and December 2015. Children referred to the service were either resident in Bristol and referred from local medical services (primary referrals) or lived outside Bristol and were referred from surrounding ophthalmology services(tertiary referrals).

Data collection

Data was collected retrospectively at standard time intervals; diagnosis, and 1, 3, 5 and 10 years. The appointment closest to the time interval was selected for analysis. Demographic data included age at diagnosis, gender and ethnicity. Clinical uveitis details included aetiology, laterality, anatomical location using Standardization of Uveitis Nomenclature (SUN) criteria [21] and structural complications. Elevated intraocular pressure (IOP) was defined as > 21 mmHg and hypotony as < 5 mmHg. Pharmacological and surgical treatments were documented. Visual acuity was recorded in logMAR. LogMAR is the logarithmic representation of visual acuity. It is the accepted standard of representing visual acuity in research as it is recognised to be more reliable, discriminative and repeatable when compared to the classic Snellen's chart [22]. Visual impairment was stratified by severity as logMAR > 0.3 (worse than 6/12) or ≥ 1.0 (6/60 or worse) [21].

Statistical analysis

The incidence rates of visual impairment and structural ocular complications were calculated for the whole population, and for the JIA-U and idiopathic uveitis cohorts. Not all patients contributed at all time points. Incidence rates were calculated per at risk eye year using longitudinal data analysis to account for variable length of follow up [23]. Year of complication onset was not recorded for 20 out of a total of 247 events (band keratopathy $n = 5$, cataracts $n = 8$, glaucoma $n = 3$, posterior synechiae $n = 1$, elevated IOP $n = 3$). A year of onset of 4 years was used for these events as this was the nearest whole year to the study cohort's mean years of follow-up (range from 3.8 to 4.5 years). The association between various baseline characteristics and later visual impairment was investigated using logistic regression (crude and adjusting for age and sex). Analyses allowed for intragroup correlation between eyes in patients with bilateral events. Analyses were performed using Stata 14 statistical software (Stata Corp, College Station, Texas).

Data collection was approved by the hospital trust and ethics committee approval was not required.

Results

Patient demographics and clinical characteristics of the 166 patients included in the study are outlined in Table 1. Of the 50 children with unilateral uveitis on presentation, 11 progressed to bilateral disease. A total of 293 affected eyes were included in the study. Baseline information was available for 234 eyes in total. 60.2% of patients had an underlying systemic disease association (Fig. 1). JIA was the primary associated systemic disease, however Tubulointerstitial Nephritis and Uveitis (TINU; 4 patients, 6 eyes), Blau (3 patients; 6 eyes), Behcet (1 patient; 1 eye) and undifferentiated inflammatory disease (1 patient; 2 eyes) was also present. Anterior uveitis was the most common form of uveitis occurring in 125 patients (75.3%). In JIA 89 out of 91 patients (97.8%) had anterior uveitis. Unfortunately time to diagnosis data was not available for the cohort. Of the 93 tertiary referral patients (i.e. referred from surrounding ophthalmology services for subspecialist opinion); 64.5, 8.6, 10.8, 6.5 and 9.7% were seen at the tertiary centre within 3 months, 1 year, 3 years, 5 years and 10 years of diagnosis respectively.

Medications are recorded in Table 1. The first line systemic immunosuppressive agent for all children was methotrexate. Of the 166 patients, 39 (23.5%) children received additional conventional DMARD therapy; either as monotherapy or in combination with Methotrexate (20/91 JIA patients, 17/66 idiopathic uveitis patients and 2/9 patients with other systemic diseases). 58 children (34.4%) received a biologic agent and 14 children (8.4%) required ≥2 biologics over the follow up period. No child received a biologic agent at baseline. Biologics were more likely to be delivered to children with JIA-U (43 children; 47.3%) than those with idiopathic uveitis (10 children; 15.2%). 7 (10.6%) children with idiopathic uveitis did not require treatment ($p = < 0.001$).

A total of 678 person years and 1216 eye years (EY) of follow up were available. For the total population the

Table 1 Patient Demographic and Clinical Characteristics

	Cohort (%)	JIA (%)	Other Associated Systemic Disease(%)	Idiopathic (%)
No. of Patients	166	91 (54.8)	9 (5.4)	66 (39.8)
Female	99 (59.6)	62 (68.1)	2 (22.2)	35 (53)
Age at diagnosis				
Average	8.03y	5.9y	10.5y	10.7y
Median	7y	5y	12y	11y
Referral type				
Tertiary	93 (56)	56 (61.5)	6 (66.7)	31 (47)
Ethnicity				
Caucasian	128 (77.1)	73(80.2)	6 (66.7)	49 (74.2)
Asian	8 (4.8)	2 (2.2)	2 (22.2)	4 (6)
African	1 (0.6)	0	0	1 (1.5)
Other	7 (4.2)	2 (2.2)	1 (11.1)	4 (6)
Unknown	22 (13.3)	14 (15.4)	0	8 (12.1)
Laterality on presentation				
Bilateral	116 (69.9)	62 (68.1)	5 (55.6)	49 (74.2)
Anatomic Localisation				
Anterior	125 (75.3)	89 (97.8)	5 (55.6)	31 (47)
Intermediate	29 (17.5)	0	1 (11.1)	28 (42.4)
Posterior	1 (0.6)	0	0	1 (1.5)
Panuveitis	11 (6.6)	2 (2.2)	3 (33.3)	6 (9.1)
Visual Impairment at baseline (per eye)				
> 0.3logMAR	43 (18.4)	22 (18.6)	3 (27.3)	18 (17.1)
≥ 1.0 logMAR	10 (4.3)	7 (5.9)	0	3 (2.9)
Medication use over study				
Corticosteroids				
Topical CS	155 (93.4)	91 (100)	8 (88.9)	56 (84.8)
Systemic CS	58 (34.9)	28 (30.8)	7 (77.8)	23 (34.8)
Peri/Intraocular Steroids	12 (7.2)	6 (6.6)	3 (33.3)	6 (9.1)
Conventional DMARD	121 (72.9)	82 (90.1)	6 (66.7)	33 (50)
Methotrexate	121 (72.9)	82 (90.1)	6 (66.7)	33 (50)
Only Methotrexate	47 (28.3%)	35 (38.5)	1 (11.1)	11 (16.7)
Mycophenolate mofetil	36 (21.7)	19 (20.9)	2 (22.2)	15 (22.7)
Tacrolimus	6 (3.6)	3 (3.3)	0	3 (4.5)
Ciclosporin	3 (1.8)	2 (2.2)	0	1 (1.5)
Biologics	58 (34.9)	43 (47.3)	5 (55.6)	10 (15.2)
Adalimumab	52 (31.3)	38 (41.8)	5 (55.6)	9 (13.6)
Infliximab	19 (11.4)	14 (15.4)	4 (44.4)	1 (1.5)
Abatacept	3 (1.8)	3 (1.8)	0	0
Tocilizumab	2 (1.2)	2 (1.2)	0	0

At presentation 118 eyes JIA, 11 other associated systemic diseases and 105 idiopathic

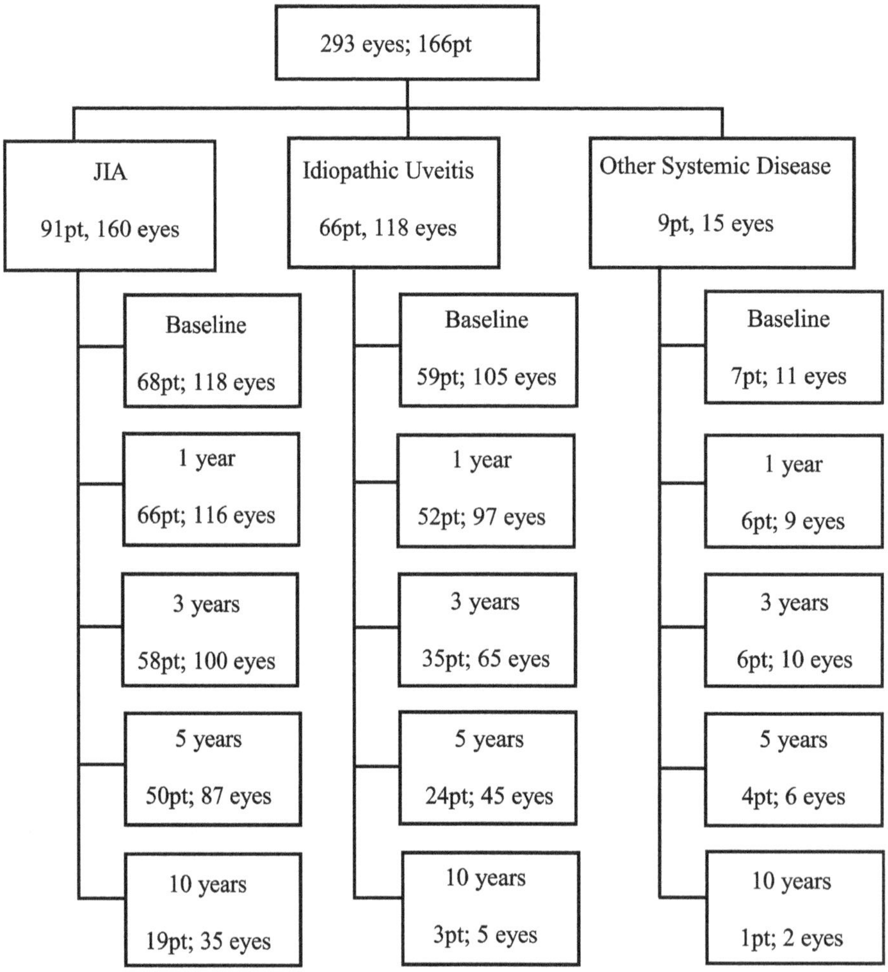

Fig. 1 Data Available at Standard Time Intervals Detailed information of the number of patients and affected eyes per aetiology at baseline, 1 year, 3 years, 5 years and 10 years post diagnosis

median duration of follow up was 5 years. Children with JIA-U had a longer duration of follow up when compared to children with idiopathic uveitis (median 5 years vs 3 years). Availability of follow up data is outlined in Fig. 1. 34 children contributed only 1 visit; the majority of these children (21 children) were tertiary referrals seen at least 1 year post diagnosis. The median number of evaluation visits per patient was 3. Rates of complications at presentation and incidence rates of newly diagnosed complications are summarised in Table 2. The rates of visual acuity loss over the period of observation to > 0.3 LogMAR and to ≥1.0 LogMAR among affected eyes were 0.05/EY and 0.01/EY, respectively. At presentation 81/234 eyes (34.6%) had at least one ocular uveitis associated complication, of which posterior synechiae was the most common (43 eyes; 18.4%). The rate of newly diagnosed band keratopathy and posterior synchiae was 0.02/EY. Children with JIA-U were more likely to develop raised IOP ($p = 0.05$) and glaucoma ($p = 0.002$) when compared to children with idiopathic uveitis, while children with idiopathic uveitis were more likely to developed macular oedema ($p = 0.01$) over the period of follow up. Cataract was the frequent complication to occur over the follow up period with an incidence rate of 0.05/EY.Three eyes (3 children) had amblyopia. All three eyes had visual impairment, 2 eyes had ≥1.0 logMAR and one had > 0.3logMAR. There was no statistical difference between the rate of visual impairment between children with anterior uveitis versus children with intermediate uveitis. The incidence rate of visual impairment > 0.3 logMAR for anterior uveitis was 0.04/EY (CI95% 0.03–0.06) compared to 0.05/EY (CI95% 0.02–0.11) for children with intermediate uveitis ($p = 0.80$). No child with intermediate uveitis developed a visual impairment of ≥1.0logMAR over the study period whereas the incidence in children with anterior uveitis was 0.01/EY (CI95% 0.01–0.02) ($p = 0.13$). Additionally, there was no significant difference between rates of visual impairment in those children with JIA-U anterior uveitis and non-JIA-U anterior uveitis. Children with JIA-U

Table 2 Complication Incidence Rates

	Total Cohort			JIA-Uveitis			Idiopathic Uveitis			
	Eyes On Presentation $n = 234$^ (%)	n/EY*	Incidence Rate/EY (CI 95%)	Eyes On Presentation $n = 118$^ (%)	n/EY	Incidence Rate/EY (CI 95%)	Eyes On Presentation $n = 105$^ (%)	n/EY	Incidence Rate/EY (CI 95%)	IU vs JIA-U Incidence $p = 0.05$
Visual Impairment										
> 0.3 LogMAR	43 (18.4%)	39/830	0.05 (0.03–0.06)	22 (18.6%)	27/529	0.05 (0.04–0.07)	18 (17.1%)	11/260	0.04 (0.02–0.08)	0.69
≥ 1.0 LogMAR	10 (4.3%)	14/1034	0.01 (0.01–0.02)	7 (5.9%)	10/652	0.02 (0.01–0.03)	3 (2.9%)	2/335	0.01 (0.00–0.02)	0.15
Ocular Complication										
Cataract	17 (7.3%)	47/939	0.05 (0.04–0.07)	11 (9.3%)	31/578	0.05 (0.04–0.08)	5 (4.8%)	12/317	0.04 (0.02–0.07)	0.24
Raised IOP	19 (8.1)	22/986	0.02 (0.02–0.04)	13 (11%)	17/606	0.03 (0.02–0.05)	6 (5.7%)	3/327	0.01 (0.00–0.03)	**0.05**
Glaucoma	0	15/1062	0.01 (0.01–0.02)	0	15/657	0.02 (0.01–0.04)	0	0/352		**0.002**
Posterior Synechiae	43 (18.4%)	21/860	0.02 (0.02–0.04)	23 (19.5%)	17/524	0.03 (0.02–0.05)	18 (17.1%)	4/296	0.01 (0.01–0.04)	0.14
Macular Oedema	7 (3%)	14/1027	0.01 (0.01–0.02)	3 (2.5%)	4/681	0.01 (0.00–0.02)	4 (3.8%)	9/293	0.02 (0.02–0.06)	**0.01**
Band Keratopathy	19 (8.1%)	20/938	0.02 (0.01–0.03)	15 (12.7%)	12/586	0.02 (0.01–0.04)	3 (2.9%)	6/314	0.02 (0.01–0.04)	0.77
Hypotony	4 (1.7%)	3/1084	0.00 (0.00–0.01)	3 (2.5%)	2/686	0.00 (0.00–0.01)	1 (1%)	0/347		0.31
Optic Disc Swelling	23 (9.8%)	3/1012	0.00 (0.00–0.01)	2 (1.7%)	2/690	0.00 (0.00–0.01)	19 (18.1%)	1/279	0.00 (0.00–0.03)	0.81
Vitreous Haemorrhage	0	1/1108	0.00 (0.00–0.01)	0	1/703	0.00 (0.00–0.01)	0	0/352		0.68
Epiretinal Membrane	1 (0.4%)	1/1107	0.00 (0.00–0.01)	0	0/707	0.00	1 (1%)	0/349		0.68
Surgical Procedure										
Cataract Removal	2 (0.9%)	22/1038	0.02 (0.01–0.03)	2 (1.7%)	18/639	0.03 (0.02–0.04)	0	3/350	0.01 (0.00–0.03)	**0.04**
Trabeculectomy	0	11/1087	0.01 (0.01–0.02)	0	11/682	0.02 (0.01–0.03)	0	0/352		**0.01**
Vitrectomy	2 (0.9%)	8/1074	0.01 (0.00–0.01)	2 (1.7%)	4/673	0.01 (0.00–0.02)	0	4/348	0.01 (0.00–0.03)	0.32
Laser Capsulotomy	0	3/1112	0.00 (0.00–0.01)	0	3/707	0.00 (0.00–0.01)	0	0/352		0.32
Iridectomy	0	2/1107	0.00 (0.00–0.01)	0	2/702	0.00 (0.00–0.01)	0	0/352		0.47

*n/EY – Number of new events/Number of Eye Years of Follow up

^ Within the cohort 293 eyes were affected. However, not all children had baseline presentation data available anterior uveitis had an incidence rate of visual impairment > 0.3logMAR of 0.05/EY (CI95% 0.03–0.07) compared to 0.02/EY (CI95% 0.01–0.07) in the non-JIA-U anterior group ($p = 0.19$). The rate of visual impairment ≥1.0logMAR between the JIA-U anterior uveitis and the non-JIA-U anterior uveitis cohort was 0.01/EY (CI95% 0.00–0.05) and 0.01/EY (CI95% 0.01–0.03) respectively ($p = 0.5$).

Surgical procedures were required in 38 eyes and in some cases one eye received multiple procedures. Cataract extraction was the most common procedure, performed in 24 eyes (0.9% within 3 months of presentation; Incidence rate 0.02/EY). 20 eyes received an intraocular lens implant and 3 remained aphakic. Lens insertion data was not available for 1 eye. Trabeculectomy was required in 11 eyes (0.01/EY) and vitrectomy in 10 eyes (0.9% within 3 months of presentation; 0.01/EY). Indication for vitrectomy is as follows; uncontrolled inflammation despite aggressive therapy (3 eyes), vitreal debris (3 eyes), cyclitic membrane (1 eye) and undocumented reasons (3 eyes) Patients with JIA were more likely to require cataract removal and trabeculectomy than those with idiopathic uveitis ($p = 0.04$ and $p = 0.01$ respectively) over the period of follow up. Two children required an enucleation at 5 and 10 years follow up. Both eyes had severe sight loss and required removal due to chronic pain.

Using logistic regression, demographic and clinical characteristics on presentation were analysed to determine whether they were predictive of visual impairment. These characteristics are detailed in Table 3. Tertiary referral patients were statistically more likely to develop a visual impairment of logMAR > 0.3 ($p = 0.03$) and ≥ 1.0 ($p = 0.05$). The presence of posterior synechiae at presentation was also a risk factor for visual impairment ≥1.0 logMAR ($p = 0.01$).

Discussion

We report a large cohort of children with non-infectious uveitis managed in a UK tertiary unit. Use of systemic immunosuppression was high with 72.9% of children receiving methotrexate and 34.9% receiving a biologic agent. The recent publication of the SYCAMORE trial [20] has supported the efficacy of rapid escalation to biologics in the management of children with JIA-U refractory to conventional immunosuppressive therapy.

Despite published evidence that up to 73% of children experience improvement in intraocular inflammation with methotrexate [14], in this population methotrexate refractory disease was common. Of the 121 children

Table 3 Patient Risk Factors at Baseline for Visual Impairment

	Risk of Visual Impairment > 0.3logMAR		Risk of Visual Impairment ≥1.0 logMAR	
	OR (95%CI)	p (0.05)		p (0.05)
Demographics				
Age at uveitis diagnosis	0.97 (0.87–1.08)	0.56	1.02 (0.88–1.19)	0.76
Bilateral Disease	1.23 (0.46–3.34)	0.68	0.45 (0.12–1.65)	0.23
Female	1.43 (0.61–3.36)	0.41	1.24 (0.38–4.12)	0.72
Tertiary Referral	2.71 (1.12–6.56)	0.03	4.59 (0.98–21.47)	0.05
Aetiology				
JIA	2.05 (0.88–4.77)	0.10	2.15 (0.62–7.43)	0.23
Idiopathic	0.54 (0.23–1.29)	0.16	0.23 (0.05–1.09)	0.07
Uveitis Characteristics				
Anterior Uveitis	0.89 (0.37–2.14)	0.80	0.89 (0.26–3.07)	0.85
Bilateral Disease	1.23 (0.46–3.34)	0.68	0.45 (0.12–1.65)	0.23
Complications at Baseline				
Band keratopathy	1.24 (0.24–6.37)	0.80	1.12 (0.15–8.53)	0.92
Cataracts	1.43 (0.29–6.99)	0.66	5.16 (0.91–29.23)	0.06
Posterior synechiae	0.84 (0.26–2.71)	0.77	4.91 (1.38–17.39)	0.01
Elevated IOP	0.35 (0.05–2.51)	0.29	1.00	
Macular oedema	1.09 (0.12–10.07)	0.94	1.00	
Hypotony	2.20 (0.19–25.31)	0.53	7.08 (0.64–78.00)	0.11
Optic disc swelling	0.98 (0.29–3.30)	0.97	2.05 (0.47–8.88)	0.34

started on methotrexate, 58 (47.9%) required third line therapy in the form of one or more biologic agent. Tertiary referral patients were 1.6 times more likely to be treated with a biologic when compared to primary referral patients (41.9% vs 26%). This difference was statistically significant ($p = 0.03$). Children with an associated systemic disease were statistically more likely to receive a biologic than those with idiopathic uveitis (48% vs 15.2% $p = < 0.001$). However the rates of visual impairment were similar in the JIA-U and idiopathic uveitis cohorts and so the difference in treatment may represent a milder disease course of idiopathic uveitis or the longer median duration of follow up of the JIA-U cohort. Overall rates of biologic use are higher than previous reports. The rate of biologic use in the idiopathic uveitis cohort (15.2%) is slightly lower than reported in Sardar et al. [24] where 21% of patients required third line therapy. However, the proportion of children with idiopathic panuveitis and posterior uveitis was slightly higher in the French cohort, which may explain the slightly higher rate of biologic use. In 2007 Saurenmann et al. [25] reported that 11% of children with JIA-U received an anti-TNF agent but over the last 10 years biologics have become more widely available and accepted practice for refractory JIA-U.

Visual outcomes in this cohort are an improvement on previously published data. Thorne et al. [10] reported in a population of children with JIA-U rates of visual impairment of 6/15 or worse (≥0.4 logMAR) and 6/60 or worse (≥1.0 logMAR) of 0.10/UEY and 0.08/EY respectively. In our study, the incidence rate of visual impairment in those children with JIA-U was 0.05/EY (> 0.3logMAR) and 0.02/EY (≥1.0logMAR). While JIA-U had a higher incidence rate of visual impairment compared to idiopathic uveitis, the difference was not significant. Comparison between rates of ocular complications within our study population and previous published data is outlined in Table 4. In this study eight children developed bilateral visual impairment > 0.3 logMAR and only one child had bilateral visual impairment ≥1.0logMAR at final documented contact.

Uncertainties remain on the optimum time to initiate systemic therapy and the duration of systemic treatments for children with uveitis as well as the visual outcomes of those children with uveitis moving on to adulthood. Evidence for biologic treatments other than Adalimumab remains limited in childhood uveitis. A trial of subcutaneous tocilizumab for JIA-U is currently underway which hopefully will provide further evidence for the use of IL-6 blockade (APTITUDE) [26]. Biologic agents are expensive and carry an increased risk of infection and other side effects [27–30] which needs to be balanced against the potential benefits in reducing sight loss. We also recognise the burden to children and their families managing frequent hospital appointments, eye drops and immunosuppression regimes. Even in the absence of long term complications, uveitis can have emotional and psychological consequences for the child and family encompassing anxiety, anger and fear of the future [31].

As a retrospective study we acknowledge certain limitations to the study. The duration of follow up within the patient cohort was unequal in some cases, and as a result data is not available for all patients at all time points. Additionally, in a tertiary centre there may be overrepresentation of severe cases, and children who had mild disease may have not had been included as they are no longer managed by the service. Unfortunately therapy adverse events were not captured in this study. The era of biologic therapy has brought improvements in visual outcomes for children with uveitis but

Table 4 JIA-U Ocular Outcomes per affected eyes

	JIA -U				Idiopathic Uveitis/Pars Plantis			
	Current Study ($n = 91$)	Tugal-Tutkun [9] 1996 ($n = 100$)	Kadayifçilar [33] 2003 ($n = 55$)	Kump7 2005 ($n = 165$)	Current Study (n = 118)	Tugal-Tutkun[9] 1996 ($n = 88$)	Kadayifçilar [33] 2003 ($n = 134$)	Kump[7] 2005 ($n = 202$)
Cataract	42 (26.3%)	71 (71%)	16 (32.7%)	105 (64%)	17 (14.4%)	33 (37.5%)	41 (30.6%)	60 (29.6%)
Glaucoma	15 (9.4%)	30 (30%)	1 (2%)	33 (20%)	0	2 (2.3%)	7 (5.2%)	29 (14.4%)
Band Keratopathy	27 (16.9%)	66 (66%)	5 (10%)	76 (46%)	9 (7.6%)	16 (18.2%)	13 (9.7%)	24 (11.9%)
Post. Synechiae	40 (25%)	–	–	96 (58%)	22 (18.6%)	–	–	49 (24.3%)
Optic Disc Swelling	4 (2.5%)	6 (6%)	1 (2%)	5 (3%)	20 (16.9%)	10 (11.4%)	6 (4.5%)	14 (6.9%)
Hypotony	5 (3.1%)	19 (19%)	3 (5.5%)	17 (10%)	1 (0.8%)	2 (2.3%)	1 (0.7%)	1 (0.5%)
Macular Oedema	7 (4.4%)	–	–	–	13 (11%)	–	–	–
Vitreous Haemorrhage	1 (0.6%)	3 (3%)	0	0	0	8 (5%)	2 (1.5%)	3 (1.5%)
Epiretina Membranel	0	–	1 (2%)	17 (10%)	1 (0.8%)	–	–	20 (9.9%)

there is still potential for ongoing improvement in outcomes in the future.

Improved visual outcomes may be a result of a combination of factors. New therapies are capable of controlling inflammation refractory to conventional immunosuppressive therapy [20]. However clinical practice has evolved over the past decade to include robust and audited JIA uveitis screening standards [32], early treatment and close monitoring of affected children within a multidisciplinary team. The establishment of a combined paediatric rheumatology and uveitis clinic with specialist nurses at the Bristol Eye Hospital has been crucial in providing timely and effective monitoring and management for children with complex uveitis. The implementation of these practices may have contributed to improved outcomes.

Conclusion

This study has demonstrated an encouraging improvement in the rate of ocular complications and visual impairment in children with non-infectious uveitis when compared to previous publications. Notably, the rate of biologic use was high (34.9%), reflecting their increasing importance in modern immunomodulation. Visual outcomes between the JIA-U and idiopathic uveitis cohorts were not significant. Cataract development was the most common ocular complication within the cohort.

Abbreviations

CI: Confidence Interval; DMARD: Disease Modifying Antirheumatic Drug; EY: Eye Year; IOP: Intraocular Pressure; JIA: Juvenile Idiopathic Arthritis; JIA-U: Juvenile Idiopathic Arthritis associated Uveitis; mmHg: Millimeter of mercury; Pt: Patient; RCT: Randomised Control Trial; SUN: Standardization of Uveitis Nomenclature; TINU: Tubulointerstitial Nephritis and Uveitis

Authors' contributions

MC engaged in data collection, data analysis and interpretation and drafting of the submitted article, AVR was involved in the conception and design of the study, data interpretation and engaged in critical revision of the article, AC provided statistical analysis of the data and engaged in critical revision of the article,.AD was involved in the conception and design of the study, data interpretation and engaged in critical revision of the article, SC was involved in the conception and design of the study, data interpretation and engaged in critical revision of the article, FR engaged in data collection and study design,CG was involved in the conception and design of the study, data interpretation and engaged in critical revision of the article, All authors read and approved the final manuscript.

Competing interests

MC has received financial support from Abbvie to attend one conference, AD has received consultancy for Abbvie, Sanofi, Gyroscope, Roche. AVR has received honoria from Abbvie and is Co-Chief Investigator of Sycamore Study which was funded by NIHR and Arthritis Research UK. CG has received fees from Abbvie SC, FR, and AC have no conflicts to declare.

Author details

[1]University Hospitals Bristol NHS Foundation Trust, Bristol, UK. [2]Translational Health Sciences, Bristol Medical School, Faculty of Health sciences, Bristol, UK. [3]BHF Centre for Cardiovascular Science, Queen's Medical Research Institute, University of Edinburgh, Edinburgh, UK. [4]MRC Integrative Epidemiology Unit, Population Health Sciences, University of Bristol, Bristol, UK. [5]National Institute for Health Research (NIHR) Biomedical Research Centre at Moorfield Eye Hospital, London, UK. [6]University College London Institute of Ophthalmology, London, UK.

References

1. Päivönsalo-Hietanen T, Tuominen J, Saari KM. Uveitis in children: population-based study in Finland. Acta Ophthalmol Scand. 2000 Feb; 78(1):84–8.
2. Zierhut M, Michels H, Stubiger N, Besch D, Deuter C, Heiligenhaus A. Uveitis in Children. Int Ophthalmol Clin. 2005 Spring;45(2):135–56.
3. Smith JA, Mackensen F, Sen HN, Leigh JF, Watkins AS, Pyatetsky D, Tessler HH, Nussenblatt RB, Rosenbaum JT, Reed GF, Vitale S, Smith JR, Goldstein DA. Epidemiology and course of disease in childhood uveitis. Ophthalmology. 2009 Aug;116(8):1544–51.
4. de Boer J, Wulffraat N, Rothova A. Visual loss in uveitis of childhood. Br J. Ophthalmol. 2003;87:879–84.
5. Hettinga YM, de Groot-Mijnes JD, Rothova A, de Boer JH. Infectious involvement in a tertiary center pediatric uveitis cohort. Br J Ophthalmol. 2015;99(1):103–7.
6. Paroli MP, Spinucci G, Liverani M, Monte R, Pezzi PP. Uveitis in childhood: an Italian clinical and epidemiological study. Ocul Immunol Inflamm. 2009; 17(4):238–42.
7. Kump LI, Cervantes-Castaneda RA, Androudi SN, Foster CS. Analysis of pediatric uveitis cases at a tertiary referral center. Ophthalmology. 2005; 112(7):1287–92.
8. Edelsten C, Reddy MA, Stanford MR, Graham EM. Visual loss associated with pediatric uveitis in English primary and referral centers. Am J Ophthalmol. 2003;135(5):676–80.
9. Tugal-Tutkun I, Havrlikova K, Power WJ, Foster CS. Changing patterns in uveitis of childhood. Ophthalmology. 1996;103(3):375–83.
10. Thorne JE, Woreta F, Kedhar SR, Dunn JP, Jabs DA. Juvenile idiopathic arthritis-associated uveitis: incidence of ocular complications and visual acuity loss. Am J Ophthalmol. 2007;143(5):840–6.
11. Thorne JE, Woreta FA, Dunn JP, Jabs DA. Risk of cataract development among children with juvenile idiopathic arthritis-related uveitis treated with topical corticosteroids. Ophthalmology. 2010 Jul;117(7):1436–41.
12. Sen ES, Dick AD, Ramanan AV. Uveitis associated with juvenile idiopathic arthritis. Nat Rev Rheumatol. 2015 Jun;11(6):338–48.
13. Heiligenhaus A, Michels H, Schumacher C, Kopp I, Neudorf U, Niehues T, et al. Evidence-based, interdisciplinary guidelines for anti-inflammatory treatment of uveitis associated with juvenile idiopathic arthritis. Rheumatol Int. 2012;32(5):1121–33.
14. Simonini G, Paudyal P, Jones G, Cimaz R, Macfarlane G. Current evidence of methotrexate efficacy in childhood chronic uveitis: a systematic review and meta-analysis approach. Rheumatology. 2013;2013(52):825–31.
15. Gangaputra S, Newcomb CW, Liesegang TL, Kacmaz RO, Jabs DA, LevyClarke GA, Nussenblatt RB, Rosenbaum JT, Suhler EB, Thorne JE, Foster CS, Kempen JH. Methotrexate for ocular inflammatory diseases. Ophthalmology. 2009;116:2188–98.
16. Samson CM, Waheed N, Baltatzis S, Foster CS. Methotrexate therapy for chronic noninfectious uveitis: analysis of a case series of 160 patients. Ophthalmology. 2001;108(6):1134–9.
17. Richards JC, Tay-Kearney ML, Murray K, Manners P. Infliximab for juvenile idiopathic arthritis-associated uveitis. Clin Exp Ophthalmol. 2005;33(5):461–8.
18. Vazquez-Cobian LB, Flynn T, Lehman TJ. Adalimumab therapy for childhood uveitis. J Pediatr. 2006 Oct;149(4):572–5.
19. Jaffe GJ, Dick AD, Brézin AP, Nguyen QD, Thorne JE, Kestelyn P, Barisani-Asenbauer T, Franco P, Heiligenhaus A, Scales D, Chu DS, Camez A, Kwatra NV, Song AP, Kron M, Tari S, Suhler EB. Adalimumab in patients with active noninfectious uveitis. N Engl J Med. 2016 Sep 8;375(10):932–43.
20. Ramanan AV, Dick AD, Jones AP, McKay A, Williamson PR, Compeyrot-Lacassagne S, Hardwick B, Hickey H, Hughes D, Woo P, Benton D, Edelsten C, Beresford MW, SYCAMORE Study Group. N Engl J Med. 2017;376(17):1637–46.

21. Jabs DA, Nussenblatt RB, Rosenbaum JT; Standardization of uveitis nomenclature (SUN) working group. Standardization of uveitis nomenclature for reporting clinical data. Results of the first international workshop. Am J Ophthalmol 2005;140(3):509–516.
22. Elliott DB. The good (logMAR), the bad (Snellen) and the ugly (BCVA, number of letters read) of visual acuity measurement. Ophthalmic Physiol Opt. July;36(4):355–8.
23. Jabs DA. Improving the reporting of clinical case series. Am J Ophthalmol. 2005;139(5):900–5.
24. Sardar E, Dusser P, Rousseau A, Bodaghi B, Labetoulle M, Koné-Paut I. Retrospective study evaluating treatment decisions and outcomes of childhood uveitis not associated with juvenile idiopathic arthritis. J Pediatr. 2017;186:131–7.
25. Saurenmann RK, Levin AV, Feldman BM, Rose JB, Laxer RM, Schneider R, Silverman ED. Prevalence, risk factors, and outcome of uveitis in juvenile idiopathic arthritis: a long-term followup study. Arthritis Rheum. 2007;56(2):647–57.
26. A phase II trial of tocilizumab in anti-TNF refractory patients with JIA associated uveitis (APTITUDE study) [Internet]. BioMed Central. 2015 [cited 22 Dec 2015]. Available from: http://www.isrctn.com/ISRCTN95363507.
27. Davies R, Southwood TR, Kearsley-Fleet L, Lunt M, Hyrich KL. British Society for Paediatric and Adolescent Rheumatology Etanercept Cohort Study. Medically significant infections are increased in patients with juvenile idiopathic arthritis treated with etanercept: results from the British Society for Paediatric and Adolescent Rheumatology Etanercept Cohort Study. Arthritis Rheum. 2015;67(9):2487–94.
28. Beukelman T, Xie F, Chen L, Baddley JW, Delzell E, Grijalva CG, et al. Rates of hospitalized bacterial infection associated with juvenile idiopathic arthritis and its treatment. Arthritis Rheum. 2012;64(8):2773–80.
29. Beukelman T, Xie F, Baddley J, Chen L, Mannion ML, Saag KG, Zhang J, Curtis JR. The Risk of Hospitalized Infection Following Initiation of Biologic Agents Versus Methotrexate in the Treatment of Juvenile Idiopathic Arthritis. Arthritis Res Ther. 2016;18:210.
30. Lee HH, Song IH, Friedrich M, Gauliard A, Detert J, Röwert J, Audring H, Kary S, Burmester GR, Sterry W, Worm M. Cutaneous side-effects in patients with rheumatic diseases during application of tumour necrosis factor-alpha antagonists. Br J Dermatol. 2007 Mar;156(3):486–91.
31. Sen ES, Morgan MJ, MacLeod R, Strike H, Hinchcliffe A, Dick AD, Muthusamy B, Ramanan AV. Cross sectional, qualitative thematic analysis of patient perspectives of disease impact in juvenile idiopathic arthritis-associated uveitis. Pediatr Rheumatol Online J. 2017;15(1):58.
32. BSPAR and RCOphth Guidelines for screening for uveitis in juvenile idiopathic arthritis 2006 http://www.bspar.org.uk/downloads/clinical_guidelines/BSPAR_guidelines_eye_screening_2006.pdf
33. Kadayifçilar S, Eldem B, Tumer B. Uveitis in childhood. J Pediatr Ophthalmol Strabismus. 2003;40(6):335–40.

2

Amendment of the OMERACT ultrasound definitions of joints' features in healthy children when using the DOPPLER technique

P. Collado[1*], D. Windschall[2], J. Vojinovic[3], S. Magni-Manzoni[4], P. Balint[5], G. A. W. Bruyn[6], C. Hernandez-Diaz[7], J. C. Nieto[8], V. Ravagnani[9], N. Tzaribachev[10], A. Iagnocco[11], M. A. D'Agostino[12], E. Naredo[13] and on behalf of the OMERACT ultrasound subtask force on pediatric

Abstract

Background: Recently preliminary ultrasonography (US) definitions, in B mode, for normal components of pediatric joints have been developed by the OMERACT US group. The aim of the current study was to include Doppler findings in the evaluation and definition of normal joint features that can be visualized in healthy children at different age groups.

Methods: A multistep approach was used. Firstly, new additional definitions of joint components were proposed during an expert meeting. In the second step, these definitions, along with the preliminary B-mode-US definitions, were tested for feasibility in an exercise in healthy children at different age groups. In the last step, a larger panel of US experts were invited to join a web-based consensus process in order to approve the developed definitions using the Delphi methodology. A Likert scale of 1–5 was used to assess agreement.

Results: Physiological vascularity and fat pad tissue were identified and tested as two additional joint components in healthy children. Since physiological vascularity changes over the time in the growing skeleton, the final definition of Doppler findings comprised separate statements instead of a single full definition. A total of seven statements was developed and included in a written Delphi questionnaire to define and validate the new components. The final definitions for fat pad and physiological vascularity agreed by the group of experts reached 92.9% and 100% agreement respectively in a web survey.

Conclusion: The inclusion of these two additional joints components which are linked to detection of Doppler signal in pediatric healthy joints will improve the identification of abnormalities in children with joint pathologies.

Keywords: Ultrasonography, Power-Doppler, Pediatric rheumatology, Joint anatomy

Background

Musculoskeletal ultrasonography (US) has been shown to be a reliable, widely available, and child-friendly technique in the routine practice, particularly to detect joint inflammation in children with juvenile idiopathic arthritis (JIA) [1–5]. In adults with rheumatoid arthritis, both grey-scale (GS) and power Doppler (PD) US have been shown to be sensitive to change and predictive of developing arthritis and radiographic structural damage [6]. However, despite its great utility in adults, a systematic review concluded that the basis for the use of US in pediatric rheumatology has not been established yet [7]. In fact, the review showed that very few publications collected information on PD US. Given the unique anatomy of the growing child, it was not surprising that questions related to the presence of joint Doppler signals in the pediatric population were more difficult to answer than in adults. Moreover, several studies have shown that Doppler

* Correspondence: paxko10@gmail.com
[1]Hospital Universitario Severo Ochoa., Madrid, Spain
Full list of author information is available at the end of the article

signal within joints is detectable in healthy children [8, 9]. To understand it, we have to take into account that normal growth and ossification in the developing skeleton is intimately related to the vascularity of the unossified epiphyseal and physeal cartilage [10–14] (Fig. 1).

The Outcome Measures in Rheumatology (OMERACT) US Pediatric Task Force was formed to standardize the use of US in juvenile arhritis. It has developed preliminary B-mode US definitions (or GS-US definitions) for joint components in healthy children [15], as well as, a standardized US scanning procedure specifically adapted to children [9]. However, vascularity of the unossified epiphyseal and physeal cartilage has not been described in detail yet [15]. At that point, some obstacles have been found (i.e., the features of this imaging modality, operator-dependent on expert and equipment, and the unclear terminology that is used to refer to physis, also known as "the growth plate" or "the epiphyseal growth plate") [10–15].

Besides unossified cartilage, fat pads, particularly in the knee and ankle joints, can show Doppler signal (physiological vascularity). Small masses of fat are enveloped by the fibers of the joint capsule, which separate the fat pads from the synovial lining, making the fat pads intracapsular and extrasynovial in location. This anatomic arrangement is the basis for understanding the role of fat pad in development of inflammation at joint level [16, 17] (Fig. 2).

To describe the vascularity in healthy joints and develop its definition to add to the preliminary B-mode US definitions of joint components, would therefore improve the performance of US as an outcome measure in JIA clinical trials.

Methods

Study design

The new additional definitions were developed through a Delphi process involving three steps (Additional file 1 shows the workflow outlining the consensus process to develop and validate the new additional definitions). It was based on the OMERACT methodology previously described [15].

The first step was a face-to-face meeting among ten US experts in Germany. Most of them have been involved in development of the previous B-mode US definitions [15]. The aim was to identify the relevant joint components showing Doppler signal and the terminology used to describe them with the objective to use the results of this first step to draft actual definitions. The group reviewed and discussed a set of US images from pediatric healthy joints and literature review focusing on the vascularity of the unossified epiphyseal cartilage and fat pad [9–14, 18–20]. This set comprised 40 representative US images (12 knees, 12 ankles, 10 wrists, 6 metacarpophalangeal joints) of variously aged children from previous studies [9]. Several questions regarding PD findings located in the unossified epiphyseal and physeal cartilage and fat pad of the joint were discussed in order to plan the Delphi process. While ephyseal cartilage can be detected in the four joints, finger joint does not contain fat pad. Given that the secondary ossification centre fills in and replaces epiphyseal cartilage in bone throughout the growth of child, the process of ossification in the joint was analysed because of its relevance in the definition of the PD findings detected. The second step was to test the applicability of the previous B-mode and new PD-mode proposed US definitions (i.e., non-

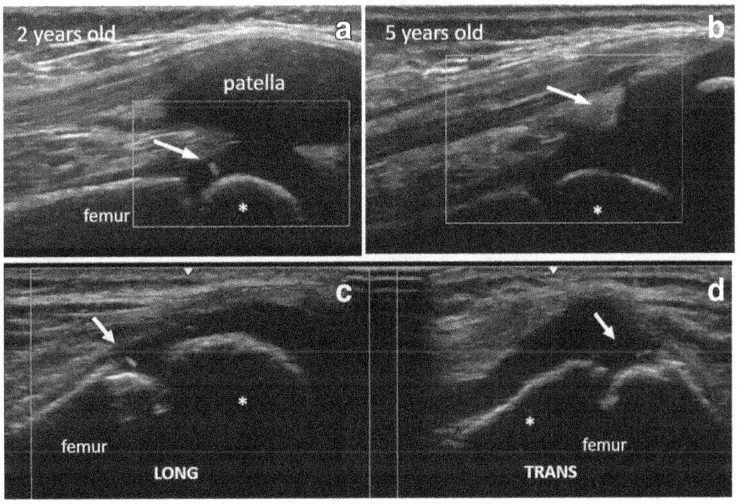

Fig. 1 US images show normal anatomy of the knee joint. The upper images (**a**, **b**). We see the distal epiphyseal end of the femur with its secondary ossification centre (asterisk). Note a physiological vessel (arrow) in the epiphyseal cartilage of the femoral condyle (**a**) and in the quadriceps fat pad (**b**). Every vessel should be proved in longitudinal (**c**) and transverse view (**d**)

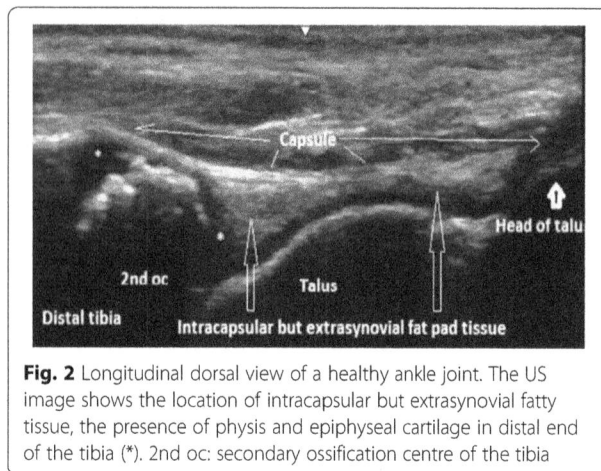

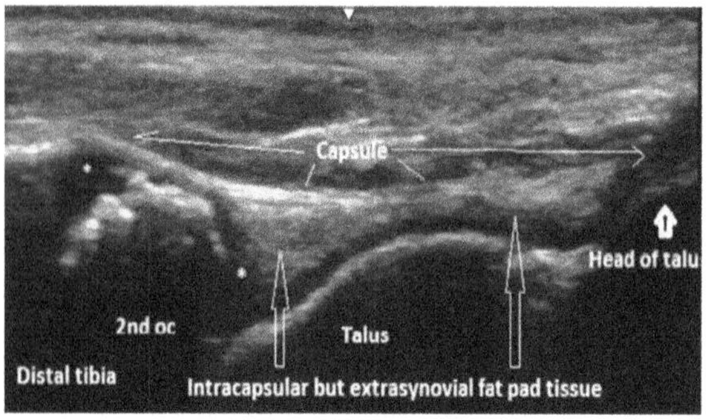

Fig. 2 Longitudinal dorsal view of a healthy ankle joint. The US image shows the location of intracapsular but extrasynovial fatty tissue, the presence of physis and epiphyseal cartilage in distal end of the tibia (*). 2nd oc: secondary ossification centre of the tibia

ossified hyaline cartilage, ossification center, joint capsule, synovial membrane, ossified bone, fat pad tissue, intra-articular vascularity) in an exercise involving 12 healthy children. The same ten US experts previously involved in the step 1 participated in the workshop. All experts were experienced (variable experience from 2 to 15 years) in musculoskeletal US in children. Four joints (i.e. knee, ankle, wrist, and second metacarpophalangeal (MCP II) joints) were examined in four different age groups (toddler and preschool ages 2–4 years, young children ages 5–8 years, preadolescent ages 9–12 years, and teenager ages 13–16 years) following standardized image acquisition and machine setting protocols [9]. Joint selection was based on previous studies and its common involvement in JIA [5, 9, 15, 20, 21]. The study was approved by the Ethics Committee of the Medical Board of Saxony-Anhalt (43/15) in Halle, Germany and was conducted in compliance with the Helsinki Agreement. Written consent was obtained from all parents and children prior to the exercise.

The examinations were performed on the same day, in the same room, using three different machines but identical brand (Logiq E, Logiq S8 and Logiq E9; General Electric Medical Systems, Waukesha, WI, USA) equipped with a 5–13 MHz broadband linear array transducer in the Logiq E and a 4–15 MHz broadband linear array transducer in the Logiq S8 and Logiq E9. PD was selected instead of colour Doppler based on the experience and daily use of the experts. The machines were calibrated with identical B-mode settings (frequency of 10–15 MHZ), but PD setting was optimized in the three US machine adjusting for the knee joint, wrist and tibiotalar joints, and MCP II joint as follows: pulse repetition frequency [PRF] 0.6, 0.8 and 0.8 MHZ respectively, and Doppler frequency [DF] 5, 7 and 10 MHZ respectively. It was emphasised the importance of correct size of the Doppler box, i.e. the Doppler box had to include the relevant joint structures and extend to the top of the image.

For each joint, participants were asked to assess the applicability of US definition (definition applicable: 1, yes or 0, not) attributed to each of joint components. Each participant evaluated real US images for applicability according to the following quality parameters (i) an image with appropriate magnification of the target structures and (ii) correctly displaying the wording of that relevant structure developed by the group consensus. The results were recorded on a preprinted data collection sheet.

The final step was to formulate a proposal wording of the new definitions considering the results obtained in the two previous steps in order to be presented to a larger panel of experts. Sixteen international experts were invited to join a web-based consensus process in order to reach consensus on the proposed definitions using the Delphi methodology. Most experts had participated in tasks of validation of US in adults or in children within the OMERACT US group at some time. The first online questionnaire comprised seven statements regarding definitions of interest. Expert agreement for each statement was rated using a 1–5 Likert scale [15]. If successive rounds were needed, it would include the statement that required modifications according to participant suggestions during the previous round interaction.

Statistical analysis

Statistical analysis was performed using the software package SPSS, version 22 (IBM, Armonk, US) and the software package R (R Foundation for Statistical Computing, Austria). Applicability of the US definitions on each joint was calculated as the percentage of rates that scored it as yes (percentage of agreement on the applicability).

In the web based consensus process, the agreement was scored using a 1–5 Likert scale as follows: 1 = strongly disagree, 2 = disagree, 3 = neutral, 4 = agree, and 5 = strongly agree. An agreement ≥80% was considered mandatory for accepting the definition as appropriated.

Results

Step 1. Nominal group consensus

Comments of the group showed the challenge to define physiological vascularity (normal Doppler signal) as a single item. Particularly applied to the epiphyseal cartilage and the ossification centre, which undergo significant changes throughout the maturation of the child. Therefore, they had to do a more cautious wording in this new definition. The new proposed US definitions for Doppler features were: 1) Doppler signal within the pediatric healthy joint can be detected as physiological vascularity of the unossified epiphyseal and physeal cartilage and the fat pads at any age during the growth, but since synovial membane is undetectable under normal circumstances, any Doppler signal observed in a synovial thickening should be considered an abnormality, 2) fat pad tissue can be present as an intraarticular structure, in a proper anatomical location, with heterogeneous echogenicity (similar to the US appearance of fat in the tissues below the skin) which might show Doppler signal (Fig. 3). Epiphyseal cartilage was not defined in this step, since the hyaline cartilage and the epiphyseal secondary ossification centre were included in the preliminary B-mode definitions.

Step 2. Practical exercise

The applicability of the preliminary and new US definitions were assessed on a total of 48 joints within the different age groups by all 10 participants. A perfect agreement (100%) was reached on the preliminary GS-US definitions (i.e., the hyaline cartilage, the epiphyseal secondary ossification centre, the normal joint capsule, the normal synovial membrane, the ossified portion of articular bone) for each joint. The percentage agreement was 100% in the definition for fat pad for each joint, whereas agreement in physiological vascularity was variable depending on the kind of joint. A 100% agreement was reached in the wrist, but it was lower in the rest of joints. It was a 69.5% [mean 69.5%; range 67%–72%] in the MCP II, 83.3% [range 83.1%–88%] in the knee and 86.1% [range 83%–89%] in the tibiotalar joint.

Step 3. Delphi consensus results

Taking into account the results of the practical exercise, definitions were reworded. It was suggested to provide separate statements instead of a full definition in order to identify components that would require further modification before their validation. Seven statements were therefore circulated to the panel of experts. The web based consensus process involved two rounds. In the second round the final version of the definitions obtained approval. This final version is shown in Table 1.

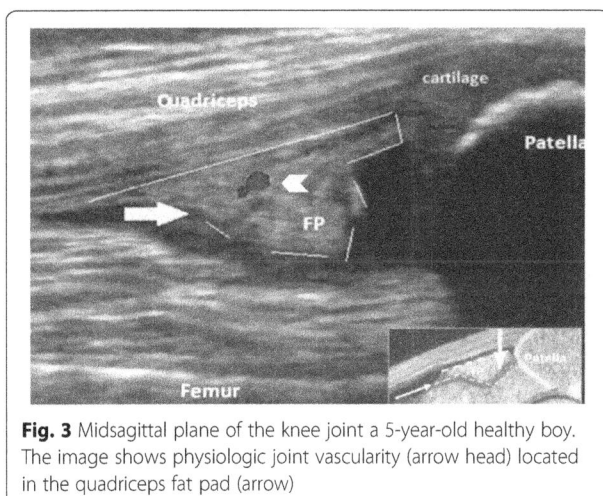

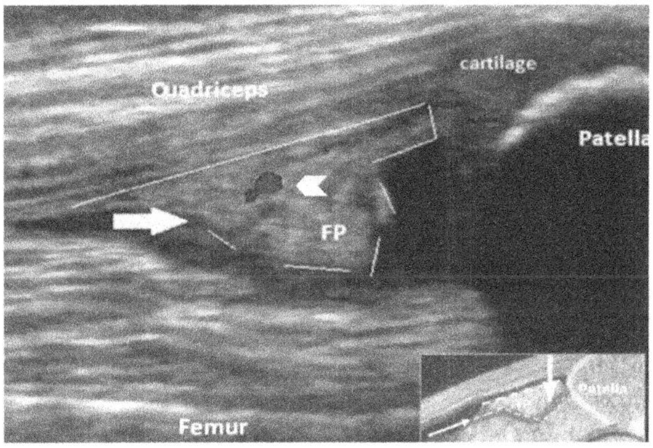

Fig. 3 Midsagittal plane of the knee joint a 5-year-old healthy boy. The image shows physiologic joint vascularity (arrow head) located in the quadriceps fat pad (arrow)

All invited participants responded to the first and the second round of the Delphi questionnaire (100% response rate). In the first round, consensus for fat pad and physiological joint vascularity (92.9% and 100%, respectively) was reached (Table 1). Nevertheless, as the challenge for scanning children is to ensure the general applicability (i.e., the wide age range and all kind of joints), aiming to avoid specific age descriptions, the final wording for the definition of joint vascularity was adjusted to be applicable to all age ranges. Hence, the actual definition for sonographic features of physiological vascularity comprises several statements (i.e., statements 1–4).

Due to PD US was not used in preliminary definitions of joint components, physis was not described in detail [15]. Physis is a relevant structure that might show Doppler signal, but physis is not detectable in the fully ossified bone of an adolescent. One statement related to physis was included in the survey too. No consensus was found for physis in the first round (57%), but it was reached in the second (85.7%) when the statement was reworded clarifing that this structure could be intra- or extra-articular according to its anatomical location (Table 1). Similarly, the agreement for statement 3 was low in the first round (50%), but could exceed the threshold of 80% when the statement was rephrased. Here, the panel of experts suggested to clarify that detection and anatomical location of Doppler signal are mostly age dependent (Table 1).

Despite the ossification process was not considered as a joint component to define, its description was included in the survey. The statement number 6 and 7 are related to the ossification and reached almost 100% of agreement in the first round.

Discussion

Without clear definitions of physiologic Doppler US findings in normal joints of children, it will be difficult to discriminate minimal active arthritis from physiologic growth patterns of joints. The interpretation of the Doppler signal in the pediatric joint is still being the most challenging and the least researched joint component.

We have used Doppler US to complete definitions of joints' features in healthy children. We have successfully developed, tested and validated two additional definitions through the Delphi method used in previous OMERACT studies.

Despite the OMERACT US Pediatric Task Force has been working on definitions of B-mode US findings of the healthy joint [15], standardization of US scanning in children, and definitions for the US appearance of synovitis in children [22], none of those studies included systematically a definition of normal Doppler signal. Indeed, the main concern showed in the development of

Table 1 Final statements and group agreement (percentage agreement) achieved for each statement of the second round

N.	Definition Statement	Percentage agreement, %
1	Physiological vascularity can be detected by PD as Doppler signal in the joint structures at any age during growth	100
2	Physiological intraarticular vascularity can be detected in children within the fat pads and unossified joint structures (i.e., the physis, the cartilage of epiphysis and the short bones cartilage)	85.7
3	Detection of physiological vascularity and its intraarticular anatomical position is joint and age (particularly in the youngest children) dependent	85.7
4	Physis can be detected in children as an anechoic unossified structure, intra- or extra-articular according to its anatomical location	85.7
5	Fat pad can be detected as an intra-articular structure with heterogeneous echotexture (similar to the subcutaneous tissue) which might show vascularity	92.9
6	In different age groups of children, due to the skeletal development, ossification centers can be detected with different maturation state	100
7	Ossification grade is age and joint dependent	92.9

the definition of synovitis was the difficulty on how to define abnormal Doppler signal.

Because of the limitations identified in the previous studies [15, 22], our research activity started with a face to face meeting that permitted to clarify several issues with regard to what joint components and anatomical locations of Doppler signals should be considered taking into account the preliminary five definitions (the hyaline cartilage, the epiphyseal secondary ossification centre, the normal joint capsule, the normal synovial membrane, the ossified portion of articular bone) [15]. Besides the Doppler signal, it suggested to include the description of fat pad and physis in the present study in which Doppler signal might be detected and they were not define previously.

The practical exercise permitted the assessment of potential variation in image acquisition. As expected, we found a very good applicability of definition between experts when applying the preliminary OMERACT definitions for GS-US (namely, B-mode US) joint components. These findings enhance the results of previous study [15]. The disagreement between experts was related to the applicability of definition for Doppler signal; we found a good but variable

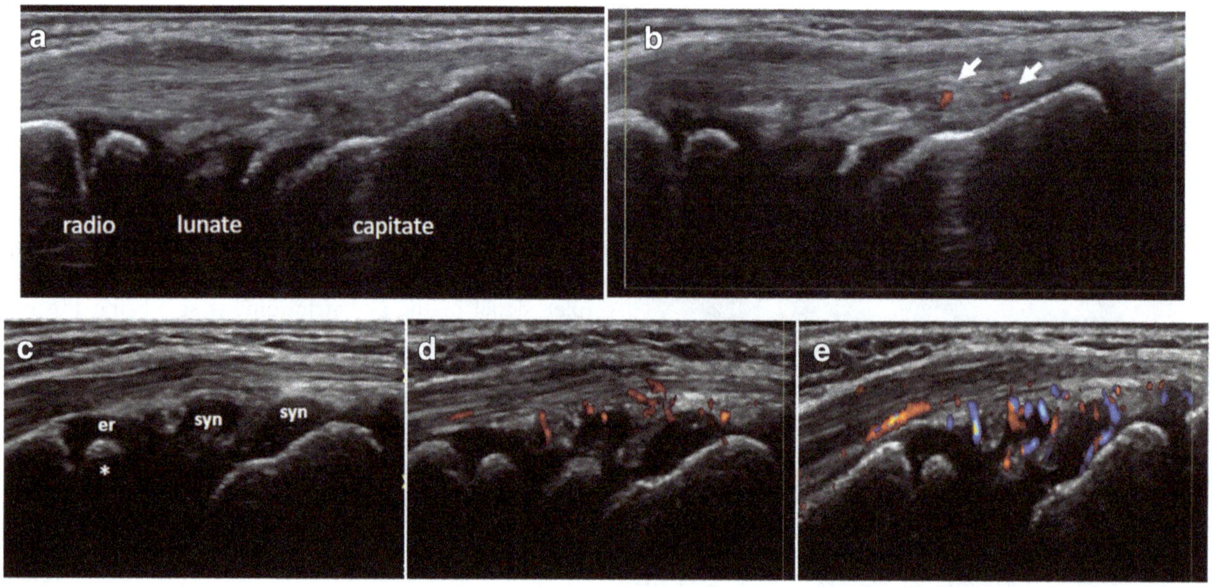

Fig. 4 Longitudinal view of the dorsal aspect of the wrist joint in a 6-year-old child. The upper images (**a**, **b**) show the normal sonoanatomy on Grey-scale US (**a**) and power-Doppler US (**b**) showing single vessels close to os capitate. The lower images (**c**, **d**, **e**) show synovitis of the wrist joint in a patient with JIA. Synovial vascularity detected in the joint recesses by Doppler (image **d**, power Doppler and image **e**, color Doppler) reflects active inflammation. The distal epiphyseal cartilage of radius (er) is visible as an anechoic structure surrounding the secondary ossification nucleus (*). Dynamic examination let distinguish the epiphyseal cartilage of radius from effusion/synovitis (syn)

agreement in all joints except for MCP joint. The disagreement for MCP was not later discussed during the consensus process, hence further investigation is needed. We are aware that several factors might contributed to that variability. First, as different PD settings were used depending on machine and joint, the impact of machines on the results could not have been minimised enough. Second, patient factors such as the small size of the MCP joint with slow blood flow velocity and restless children, may contribute to a lesser accurate assessment.

Doppler signal within joint or peri-articular is a source of uncertainty or misinterpretation for pediatric rheumatologist who infrequently perform the musculoskeletal US (Fig. 4). In addition, taking into account unclear meaning of Doppler signals in asymptomatic joints of children having JIA, it seems mandatory to include Doppler mode in the definitions of pediatric joint in order to enhance the validity of US in children [7, 23–25].

Seven separate statements were provide instead of a full definition, and most of them regarding physiological vascularity as a reflexion of its complexity. This complexity might be explained by (i) the availability of only a basic knowledge in Doppler findings in healthy children [9], (ii) a scarce validation in Doppler US assessment of pediatric joints [7] and (iii) the difficulty in the interpretation of the Doppler findings in children, particularly at the level of cartilaginous structures [26].

Two rounds of the Delphi exercise were needed to reach an agreement on US definitions of these additional joint components. Because of the fat pad tissue has already been considered in adults [27], its definition reached the agreement easier than expected. Nevertheless, a recent reliability study on MRI in JIA showed some discrepancies in the assessment of the knee fat pads [28].

Despite the fact that ossification is not a structural component of joint, we had to describe it for two important reasons: first, because bone landmarks are important for proper image acquisition during US scanning and second, because the appearance of physeal and epiphyseal cartilages changes through childhood; indeed, the physis (or the growth plate) should be considered in the oldest children as the unique cartilaginous structure of the growing skeleton which is displayed on US as an anechoic gap in the bone cortex [15].

Using the Doppler modality, we have produced additional US definitions for joint components that should be used in combination with the five published previously. Despite the present study represents an essential step toward a more reliable use of the Doppler technique in children, the Delphi approach has showed that the issue regarding physiological vascularity (i.e., normal Doppler signal) requires further investigations. Besides the expertise of sonographer, the potential effect of transducer pressure in small pediatric joints and the variation in Doppler sensitivity in different machines [29], may influence on acquiring of images and make difficult to provide a unique definition of the physiological vascularity. Since the aim of the study was to define components of the healthy joint as displayed on Doppler US, none validation of these definitions using a comparison imaging technique was done.

Our results are in line with others studies that show how the Doppler US can detect early inflammatory lesions and display an enhancement of physiological joint vascularity in JIA patients [30], and it can also show a increased physiological blood flow adjacent to the distal metaphysis and epiphysis of a long bone in acute osteomyelitis [31].

Although these definitions should be considered when US is applied on children with arthritis in daily practice, further studies are required to evaluate the applicability of these new PD definitions to other joints and to explore their potential use in clinical trials.

Conclusion

The inclusion of these two additional joints components which are linked to detection of Doppler signal in pediatric healthy joints will improve the identification of joint abnormalities in pediatric rheumatic diseases.

Abbreviations

DF: Doppler frequency; GS: Grey-scale; JIA: juvenile idiopathic arthritis; MCP II: second metacarpophalangeal; OMERACT: Outcome Measures in Rheumatology; PD: Power Doppler; PRF: Pulse repetition frequency; US: Ultrasonography

Acknowledgments

The authors thank all volunteers and their parents who participated in this study.

Funding

There was no funding.

Authors' contributions

All authors participated in the three steps of the study. PC and EN were major contributors in writing the manuscript. All authors read and approved the final manuscript.

Competing interests

The authors declare that they have no competing interests.

Author details
[1]Hospital Universitario Severo Ochoa., Madrid, Spain. [2]Department of Pediatrics, Asklepios Hospital Weissenfels, Weissenfels, Germany. [3]Department of Pediatrics, Clinical Center, Faculty of Medicine, University of Nis, Nis, Serbia. [4]Rheumatology Division, IRCCS Ospedale Pediatrico Bambino Gesù, Rome, Italy. [5]3rd Department of Rheumatology, National Institute of Rheumatology and Physiotherapy, Budapest, Hungary. [6]Department of Rheumatology, MC Groep, Lelystad, the Netherlands. [7]Instituto Nacional de Rehabilitación, Mexico City, Mexico. [8]Department of Rheumatology, Hospital Universitario Gregorio Marañon, Madrid, Spain. [9]Department of Internal Medicine, ASST Mantova, C. Poma Hospital, Mantova, Italy. [10]Pediatric Rheumatology Research Institute, Bad Bramstedt, Germany. [11]Rheumatology Unit, Sapienza Università di Roma, Rome, Italy. [12]Rheumatology Department, Hôspital Ambroise Paré, Boulogne Billancourt; INSERM U1173, Laboratoire d'Excellence INFLAMEX, UFR Simone Veil, Versailles-Saint-Quentin University, Yvelines, France. [13]Department of Rheumatology, Hospital Universitario Fundación Jimenez Díaz and Autonoma University, Madrid, Spain.

References

1. Laurell L, Court-Payen M, Nielsen S, Zak M, Boesen M, Fasth A. Ultrasonography and color Doppler in juvenile idiopathic arthritis: diagnosis and follow-up of ultrasound- guided steroid injection in the ankle region. A descriptive interventional study. Pediatr Rheumatol Online J. 2011;9:4.
2. Laurell L, Court-Payen M, Nielsen S, Zak M, Fasth A. Ultrasonography and color Doppler in juvenile idiopathic arthritis: diagnosis and follow-up of ultrasound-guided steroid injection in the wrist region. A descriptive interventional study. Pediatr Rheumatol Online J. 2012;10:11.
3. Jousse-Joulin S, Breton S, Cangemi C, Fenoll B, Bressolette L, de Parscau L, et al. Ultrasonography for detecting enthesitis in juvenile idiopathic arthritis. Arthritis Care Res. 2011;63:849–5.
4. Breton S, Jousse-Joulin S, Cangemi C, de Parscau L, Colin D, Bressolette L, et al. Comparison of clinical and ultrasonographic evaluations for peripheral synovitis in juvenile idiopathic arthritis. Semin Arthritis Rheum. 2011;41:272–8.
5. Filippou G, Cantarini L, Bertoldi I, Picerno V, Frediani B, Galeazzi M. Ultrasonography vs. clinical examination in children with suspected arthritis. Does it make sense to use poliarticular ultrasonographic screening? Clin Exp Rheumatol. 2011;29:345–50.
6. Naredo E, Collado P, Cruz A, et al. Longitudinal power Doppler ultrasonographic assessment of joint inflammatory activity in early rheumatoid arthritis: predictive value in disease activity and radiologic progression. Arthritis Rheum. 2007;57:116–24.
7. Collado P, Jousse-Joulin S, Alcalde M, Naredo E, D'Agostino MA. Is ultrasound a validated imaging tool for the diagnosis and management of synovitis in juvenile idiopathic arthritis? A systematic literature review. Arthritis Care Res. 2012;64:1011–9.
8. Bearcroft P, Berman L, Robinson A, Butler G. Vascularity of the neonatal femoral head: in vivo demonstration with power Doppler US. Radiology. 1996;200:209–11.
9. Collado P, Vojinovic J, Nieto JC, Windschall D, Magni-Manzoni S, Bruyn GAW, et al. Toward standardized musculoskeletal ultrasound in pediatric rheumatology: normal age-related ultrasound findings. Arthritis Care Res. 2016;68:348–56.
10. McCarthy EF, Frassica FJ. Anatomy and Physiology of bone. In: Pathology of bone and joint disorders. Philadelphia: WB Saunders; 1998. p. 25–50.
11. Floyd WE, Zaleske DJ, Schiller AL, Trahan C, Mankin HJ. Vascular events associated with the appearance of the secondary center of ossification in the murine distal femoral epiphysis. J Bone Joint Surg Am. 1987;69:185–90.
12. Shapiro F. Epiphyseal and Physeal cartilage vascularization: a light microscopic and Tritiated thymidine autoradiographic study of cartilage canals in newborn and young postnatal rabbit bone. Anat Rec. 1998;252:140–8.
13. Varich LJ, Laor T, Jaramillo D. Normal maturation of the distal femoralepiphyseal cartilage: age-related changes at MR imaging. Radiology. 2000;214:705–9.
14. Ho-Fung VM, Jaramillo D. Cartilage imaging in children: current indications,magnetic resonance imaging techniques, and imaging findings. Radiol Clin North Am. 2013;51:689–702.
15. Roth J, Jousse-Joulin S, Magni-Manzoni S, Rodriguez A, Tzaribachev N, Iagnocco A, et al. Definitions for the sonographic features of joints in healthy children. Arthritis Care Res. 2015;67:136–42.
16. Caspar-Bauguil S, Cousin B, Galinier A, Segafredo C, Nibbelink M, Andre M, et al. Adipose tissues as an ancestral immune organ: site-specific change in obesity. FEBS Lett. 2005;579:3487–92.
17. Šenolt L. Adipokines: role in local and systemic inflammation of rheumatic diseases. Expert Rev Clin Immunol. 2017;13(1):1–3. https://doi.org/10.1080/1744666X.2017.1249850.
18. Jacobson JA, Lenchic L, Ruboy MK, Schweizert ME, Resnick D. MR imaging of the infrapatellar fat pad of Hoffa. Radiographics. 1997;17:675–91.
19. Ng JM, Rosenberg ZS, Bencardino JT, Restrepo-Velez Z, Ciavarra GA, Adler RS. US and MR imaging of the extensor compartment of the ankle. Radiographics. 2013;33:2047–64.
20. Collado P, Naredo E, Calvo C, MI G, Calvo I, MI G-V, et al. Reduced joint assessment versus comprehensive assessment for ultrasound detection of synovitis in juvenile idiopathic arthritis. Rheumatology. 2013;52:1477–84.
21. Selvaag AM, Flato B, Dale K. Radiographic and Clinical outcome in early juvenile rheumatoid arthritis and juvenile spondylarthropathy: a 3-year prospective study. J Rheumatol. 2006;33:1382–91.
22. Roth J, Ravagnani V, Backhaus M, Balint P, Bruns A, Bruyn GA, et al. Preliminary definitions for the Sonographic features of Synovitis in children. Arthritis Care Res. 2017;69:1217–23.
23. Colebatch-Bourn AN, Edwards CJ, Collado P, D'Agostino M-A, Hemke R, Jousse-Joulin S, et al. EULAR-PReS points to consider for the use of imaging in the diagnosis and management of juvenile idiopathic arthritis in clinical practice. Ann Rheum Dis. 2015;74:1946–57.
24. Magni-Manzoni S, Scirè CA, Ravelli A, Klersy C, Rossi S, Muratore V, et al. Ultrasound-detected synovial abnormalities are frequent in clinically inactive juvenile idiopathic arthritis, but do not predict a flare of synovitis. Ann Rheum Dis. 2013;72:223–8.
25. Collado P, Gamir ML, López-Robledillo JC, Merino R, Modesto C, Monteagudo I. Detection of synovitis by ultrasonography in clinically inactive juvenile idiopathic arthritis on and off medication. Clin Experimental. 2014;32:597–603.
26. Barnewolt CE, Shapiro F, Jaramillo D. Normal gadolinium-enhanced MR images in the developing appendicular skeleton. Part 1: cartilaginous epiphysis and physis. AJR. 1997;169:183–9.
27. Mandl P, Benis S, Patonay L, Balint PV. The normal joint. In: Wakefield RJ, D'Agostino MA, editors. Essential applications of ultrasound in rheumatology. 1st ed. Philadelphia: SAUNDERS. Elsevier; 2010. p. 51–64.
28. Henke R, Tzaribachev N, Nusman CM, van Rossum MAJ, Maas M, Doria AS. Magnetic resonance imaging (MRI) of the knee as at outcome mesure in juvenile idiopathic arthritis: an OMERACT reliability study on MRI scales. J Rheumatol. 2017;44:1224–30.
29. Torp-Pedersen S, Christensen R, Szkudlarek M, et al. Power and color Doppler ultrasound settings for inflammatory flow: impact on scoring of disease activity in patients with rheumatoid arthritis. Arthritis Rheumatol. 2015;67:386–95.
30. Karmazyn B, Bowyer SL, Schmidt KM, et al. US findings of metacarpophalangeal joints in children with idiopathic juvenile arthritis. Pediatr Radiol. 2007;37:475–82.
31. Collado P, Naredo E, Calvo C, Crespo M. Role of power Doppler sonography in early diagnosis of osteomyelitis in children. J Clin Ultrasound. 2008;36:251–3.

3

Dealing with Chronic Non-Bacterial Osteomyelitis: a practical approach

Andrea Taddio[1,2*], Giovanna Ferrara[2], Antonella Insalaco[3], Manuela Pardeo[3], Massimo Gregori[1], Martina Finetti[4], Serena Pastore[1], Alberto Tommasini[1], Alessandro Ventura[1,2] and Marco Gattorno[4]

Abstract

Background: Chronic Non-Bacterial Osteomyelitis (CNO) is an inflammatory disorder that primarily affects children. Although underestimated, its incidence is rare. For these reasons, no diagnostic and no therapeutic guidelines exist. The manuscript wants to give some suggestions on how to deal with these patients in the every-day clinical practice.

Main body: CNO is characterized by insidious onset of bone pain with local swelling. Systemic symptoms such as fever, skin involvement and arthritis may be sometimes present. Radiological findings are suggestive for osteomyelitis, in particular if multiple sites are involved. CNO predominantly affects metaphyses of long bones, but clavicle and mandible, even if rare localizations of the disease, are very consistent with CNO diagnosis. CNO pathogenesis is still unknown, but recent findings highlighted the crucial role of cytokines such as IL-1β and IL-10 in disease pathogenesis. Moreover, the presence of non-bacterial osteomyelitis among autoinflammatory syndromes suggests that CNO could be considered an autoinflammatory disease itself. Differential diagnosis includes infections, malignancies, benign bone tumors, metabolic disorders and other autoinflammatory disorders. Radiologic findings, either with Magnetic Resonance or with Computer Scan, may be very suggestive. For this reason in patients in good clinical conditions, with multifocal localization and very consistent radiological findings bone biopsy could be avoided. Non-Steroidal Anti-Inflammatory Drugs are the first-choice treatment. Corticosteroids, methotrexate, bisphosphonates, TNFα-inhibitors and IL-1 blockers have also been used with some benefit; but the choice of the second line treatment depends on bone lesions localizations, presence of systemic features and patients' clinical conditions.

Conclusion: CNO may be difficult to identify and no consensus exist on diagnosis and treatment. Multifocal bone lesions with characteristic radiological findings are very suggestive of CNO. No data exist on best treatment option after Non-Steroidal Anti-Inflammatory Drugs failure.

Keywords: Chronic Non-Bacterial Osteomyelitis, Chronic recurrent multifocal Osteomyelitis, Autoinflammatory syndrome, Magnetic resonance, Treatment, Bisphosphonate, Anti-TNFα treatment

Background

Chronic Non-Bacterial Osteomyelitis (CNO) is a rare inflammatory disorder not related to infectious disease [1]. It was first described in 1972 by Giedion et al. [2] as a symmetric multifocal bone lesions; later, in 1980, Bjorksten B et al. [3] first used the term CNO in order to identify a clinical condition which is characterized by recurring episodes or persisting presence of chronic sterile osteomyelitis [4–6]. Multiple names have been used in literature to describe this disorder; these include chronic recurrent multifocal osteomyelitis (CRMO) in cases with extended multifocal involvement (often symmetric) and synovitis, acne, pustulosis, hyperostosis, and osteitis syndrome (SAPHO), which usually manifests in adolescent and adult patients and which distinguishes for skin involvement [7]. The terms CRMO and CNO are often used interchangeably. Although CNO is still considered a rare disorder, its incidence is probably underestimated. In fact, in a single center retrospective study, it has been recently demonstrated that the incidence of CNO is similar to infectious osteomyelitis [8]. For these reasons, in absence of standardized diagnostic work out and treatment guidelines, it is important to provide some

* Correspondence: andrea.taddio@burlo.trieste.it
[1]Institute for Maternal and Child Health, IRCCS "Burlo Garofolo", Trieste, Italy
[2]University of Trieste, Via dell'Istria 65/1, 34100 Trieste, Italy
Full list of author information is available at the end of the article

clinical practical suggestion about the every-day clinical management of CNO patients.

Main Text

Pathogenesis

Since this is not the main aim of the manuscript, CNO pathogenesis will be only briefly discussed. Although CNO pathogenesis is still not clear, the hypothesis that the disorder could be sustained by infections was not confirmed by extensive microbiological analyses and uselessness of antibiotic treatment [4]. Findings indicate that pro-inflammatory cytokines such as IL-6 and TNF-a as well as anti-inflammatory (IL-10) [4, 9], IL-1β [10] and IL-10 [11] may play an important role in disease pathogenesis of CNO. In the last years, the hypothesis that CNO might be a genetic disease in the spectrum of autoinflammatory disorders has acquired even more importance. The strongest evidence comes from the so called syndromic forms of CNO: Majeed syndrome [12, 13], Cherubism [14], Hypophosphatasia [15] and Primary Hypertrophic Osteoarthropathy [16]. In addition, chronic osteomyelitis is a typical feature of two monogenic diseases caused by mutations of genes involved in the activation of the NLRP3 inflammasome or in the homeostasis of IL-1, namely pyogenic arthritis, pyoderma gangrenosum and acne (PAPA) syndrome [17] and the deficiency of IL-1 receptor antagonist (DIRA), [18] respectively. There is also some evidence for a genetic basis in non-syndromic or sporadic CNO [19]. Moreover, in largest cohorts of CNO patients, the prevalence of the disease among patients' relatives was higher [20] and some reports have described families with multiple affected members [21] or have reported a high incidence of psoriasis, inflammatory bowel disease, and other chronic inflammatory conditions in first-degree family members of individuals with CNO suggesting that there is a significant genetic component to disease susceptibility [3, 6]. In mice, homozygous mutation of *PSTIPI2* gene results in an autoinflammatory disease very similar to CNO [22, 23].

Clinical features

The clinical manifestations of CNO are highly variable. CNO typically presents with bone pain that is worse at night and occurs in the presence or absence of fever [20, 24]. The onset is typically insidious, and most children appear well.

Swelling and heat of the involved bone are not necessarily always present. In 30% of cases CNO involves the adjacent joint with the presence of exudate, synovial thickening and/or damage to the articular cartilage. The lesions may affect any bone segment. One to 20 sites can be affected at one time. The main sites of involvement in order of decreasing frequency are the lower extremities, pelvis, clavicle and spine [6, 20, 24]. Metaphyseal area is the most common bone site localization as well as the involvement of clavicle, mandible and sternum which is particularly suggestive of CNO [20]. The skull involvement has been described in the occipital bone in only one case. In this patient, however, the lesion was not present at time of diagnosis, but it developed after 1 year from diagnosis [25]. Skull involvement should always be considered a potential malignancy; in this case bone biopsy is mandatory.

Systemic symptoms are subtle and may be present in the form of low-grade fever, malaise, or poor growth. In this case, malignancies, most of all acute lymphoblastic leukemia, and inflammatory bowel disease must be ruled out. Current estimates suggest that approximately 25% of individuals with CNO have manifestations involving organ/systems other than bone [20]. The extra - articular manifestations include the skin (especially Psoriasis, Palmoplantar Pustulosis, Acne, Pyoderma Gangrenosum and Sweet Syndrome) and the bowel (Crohn Disease, Ulcerative Colitis, Celiac Disease) [26]. Renal involvement has been demonstrated in almost 10% of patients [27].

The disease may follow a chronic or recurrent disease course, often the course is prolonged over several years with periodic exacerbations [1–6]. The prognosis is generally good and provides self-resolution in a time ranging from months to years. However, recently complications of entity variable from mild to incapacitating have been described in a considerable percentage of cases (30 to 50%). In particular asymmetries of limb length, kyphosis, chronic spondylo-arthropathy, vertebral collapse and stunting for early closure of the growth-cartilages have been reported [6, 7, 24]. Monophasic disease is usually less severe and prognosis is excellent being, in most cases, almost a cosmetic problem.

Diagnosis

CNO is a diagnosis of exclusion. Differential diagnoses include infections (septic osteomyelitis, typical and atypical mycobacterial infections, etc.), malignancies (primary bone tumors and leukemia/lymphoma), benign bone tumors (osteoid osteoma), trauma, metabolic disorders (including hypophosphatasia), other autoinflammatory disorders (DIRA, PAPA, Cherubism, etc.), osteonecrosis and osteopetrosis.

The most common clinical challenge is with acute bacterial osteomyelitis; in this case, however, pain and fever are usually present and, except for some rare circumstances, such as severe immunodeficiencies, the disease is always monofocal. In early stage of the disease, and in the monofocal course, the radiological assays may be undistinguishable and a trial with antibiotics is indicated. If there will be no response to antibiotic treatment, once ruled out infective complication (e.g. bone abscess), CNO should be taken into account. Malignancies should be considered in any patients with poor clinical conditions, with systemic features, with skull involvement or with suggestive radiologic lesions. Osteoma Osteoid has a very typical radiological pattern (nidus surrounded by dense bone) and nocturnal pain is almost even present. Hypophosphatasia is an inherited disorder that affects the development of bones and teeth. This condition disrupts bone mineralization, causing skeletal abnormalities similar to rickets. However, the forms of hypophosphatasia that appear in childhood or adulthood are typically less severe than those that appear in infancy and may present as genu varum or genu valgum, enlarged wrist and ankle joints, and an abnormal skull shape leading to CNO diagnosis. CNO may be present in other autoinflammatory disorders; however, in this case, many other clinical features may prevail such as arthritis, pustulosis, hepatomegaly, interstitial pneumonia, splenomegaly, fever and etc. Differential diagnosis are summarized in Table 1.

Laboratory investigations may reveal mild elevation in white blood cell count and in inflammatory parameters (C-Reactive Protein; Erythrocyte Sedimentation Rate), but often these abnormalities are absent in CNO patients [20, 24]. Cultures of blood and bone are invariably negative, and sophisticated assays to identify evidence of a microbial etiology have been unsuccessful. Autoantibodies (antinuclear antibodies, rheumatoid- factor), as well as carriage of the HLAB27 allele, have the same prevalence in CNO patients when compared to healthy individuals. At present, no specific biomarkers are available for the diagnosis or prediction of flares in CNO patients. In 2007 Jansson et al. [24] proposed diagnostic criteria for CNO according to which diagnosis could be formulated if present 2 majors and one minor criteria or one major and three minors criteria. However, these criteria are not still internationally validated and accepted so far. A crucial role in the diagnosis of this condition is provided by imaging and biopsy.

The role of radiology

Standard radiography of bones could not reveal characteristic changes in early CNO, while the presence of osteolytic lesions with a sclerotic edge in X-ray imaging is the key feature later. Clavicular lesions and mandibular often have a more prominent sclerotic appearance [28].

Cortical bone is usually unaffected and thickened but there are also reports of cortical defect mimicking tumor. The involvement of the mandible is often associated with mandibular nerve canal enlargement (Fig. 1). CNO is a systemic disorder that can affect multiple skeletal sites. Isotopic bone scan and/or whole-body Magnetic Resonance (MR) are the cornerstone for confirming the multifocal pattern of CNO, even if bone scan may be falsely negative in some cases. However, if isotopic bone scan may just confirm the presence of one or more foci of inflammation, MR may also add more information concerning the types of lesions being the more sensitive and accurate radiological examination at CNO diagnosis.

The typical MR findings are the presence of bone cortical thickening, lytic lesions with sclerosis and bone edema. Moreover, MR is particularly important in the early stages of the disease for its ability to detect bone edema and also asymptomatic bone lesions [29], before osteolysis and/or sclerosis can be detected. On the other hand, it should be mentioned that, due to its high sensitivity, this technique might lead to an over-interpretation of some bone lesions that, especially in pediatric age, can be related to normal bode growth or accidental traumatic events. This issue should be taken into careful consideration if the site of the bone biopsy is chosen on the basis of the MR images. Due to the lack of ionizing radiation, total body MR (with STIR sequences) is currently used to monitor the evolution of the bone lesions during the follow-up. Again, due to its

Table 1 Clinical characteristics of CNO compared with other bone diseases

	CNO	Bacterial Osteomyelitis	Malignancy	Osteoid Osteoma	DIRA	PAPA	Cherubism	Osteopetrosis
Multifocal Involvement	+++	–	+	–	+	–/+	+	+++
Pain	++++	++++	++++	++++	++	+++	++	++
Fever	+	+++	–/+	–	–/+	–/+	–	–
Skin Involvement	+	–	–	–	++++	+++	–	–
Articular Involvement	+	++	–	–	++++	++++	–	–
Bone Swelling	+++	–/+	++	–	++	++	++++	++
Renal Involvement	+	–	–/+	–	–	+	–	–
Hepatosplenomegaly	–	–	+	–	++++	–	–	++
Early Age of onset	–/+	+	–/+	–	++++	–	–	++
ESR/CRP elevation	+	+++	–/+	–	++++	++++	–	–
Leukocytosis	–/+	+++	–/+	–	++++	++++	–	–

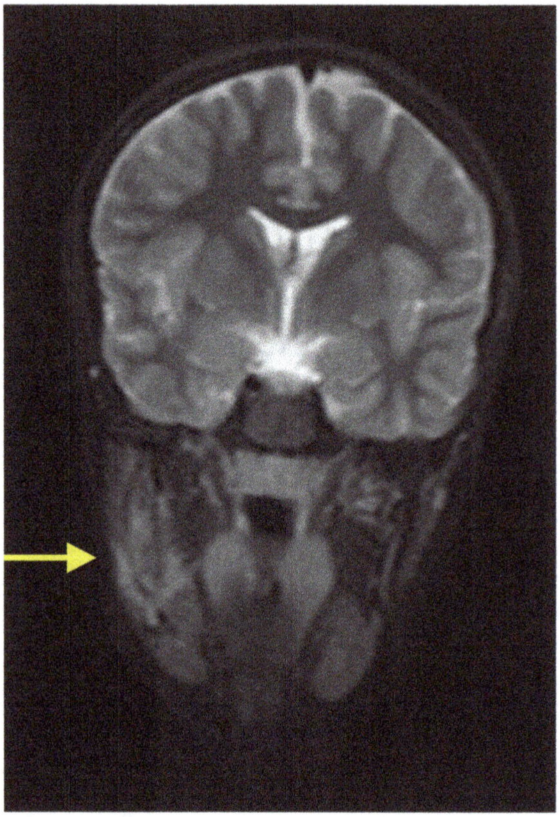

Fig. 1 MR of mandible. Mandible edema and mandibular nerve canal enlargement (arrow) in a CNO patient

high sensitivity MR might provide signs of possible bone activity in a subgroup of patients which did not complain any clinical manifestation or bone pain and could be considered in clinical remission [30]. For this reason it is not clear if the evidence of radiological disease activity in spite of a persistent clinical and laboratoristic, remission should be taken into consideration for patient's treatment strategy or, vice versa, if it could lead to an over-treatment in some patients. For this reason, longitudinal MR control could be useful in particular among patients with a more severe disease course and resistant to ongoing treatments, and in case of the involvement of some specific sites, such as the mandible or the spine, which is traditionally characterized by a higher rate of complication such as scoliosis or kyphosis.

The role of biopsy

Although no formal guidelines are so far available, a biopsy of the bone lesion is usually performed, mainly to exclude other causes. In CNO bone biopsy shows signs of inflammation in the absence of infection. The composition of cellular infiltrates at the sites of inflammation is strictly correlated to the "age" of biopsied lesions. Neutrophils are predominant in early lesions, whereas lymphocytes, macrophages and plasma cells can be detected during the later course of the inflammatory. The final stage of the lesion is characterized by the predominance of fibrosis. The cultures of the biopsy are always negative [4].

Although histological findings are specific, the main role of the biopsy is to rule out malignancy such as histiocytosis, Ewing sarcoma, osteosarcoma, leukemia and lymphoma. All these disorders should be considered in the differential diagnosis of persistent bone pain in all age groups.

Recently, Jansson et al. proposed a clinical score that could facilitate the diagnosis and treatment process, especially with respect to the decision on whether to carry out invasive procedures required for diagnosis of these diseases [31]. Even if the Jansson Score is not still widely validated, it is suggested that patients with a score > 39 could not undergo biopsy. Our practical approach is to perform a biopsy in all patients with poor general conditions, persistent and significant elevation of acute phase reactants and/or hematological abnormalities (anemia, alteration in leukocyte or platelet counts), and all those patients with unifocal or atypical (i.e. skull) bone involvement. In these cases, the biopsy may be performed in the most accessible lesion. On the contrary, the decision to perform the biopsy can be postponed in those patients with good general conditions, with slight elevation of acute phase reactants, involvement of multiple and/or typical and bone sites, typical radiological findings and favorable response to Non-Steroidal Anti-Inflammatory Drugs (NSAIDs) treatment (Fig. 2). In any case, further studies are needed to clarify the role of biopsy; to now the decision to perform the biopsy remains a physician related decision based on his expertness and knowledge toward CNO diagnosis.

Treatment

Generally accepted treatment protocols for CNO do not exist and the treatment of CNO has been largely empiric. A number of retrospective assessments of response to treatment in case reports or small series are available in the literature. Neither Guidelines nor expert consensus treatment do exist for CNO so far; however our group has recently proposed a suggested treatment protocol base exclusively on their clinical expertise [32].

The first line treatment is usually NSAIDs, which have been demonstrated useful for pain control and inducing remission in a percentage of patients varying from 43 to 83% [24, 33]. The NSAIDs more frequently used are naproxen, indomethacin and, especially, in those patients with concomitant inflammatory bowel disease, sulfasalazine. The prospective use of NSAIDs has been evaluated in a single study performed in thirty-seven CNO patients. A favourable clinical course identified as

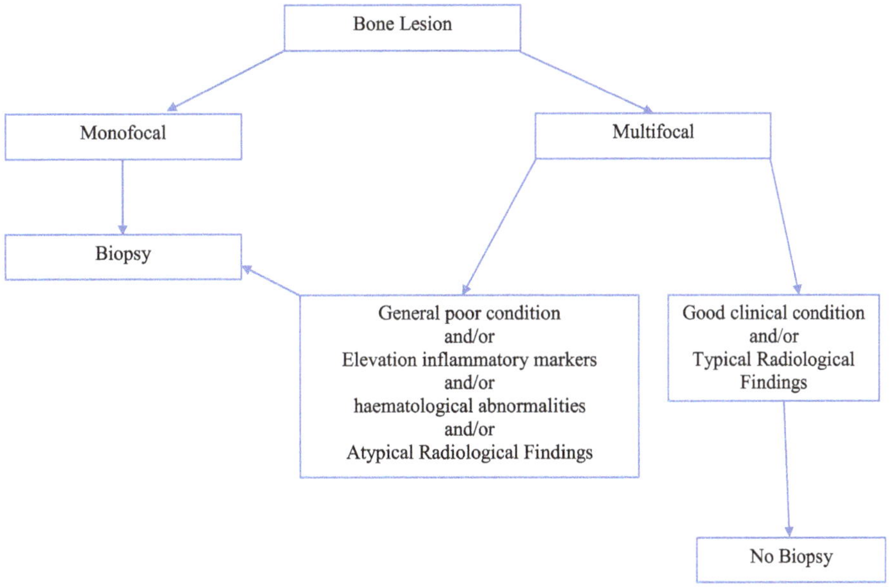

Fig. 2 Suggested diagram to perform or not perform bone biopsy in a patient with suspected CRMO

symptoms free status was reported in 43% of patients taking naproxen at 1 year of follow-up; moreover, the total number of clinical detectable lesions was significantly reduced. Mean disease activity estimated by the patient/physician and the physical aspect of health-related quality of life including functional ability (global assessment/childhood health assessment questionnaire and childhood health assessment questionnaire) and pain improved significantly [33]. At least 1 month trial is needed in order to determine their failure. However, it is important to underline that NSAIDs did not seem to be sufficient for vertebral involvement or in case of peripheral arthritis. In case of NSAIDs failure, a single course of corticosteroids could be beneficial at the beginning of the disease; some others suggest their use only in those cases unresponsiveness to NSAIDs, in relapsing diseases or in severe clinical involvement [33, 34]. In this case, a bone biopsy should precede the use of steroid; prednisolone is usually the drug of choice.

TNF-alfa inhibitors have also been used in CNO patients. Infliximab was the first biologic treatment used [35] in an 18-years old with relapsing CNO. Etanercept has also been demonstrated effective in a patient with active disease despite previous treatment options, together with Methotrexate (MTX) [36]. Some large cohorts of patients report their use in a small sample of patients, usually <10%, who did not achieve clinical remission with previous treatment. In these patients, their use was usually of benefit [20, 24].

In the last years, the use of bisphosphonate was found to be effective and safe in the treatment of CNO. Most part of data about bisphosphonate use is based on case reports or small case series [37]. The most common used molecule is pamidronate, but alendronate has been reported to be safe and useful as well [38]. Bisphosphonates have demonstrated to be effective not only in controlling pain, [39] but recently it has also been demonstrated their efficacy in the resolution of bone lesions assessed by whole body magnetic resonance imaging [40]. At the moment it is not clear whether treatment option is better. Wipff et al. suggested that CNO patients may be divided into three categories of clinical severity. The patients with a mild phenotype presented a high remission rate irrespectively from treatment and use of pamidronate or TNF inhibitors; on the contrary, among the severe phenotype, the rate of clinical remission was lower despite high percentage of patients undergoing treatment with biphosphonate or TNF inhibitors [20]. In our experience bisphosphonate were the most useful treatment option irrespectively of previous treatment or clinical features [27]; in fact we have demonstrated that bisphosphonates may lead to remission the 73% of CNO patients after NSAIDs and steroids failure. For this reason, we would suggest that bisphosphonate could be considered the first treatment options for CNO patients when NSAIDs failed, especially when the spine is involved. Their safety is debated. Although to date, jaw osteonecrosis has never been reported in pediatric patients with CNO, periodic oral controls are recommended. In patients with concomitant gastro-intestinal or articular involvement (synovitis, spondylitis), sulfasalazine, MTX or anti-TNF treatment can be considered as treatments of choice. Data reporting clinical studies on CNO treatment are summarized in Table 2.

Table 2 List of manuscripts reporting data about response to treatment of patients with CNO

Reference	Nr. patients	Treatment	Response to treatment
Wipff J et al., 2015 [20]	178	NSAIDs	126/178 (71%): clinical response
		Sulfasalazine	7/17 (41%): clinical response
		Methotrexate	3/8 (37%): clinical response
		Bisphosphonates	6/8 (75%): clinical response
		Anti-TNFα	8/9 (89%): clinical response
Jansson A et al., 2007 [24]	89	NSAIDs	64/77 (83%): clinical response
		Steroids	13/13 (100%): transient response
		DMARDs	6/6 (100%): no response
		PAM	1/4 (25%): clinical response
			1/4 (25%:) partial response
			2/4 (50%): no response
Kaiser D et al., 2015 [45]	41	NSAIDs	21/37 (57%): clinical response
		Methotrexate	6/7 (86%): no response
		Bisphosphonates	1/5 (20%): clinical response
			1/5 (20%): partial response
		Etanercept	2/8 (25%): clinical response
Beck C et al., 2010 [33]	37	Naproxene	16/37 (43%) clinical response
		Indomethacin	4/7 (57%) clinical response
		Diclofenac	9/12 (75%) clinical response
		Others NSAIDs	6/19 (32%) clinical response
		Sulfasalazine	4/5 (80%) clinical response
		Steroids	4/4 (100%) clinical response but recurrence during dosage tapering
Roderick M et al., 2014 [40]	11	PAM	8/11 (73%) clinical response
Miettunen PM et al., 2009 [46]	9	PAM	9/9 (100%) clinical and radiological response
Gleeson H et al., 2008 [39]	7	PAM	6/7 (86%) clinical response
Hospach T et al., 2010 [47]	7	PAM	7/7 (100%) clinical response and radiological improvement
Kerrison C et al., 2004 [48]	7[a]	PAM	7/7 (100%) clinical remission
Batu ED, et al., 2015 [49]	5	Etanercept	5/5 (100%) clinical response
Simm PJ et al., 2008 [37]	5	PAM	4/5 (80%) clinical response and radiological improvement
Eleftheriou D et al., 2010 [50]	4	anti-TNFα	2/3 clinical response to infliximab, 1/3 response to adalimumab

DMARDS Disease-modifying anti-rheumatic drugs (Methotrexate or Azathioprine), *NSAIDs* Non-steroidal anti-inflammatory drugs, *PAM* Pamidonate
[a]patients with SAPHO

All monogenic forms of CNO (DIRA, Majeed syndrome and PAPA) respond really well to anti-IL1 blockade, [41–43] and, even if its role it is not clear in CNO, it has been recently demonstrated that Anakinra may be a possible therapeutic alternative in patients with refractory CNO [44].

The lack of longitudinal, placebo-control large studies on the different possible therapeutic strategies unable us to indicate an evidence-based approach to the treatment of this enigmatic and protean condition. Thus, the optimal treatment strategy for CNO remains to be determined.

Conclusions

CNO is a rare disorder and many considerations about diagnosis and treatment remain to be clarified. However, clinical features, the presence of multifocal lesions and radiologic features may help in diagnosis avoiding bone biopsy. NSAIDs remain the first treatment option, while bisphosphonates and TNF-alpha inhibitors could be considered the best second line treatment option. Even if CNO is often a benign disease, it can lead to severe and persistent complications.

Abbreviations

CNO: Chronic non-bacterial osteomyelitis; CRMO: Chronic recurrent multifocal osteomyelitis; DIRA: Deficiency of IL-1 receptor antagonist; MR: Magnetic resonance; NSAIDS: Non-steroidal anti-inflammatory drugs; PAPA: Pyogenic arthritis, Pyoderma gangrenosum and acne syndrome; SAPHO: Synovitis, Acne, Pustulosis, Hyperostosis, and Osteitis syndrome

Acknowledgements
Not applicable.

Funding
No funds to declare.

Authors' contributions
AT and SP conceptualized and designed the study, drafted the initial manuscript, and approved the final manuscript as submitted. GF, AT, MG, MF and MP carried out the initial analyses and reviewed the literature, reviewed and revised the manuscript, and approved the final manuscript as submitted. AI, AV and MG designed the data collection and the paper form, and coordinated and supervised data informations from the three different sites, critically reviewed the manuscript, and approved the final manuscript as submitted. All authors approved the final manuscript as submitted and agree to be accountable for all aspects of the work.

Competing interest
AT had speaking fees from Pfizer <10,000$; MG had speaking fees form Novartis, SOBI <10,000$.

Author details
[1]Institute for Maternal and Child Health, IRCCS "Burlo Garofolo", Trieste, Italy. [2]University of Trieste, Via dell'Istria 65/1, 34100 Trieste, Italy. [3]Division of Rheumatology, Department of Paediatric Medicine, Bambino Gesù Children's Hospital, IRCCS, Piazza di Sant'Onofrio, 4, 00165 Rome, Italy. [4]Pediatria 2, Istituto Gaslini, Via Gerolamo Gaslini, 5, 16148 Genoa, Italy.

References
1. Solheim LF, Paus B, Liverud K, Støen E. Chronic recurrent multifocal osteomyelitis. A new clinical-radiological syndrome. Acta Orthop Scand. 1980;51:37–41.
2. Giedion A, Holthusen W, Masel LF, Vischer D. Subacute and chronic "symmetrical" osteomyelitis. Ann Radiol (Paris). 1972;15:329–42.
3. Bjorksten B, Boquist L. Histopathological aspects of chronic recurrent multifocal osteomyelitis. J Bone Joint Surg Br. 1980;62:376–80.
4. Gamble JG, Rinsky LA. Chronic recurrent multifocal osteomyelitis: a distinct clinical entity. J Pediatr Orthop. 1986;6:579–84.
5. Robertson LP, Hickling P. Chronic recurrent multifocal osteomyelitis is a differential diagnosis of juvenile idiopathic arthritis. Ann Rheum Dis. 2001;60:828–31.
6. Huber AM, Lam PY, Duffy CM, Yeung RS, Ditchfield M, Laxer D, et al. Chronic recurrent multifocal osteomyelitis: clinical outcomes after more than five years of follow-up. J Pediatr. 2002;141:198–203.
7. Beretta-Piccoli BC, Sauvain MJ, Gal I, Schibler A, Saurenmann T, Kressebuch H, et al. Synovitis, acne, pustulosis, hyperostosis, osteitis (SAPHO) syndrome in childhood: a report of ten cases and review of the literature. Eur J Pediatr. 2000;159:594–601.
8. Schnabel A, Range U, Hahn G, Siepmann T, Berner R, Hedrich CM. Unexpectedly high incidences of chronic non-bacterial as compared to bacterial osteomyelitis in children. Rheumatol Int. 2016;36(12):1737–45.
9. Hamel J, Paul D, Gahr M, Hedrich CM. Pilot study: possible association of IL10 promoter polymorphisms with CRMO. Rheumatol Int. 2012;32:555–6.
10. Scianaro R, Insalaco A, Bracci Laudiero L, De Vito R, Pezzullo M, Teti A, et al. Deregulation of the IL-1β axis in chronic recurrent multifocal osteomyelitis. Pediatr Rheumatol Online J. 2014;12:30.
11. Hofmann SR, Morbach H, Schwarz T, Rösen-Wolff A, Girschick HJ, Hedrich CM. Attenuated TLR4/MAPK signaling in monocytes from patients with CRMO results in impaired IL-10 expression. Clin Immunol. 2012;145:69–76.
12. Majeed HA, Kalaawi M, Mohanty D, Teebi AS, Tunjekar MF, al-Gharbawy F, et al. Congenital dyserythropoietic anemia and chronic recurrent multifocal osteomyelitis in three related children and the association with sweet syndrome in two siblings. J Pediatr. 1989;115(5 Pt 1):730–4.
13. Ferguson PJ, Chen S, Tayeh MK, Ochoa L, Leal SM, Pelet A, et al. Homozygous mutations in LPIN2 are responsible for the syndrome of chronic recurrent multifocal osteomyelitis and congenital dyserythropoietic anaemia (Majeed syndrome). J Med Genet. 2005;42:551–7.
14. Papadaki ME, Lietman SA, Levine MA, Olsen BR, Kaban LB, Reichenberge EJ. Cherubism: best clinical practice. Orphanet J Rare Dis. 2012;7(1):S6.
15. Whyte MP. Physiological role of alkaline phosphatase explored in hypophosphatasia. Ann N Y Acad Sci. 2010;1192:190–200.
16. Castori M, Sinibaldi L, Mingarelli R, Lachman RS, Rimoin DL, Dallapiccola B. Pachydermoperiostosis: an update. Clin Genet. 2005;68:6477–86.
17. Smith EJ, Allantaz F, Bennett L, Zhang D, Gao X, Wood G, et al. Clinical, molecular, and genetic characteristics of PAPAsyndrome: a review. Curr Genomics. 2010;11:519–27.
18. Aksentijevich I, Masters SL, Ferguson PJ, Dancey P, Frenkel J, van Royen-Kerkhoff A, et al. An autoinflammatory disease with deficiency of the interleukin-1-receptor antagonist. N Engl J Med. 2009;360:2426–37.
19. Golla A, Jansson A, Ramser J, Hellebrand H, Zahn R, Meitinger T, et al. Chronic recurrent multifocal osteomyelitis (CRMO): evidence for a susceptibility gene located on chromosome 18q21.3-18q22. Eur J Hum Genet. 2002;10:217–21.
20. Wipff J, Costantino F, Lemelle I, Pajot C, Duquesne A, Lorrot M, et al. A large national cohort of French patients with chronic recurrent multifocal osteitis. Arthritis Rheumatol. 2015;67:1128–37.
21. Ben Becher S, Essaddam H, Nahali N, Ben Hamadi F, Mouelhi MH, Hammou A, et al. Recurrent multifocal periostosis in children. Report of a familial form. Ann Pediatr (Paris). 1991;38:345–9.
22. Ferguson PJ, Bing X, Vasef MA, Ochoa LA, Mahgoub A, Waldschmidt TJ, et al. A missense mutation in pstpip2 is associated with the murine autoinflammatory disorder chronic multifocal osteomyelitis. Bone. 2006;38:41–7.
23. Grosse J, Chitu V, Marquardt A, Hanke P, Schmittwolf C, Zeitlmann L, et al. Mutation of mouse Mayp/Pstpip2 causes a macrophage autoinflammatory disease. Blood. 2006;107:3350–8.
24. Jansson A, Renner ED, Ramser J, Mayer A, Haban M, Meindl A, et al. Classification of non-bacterial osteitis: retrospective study of clinical, immunological and genetic aspects in 89 patients. Rheumatology (Oxford). 2007;46:154–60.
25. Watanabe T, Ono H, Morimoto Y, Otsuki Y, Shirai M, Endoh A, et al. Skull involvement of a pediatric case of chronic recurrent multifocal Ostemyelitis. Nagoya J Med Sci. 2015;77:493–500.
26. Bousvaros A, Marcon M, Treem W, Waters P, Issenman R, Couper R, et al. Chronic recurrent multifocal osteomyelitis associated with chronic inflammatory bowel disease in children. Dig Dis Sci. 1999;44:2500–7.
27. Pastore S, Ferrara G, Monasta L, Meini A, Cattalini M, Martino S, et al. Chronic nonbacterial osteomyelitis may be associated with renal disease and bisphosphonates are a good option for the majority of patients. Acta Paediatr. 2016;105:e328–33.
28. Khanna G, Sato TS, Ferguson P. Imaging of chronic recurrent multifocal osteomyelitis. Radiographics. 2009;29:1159–77.
29. Fritz J, Tzaribatchev N, Claussen CD, Carrino JA, Horger MS. Chronic recurrent multifocal osteomyelitis: comparison of whole-body MR imaging with radiography and correlation with clinical and laboratory data. Radiology. 2009;252:842–51.
30. Voit AM, Arnoldi AP, Douis H, Bleisteiner F, Jansson MK, Reiser MF, et al. Whole-body magnetic resonance imaging in chronic recurrent multifocal Osteomyelitis: clinical Longterm assessment may underestimate activity. J Rheumatol. 2015;42:1455–62.
31. Jansson AF, Müller TH, Gliera L, Ankerst DP, Wintergest U, Belohradsky BH, et al. Clinical score for nonbacterial osteitis in children and adults. Arthritis Rheum. 2009;60:1152–9.
32. Taddio A, Zennaro F, Pastore S, Cimaz R. An update on the pathogenesis and treatment of chronic recurrent multifocal Osteomyelitis in children. Paediatr Drugs. 2017;19:165–72.
33. Beck C, Morbach H, Beer M, Stenzel M, Tappe D, Gattenlöhner S, et al. Chronic nonbacterial osteomyelitis in childhood: prospective follow-up during the first year of anti-inflammatory treatment. Arthritis Res Ther. 2010;12:R74.
34. Walsh P, Manners PJ, Vercoe J, Burgner D, Murray KJ. Chronic recurrent multifocal osteomyelitis in children: nine years' experience at a statewide tertiary paediatric rheumatology referral centre. Rheumatology (Oxford). 2015;54:1688–91.

35. Deutschmann A, Mache CJ, Bodo K, Zebedin D, Ring E. Successful treatment of chronic recurrent multifocal osteomyelitis with tumor necrosis factor-alpha blockage. Pediatrics. 2005;116:1231–3.
36. Eisenstein EM, Syverson GD, Vora SS, Williams CB. Combination therapy with methotrexate and etanercept for refractory chronic recurrent multifocal osteomyelitis. J Rheumatol. 2011;38:782–3.
37. Simm PJ, Allen RC, Zacharin MR. Bisphosphonate treatment in chronic recurrent multifocal osteomyelitis. J Pediatr. 2008;152:571–5.
38. De Cunto A, Maschio M, Lepore L, Zennaro F. A case of chronic recurrent multifocal osteomyelitis successfully treated with neridronate. J Pediatr. 2009;154:154–5.
39. Gleeson H, Wiltshire E, Briody J, Hall J, Chaitow J, Sillence D, et al. Childhood chronic recurrent multifocal osteomyelitis: pamidronate therapy decreases pain and improves vertebral shape. J Rheumatol. 2008;35:707–12.
40. Roderick M, Shah R, Finn A, Ramanan AV. Efficacy of pamidronate therapy in children with chronic non-bacterial osteitis: disease activity assessment by whole body magnetic resonance imaging. Rheumatology (Oxford). 2014;53:1973–6.
41. Herlin T, Fiirgaard B, Bjerre M, Kerndrup G, Hasle H, Bing X, et al. Efficacy of anti-IL-1 treatment in Majeed syndrome. Ann Rheum Dis. 2013;72:410–3.
42. Schnellbacher C, Ciocca G, Menendez R, Aksentijevich I, Goldbach-Mansky R, Duarte AM, et al. Deficiency of interleukin-1 receptor antagonist responsive to anakinra. Pediatr Dermatol. 2013;30:758–60.
43. Dierselhuis MP, Frenkel J, Wulffraat NM, Boelens JJ. Anakinra for flares of pyogenic arthritis in PAPA syndrome. Rheumatology (Oxford). 2005;44:406–8.
44. Pardeo M, Pires Marafon D, Messia V, Garganese MC, De Benedetti F, Insalaco A. Anakinra in a cohort of children with chronic nonbacterial Osteomyelitis. J Rheumatol. 2017;44:1231–8.
45. Kaiser D, Bolt I, Hofer M, Relly C, Berthet G, Bolz D, et al. Chronic nonbacterial osteomyelitis in children: a retrospective multi center study. Pediatr Rheumatol Online J. 2015;13:25.
46. Miettunen PM, Wei X, Kaura D, Reslan WA, Aguirre AN, Kellner JD. Dramatic pain relief and resolution of bone inflammation following pamidronate in 9 pediatric patients with persistent chronic recurrent multifocal osteomyelitis (CRMO). Pediatr Rheumatol Online J. 2009;7:2.
47. Hospach T, Langendoerfer M, von Kalle T, Maier J, Dannecker GE. Spinal involvement in chronic recurrent multifocal osteomyelitis (CRMO) in childhood and effect of pamidrnate. Eur J Pediatr. 2010;169:1105–11.
48. Kerrison C, Davidson JE, Cleary AG, Beresford MW. Pamidronate in the treatment of childhood SAPHO syndrome. Rheumatology (Oxford). 2004;43:1246–51.
49. Batu ED, Fergen FB, Gulhan B, Topaloglu R, Aydingoz U, Ozen S. Etanercept treatment in five cases of refractory chronic recurrent multifocal osteomyelitis (CRMO). Joint Bone Spine. 2015;82:471–3.
50. Eleftheriou D, Gerschman T, Sebire N, Woo P, Pilkington CA, Brogan PA. Biologic therapy in refractory chronic non-bacterial osteomyelitis of childhood. Rheumatology (Oxford). 2010;49:1505–12.

4

Clinical predictors of proteinuric remission following an LN flare - evidence from the UK JSLE cohort study

Eve M. D. Smith[1,2*], Peng Yin[3], Andrea L. Jorgensen[4], Michael W. Beresford[1,5] and on behalf of the UK JSLE Study Group

Abstract

Background: Proteinuria is a well-known risk factor for progression of renal dysfunction in a variety of chronic kidney diseases. In adult-onset Systemic Lupus Erytematosus (SLE) patients with lupus nephritis (LN), proteinuria takes a significant period of time to normalise, with proteinuric remission being associated with improved renal survival and reductions in mortality. The length of time required to attain proteinuric remission has not previously been investigated in Juvenile-onset SLE (JSLE). The aim of this study was to elucidate when proteinuric remission occurs, and whether clinical/demographic factors at LN onset bear influence on the time to proteinuric remission.

Methods: Participants of the UK JSLE Cohort Study and Repository were included if they had active LN (renal biopsy and/or renal British Isles Lupus Assessment Grade (BILAG) score defined active LN) and proteinuria. Univariate Cox proportional hazard regression modelling was used to explore factors associated with time to proteinuric recovery. Covariates with *p*-value < 0.2 were included in a multivariable Cox regression model, and backward stepwise variable selection applied.

Result: 64/350 (18%) of UK JSLE Cohort Study patients fulfilled the study inclusion criteria. 25 (39%) achieved proteinuric remission within a median of 17 months (min 2.4, max 78). Within a multivariate Cox proportional hazard regression model, age at time of LN flare ($p = 0.007$, HR 1.384, CI 1.095–1.750), eGFR ($p = 0.035$, HR 1.016, CI 1.001–1.030) and haematological involvement ($p = 0.016$, HR 0.324, CI 0.129–0.812) at the time of LN onset were found to be significantly associated with time to proteinuric recovery.

Conclusions: A significant proportion of children with LN have on-going proteinuria approximately two years after their initial flare. Poor prognostic factors all at time of LN onset include younger age, low eGFR, and concomitant haematological involvement.

Keywords: Juvenile-onset systemic lupus erythematosus, JSLE, Lupus nephritis, Active LN, Proteinuria, Prognosis

Background

Following a lupus nephritis (LN) flare, proteinuria has been shown to take a significant period of time to normalise in adults with systemic lupus erythematosus (SLE), with 53% of patients requiring up to 2 years to recover and only 74% recovering by 5 years [1]. Several adult SLE studies have shown that an early reduction in proteinuria following initiation of immunosuppressive therapy is associated with improved longer term renal outcomes [2–5]. Whilst proteinuria is on-going, differentiating between proteinuria due to on-going LN flare or chronic renal damage can be problematic. This leads the clinician to consider repetition of the renal biopsy, despite a lack of agreement as to the appropriate timing and indications for a repeat renal biopsy, particularly in children [6, 7].

Time to recovery from proteinuria in children with active LN receiving standard treatment has not been described to date. It is therefore of great interest to

* Correspondence: esmith8@liverpool.ac.uk
[1]Department of Women's & Children's Health, University of Liverpool, Institute In The Park, Alder Hey Children's Hospital, East Prescott Road, Liverpool L14 5AB, UK
[2]Department of Paediatric Rheumatology, Alder Hey Children's NHS Foundation Trust, Liverpool, UK
Full list of author information is available at the end of the article

explore this within the national UK JSLE Cohort Study, to appreciate how long proteinuria persists for within a real world clinical setting (in contrast for example to a clinical trial setting). Identification of clinical and demographic factors at the onset of LN which are predictive of longer duration to resolution of proteinuria would be useful for stratifying patients as having high or low risk for achieving proteinuric remission, and helping to modify the intensity and duration of early immunosuppressive therapy.

Methods

Aim

The main aim of this study was to use data arising from the UK JSLE Cohort Study (a UK-wide multicentre longitudinal cohort study collecting data as part of routine care) [8] between 1995 and 2015 to assess whether clinical and demographic factors can be used to predict time to proteinuric remission following an LN flare.

Patients

Participants of the UK JSLE Cohort Study [8], aged < 16 years at the time of diagnosis and with ≥4 American College of Rheumatology (ACR) SLE classification criteria, were included in the current study if they had the following:

1. Active LN - defined in terms of having either renal biopsy defined active LN (International Society of Nephrology / Renal Pathology Society 2003 score, ISN/RPS classification score [9]), or renal British Isles Lupus Assessment Grade (BILAG) domain score of A or B [10].
2. Significant proteinuria - defined as a urine protein creatinine ratio (UPCR) or urine albumin creatinine ratio (UACR) of > 50 mg/mmol or a 24-h urine protein of ≥0.5 g.
3. At least two consecutive follow-up visits with significant proteinuria following its initial proteinuria onset.

Patients were therefore excluded if they did not have BILAG (renal domain score of C-E) or renal biopsy defined active LN, if their UPCR was ≤50 mg/mmol or 24-h urine protein was < 0.5 g, or if they had < two follow-up visits following the onset of proteinuria (as this precluded the ability for longitudinal follow-up). The proteinuria cutoff was chosen on the basis of the renal BILAG score, where a UPCR or UACR ratio of > 50 mg/mmol or a 24-h urine protein of ≥0.5 g is required for at least a score of B to be achieved, signifying moderate LN activity [10]. Further practical information on the BILAG score is detailed within a review by Lattanzi et al., comparing the BILAG score to other scores such as the SLEDAI score [11].

Potential predictors of proteinuric recovery

Clinical and demographic factors (at the time of LN onset) were assessed as predictors within the analyses. Disease activity data was collected using the BILAG disease activity score at each routine clinic visit (approximately 3 monthly) [10]. Demographic details were collected using a standardized UK JSLE Cohort study case report form [8]. The demographic factors included gender, age at LN onset, ethnicity (caucasian/non-caucasian) and length of disease since diagnosis. Clinical renal factors consisted of proteinuria (spot UPCR or UACR), severe hypertension (blood pressure rising to > 170/110 mmHg within 1 month with grade 3 or 4 Keith-Wagener-Barker retinal changes), nephrotic syndrome (heavy proteinuria ≥3.5 g/day or protein-creatinine ratio of ≥350 mg/mmol or albumin-creatinine ratio of ≥350 mg/mmol, with hypoalbuminaemia and oedema), serum creatinine, presence of active urine sediment and estimated glomerular filtration rate (eGFR). Haematological features included haemoglobin, white cell count, neutrophils, lymphocytes and platelets. Immunological features consisted of complement factors 3 and 4 (C3/C4), anti-double-stranded DNA antibodies (anti-dsDNA), immunoglobulins (IgG, IgA, IgM), erythrocyte sedimentation rate (ESR) and c-reactive protein (CRP). Data on Coomb's positivity was not included as the dataset was incomplete.

The physician global assessment, total numerical BILAG score and concomitant active involvement of different BILAG domains were also considered (score of A or B for a given organ domain) in the analyses, including constitutional, mucocutaneous, neuropsychiatric, musculoskeletal, cardiorespiratory, gastrointestinal, opthalmological and haematological domain involvement. Medication use at the time of LN onset was also recorded (hydroxychloroquine, azathioprine, mycophenelate mofetil, prednisolone, intra-venous immunoglobulin (IVIG), angiotensin inhibitor or angiotensin receptor blocker, previous rituximab or cyclophosphamide use) for the analyses.

Study outcomes

Patients were categorised as having attained proteinuric recovery if their spot UPCR or UACR ratio was < 25 mg/mmol at two consecutive visits, or not recovered if the spot UPCR or UACR ratio was > 25 mg/mmol. The proteinuria cut off levels were chosen on the basis of the renal BILAG score as a spot UPCR or UACR ratio of < 25 mg/mmol would lead to a renal BILAG score of D, signifying inactive LN but previous renal involvement.

Statistical analysis

The study was undertaken using retrospective data from a longitudinal patient cohort. The outcome for each patient was defined as time to the date of proteinuric recovery, or to the date of the last visit date if they had not achieved proteinuric recovery and were censored. Cox proportional hazard regression modelling was used to univariately test the association between each clinical/demographic variable of interest and outcome. Variables with missing data were tested with complete cases only univariately. Covariates with $p < 0.2$ on univariate analysis were included in a multiple Cox regression model. Where > 10% of the data was missing for an included covariate, 'MICE' package in R version 3.2.0 was used to undertake multiple imputation [12]. Covariates to be retained in the final model were chosen by using a backward stepwise model selection procedure (threshold $p < 0.05$). Hazard ratios (HRs), 95% confidence intervals (CIs) and *p-values* were summarised for covariates present in the final model. The results were displayed graphically with Kaplan-Meier curves and risk tables. All analysis was undertaken with R version 3.2.0 [13].

Results

The study cohort consisted of 350 UK JSLE Cohort Study patients, of which 64/350 (18%) met the study's inclusion criteria and were therefore considered within these analyses. 43/64 (67%) had renal biopsy defined LN (class II $n = 4$, class III $n = 10$, class IV $n = 28$, class V n = 1) and 21/64 (33%) had renal BILAG defined LN (A = 3, B = 18). 55/350 patients met some but not all of the inclusion criteria and were therefore excluded (see Fig. 1 for further details). 54/64 patients had LN at the time of their initial diagnosis and 10/64 had a subsequent recurrent episode of LN. During the study follow-up period, proteinuric remission was achieved in 25/64 (39%) patients, within a median of 17 months (interquartile range, IQR 3.5–49.2).

Clinical / demographic factors influencing time to proteinuric recovery?

Using univariate Cox proportional hazard regression modelling, age at LN onset, serum creatinine, eGFR, neutrophil count, physician global assessment and BILAG defined haematological involvement all gave *p values* of < 0.2 (see Table 1), and therefore were considered within a multiple Cox regression model. There was no statistical difference in the distribution of renal biopsy subclasses, or whether patients had LN at diagnosis or recurrent LN, amongst the recovered and not-recovered groups ($p = 0.388$ and $p = 0.0784$ respectively).

After applying stepwise backward variable selection to the multivariable Cox regression model, it was identified that those who were older, or had higher eGFR values at the time of LN onset, were more likely to achieve proteinuric recovery. Further, those with haematological involvement at the time of LN onset were less likely to achieve proteinuric recovery (see Table 2).

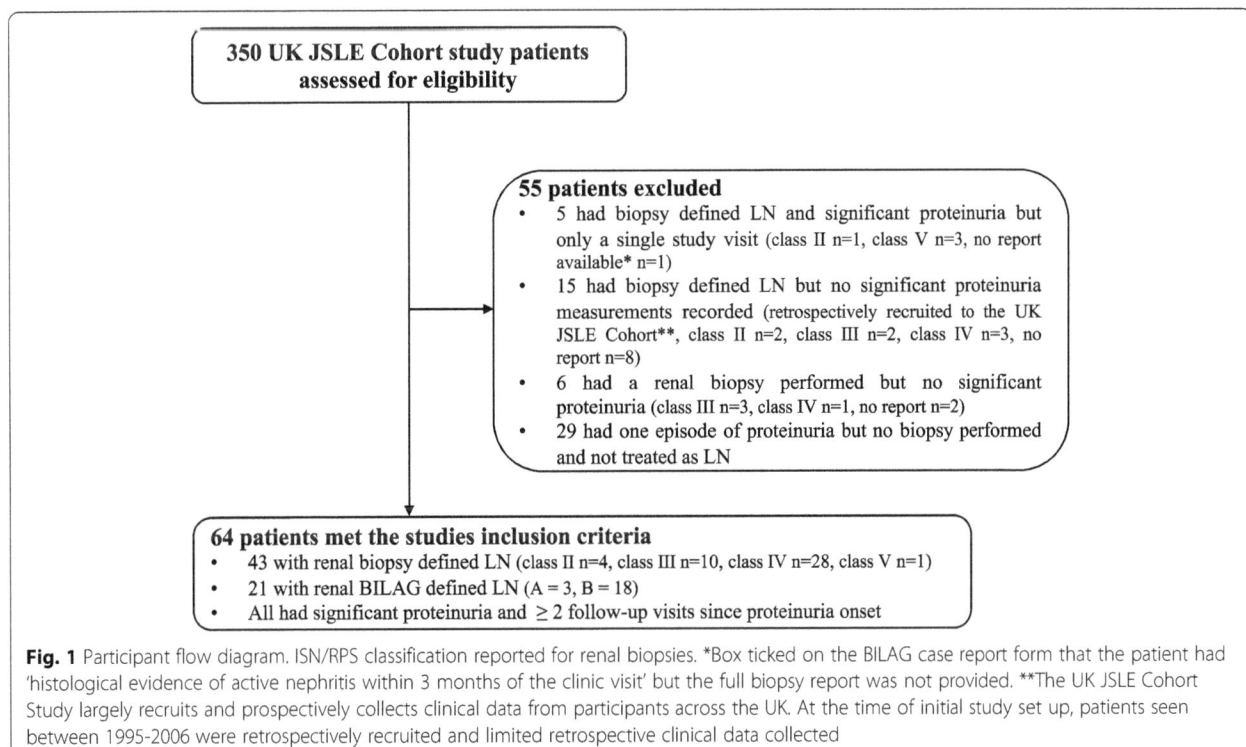

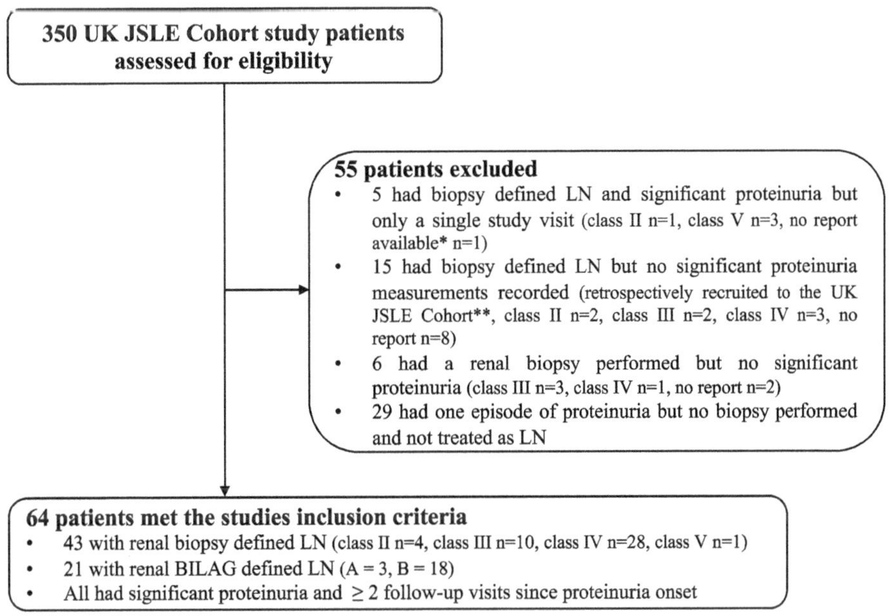

Fig. 1 Participant flow diagram. ISN/RPS classification reported for renal biopsies. *Box ticked on the BILAG case report form that the patient had 'histological evidence of active nephritis within 3 months of the clinic visit' but the full biopsy report was not provided. **The UK JSLE Cohort Study largely recruits and prospectively collects clinical data from participants across the UK. At the time of initial study set up, patients seen between 1995-2006 were retrospectively recruited and limited retrospective clinical data collected

Table 1 Univariate Cox proportional hazard regression modelling looking at time to proteinuric remission

	Clinical and demographic factors at LN onset	Not recovered ($n = 39$)[a]	Recovered ($n = 25$)[b]	Hazard Ratio (95% CI)	*p-value*
Factors included within the multivariate model	Age at LN onset (yrs)	13.9 (6.4, 17.7)	13.6 (8.1, 17.9)	1.0007 (1.0001, 1.0013)	*0.013*
	S creatinine (micromol/l, NA = 8)	61 (34, 234)	50 (36, 177)	0.991 (0.976, 1.005)	*0.184*
	eGFR (ml/min/m^{2,} NA = 2)	104 (29, 159)	121 (29,153)	1.014 (0.999, 1.028)	*0.060*
	Neutrophil count (× 10^9/L, NA = 2)	3.4 (1.1, 17.8)	3.44 (0.4, 12.33)	0.932 (0.837, 1.037)	*0.197*
	Physicians global assessment	23 (0, 75)	41 (1, 71)	1.027 (0.994, 1.061)	*0.107*
	Haematological involvement[c]	Y: 33, N: 6	Y: 13, N: 12	0.421 (0.187, 0.952)	*0.038*
Demographics, clinical features and laboratory investigations	LN ISN/RPS renal biopsy class[d]	Class II: 1 Class III: 5 Class IV: 15 Class V: 2	Class II: 3 Class III: 5 Class IV: 10 Class V: 2	0.769 (0.429, 1.378)	*0.388*
	LN at diagnosis or recurrent LN	Diagnosis: 33 Recurrent: 6	Diagnosis: 21 Recurrent: 4	0.320 (0.090, 1.138)	*0.078*
	Female gender	32/39 (82%)	18/25 (72%)	1.572 (0.642, 3.852)	*0.322*
	Caucasian ethnicity[e]	13/39 (33%)	13/25 (52%)	1.404 (0.637, 3.091)	*0.421*
	Length of disease at LN onset (days)	225 (0, 4857)	27 (0, 2679)	0.9999 (0.9994, 1.0005)	*0.934*
	Baseline Proteinuria[f]	149 (50, 2772)	252 (51, 1418)	0.9999 (0.9993, 1.0006)	*0.989*
	Severe hypertension (NA = 3)[g]	Y: 6, N: 31	Y: 3, N: 21	0.482 (0.140, 1.671)	*0.253*
	Nephrotic syndrome (NA = 3)[h]	Y: 7, N: 30	Y: 5, N: 19	0.853 (0.318, 2.342)	*0.765*
	Active urinary sediment (NA = 40)[i]	Y: 5, N: 9	Y: 3, N: 7	1.722 (0.402, 7.423)	*0.466*
	Haemoglobin (g/dl)	10.8 (5.6, 96)	11.3 (7.1, 14.9)	0.999 (0.949, 1.052)	*0.979*
	WCC (×10^9/L)	4.8 (2.5, 22.4)	6.4 (0.5, 9.1)	0.965 (0.885, 1.053)	*0.426*
	Lymphocytes (×10^9/L, NA = 2)	1.40 (0.1, 5.0)	1.53 (0.1, 5.42)	0.970 (0.670, 1.410)	*0.879*
	Platelets (×10^9/L)	245 (77, 589)	225 (82, 522)	0.998 (0.995, 1.002)	*0.342*
	ESR (mm/h, NA = 11)	40 (2, 170)	37.5 (4, 102)	0.994 (0.982, 1.006)	*0.353*
	CRP (mg/L, NA = 27)	5 (1, 19)	5 (1, 295)	0.998 (0.991, 1.005)	*0.601*
	C3 (g/L, NA = 7)	0.51 (0.18, 1.61)	0.71 (0.22, 1.31)	1.011 (0.301, 3.400)	*0.986*
	C4 (g/L, NA = 7)	0.06 (0.01, 0.90)	0.07 (0.02, 0.21)	0.282 (0.005, 15.171)	*0.537*
	Anti-dsDNA titres (IU/L, NA = 22)	119 (0, 3503)	220 (42, 3770)	0.999 (0.999, 1.000)	*0.577*
	IgG (g/L, NA = 27)	14.6 (0.9, 70.2)	11.8 (2.8, 33.1)	0.957 (0.895, 1.022)	*0.296*
	IgA (g/L, NA = 28)	2.06 (0.8, 4.9)	2.36 (0.3, 3.7)	0.870 (0.493, 1.542)	*0.636*
	IgM (g/L, NA = 28)	1.11 (0.4, 9.6)	(0.07, 2.5)	0.614 (0.271, 1.412)	*0.252*
Medications at LN onset	Hydroxychloroquine[j]	Y: 21, N: 18	Y: 12, N: 13	1.514 (0.663, 3.411)	*0.328*
	Azathioprine	Y: 8, N: 31	Y: 2, N: 23	0.520 (0.123, 2.222)	*0.377*
	Mycophenolate Mofetil	Y: 10, N: 29	Y: 6, N: 19	1.400 (0.550, 3.590)	*0.475*
	Prednisolone	Y: 24, N: 15	Y: 14, N: 11	1.260 (0.560, 2.860)	*0.581*
	Intravenous immunoglobulin	Y: 2, N: 37	Y: 2, N: 23	0.790 (0.170, 3.640)	*0.762*
	Rituximab ever	Y: 2, N: 37	Y: 1, N: 14	0.373 (0.046, 2.982)	*0.351*
	Cyclophosphamide ever	Y: 3, N: 36	Y: 2, N: 23	0.574 (0.132, 2.563)	*0.463*
	ACEi or AT2i[k]	Y: 11, N: 28	Y: 4, N: 21	0.753 (0.263, 2.222)	*0.607*
Concomitant BILAG defined organ involvement	Constitutional involvement	Y: 15, N: 24	Y: 15, N: 10	1.410 (0.621, 3.183)	*0.411*
	Mucocutaneous involvement	Y: 23, N: 16	Y: 15, N: 10	0.971 (0.431, 2.182)	*0.936*
	Neuropsychiatric involvement	Y: 3, N:36	Y: 3, N: 22	0.920 (0.261, 3.231)	*0.901*
	Musculoskeletal involvement	Y: 19, N: 20	Y: 14, N: 11	0.612 (0.251, 1.473)	*0.272*

Table 1 Univariate Cox proportional hazard regression modelling looking at time to proteinuric remission *(Continued)*

Clinical and demographic factors at LN onset	Not recovered ($n = 39$)[a]	Recovered ($n = 25$)[b]	Hazard Ratio (95% CI)	*p-value*
Cardiorespiratory involvement	Y: 3, N: 36	Y: 5, N: 20	1.253 (0.462, 3.422)	*0.663*
Gastrointestinal involvement	Y: 0, N: 39	Y: 3, N: 22	1.311 (0.361, 4.761)	*0.680*
Ophthalmological involvement	Y: 0, N: 39	Y: 2, N: 23	1.082 (0.221, 5.300)	*0.919*
Total numerical BILAG score	11 (3, 27)	11 (1, 53)	0.980 (0.951, 1.021)	*0.424*

Summary statistics used for continuous variables in the recovered and not recovered columns (median, min, max), whereas number count was detailed for discrete variables. Missing data shown in brackets with NA. *p-values* are from univariate Cox Proportion hazard models. [a]Not recovered = not attained proteinuric recovery during the follow up period. [b]Recovered = attained proteinuric recovery defined as if their spot UPCR or UACR ratio being <25mg/mmol at two consecutive visits. [c]BILAG defined active organ domain involvement (score of A or B). [d]Active LN defined in terms of having either renal biopsy defined active LN (ISN/RPS score), 32 or renal BILAG domain score of A or B. 43/64 patients had renal biopsy defined LN and 21/64 had renal BILAG defined LN. [e]Patients grouped as caucasian / non-caucasian for the purposes of the analysis. [f]Baseline Proteinuria = spot UPAC or UAUC measurements depending on hospital laboratory. [g]BILAG defined severe hypertension. [h]Nephrotic syndrome = heavy proteinuria (> 50 mg/kg/day or > 3.5 g/day or protein-creatinine ratio > 350 mg/mmol or albumin-creatinine ratio > 350mg/mmol) + hypoalbuminaemia + oedema. [i]Active urine sediment = pyuria (> 5 WCC/hpf), haematuria (> 5 RBC/hpf) or red cell casts in absence of other causes. [j]Medication use (yes) or non-use (no) considered rather than absolute drug dose. [k]ACEi or AT2i = Angiotensin inhibitor or angiotensin receptor blocker

Kaplan Meier plots for age, eGFR and BILAG defined haematological involvement are shown in Fig. 2. Figure 2a demonstrates that at a given time, patients who are older at the time of LN onset (> 14 years vs < 14 years) are more likely to achieve proteinuric recovery. The median patient age across the whole patient group was 14 years, therefore, that is why this cut-off was used to divide patients into younger or older groups. Median time to recovery was 4.95 years (95% CI: 0.33–9.09) in the younger age group and 0.65 years (95% CI: 0.29–5.31) in the older age group ($p = 0.021$). The Kaplan Meier plot for eGFR (Fig. 2b) divides patients into two clinically relevant sub-groups with an eGFR of less or greater that 80 mls/min, demonstrating that at a given time, patients with a eGFR of > 80 mls/min at LN onset are more likely to recover. Those with eGFR levels < 80 mls/min had a median time to recovery of 2.00 years (95% CI: 0.43–8.85) whilst those above 80 mls/min had median time to recovery of 1.82 years (95% CI: 0.28–7.95, $p = 0.170$). Figure 2c illustrates that at a given time, patients without haematological involvement at LN onset are more likely to attain proteinuric recovery at each time point. Median time to recovery was 1.73 years (95% CI: 0.28–8.34) in those without involvement and 2.14 years (95% CI: 0.30–8.13) in those with haematological involvement ($p = 0.038$).

Table 2 Multivariable–Cox regression model displaying factors associated with time to proteinuric recovery

Clinical and demographic factors at LN onset	HR (95% CI)	*p value*
Age at LN onset (years)	1.384 (1.095, 1.750)	*0.007*
eGFR	1.016 (1.001, 1.030)	*0.035*
Haematological involvement	0.324 (0.129, 0.812)	*0.016*

eGFR estimated glomerular filtration rate, *HR* hazard ration, *CI* confidence interval
Multivariable Cox regression model after applying variable selection

Discussion

Using data from a large national cohort of patients recruited to the UK JSLE Cohort Study, this study has demonstrated that proteinuria can be persistent following a LN flare. Clinical and demographic data have been used within this study to characterise patients who are at increased risk of having a prolonged period of proteinuria following an LN flare. Early reduction in proteinuria following initiation of immunosuppressive therapy has been shown to be associated with improved longer term renal outcomes [1, 14] and patient survival [4] in adult SLE, therefore, appreciation of those who are likely to need longer to achieve proteinuric recovery may influence monitoring and treatment decisions. Outwith a LN setting, levels of albuminuria have been shown to relate to all cause and cardiovascular mortality [15, 16], with proteinuria reduction being the main target for halting the progression of diabetic [17] and many non-diabetic kidney diseases [18].

A total of 39% of patients were shown to reach proteinuric remission following a LN flare during the study period, within a median of 17 months (IQR 3.5–49.2). This observation provides useful information on the length of time necessary to achieve proteinuric recovery following a LN flare within real world clinical practice, as opposed to a tightly regulated clinical trial setting. A similar study in adult SLE showed proteinuric recovery to occur in 53% of patients by 2 years [1], suggest that proteinuria may take longer to normalize in children than adults with SLE. In a Korean study including 193 adults with SLE and severe proliferative LN, proteinuric remission was attained in 8% of patients within 12 months, 19% between 12 and 60 months, and 16% after more than 60 months post renal biopsy, suggesting that those with the most severe LN histological subtypes may need even longer to achieve proteinuric remission [14].

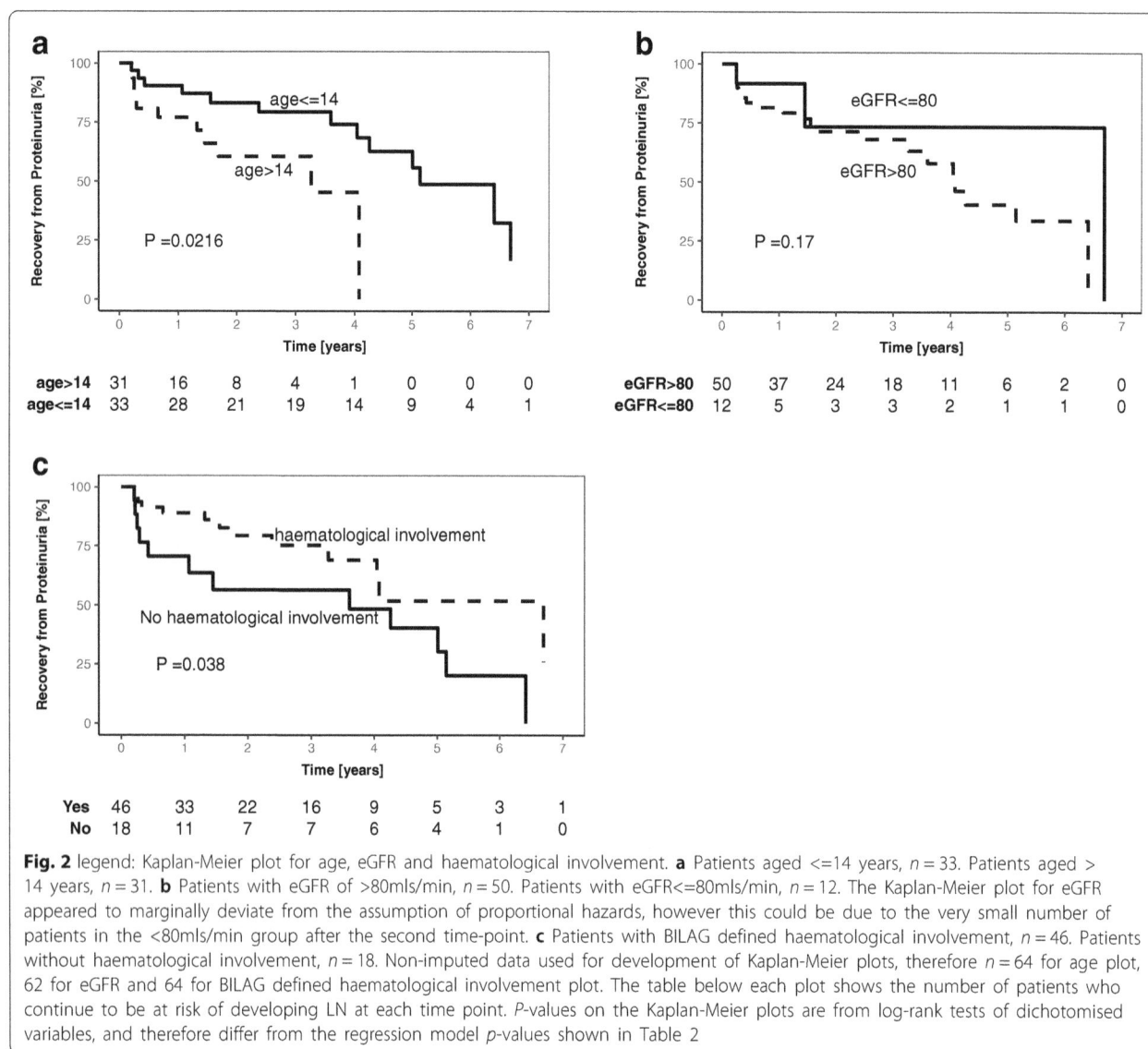

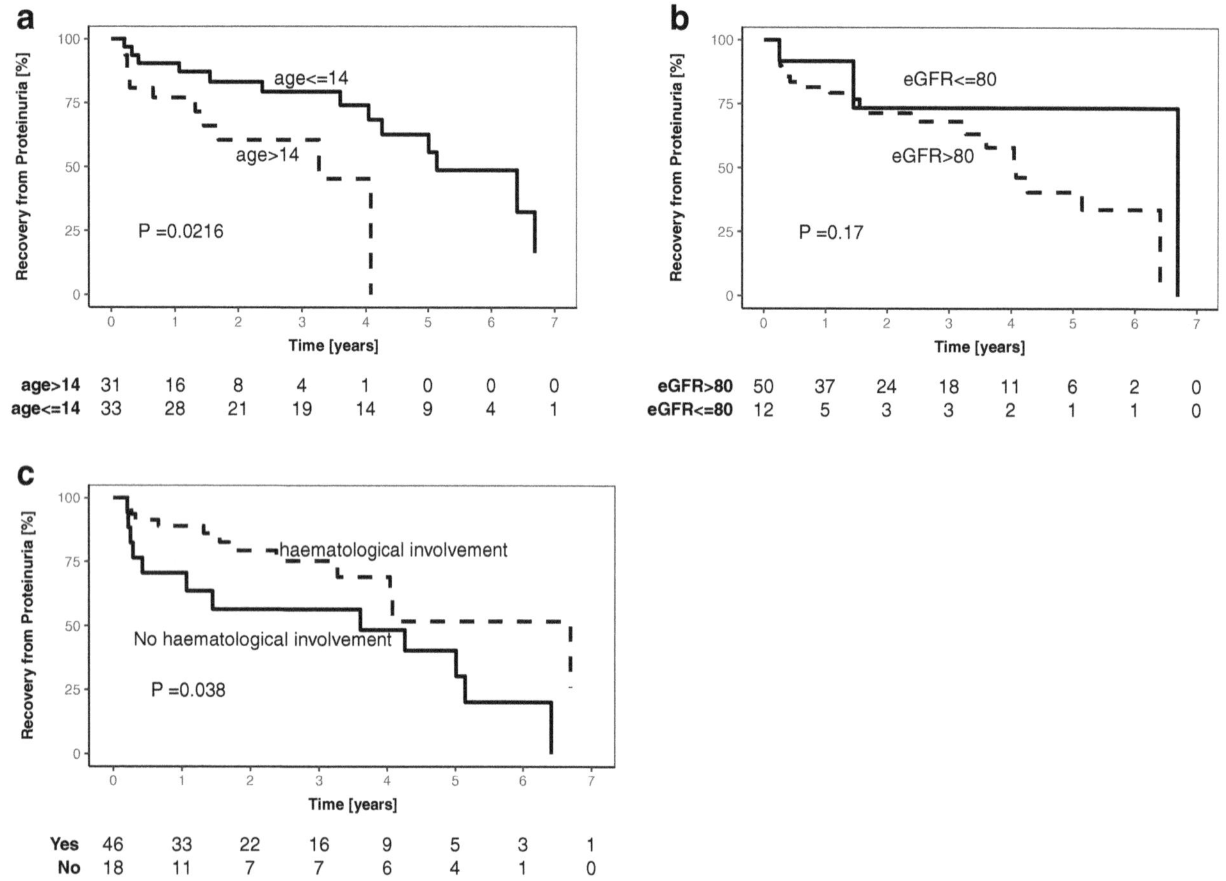

Fig. 2 legend: Kaplan-Meier plot for age, eGFR and haematological involvement. **a** Patients aged <=14 years, $n = 33$. Patients aged > 14 years, $n = 31$. **b** Patients with eGFR of >80mls/min, $n = 50$. Patients with eGFR<=80mls/min, $n = 12$. The Kaplan-Meier plot for eGFR appeared to marginally deviate from the assumption of proportional hazards, however this could be due to the very small number of patients in the <80mls/min group after the second time-point. **c** Patients with BILAG defined haematological involvement, $n = 46$. Patients without haematological involvement, $n = 18$. Non-imputed data used for development of Kaplan-Meier plots, therefore $n = 64$ for age plot, 62 for eGFR and 64 for BILAG defined haematological involvement plot. The table below each plot shows the number of patients who continue to be at risk of developing LN at each time point. *P*-values on the Kaplan-Meier plots are from log-rank tests of dichotomised variables, and therefore differ from the regression model *p*-values shown in Table 2

Younger age at the time of LN onset was shown to be the strongest predictor of having a prolonged time to proteinuric recovery, likely reflecting the more severe disease phenotype and potential genetic predisposition to JSLE/LN seen in younger patients [8, 19–24]. This study did not collect information on pubertal status, but in future work it would be useful to assess the influence of pubertal status on time to proteinuric recovery. Reductions in eGFR usually occur following significant renal damage and may be preceded by a period of hyper-filtration [25–27]. It is therefore not unexpected that low eGFR at the time of LN onset was associated with longer time to proteinuric recovery in the current study.

Haematological involvement at the time of LN onset was associated with a longer time to proteinuric recovery. It is of interest that individual haematological measures (e.g. haemoglobin, white count, platelets) were not individually associated with time to proteinuric recovery, but as reflected by the haematological domain of the BILAG score, combinations of abnormalities were found to be important. It can be speculated that concomitant haematological involvement may also affect the ability to intensify immunosuppressant treatment due to concerns about treatment toxicity, thereby influencing time to proteinuric recovery. Awareness of these factors is important for stratification of patients at the time of LN onset, and considering the intensity and duration of early immunosuppressive therapy. In future work it would also be of interest to look at whether patients were Coombs' positive and their reticulocyte counts.

The strengths of this study lie in the large real-world patient cohort receiving a multitude of treatment regimens, as opposed to a tightly regulated clinical trial. Certain limitations of this study do however warrant recognition and should be addressed in future work. The study did not include all LN patients; with five biopsy proven LN patients excluded as they only had a single follow-up visit, and a further 15 patients excluded who were retrospectively recruited to the cohort and had insufficient proteinuria measurements recorded for meaningful analysis to be undertaken. The analysis looked at treatment at baseline and did not look at the influence of on-going treatment (steroids and DMARDs) due to the number and complexity of the different treatment plans used, precluding meaningful analysis in this area. Similarly, these analyses did not consider serially collected disease activity and damage data as the aim of this work was to look at factors at the time of LN onset which predict time to proteinuric remission. Further work involving sophisticated longitudinal modelling of all data would be of interest in future work.

The definition of proteinuric remission used in this study was based on the renal BILAG score. Other cut-offs could have been chosen based on other scoring systems, e.g. the Systemic Lupus Erythematosus Disease Activity Index (SLEDAI) or the European Community Lupus Activity Measure (ECLAM), that both define proteinuric remission as < 0.5 g/24 h, and the ACR score defines it as persistently < 0.5 g/24 h or <+++ on protein dipstix if quantification not performed [28–30]. The BILAG score provides the most comprehensive assessment of renal disease activity of these disease activity scores and includes UPCR or UACR measurements which are more practical in children, less dependent on patient compliance and yield more complete longitudinal data.

The urine samples were collected at different times of the day and in future work it would be useful to standardize the time of sample collection (e.g. all early morning urine samples) to minimize the influence of orthostatic proteinuria. Within the inclusion criteria it was specified that patients must have at least two consecutive follow-up visits with significant proteinuria following its initial proteinuria onset, to minimize the inclusion of patients with one off episodes of orthostatic proteinuria. The study also did not include patients with mild LN within the active LN group (renal BILAG domain score of C) as such a BILAG score can easily be obtained by having 1+ of urine dipstick proteinuria, which may be due to orthostatic proteinuria. This study looked at medication use at the time of LN onset but could not sub-divide patients according to the LN treatment regimen received in view of the multitude of different treatment regimens used in clinical practice over time. The cohort study data is collected alongside routine clinical practice leading to missing data and the need for multiple imputation within the analyses, therefore further analysis in more complete datasets would be of interest in future work.

Conclusions

A high proportion of JSLE patients develop LN [8, 31, 32]. This study has demonstrated that proteinuria can be persistent within a real world clinical setting. This study has elucidated basic characteristics of patients who are at increased risk of having prolonged proteinuria following an LN flare, namely patients who are younger (< 14 years), have an abnormal eGFR (< 80 mls/min) and concomitant haematological involvement at the time of LN onset. These data cannot guide the clinician as to when to repeat the renal biopsy and/or intensify immunosuppressive treatment, however they do highlight at an early stage, patients who need closer surveillance as they are at increased risk of having a more prolonged period to proteinuric remission. Ideally there would be a specific biomarker or urinary biomarker panel that clinicians could easily test to highlight patients who will display persistence of proteinuria following LN flare [33]. Whilst awaiting this development, it is important to be aware of such clinical and demographic factors. Early reduction in proteinuria following initiation of immunosuppressive therapy has been shown to be associated with improved longer term renal outcomes and survival in adult SLE. Therefore, appreciation of those at risk of prolonged proteinuria may help the clinician to change or fine-tune the intensity and duration of early immunosuppressive therapy.

Abbreviations

ACR: American College of Rheumatology; anti-dsDNA: anti-double-stranded DNA antibody; BILAG: British Isles Lupus Assessment Grade; C3: complement factor 3; C4: complement factor 4; CI: confidence interval; CRP: c-reactive protein; ECLAM: European Community Lupus Activity Measure; eGFR: estimated glomerular filtration rate; ESR: erythrocyte sedimentation rate; HR: hazard ratio; Ig: immunoglobulin; IVIG: intra-venous immunoglobulin; JSLE: Juvenile Systemic Lupus Erythematosus; LN: lupus nephritis; MMF: mycophenolate mofetil; SLEDAI: Systemic Lupus Erythematosus Disease Activity Index; UACR: urine albumin creatinine ratio; UK: United Kingdom; UPCR: urine protein creatinine ratio

Acknowledgements

The authors would like to acknowledge all patients and their families for participating in this Study, as well as all the support given by the entire multi-disciplinary team within each of the paediatric centres. The study was supported by the National Institute of Health Research (NIHR) Clinical Research Network (CRN): Children and CRN Research Nurses and staff in all centres. Special acknowledgement is given to the principle investigators in each of the participating centres and lead nurse(s) for the Study, and all those who have supported the work of the UK JSLE Study Group to date including Dr. Eslam Al Abadi, Dr. Jane Tizard, Dr. Janet Gardiner Medwin, Dr. Joyce Davidson, Dr. Clarissa Pilkington, Dr. Valentina Leone, Dr. Flora McErlane, Dr. Satyapal Rangaraj, Dr. Phil Riley, Dr. Nick Wilkinson, Dr. Kate Armon, Dr. John Ioannou, Dr. Devesh Mewar, Dr. Gita Modgil, Dr. Alice Leahy, Dr. Arani Sridhar, Dr. Dan Hawley and Dr. Kirsty Haslam. We acknowledge the important work of the NIHR and other funded Clinical Research Facilities that have supported this Study, including specifically the NIHR Alder Hey Clinical Research Facility. Particular thanks to the UK's 'Experimental Arthritis Treatment Centre for Children' funded by Arthritis Research UK, the University of Liverpool, Alder Hey Children's NHS Foundation Trust and the Alder Hey Charity. Specific acknowledgement goes to Duncan Appleby for database and information technology support and Carla Roberts for co-ordination of the Cohort study.

Funding
This work was supported by the Alder Hey Children's Kidney Fund through a training fellowship [UOG10065 to ES]. Lupus UK also provides financial support for co-ordination of the UK JSLE Cohort Study. The funders have not played a role in the design of the study and collection, analysis, interpretation of data or writing of the manuscript.

Authors' contributions
All authors participated in conception, design of the study and interpretation of the data. ES and MWB participated in the acquisition of data. PY, AJ and ES performed the statistical analysis. MWB is Chief Investigator of the UK JSLE Cohort Study. All authors were involved in drafting the manuscript and revising it critically for important intellectual content. They have also all read and given final approval of the version to be published.

Competing interests
The authors declare that they have no competing interests.

Author details
[1]Department of Women's & Children's Health, University of Liverpool, Institute In The Park, Alder Hey Children's Hospital, East Prescott Road, Liverpool L14 5AB, UK. [2]Department of Paediatric Rheumatology, Alder Hey Children's NHS Foundation Trust, Liverpool, UK. [3]Research Center for Biomedical Information Technology, Shenzhen Institutes of Advanced Technology, Chinese Academy of Sciences, Shenzhen, China. [4]Department of Biostatistics, Block F, Waterhouse Building, University of Liverpool, Liverpool, UK. [5]Department of Paediatric Rheumatology, Alder Hey Children's NHS Foundation Trust, Liverpool, UK.

References
1. Touma Z, Urowitz MB, Ibanez D, Gladman DD. Time to recovery from proteinuria in patients with lupus nephritis receiving standard treatment. J Rheumatol. 2014;41:688–97.
2. Houssiau FA, Vasconcelos C, D'Cruz D, Sebastiani GD, de Ramon Garrido E, Danieli MG, Abramovicz D, Blockmans D, Mathieu A, Direskeneli H, et al. Early response to immunosuppressive therapy predicts good renal outcome in lupus nephritis: lessons from long-term followup of patients in the euro-lupus nephritis trial. Arthritis Rheum. 2004;50:3934–40.
3. Houssiau FA, Vasconcelos C, D'Cruz D, Sebastiani GD, de Ramon Garrido E, Danieli MG, Abramovicz D, Blockmans D, Cauli A, Direskeneli H, et al. The 10-year follow-up data of the euro-lupus nephritis trial comparing low-dose and high-dose intravenous cyclophosphamide. Ann Rheum Dis. 2010;69:61–4.
4. Korbet SM, Lewis EJ, Collaborative Study G. Severe lupus nephritis: the predictive value of a >/= 50% reduction in proteinuria at 6 months. Nephrol Dial Transplant. 2013;28:2313–8.
5. Dall'Era M, Cisternas MG, Smilek DE, Straub L, Houssiau FA, Cervera R, Rovin BH, Mackay M. Predictors of long-term renal outcome in lupus nephritis trials: lessons learned from the euro-lupus nephritis cohort. Arthritis Rheumatol. 2015;67:1305–13.
6. Greloni G, Scolnik M, Marin J, Lancioni E, Quiroz C, Zacariaz J, De la Iglesia Niveyro P, Christiansen S, Pierangelo MA, Varela CF, et al. Value of repeat biopsy in lupus nephritis flares. Lupus Sci Med. 2014;1:e7099.
7. Subils G, Alba P, Gobbi C, Astesana P, Babini A, Albiero E. The repeated biopsy in patients with lupus nephritis. Rev Fac Cien Med Univ Nac Cordoba. 2014;71:165–70.
8. Watson L, Leone V, Pilkington C, Tullus K, Rangaraj S, McDonagh JE, Gardner-Medwin J, Wilkinson N, Riley P, Tizard J, et al. Disease activity, severity, and damage in the UK juvenile-onset systemic lupus erythematosus cohort. Arthritis Rheum. 2012;64:2356–65.
9. Weening JJ, D'Agati VD, Schwartz MM, Seshan SV, Alpers CE, Appel GB, Balow JE, Bruijn JA, Cook T, Ferrario F, et al. The classification of glomerulonephritis in systemic lupus erythematosus revisited. J Am Soc Nephrol. 2004;15:241–50.
10. Isenberg DA, Rahman A, Allen E, Farewell V, Akil M, Bruce IN, D'Cruz D, Griffiths B, Khamashta M, Maddison P, et al. BILAG 2004. Development and initial validation of an updated version of the British isles lupus assessment Group's disease activity index for patients with systemic lupus erythematosus. Rheumatology (Oxford). 2005;44:902–6.
11. Lattanzi B, Consolaro A, Solari N, Ruperto N, Martini A, Ravelli A. Measures of disease activity and damage in pediatric systemic lupus erythematosus: British isles lupus assessment group (BILAG), European consensus lupus activity measurement (ECLAM), systemic lupus activity measure (SLAM), systemic lupus erythematosus disease activity index (SLEDAI), Physician's global assessment of disease activity (MD global), and systemic lupus international collaborating clinics/American College of Rheumatology Damage Index (SLICC/ACR DI; SDI). Arthritis Care Res (Hoboken). 2011;63(Suppl 11):S112–7.
12. MICE package in R [https://cran.r-project.org/web/packages/mice/index.html]. Accessed 19 Feb 2018.
13. R: A language and environment for statistical computing version 3.3.3 [https://www.r-project.org//]. Accessed 19 Feb 2018.
14. Koo HS, Kim S, Chin HJ. Remission of proteinuria indicates good prognosis in patients with diffuse proliferative lupus nephritis. Lupus. 2016;25:3–11.
15. Oh SW, Baek SH, Kim YC, Goo HS, Heo NJ, Na KY, Chae DW, Kim S, Chin HJ. Mild decrease in estimated glomerular filtration rate and proteinuria are associated with all-cause and cardiovascular mortality in the general population. Nephrol Dial Transplant. 2012;27:2284–90.
16. Oh SW, Kim S, Na KY, Kim KW, Chae DW, Chin HJ. Glomerular filtration rate and proteinuria: association with mortality and renal progression in a prospective cohort of a community-based elderly population. PLoS One. 2014;9:e94120.
17. Strippoli GF, Bonifati C, Craig M, Navaneethan SD, Craig JC. Angiotensin converting enzyme inhibitors and angiotensin II receptor antagonists for preventing the progression of diabetic kidney disease. Cochrane Database Syst Rev. 2006:CD006257.
18. Remuzzi G1, Chiurchiu C, Ruggenenti P. Proteinuria predicting outcome in renal disease: nondiabetic nephropathies (REIN). Kidney Int Suppl. 2004;(92): S90-6. https://www.ncbi.nlm.nih.gov/pubmed/15485427.
19. Brunner HI, Gladman DD, Ibañez D, Urowitz MD, Silverman ED. Difference in disease features between childhood-onset and adult-onset systemic lupus erythematosus. Arthritis Rheum. 2008;58:556–62.
20. Hoffman IE, Lauwerys BR, De Keyser F, Huizinga TW, Isenberg D, Cebecauer L, Dehoorne J, Joos R, Hendrickx G, Houssiau F, Elewaut D. Juvenile-onset systemic lupus erythematosus: different clinical and serological pattern than adult-onset systemic lupus erythematosus. Ann Rheum Dis. 2009;68:412–5.
21. Stegert M, Bock M, Trendelenburg M. Clinical presentation of human C1q deficiency: how much of a lupus? Mol Immunol. 2015;67:3–11.
22. Gargiulo Mde L, Gomez G, Khoury M, Collado MV, Suarez L, Alvarez C, Sarano J. Association between the presence of anti-C1q antibodies and active nephritis in patients with systemic lupus erythematosus. Medicina (B Aires). 2015;75:23–8.
23. van Schaarenburg RA, Schejbel L, Truedsson L, Topaloglu R, Al-Mayouf SM, Riordan A, Simon A, Kallel-Sellami M, Arkwright PD, Ahlin A, et al. Marked variability in clinical presentation and outcome of patients with C1q immunodeficiency. J Autoimmun. 2015;62:39–44.
24. Orbai AM, Truedsson L, Sturfelt G, Nived O, Fang H, Alarcon GS, Gordon C, Merrill J, Fortin PR, Bruce IN, et al. Anti-C1q antibodies in systemic lupus erythematosus. Lupus. 2015;24:42–9.
25. Cottiero RA, Madaio MP, Levey AS. Glomerular filtration rate and urinary albumin excretion rate in systemic lupus erythematosus. Nephron. 1995;69:140–6.
26. Park M, Yoon E, Lim YH, Kim H, Choi J, Yoon HJ. Renal hyperfiltration as a novel marker of all-cause mortality. J Am Soc Nephrol. 2015;26:1426–33.
27. Altay S, Onat A, Ozpamuk-Karadeniz F, Karadeniz Y, Kemaloglu-Oz T, Can G. Renal "hyperfiltrators" are at elevated risk of death and chronic diseases. BMC Nephrol. 2014;15:160.
28. Bencivelli W, Vitali C, Isenberg DA, Smolen JS, Snaith ML, Sciuto M, Bombardieri S. Disease activity in systemic lupus erythematosus: report of the consensus study Group of the European Workshop for rheumatology research. III. Development of a computerised clinical chart and its application to the comparison of different indices of disease activity. The European consensus study Group for Disease Activity in SLE. Clin Exp Rheumatol. 1992;10:549–54.

29. Vitali C, Bencivelli W, Isenberg DA, Smolen JS, Snaith ML, Sciuto M, d'Ascanio A, Bombardieri S. Disease activity in systemic lupus erythematosus: report of the consensus study Group of the European Workshop for rheumatology research. I. A descriptive analysis of 704 European lupus patients. European consensus study Group for Disease Activity in SLE. Clin Exp Rheumatol. 1992;10:527–39.
30. Vitali C, Bencivelli W, Isenberg DA, Smolen JS, Snaith ML, Sciuto M, Neri R, Bombardieri S. Disease activity in systemic lupus erythematosus: report of the consensus study Group of the European Workshop for rheumatology research. II. Identification of the variables indicative of disease activity and their use in the development of an activity score. The European consensus study Group for Disease Activity in SLE. Clin Exp Rheumatol. 1992;10:541–7.
31. Tucker LB, Menon S, Schaller JG, Isenberg DA. Adult- and childhood-onset systemic lupus erythematosus: a comparison of onset, clinical features, serology, and outcome. Br J Rheumatol. 1995;34:866–72.
32. Hiraki LT, Benseler SM, Tyrrell PN, Hebert D, Harvey E, Silverman ED. Clinical and laboratory characteristics and long-term outcome of pediatric systemic lupus erythematosus: a longitudinal study. J Pediatr. 2008;152:550–6.
33. Smith EMD, Beresford MW. Urinary biomarkers in childhood lupus nephritis. Clin Immunol. 2017;185:21–31.

5

The safety of live-attenuated vaccines in patients using IL-1 or IL-6 blockade: an international survey

Jerold Jeyaratnam[1†], Nienke M. ter Haar[2†], Helen J. Lachmann[3], Ozgur Kasapcopur[4], Amanda K. Ombrello[5], Donato Rigante[6], Fatma Dedeoglu[7], Ezgi H. Baris[7], Sebastiaan J. Vastert[8], Nico M. Wulffraat[8] and Joost Frenkel[1*]

Abstract

Background: Withholding live-attenuated vaccines in patients using interleukin (IL)-1 or IL-6 blocking agents is recommended by guidelines for both pediatric and adult rheumatic diseases, since there is a risk of infection in an immune suppressed host. However, this has never been studied. This retrospective, multicenter survey aimed to evaluate the safety of live-attenuated vaccines in patients using IL-1 or IL-6 blockade.

Methods: We contacted physicians involved in the treatment of autoinflammatory diseases to investigate potential cases. Patients were included if a live-attenuated vaccine had been administered while they were on IL-1 or IL-6 blockade.

Results: Seventeen patients were included in this survey (7 systemic juvenile idiopathic arthritis (sJIA), 5 cryopyrin associated periodic syndrome (CAPS), 4 mevalonate kinase deficiency (MKD) and 1 familial Mediterranean fever (FMF). Three patients experienced an adverse event, of which two were serious adverse events (a varicella zoster infection after varicella zoster booster vaccination, and a pneumonia after MMR booster). One additional patient had diarrhea after oral polio vaccine. Further, seven patients experienced a flare of their disease, which were generally mild. Eight patients did not experience an adverse event or a flare.

Conclusion: We have described a case series of seventeen patients who received a live-attenuated vaccine while using IL-1 or IL-6 blocking medication. The findings of this survey are not a reason to adapt the existing guidelines. Prospective trials are needed in order to acquire more evidence about the safety and efficacy before considering adaptation of guidelines.

Keywords: Autoinflammatory diseases, Live-attenuated vaccines, Biologicals, IL-1 blockade, IL-6 blockade

Background

Vaccines have contributed greatly to public health, protecting children and adults from serious infectious diseases [1]. Besides inactivated vaccines there are several live-attenuated vaccines.

Autoinflammatory diseases, such as systemic juvenile idiopathic arthritis (sJIA), familial Mediterranean fever (FMF), mevalonate kinase deficiency (MKD), cryopyrin associated periodic syndrome (CAPS) and tumor necrosis factor (TNF)-receptor associated periodic syndrome (TRAPS) exhibit systemic inflammation or organ specific inflammation caused by dysregulation of the innate immune system. Interleukin (IL)-1 blockade (anakinra, canakinumab and rilonacept) and IL-6 blockade (tocilizumab) have greatly improved the outcome of these patients [2]. However, patients with autoinflammatory diseases potentially face long-term or lifelong immunosuppression thus raising the dilemma if and when vaccinations could be given.

Although vaccination is generally considered safe in the healthy population, existing guidelines for both pediatric and adult rheumatic diseases recommend to withhold live-attenuated vaccines in patients using IL-1 or IL-6 blocking

* Correspondence: J.Frenkel@umcutrecht.nl
†Equal contributors
[1]Department of General Pediatrics, University Medical Center Utrecht, Room KE 04 133 1, PO-Box 85090, 3508, AB Utrecht, The Netherlands
Full list of author information is available at the end of the article

agents, because of lack of safety data and the (theoretical) risk of introducing infection in an immune suppressed host [3–5]. On the other hand, patients with autoinflammatory diseases might especially benefit from protection against infectious diseases, as the immunosuppressive therapy renders them more susceptible to infections [6, 7]. In clinical practice, vaccination can be considered on a case-to-case basis weighing the risk of natural infection versus the risk of vaccination, e.g. measles mumps and rubella (MMR) vaccination during measles outbreaks or yellow fever vaccine before travelling to endemic regions.

In this retrospective survey, we aimed to evaluate the safety and efficacy of live-attenuated vaccines in patients using IL-1 or IL-6 blockade.

Methods

Via the Paediatric Rheumatology European Society and the International Society for Systemic Auto Inflammatory Diseases pediatric and adult rheumatologists and immunologists were contacted by e-mail in January 2016 in order to recruit potential cases. A reminder was sent up to three times, if no response was obtained. Patients were included if they had received a live-attenuated vaccine while using IL-1 blockade or IL-6 blockade.

Ethical approval was obtained by the institutional ethical committee in accordance with local ethical regulations; the survey was conducted in accordance with the ethical principles of the declaration of Helsinki. Written informed consent was obtained from the patient or the legal guardians in case of minors according to local requirements. Demographic and clinical data were collected by local physicians and were anonymized. Adverse events were categorized as adverse events and serious adverse events. Serious adverse events were defined as events leading to death, life-threatening events, events leading to hospitalization, prolonged hospitalization and events leading to severe and/or permanent disability [8]. A flare was defined as the presence of any symptoms of the disease, e.g. fever, rash, abdominal pain and diarrhea.

Results

In total 85 physicians from 23 countries were contacted. In total, seventeen patients were included: 7 sJIA, 5 CAPS, 4 MKD and 1 FMF. The median age at vaccination was 9 years (1–58 years), 11 patients were female. Most patients received a booster vaccine for MMR, but patients also received varicella zoster, yellow fever and oral polio vaccines. Patient characteristics are listed in Table 1. The patients are discussed in more detail below.

Adverse events

Three patients reported an adverse event after vaccination, of whom two were categorized as severe due to the need for hospitalization.

Patient 1 was a seven-year-old girl with sJIA, who was treated with multiple immunosuppressive agents at the same time, including prednisone, methotrexate (MTX), thalidomide, leflunomide and anakinra. Sixteen days after she received a varicella zoster booster vaccination, she developed vesicles on her trunk and a few on her scalp and extremities. The diagnosis of varicella zoster infection was made on the clinical phenotype; the virus could not be isolated. Because of suspected varicella in an immunocompromised host, she was admitted to hospital for 4 days and was discharged with a 10-day course of intravenous acyclovir. As there was no known exposure to other varicella cases, the infection in this child was considered to be caused by the vaccination itself.

Patient 2 suffered from sJIA and was treated with canakinumab. She was accidentally vaccinated with MMR booster by the vaccination campaign in Turkey. One week after vaccination she was diagnosed with pneumonia, which was confirmed by X-ray. As it was considered to be a bacterial pneumonia, treatment with cefuroxime axetil was started. The patient was hospitalized for 5 days. Besides the pneumonia, she had a sJIA flare with fever and rash during the same period. This flare was treated with low-dose prednisone with good response. The impression of the physicians in charge was that this was a flare of her sJIA. Although extremely unlikely, the coincidence of fever, rash and pneumonia could also be ascribed to measles, introduced by vaccination.

The last patient (patient 3) with an adverse event was a sJIA patient treated with tocilizumab. One week after vaccination with oral polio vaccine, the patient experienced diarrhea, which was treated with oral fluid replacements, co-trimoxazol and probiotics. This adverse event was thought to be caused by the vaccine, especially since other family members did not suffer from diarrhea.

Flares

In total seven patients reported a flare of their disease after vaccination. A MKD patient (patient 4) received 100 mg anakinra daily, which was stopped 3–4 days before booster vaccination with varicella zoster and restarted 1 day after vaccination. He experienced fever after vaccination. Since the fever was thought to be caused by a flare, the patient was treated with the normal dose of anakinra. Patient 5 used anakinra (150 mg) during MKD flares only, since the disease was relatively quiescent. The days before and after vaccination with varicella zoster, anakinra was not administered. After vaccination he experienced fever, which was treated with anakinra. Patient 6 was 4 years old when she received her first MMR and varicella zoster vaccines. Her disease was incompletely controlled under treatment with canakinumab 4 mg/kg every 6 weeks. Canakinumab was stopped 3 months before and restarted 3 months after vaccination. Before vaccination she experienced low grade

Table 1 Characteristics of all vaccinated patients

Pt	Gender	Age (y)	Country	Disease	Disease activity	Biological	Other DMARDs	Vaccination	Adverse events	Flare
1	Female	7	USA	sJIA	Inactive	Anakinra 4 mg/kg/day	Prednisone (0.12 mg/kg/day) Methotrexate Leflunomide Thalidomide	Varicella zoster (booster)	Varicella zoster infection	–
2	Female	1	Turkey	sJIA	Inactive	Canakinumab 4 mg/kg/ 2 months	Prednisone (5 mg/day) Methotrexate	MMR booster	Pneumonia	Yes
3	Male	2	Turkey	sJIA	Inactive	Tocilizumab 12 mg/kg/ monthly	Prednisone (2.5 mg/day)	Oral polio vaccine	Diarrhea	–
4	Male	12	USA	MKD	Inactive	Anakinra[a] 100 mg/day (STOP 3-4D-1D)	–	Varicella zoster (booster)	–	Yes
5	Male	9	USA	MKD	Inactive	Anakinra[a] 150 mg during flare (STOP 2D-1D)	–	Varicella zoster (booster)	–	Yes
6	Female	4	USA	MKD	Partially active	Canakinumab[a] 4 mg/kg/6 weeks (STOP 3 M–3 M)		Varicella zoster (first vaccine) and MMR first vaccine	–	Yes
7	Female	2	Turkey	FMF	Inactive	Canakinumab 4 mg/kg/ monthly	Prednisone (2.5 mg/day) Colchicine	MMR booster	–	Yes
8	Female	9	Netherlands	sJIA	Inactive	Anakinra[a] 1.7 mg/kg/ 2 days (STOP 2D-3D)	Methotrexate	MMR booster	–	Yes
9	Male	3	Netherlands	sJIA	Inactive	Tocilizumab 132 mg/14 days)	Prednisone (2.5 mg/day)	Varicella zoster (first vaccine)	–	Yes
10	Male	12	Italy	CAPS	Inactive	Anakinra[a] 1.5 mg/kg/ day (STOP 3D-14D)	Methylprednisolone (0.06 mg/kg/day)	MMR booster	–	–
11	Female	12	Italy	MKD	Partially active	Anakinra[a] 1.4 mg/kg/ day (STOP 3D-28D)	–	MMR booster	–	–
12	Female	9	Netherlands	sJIA	Inactive	Anakinra 40 mg/3 days	–	MMR booster	–	–
13	Male	9	Netherlands	sJIA	Inactive	Tocilizumab 8 mg/kg/ 2 weeks	Methotrexate	MMR booster	–	–
14	Female	58	United Kingdom	CAPS	Inactive	Anakinra[a] 100 mg/day (STOP 3D-3D)	–	Yellow fever (first vaccine)	–	–
15	Female	28	United Kingdom	CAPS	Inactive	Anakinra[a] 100 mg/day (STOP 3D-3D)	–	Yellow fever (first vaccine)	–	–
16	Female	26	United Kingdom	CAPS	Inactive	Anakinra[a] 100 mg/day (STOP 3D-3D)	–	Yellow fever (first vaccine)	–	–
17	Female	44	United Kingdom	CAPS	Inactive	Canakinumab (150 mg/ 2 months)	–	Yellow fever (first vaccine)	–	–

[a]Biological stopped prior to vaccination and restarted after vaccination. The period of discontinuation before and after vaccination is indicated in brackets.
D days before or after vaccination, *M* months before or after vaccination

fevers every week. After vaccination she had a mild flare with fever, vomiting, diarrhea and headache. This flare was treated with acetaminophen and ibuprofen. Patient 7 was treated with canakinumab due to colchicine resistant FMF. Besides FMF, she also suffered from inflammatory bowel disease. The vaccination with MMR booster was administered accidentally by the primary health service in Turkey. Due to this vaccination the next dose of canakinumab was withheld; the following dose was given 2 months after vaccination. One week after vaccination the patient had an FMF attack with fever and abdominal pain, which led to hospitalization. During hospitalization she was treated with low-dose prednisone (2.5 mg/day) and colchicine (0.5 mg/day) with good response. After 8 days she was discharged in good condition.

In another patient (patient 8) who suffered from sJIA, anakinra was stopped 2 days before and restarted 3 days after vaccination. After MMR booster vaccination she experienced a mild flare with some exanthema, but without fever, which was probably due to the stop of anakinra. This flare did not require any additional treatment.

Patient 9 was a young boy with Down syndrome and sJIA complicated by macrophage activation syndrome. He was initiated on tocilizumab treatment at a very young age, before experiencing varicella zoster infection; therefore, he was vaccinated with a first varicella zoster vaccine, in order to acquire immunity in a controlled setting. After vaccination he suffered from a mild flare with subfebrile temperature, exanthema and malaise. After this flare, the physician and parents decided not to repeat varicella vaccination.

Patients without flares or adverse events

Eight patients did not experience a flare or an adverse event. Patient 10 suffered from Chronic Infantile Neurological Cutaneous Articular (CINCA) syndrome, the most severe form of CAPS, which was treated with anakinra. At the age of 12 years he received MMR vaccination as a routine administration of the booster vaccine. Treatment with anakinra was stopped 3 days before vaccination and restarted 2 weeks afterwards. He did not have any adverse events. Patient 11 who had MKD was in partial remission at the time of vaccination. The treatment of anakinra was stopped 3 days before vaccination and restarted 4 weeks afterwards. The last two patients were Dutch sJIA patients with inactive disease on anakinra (patient 12) or tocilizumab and MTX (patient 13). They received the MMR booster vaccine through the national vaccination program, and reported no symptoms afterwards. Patients 14–16 concerned a mother and two daughters all suffering from CAPS, which was treated with anakinra. In order to be protected against yellow fever during travel, they were all vaccinated without any problems. The three of them suspended anakinra for 3 days prior and 3 days after vaccination. The last patient (patient 17) was treated with canakinumab and received a yellow fever vaccination. The vaccine was given 8 weeks after the last dose and the next dose was given 3 weeks after vaccination.

Discussion

This survey describes the safety of live-attenuated vaccine in a case series of patients using IL-1 or IL-6 blocking medication. The seventeen patients in our series reported three adverse events, of which two were categorized as severe, and seven flares, while eight patients did not report any complaints after vaccination. Although adverse events occurred soon after vaccination, coincidence cannot be ruled out. Flares were associated with discontinuation of IL-1 blockade before vaccination in four of the seven patients.

The retrospective design of this survey comes with a number of limitations. Due to this design, information on antibody titers is lacking as these are not routinely measured after vaccination. Therefore, we cannot draw any conclusions about the vaccine efficacy. Further, the small number of patients and the variety in diseases, age, medication and vaccines hampers conclusions on the safety of live-attenuated vaccines in general. Immunological characterization of patients before or after vaccination was not possible due to the retrospective design. The small number and the heterogeneity of the group precluded statistical analysis. The small number of patients included, however, reflects the reluctance of physicians to administer live-attenuated vaccines to patients using these biologicals.

A substantial number of patients in this series were vaccinated inadvertently through national vaccination programs, which has also led to a lack of follow-up data since patients were not monitored by their physician during and after vaccination. Live-attenuated vaccines cannot be considered entirely safe in patients using IL-1 or IL-6 blockade since up to three patients experienced an adverse event, while seven patients experienced a flare to some extent. This should be taken into consideration before administering live-attenuated vaccines in patients using IL-1 or IL-6 blockade.

At least one adverse event was considered to be caused by the micro-organism of the vaccine (patient 2, varicella). However, rash and in particular vesicles are also seen in 3% of healthy children after vaccination with varicella zoster vaccine [9]. Thus, the reported vesicles after vaccination might also be explained by a common vaccination reaction. In the two other patients with an adverse event it cannot be established with certainty that vaccination led to the symptoms of these patients, as pneumonia and diarrhea are common infections in childhood.

In our series, three of four MKD patients reported a flare after vaccination. It is already known that vaccination is a well-known trigger of fever episodes in MKD [10]. However, in these three patients the biological was stopped around the vaccination, as was the case in a child with another disorder who flared. The discontinuation might have contributed to the flares as well. Further, fever and rash are also quite common symptoms after vaccination in healthy children and adults. For example, fever is noted in 10–15% of children receiving varicella zoster vaccine [9]. After MMR vaccination 17% of healthy children and adults reported fever and 5% mentioned a rash [11].

Several studies have described the safety and efficacy of inactivated vaccines in patients using IL-1 blocking agents [12–15]. Two studies on canakinumab showed no difference in antibody titers between groups on canakinumab and subjects not on canakinumab [12, 13]. A study on anakinra also did not show a significant difference in antibody responses [14].

The data on disease flares and adverse events after vaccination are conflicting. In the phase-III trial of canakinumab in 109 CAPS patients, fifteen patients received influenza vaccination, five patients pneumococcal vaccination and one patient received MMR vaccine [16]. None of these patients reported an adverse event. Also in the study of 17 CAPS patients on canakinumab, no flares were described. Adverse events included predominantly upper respiratory tract infections. However, a recent study showed that CAPS patients treated with canakinumab reacted severely after pneumococcal vaccination [17]. Twelve of 18 patients who received pneumococcal immunizations developed vaccine reactions (fever, swelling, erythema, pain), usually within hours after vaccination. Reactions lasted up to 3 weeks. In two patients pneumococcal vaccination triggered CAPS reactivation with systemic inflammation.

Conclusions

In conclusion, we have described a retrospective case series of seventeen patients who received live-attenuated vaccines while using IL-1 or IL-6 blocking medication. The current data are insufficient to draw any conclusions about the safety of these vaccines in patients using IL-1/IL-6 blockade. Therefore, more safety and efficacy data are needed before considering adaptation of guidelines. Until that time, physicians should still balance the risk of natural infection versus the risk of vaccination, including disease flares and other adverse events, for each individual patient.

Acknowledgements
Not applicable

Funding
This study did not receive any funding.

Authors' contributions
All authors made substantial contributions to conception and design, or acquisition of data, or analysis and interpretation of data. JJ, NMtH and JF were involved in drafting the manuscript. All authors read and approved the final manuscript.

Competing interests
The authors declare that they have no competing interests.

Author details
[1]Department of General Pediatrics, University Medical Center Utrecht, Room KE 04 133 1, PO-Box 85090, 3508, AB Utrecht, The Netherlands. [2]Laboratory for Translational Immunology, University Medical Center Utrecht, Utrecht, the Netherlands. [3]University College Medical School, National Amyloidosis Center, Royal Free Campus, London, UK. [4]Department of Pediatric Rheumatology, Cerrahpasa Medical School-Istanbul University, Istanbul, Turkey. [5]Inflammatory Disease section, National Human Genome Research Institute, Bethesda, MA, USA. [6]Institute of Pediatrics, Università Cattolica Sacro Cuore, Rome, Italy. [7]Division of Immunology, Boston Children's Hospital, Boston, MA, USA. [8]Department of Pediatric Rheumatology, University Medical Center Utrecht, Utrecht, the Netherlands.

References

1. John M, Davey S. State of the world's vaccines and immunization. Third. Executive summary 2009. URL: http://apps.who.int/iris/bitstream/10665/70114/1/WHO_IVB_09.10_eng.pdf Accessed 27 Nov 2015.
2. ter Haar N, Lachmann H, Özen S, Woo P, Uziel Y, Modesto C, et al. Treatment of autoinflammatory diseases: results from the Eurofever registry and a literature review. Ann Rheum Dis. 2013;72(5):678–85.
3. Heijstek MW, Ott de Bruin LM, Bijl M, Borrow R, van der Klis F, Kone-Paut I, et al. EULAR recommendations for vaccination in paediatric patients with rheumatic diseases. Ann Rheum Dis. 2011;70(10):1704–12.
4. van Assen S, Agmon-Levin N, Elkayam O, Cervera R, Doran MF, Dougados M, et al. EULAR recommendations for vaccination in adult patients with autoimmune inflammatory rheumatic diseases. Ann Rheum Dis. 2011;70(3):414–22.
5. ter Haar NM, Oswald M, Jeyaratnam J, Anton J, Barron KS, Brogan PA, et al. Recommendations for the management of autoinflammatory diseases. Ann Rheum Dis. 2015;74(9):1636–44.
6. Doran MF, Crowson CS, Pond GR, O'Fallon WM, Gabriel SE. Frequency of infection in patients with rheumatoid arthritis compared with controls: a population-based study. Arthritis Rheum. 2002;46(9):2287–93.
7. Fessler BJ. Infectious diseases in systemic lupus erythematosus: risk factors, management and prophylaxis. Best Pract Res Clin Rheumatol. 2002;16:281–91.4.
8. Bankowski Z, Bruppacher R, Crusius I, Gallagher J, Kremer G, Venulet J. Reporting adverse drug reactions. Geneva: Councel for International Organizations of Medical Scientists; 1999.
9. CDC. Prevention of varicella updated recommendations of the advisory committee on immunization practices (ACIP). MMWR. 1999;48(RR06):1–5.
10. Ter Haar NM, Jeyaratnam J, Lachmann HJ, Simon A, Brogan PA, Doglio M, et al. The phenotype and genotype of mevalonate kinase deficiency: a series of 114 cases from the Eurofever registry. Arthritis Rheum. 2016;68(11):2795–805.
11. CDC. Understanding MMR vaccine safety. 2013. URL: https://www.cdc.gov/vaccines/hcp/patient-ed/conversations/downloads/vacsafe-mmr-color-office.pdf.
12. Chioato A, Noseda E, Felix SD, Stevens M, Del Giudice G, Fitoussi S, et al. Influenza and meningococcal vaccinations are effective in healthy subjects treated with the interleukin-1 beta-blocking antibody canakinumab: results of an open-label, parallel group, randomized, single-center study. Clin Vaccine Immunol. 2010;17(12):1952–7.
13. Brogan P, Hofer M, Kuemmerle-Deschner J, et al. Efficacy, safety, and post-vaccination antibody titer data in children with CAPS treated with Canakinumab. Pediatr Rheumatol. 2015;13(Suppl 1):P1.
14. Quartier P, Allantaz F, Cimaz R, Pillet P, Messiaen C, Bardin C, et al. A multicentre, randomised, double-blind, placebo-controlled trial with the

interleukin-1 receptor antagonist anakinra in patients with systemic-onset juvenile idiopathic arthritis (ANAJIS trial). Ann Rheum Dis. 2011;70(5):747–54.
15. Heijstek MW, Kamphuis S, Armbrust W, Swart J, Gorter S, de Vries LD, et al. Effects of the live attenuated measles-mumps-rubella booster vaccination on disease activity in patients with juvenile idiopathic arthritis: a randomized trial. JAMA. 2013;309(23):2449–56.
16. Kuemmerle-Deschner JB, Hachulla E, Cartwright R, Hawkins PN, Tran TA, Bader-Meunier B, et al. Two-year results from an open-label, multicentre, phase III study evaluating the safety and efficacy of canakinumab in patients with cryopyrin-associated periodic syndrome across different severity phenotypes. Ann Rheum Dis. 2011;70(12):2095–102.
17. Jaeger VK, Hoffman HM, van der Poll T, Tilson H, Seibert J, Speziale A, et al. Safety of vaccinations in patients with cryopyrin-associated periodic syndromes: a prospective registry based study. Rheumatology (Oxford) 2017;56(9):1484–91.

6

Orofacial symptoms and oral health-related quality of life in juvenile idiopathic arthritis: a two-year prospective observational study

Hanna Rahimi[1], Marinka Twilt[2], Troels Herlin[1], Lynn Spiegel[3], Thomas Klit Pedersen[4,5], Annelise Küseler[4,5] and Peter Stoustrup[5*]

Abstract

Background: Little is known about the chronicity of orofacial symptoms and how this influences the oral health-related quality of life in juvenile idiopathic arthritis (JIA). Therefore, our objectives were to study the long-term changes in self-reported orofacial symptoms, and to define the impact of orofacial symptoms on oral health-related quality of life in JIA.

Methods: At baseline (T0), 157 consecutive JIA patients ≤20 years completed a patient pain questionnaire that incorporates domains related to the orofacial area. At the 2 year follow-up (T1), 113 patients completed the same questionnaire (response rate 72%) in addition to the Child Perception's Questionnaire; a validated 31-item questionnaire addressing oral health-related quality of life.

Results: At T0, 53% (60/113) of patients reported the presence of orofacial pain, and 36% (41/113) of patients reported compromised orofacial function. At T1, 77% (46/60) of patients with pain at T0 reported persistent pain, and 66% (27/41) of patients with functional disability at T0 reported persistent disability. Patients with orofacial symptoms reported a significantly greater prevalence of negative impact of orofacial conditions on general quality of life and within the domains of emotional and social well-being compared to asymptomatic patients.

Conclusion: Self-reported orofacial pain and functional disability were common findings in a cohort of JIA patients followed over 2 years. These symptoms seem to persist over time in most patients, and have a significant negative impact on oral health-related quality of life.

Keywords: Juvenile idiopathic arthritis, Temporomandibular joint, Quality of life, Pain, Oral health, Orofacial symptoms, Health assessement questionaire

Background

Involvement of the temporomandibular joint (TMJ) is a common finding in patients with juvenile idiopathic arthritis (JIA) [1, 2]. Long-term arthritis of the TMJ may lead to growth dependent deformation of the joint components and reduced joint mobility, which in turn, may lead to secondary compromise of TMJ function and related muscular structures [3–7]. Arthritis-induced orofacial signs and symptoms are common entities in JIA, and are associated with young age at onset, long disease duration, involvement of upper extremities, and polyarticular and systemic JIA subtypes [3, 8, 9]. Across the literature, the reported prevalence of orofacial symptoms in JIA varies greatly, possibly due to the differences in the included cohort characteristics, retrospective character of most studies, and the type of questions asked [7].

Generally, there is a lack of knowledge of the long-term chronicity of orofacial symptoms in JIA. Although follow-up studies exist, the current knowledge of JIA-induced orofacial symptoms mainly originates from cross-sectional studies [4]. Long-term observational studies by Bakke et al. (15 year follow-up) and Engstrom et al. (25 year follow-up) have outlined a high prevalence of patients with persistent JIA-induced orofacial signs and

* Correspondence: pstoustrup@odont.au.dk
[5]Section of Orthodontics, Department of Dentistry and Oral Health, Aarhus University, Vennelyst Boulevard 9-11, 8000 Aarhus C, Denmark
Full list of author information is available at the end of the article

symptoms [10, 11]. However, these studies represent JIA cohorts from the pre-biologic era, which are incomparable to the contemporary JIA cohorts receiving targeted therapy [12]. A small prevalence of patients with persistent orofacial symptoms were described in a 5-year follow-up study by Twilt et al. in 2008 [13]. In support of that, a longitudinal study by Zwir et al. from 2015 found a baseline prevalence of orofacial symptoms of 29%, with a reduction to 12% at 1 year follow-up [14]. Therefore, only limited knowledge is available on the long-term nature of orofacial symptoms in contemporary JIA patients. Additionally, little knowledge is available of the impact of JIA-induced orofacial symptoms on quality of life specifically related to the orofacial area. Previous cross-sectional studies by Leksell et al. and Frid et al. have focused on the association between arthritis-induced orofacial symptoms and general health-related quality of life using the Childhood Health Assessment Questionnaire (CHAQ) and the Child Health Questionnaires (CHQ) [9, 15, 16]. These questionnaires assess general impact of arthritis and are not tools specifically designed to assess the impact of orofacial dysfunction on parameters related to oral health.

The purpose of this prospective observational cohort-study was: 1) To study the long-term changes in self-reported orofacial symptoms, 2) To study the impact of orofacial symptoms on oral health-related quality of life (OHRQOL). We hypothesized that the presence of orofacial symptoms would have a significant impact on the OHRQOL.

Methods

This prospective observational study was conducted at the Section of Orthodontics, Department of Dentistry and Oral Health, Aarhus University, Denmark in the period between 2014 and 2017. Patients with JIA are referred to the Aarhus University orthodontic clinic from all pediatric rheumatology hospital centers in Western Denmark and are followed longitudinally regardless of presence or absence of TMJ arthritis. Therefore, the entire cohort seen at the Section of Orthodontics is a representation of the JIA population of Denmark. In 2014 and 2015, consecutive patients were invited to participate in the study. Participants completed a self-report questionnaire that assesses orofacial symptoms in JIA. In 2017, all patients from the baseline study were invited to participate in a two-year follow-up survey. Inclusion criteria were: 1) JIA-diagnosis according to the criteria of the International League of Associations for Rheumatology (ILAR) [17], 2) cognitively capable of understanding and answering the questionnaires, 3) ≤20 years old when completing the baseline questionnaire.

The patient questionnaires

At baseline (T0), consecutive patients were asked to complete a standardized patient questionnaire concerning symptoms within the last 2 weeks. The questionnaire was created in accordance with international consensus-based recommendations for orofacial assessment in JIA [7], and incorporates the following domains: 1) orofacial pain frequency assessed by a 5 point Likert scale (0 = "never", 1 = "less than once a week", 2 = "several times a week", 3 = "several times a day", 4 = "all the time"); 2) orofacial pain intensity, for which a 100 mm VAS was used (0 = "not affected", 100 = "severely affected"); 3) orofacial pain location, assessed by letting the participant mark the area of pain on a diagram illustrating the head and neck; 4) orofacial functional disability (100 mm VAS, 0 = not affected, 100 = severely affected); and 5) characteristics of orofacial symptoms, assessed by asking participants to mark off all the statements that were applicable to them. To combine aspects of orofacial pain intensity and frequency into one single outcome measure, we calculated a composite pain index variable by multiplying pain frequency and pain intensity with a score range between 0 and 400. In addition, with reference to the pain intensity and frequency for the 2 weeks subsequent to the study visit, we asked the participants to assess their global pain score based on a 100 mm VAS (Endpoints: 0 = no pain, 100 = worst imaginable pain).

At follow-up (T1), the patients were asked to complete the same questionnaire that they had completed at T0. In addition, they were asked to complete a validated 31-item questionnaire addressing OHRQOL (Child Perception's Questionnaire) [18]. The questionnaire includes two global ratings: 1) Self-reported perception of own oral health status, 2) The extent to which the orofacial conditions affect the overall general quality of life. In addition, the questionnaire contains 29 questions related to general emotional and social well-being (see online Additional file 1). Information about medical treatment and TMJ arthritis-related treatment between T0 and T1 was collected from chart files. The study was approved by the Danish Data Protection Agency (2016–051-000001, ID:665) and conducted in agreement with Danish Health authority regulations on questionnaire-based studies and chart-files studies; Informed and signed consent was provided by all participants ≥15 years of age, and by their parents for participants below age 15.

Statistics

Graphical display revealed that numerical variables (pain intensity, pain index and functional disability) were skewed and not normal distributed. All numerical and categorical variables were analyzed using Wilcoxon's rank-sum tests for paired data variables and Mann-Whitney tests for unpaired data. Chi-square tests were used to assess changes in the prevalence of the specific characteristics of orofacial symptoms between T0 and T1. Agreement between the pain index composite variable (pain frequency x pain intensity) and patient global pain score was calculated using the Bland-Altman analysis [19]. Correlation coefficients were used to assess the correlation between the pain index variable global ratings of self-reported perception of own oral health status and the impact of orofacial conditions on general quality of life. The level of significance was 0.05. Statistical analysis was conducted using the Stata 13 software (StataCorp. 2013. Stata Statistical Software: Release 13. College Station, TX: StataCorp LP)

Results

At T0, 157 eligible consecutive patients completed the questionnaire. All 157 patients were invited to participate in the two-year follow-up questionnaire survey. At T1 (mean 25 months, SD 3.1 months), 113 patients accepted the invitation and repeated the questionnaire (response rate 72%). Only patients who completed the questionnaires at both time points were included in the present study. The characteristics of the 113 study patients are presented in Table 1. The most frequent JIA subcategories with baseline orofacial symptoms were oligo persistent JIA (48%) and polyarticular JIA (39%). In addition, Table 1 displays the treatments conducted between T0 and T1. No significant differences in mean age or disease duration at T0 were seen between patients with or without orofacial symptoms. A baseline analysis showed no inter-group differences in the reported symptoms between included patients who completed the questionnaires at both time-points and excluded patients who only completed the baseline questionnaire.

General findings

At T0, 55% of patients (62/113) reported the presence of orofacial symptoms and 45% of patients (51/113) were asymptomatic (Fig. 1a). The majority of symptomatic patients experienced both pain and functional disability (63%, 39/62). A smaller number of symptomatic patients experienced pain only (34%, 21/62) or functional disability only (3%, 2/62) (Fig. 1a).

At T1, 77% (48/62) of patients reported "persistent symptoms" indicated by a report of symptoms at both time points (T0 and T1). Between T0 and T1, 27% (14/51) of patients developed new symptoms; 7% (1/14) reported functional disability only; 50% (7/14) reported pain only; and 43% (6/14) reported both pain and functional disability. Twenty-three percent (14/62) of patients with symptoms at T0 experienced a resolution of symptoms at T1 (Fig. 1b).

Pain frequency

Orofacial pain frequencies for the different time-points are displayed in Fig. 2a. At T0, 53% (60/113) of patients reported the presence of orofacial pain. Almost half of patients with orofacial pain (29/60) reported pain on a weekly basis. Seventy-seven percent (46/60) of patients with pain at T0 also reported pain at T1 (Fig. 1b). Changes in pain frequency observed between T0 and T1 were: 30% (14/46) reported less frequent pain at T1; 39% (18/46) reported comparable pain frequency at T0 and T1; and 30% (14/46) reported more frequent pain at T1 (Fig. 2b). The remaining 23% (14/60) of patients with pain at T0 reported no pain at T1. There was no significant difference in the reported T0 pain frequencies between the 14 patients who only experienced pain at T0, when compared to the 46 patients with persistent pain complaints. At T1, patients with persistent pain ($n = 46$) reported significantly higher pain frequencies than patients with newly developed pain between T0 and T1 ($n = 13$) (Fig. 2a).

Pain intensity

A change in pain intensity between T0 and T1 was defined as a VAS scale difference ≥ 13 mm in accordance with the smallest detectable difference for average orofacial pain reports, as previously described [6]. At T0, the median and the inter-quartile ranges (IQR) between the 1st and 3rd quartiles for orofacial pain intensity was 33 mm (IQR = 12–52.5 mm, $n = 60$) (Fig. 3a). A non-significant difference in pain-intensity was observed between T0 and T1 in patients with reports of persistent pain. The change in pain intensity between T0 and T1 for patients with persistent pain was as follows: 37% (17/46) reported less intense pain at T1, 39% (18/46) reported comparable pain intensity at T0 and T1, and 24% (11/46) reported more intense pain at T1. Fourteen patients with pain at T0 reported no pain at T1. There was no significant difference in the reported pain intensities at T0, between the 14 patients with pain at T0 only, when compared to the 46 patients with pain complaints at both T0 and T1.

At T1, a non-significant higher median pain intensity of 27 mm (IQR = 13-45 mm, $n = 46$) was reported by patients with persistent pain when compared to the median pain intensity of 16 mm (IQR = 12–38 mm, $n = 13$) reported by patients with pain at T1 only (Fig. 3a).

Pain index

The correlation coefficient between the pain index composite variable (pain frequency x pain intensity) and patient global pain score was $r = 0.78$ indicating an acceptable validity of the pain index variable as a measure of the general pain perception of the patients.

At T0, the median orofacial patient pain index ($n = 60$) was 43.5 (IQR = 15–121, n = 60) (Fig. 3b). At T1, a non-significant higher median pain index of 50 (IQR = 13–94) was reported by patients with persistent pain ($n = 46$)

Table 1 Patient Characteristics

Cohort characteristics	Orofacial symptomatic group at T0	Orofacial asymptomatic group at T0
Number	62	51
Mean age at baseline, years (sd)	14.6 (2.9)	13.9 (2.4)
JIA subcategories, number		
Oligoarticular extended	4	1
Oligoarticular persistent	26	28
Polyarticular	27	17
Systemic	1	1
Psoriatic	3	4
Enthesitis related arthritis	0	0
Unknown	1	0
Disease duration		
Mean years (sd)	7.4 (4.2)	6.6 (4.4)
< 1 years	0	1
0–3	5	6
> 3	57	44
TMJ-specific treatment in the follow-up period, number		
Flat splint (night)	12	5
Flat splint (full time)	10	0
Distraction splint	4	6
Full fixed appliances	5	4
Previous full fixed appliances	12	9
Surgical osseous distraction	1	0
Activator	4	3
Intra articular TMJ steroid	3	0
Orofacial physiotherapy	8	0
Home Exercises	4	0
No treatment	12	25
Medical treatment in the follow-up period, number		
NSAID	19	4
Methotrexate	27	16
Leflunomide	4	0
Systemic steroid	1	0
Biologics	26	16
No medication	36	38
Combination of two drugs	19	6
Combination of three drugs	3	1
Change in treatment during follow-up	21	15

Characteristics of study patients. TMJ: Temporomandibular joint

when compared to a median 16 (IQR = 12–45) pain index reported by patients with pain at T1 only ($n = 13$). No significant changes in pain index values were observed between T0 and T1 in patients with persistent pain reports (Fig. 3b).

Pain location

Figure 4a illustrates the distribution of the orofacial pain at T0. Patients with pain at T0 only reported pain in TMJ and masseter muscle regions exclusively. In contrast, patients with persistent pain reported a more widespread pain distribution at T0, involving the temporal, frontal and parietal regions. Multiregional pain was reported by 46% (21/46) of patients with persistent orofacial pain and by 7% (1/14) of patients with orofacial pain at T0 only. There was no change in the distribution of pain locations seen between T0 and T1 in patients reporting persistent pain (Fig. 4b). Patients with persistent pain (n = 46) reported a significantly higher prevalence of masticatory muscle pain when compared to patients who reported pain at T1 only (n = 13): All other pain locations were involved to a comparable degree in these two groups (Fig. 4b). Generally, the most involved pain locations at both T0 and T1 were the TMJ and the masseter muscle regions.

Functional disability

At T0, the median level of VAS-reported functional disability was 27 mm (IQR = 17-46 mm, $n = 41$) (Fig. 3c). Ninety-five percent (39/41) of patients reporting T0 functional disability also reported orofacial pain (Fig. 1a). At T1, a non-significant median level of functional disability of 32 mm (IQR = 20-48 mm) was reported by patients with persistent functional complaints ($n = 27/41$) when compared to a median of 46 mm (IQR = 24-54 mm, $n = 15$) in patients reporting functional disability at T1 only (Fig. 3c). The non-significant changes in functional disability scores between T0 and T1 were as follows: 26% (7/27) reported an improvement of orofacial functional disability between T0 and T1, 48% (13/27) reported the same level of orofacial functional disability, and 26% (7/27) reported a worsening of orofacial functional disability at T1. Ninety-three percent (25/27) of patients reporting persistent orofacial function disability also reported orofacial pain at both time points.

Symptoms

The characteristics of orofacial symptoms reported at T0 and T1 are displayed in Fig. 5. The majority of patients reported pain when opening the mouth wide (63% at T0 and 56% at T1). Other frequent complaints were jaw morning stiffness (40% at T0 and 44% at T1), pain when chewing (39% at T0 and 37% at T1) as well as avoiding hard or chewy foods (40% at T0 and 37% at T1). No significant differences were found in the distribution of symptoms between T0 and T1.

OHRQOL

The global rating of self-reported perception of own oral health was significantly reduced in symptomatic as compared to asymptomatic patients at T1 (Fig. 6a). A

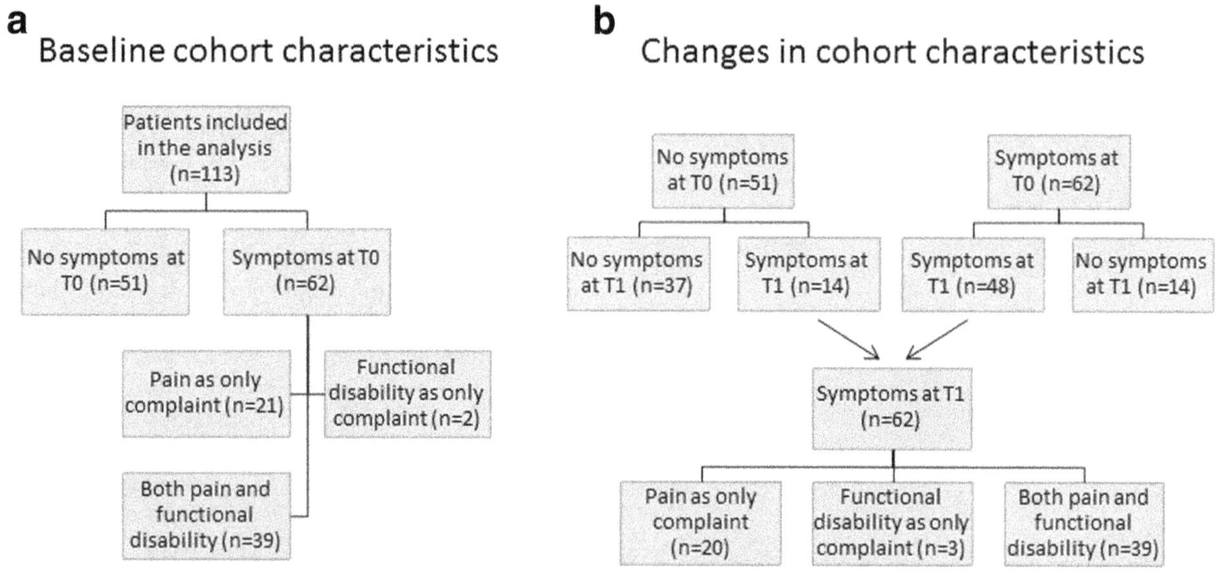

Fig. 1 **a** Description of cohort baseline (T0) orofacial symptoms. **b** Changes in orofacial symptoms between baseline (T0) and the two-year follow-up (T1)

subgroup analysis revealed that no significant differences in self-reported perception of oral health were found between patients with persistent symptoms (T0 and T1), when compared to patients who only reported symptoms at T1. Asymptomatic patients and patients with symptoms at T0 only reported comparable perceptions of oral health (Fig. 6a). A low correlation of $r = 0.32$ was found between the pain index variable and global rating of self-reported perception of own oral health in patients with symptoms at T1, indicating a limited association between the severity of orofacial pain and the self-reported rating of own orofacial health.

The impact of orofacial conditions on general quality of life was significantly higher in patients reporting symptoms as compared to asymptomatic patients at T1 (Fig. 6b). A subgroup analysis revealed a significant difference in the impact of orofacial conditions on the general quality of life in patients with persistent symptoms when compared to patients who only reported symptoms at T1. Patients with orofacial symptoms at T0

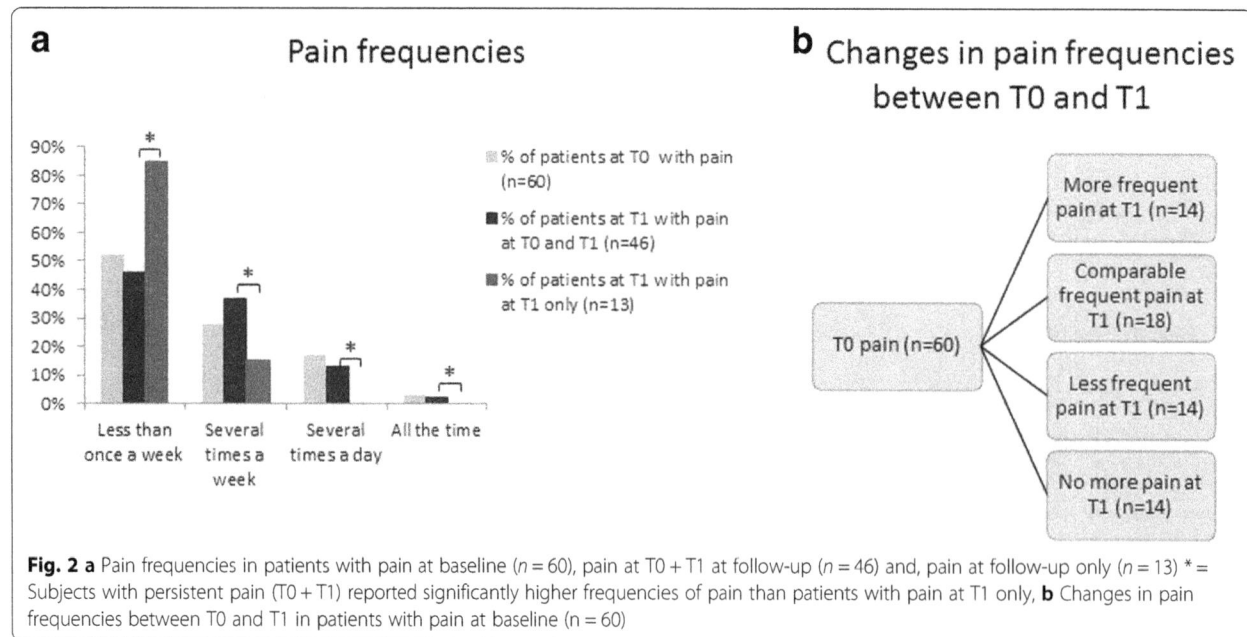

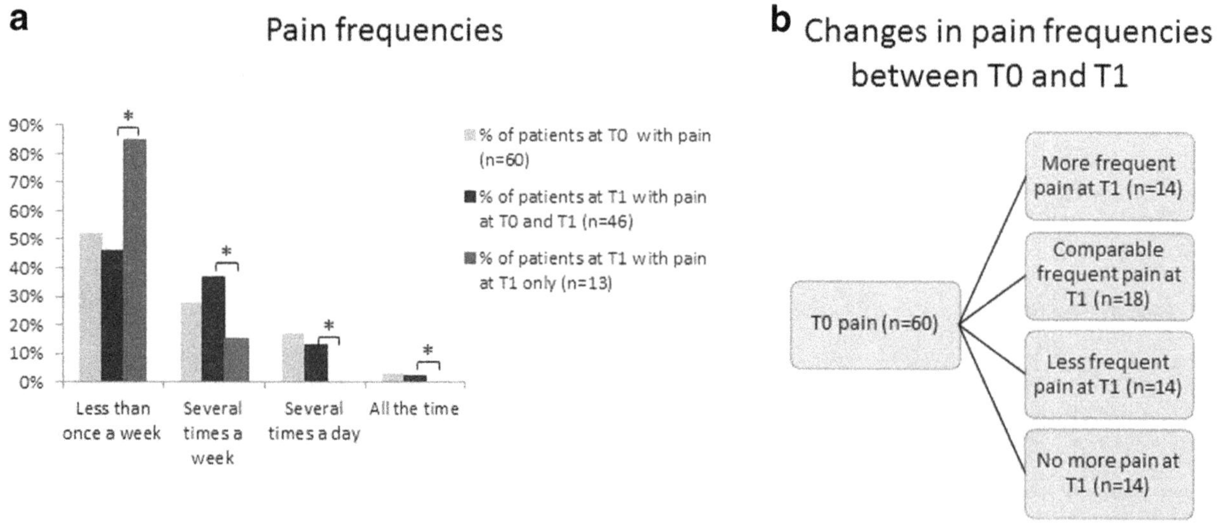

Fig. 2 **a** Pain frequencies in patients with pain at baseline ($n = 60$), pain at T0 + T1 at follow-up ($n = 46$) and, pain at follow-up only ($n = 13$) * = Subjects with persistent pain (T0 + T1) reported significantly higher frequencies of pain than patients with pain at T1 only, **b** Changes in pain frequencies between T0 and T1 in patients with pain at baseline (n = 60)

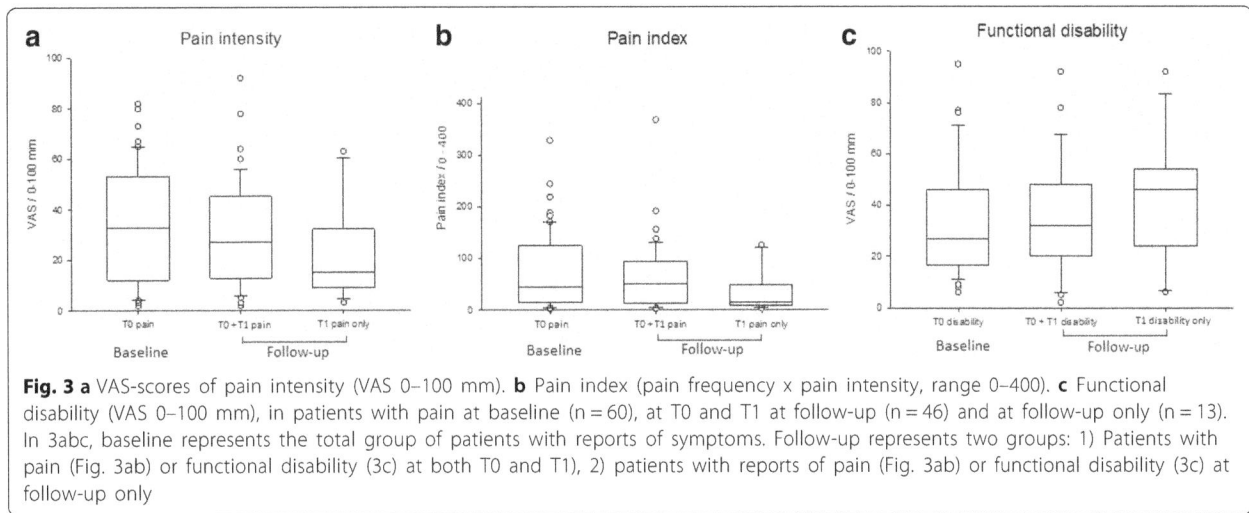

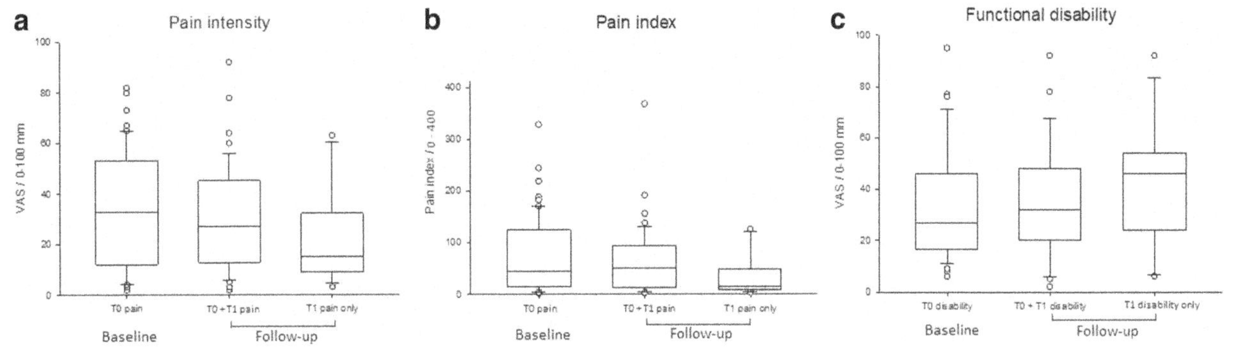

Fig. 3 **a** VAS-scores of pain intensity (VAS 0–100 mm). **b** Pain index (pain frequency x pain intensity, range 0–400). **c** Functional disability (VAS 0–100 mm), in patients with pain at baseline (n = 60), at T0 and T1 at follow-up (n = 46) and at follow-up only (n = 13). In 3abc, baseline represents the total group of patients with reports of symptoms. Follow-up represents two groups: 1) Patients with pain (Fig. 3ab) or functional disability (3c) at both T0 and T1), 2) patients with reports of pain (Fig. 3ab) or functional disability (3c) at follow-up only

and no symptoms at T1 reported a significantly higher impact of orofacial conditions on their quality of life compared to patients who were asymptomatic at both time points. Eighteen percent (11/62) of patients with orofacial pain and/or functional disability at T1 reported that the condition had "some" negative impact on the overall quality of life. Six percent (4/62) of symptomatic patients at T1 reported that the orofacial condition reduced their general quality of life "a lot" (1/62) and "very much" (3/62). A moderate correlation of $r = 0.54$ was found between pain index values and the self-reported impact of orofacial condition on general quality of life in patients with symptoms at T1.

Emotional and social well-being

The impact of items related to emotional and social well-being among patients with and without TMJ-arthritis symptoms are presented in the online Additional file 1. Patients with orofacial symptoms reported a significantly greater prevalence of negative impact on questions related to emotional and social well-being.

Discussion

To our knowledge, this is the most comprehensive longitudinal study examining orofacial symptoms in JIA. The objective of this study was to study the long-term changes in self-reported orofacial symptoms and to study the impact of orofacial symptoms on OHRQOL. The findings of this study demonstrate: Orofacial symptoms are common findings in patients with JIA, and they tend to persist with time. Furthermore, the intensity, frequency and the characteristics of orofacial symptoms do not change significantly over time. The TMJ and masseter regions are the most frequent orofacial areas affected, however, multiregional orofacial pain was seen in a substantial number of patients with persistent symptoms. Orofacial pain is associated with functional disability in the majority of patients, and it is rare

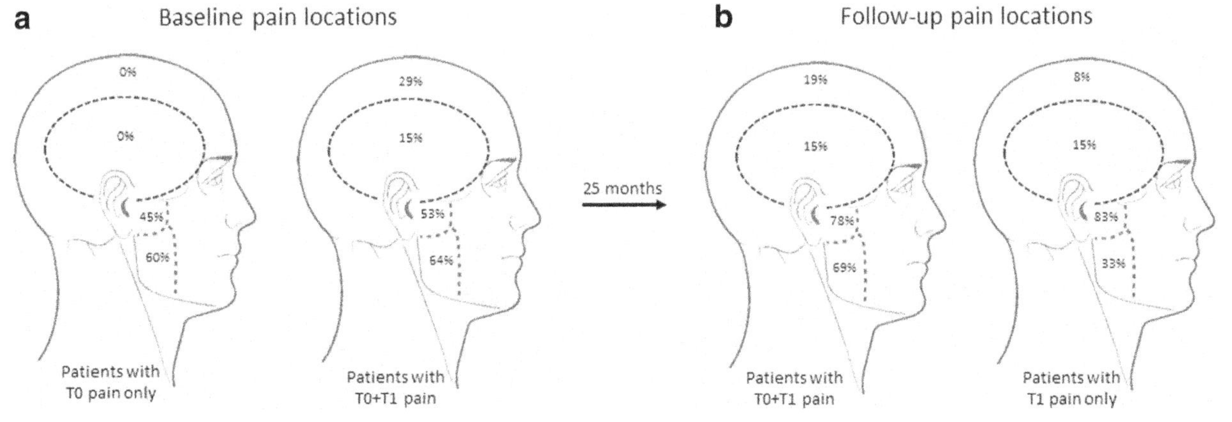

Fig. 4 **a** Distribution of orofacial pain at baseline among patients with T0 pain only and patients with pain at T0 and T1. **b** Distribution of orofacial pain at follow-up among patients with pain at T0 and T1 and patients with T1 pain only

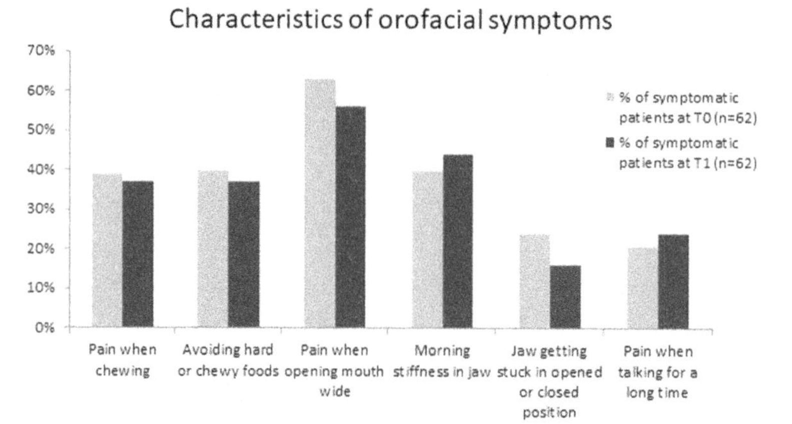

Fig. 5 Characteristics of orofacial symptoms in patients with orofacial pain and/or functional disability at T0 (*n* = 62) and T1 (n = 62). No significant difference in characteristics of orofacial symptoms between baseline and follow-up

to see functional disability in the absence of orofacial pain. We found that the pain index composite variable (pain frequency x pain intensity) is an acceptable measure of patient global pain perception. Patients with orofacial symptoms reported a significantly higher negative impact of orofacial conditions on general quality of life compared to asymptomatic patients. Finally, patients with orofacial symptoms reported a significant negative impact on emotional and social well-being.

This study found a high prevalence (55%) of JIA patients with orofacial pain and dysfunction. This is in contrast to a previous 5-year follow-up study by Twilt et al., who reported a smaller prevalence of orofacial pain (13%) and limited mandibular function (10%) [13]. In our study, 97% (60/62) of symptomatic patients at T0 experienced orofacial pain and 77% (46/60) of these patients still reported pain after 2 years (T1). This finding is in contrast with Engstrom et al. who reported a higher prevalence of orofacial symptoms over time in their 15 year follow-up study [11]. In agreement with Frid et al. we found an increased prevalence of orofacial symptoms in patients with a polyarticular disease course [9].

The nature of the questionnaire used in this study allowed for a comprehensive analysis of changes in orofacial pain characteristics in JIA over time. In the group experiencing pain at both T0 and T1, we did not observe a specific pattern for changes in pain frequency or pain intensity over time. The current literature lacks information about orofacial pain frequency in JIA [4]. This study therefore contributes valuable information by

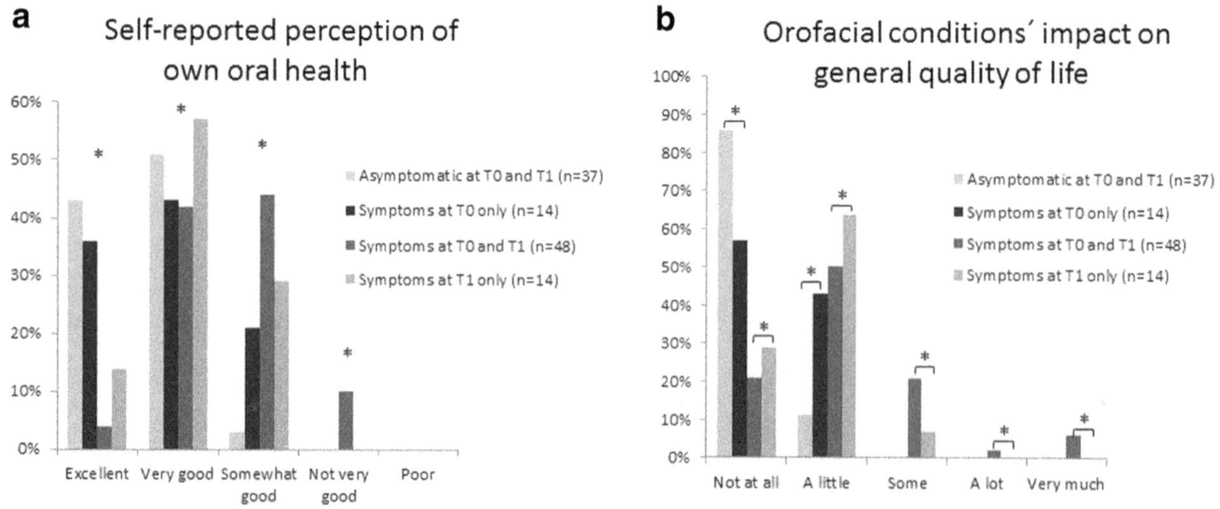

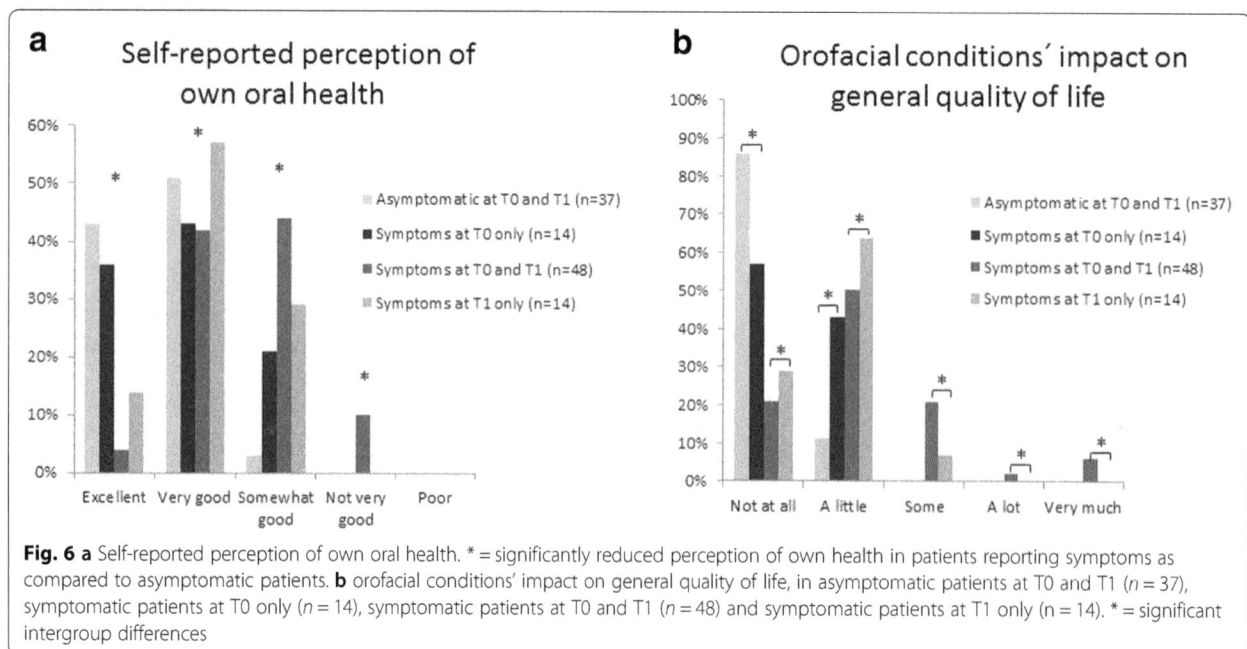

Fig. 6 a Self-reported perception of own oral health. * = significantly reduced perception of own health in patients reporting symptoms as compared to asymptomatic patients. **b** orofacial conditions' impact on general quality of life, in asymptomatic patients at T0 and T1 (*n* = 37), symptomatic patients at T0 only (*n* = 14), symptomatic patients at T0 and T1 (*n* = 48) and symptomatic patients at T1 only (n = 14). * = significant intergroup differences demonstrating that daily/weekly pain fluctuation is a characteristic finding in JIA patients who report orofacial symptoms. Many patients experienced orofacial symptoms during mastication and maximal mouth opening maneuvers. However, when asked about pain frequency, full-time symptoms were rarely reported, and the majority did not experience orofacial symptoms every day. From a clinical point of view, this is important because it conflicts with existing standardized guidelines on clinical orofacial assessment like the DC/TMD criteria, which was not exclusively developed for JIA [20]. A critical tenet of the DC/TMD criteria is the notion that arthralgia, can only be established if pain on palpation is present during the clinical examination [20]. Applied to a JIA population, this would mean an under reporting of orofacial pain, since many patients only experience pain in conjunction with functional demands like mastication. To capture the fluctuation of orofacial pain in JIA, we introduced the pain index variable (pain frequency x pain intensity). The acceptable agreement between the pain index variable and the patient global pain score of $r = 0.78$ reveals that this may be a useful variable to address the fluctuation of orofacial pain in JIA. Interestingly, the reported T0 and T1 median pain index scores were surprisingly small considering the range 0–400 of the pain index outcome measure.

In the present study, patients reporting persistent T1 pain reported more widespread pain distribution as well as higher prevalence of multiregional pain compared to those reporting pain at T0 only. Notably, the locations of the affected pain regions and the characteristics of orofacial symptoms did not significantly change over time in patients with persistent orofacial symptoms.

In this study, the presence of orofacial pain and/or functional disability significantly impacted general health related quality of life. This is in agreement with a previous study by Leksell et al. and Frid et al. [9, 15] but contrasts with findings of Twilt et al. [13] who reported no significant impact on general quality of life between patients with and without TMJ involvement. However, an only moderate association ($r = 0.54$) between the pain index variable and the impact of an orofacial condition on general quality of life demonstrates that a high level of orofacial pain may not negatively impact general quality of life and vice versa.

Patients with persistent orofacial symptoms experienced a greater impact on their general quality of life compared to patients with symptoms at T1 only. Although we do not have any information about pain related symptoms between those two observation points, this suggests that long-term symptoms impact general quality of life to a greater degree than short-term orofacial symptoms. Moreover, we also observed that patients who only had symptoms at T0 reported a significantly greater impact of orofacial conditions on general quality of life at T1 when compared to asymptomatic patients. This is an interesting finding, and may indicate that previous orofacial symptoms can impact general quality of life even after symptoms have resolved. However, the present study does not allow us to make firm conclusions in this regard. Future work with a larger patient cohort studied at more frequent time intervals could help to clarify some of these findings.

In the present study, we used a validated questionnaire to assess domains related to emotional and social well-being [18]. This is the first study to assess oral health related quality of life in JIA. We found that emotional and social well-being were significantly reduced in patients with orofacial symptoms. Currently no validated OHRQOL questionnaire exists exclusively for use in JIA which constitutes a limitation to the present study. The questionnaire used, in the present study, has been validated in non-JIA children and adolescence with "orofacial conditions" (18). This warrants a future validation of OHRQOL questionnaires exclusively to the JIA population.

Our cohort consisted of consecutively enrolled JIA patients, from the entire JIA population in Denmark, thus decreasing the risk for selection bias at T0. Although the background cohort reflects the JIA population in Denmark, it should be noted that there were no patients with enthesitis-related arthritis and undifferentiated arthritis completing the questionnaires at both time-points in the present study. Furthermore, standardized questionnaires were used assessing orofacial symptoms and OHRQOL, thus minimizing the risk of information bias. There were however some limitations to this study. The current data does not contain information about presence/absence of TMJ inflammation at the time the questionnaires were completed; this would have been important information to collect. However, this is likely of minor significance since previous studies have revealed that the presence of orofacial pain is a weak predictor of TMJ arthritis [4]. When interpreting symptoms, we typically attributed orofacial symptoms to previous TMJ arthritis leading to structural damage and impaired TMJ function. However, orofacial symptoms are also seen in non-inflammatory temporomandibular disorders, a common finding in the general population, and thus a potential confounder to the prevalence of symptoms reported in this study [21]. Therefore, a general limitation to the present study is the lack of a non-JIA control group to reflect the frequency of orofacial symptoms and OHRQOL in the background population. At this point, no validated examination methods exist to differentiate between "general temporomandibular disorders" and JIA-induced orofacial conditions and that constitute a limitation to the present study.

In addition, the degree of fluctuation of orofacial symptoms during the 25-month observation period is unknown, since we only examined two time-points (T0 and T1). Therefore, the term "persistent symptoms" in patients with reports of orofacial symptoms at both time points is somewhat vague and does not accurately characterize the degree of fluctuation or persistence of symptoms between these time points.

Conclusion

Self-reported orofacial pain and functional disability were common findings in a cohort of JIA patients followed over 2 years. These symptoms seem to persist over time in most patients, and significantly reduce OHRQOL. Based on the findings of this study, we strongly recommend incorporating a standardized orofacial examination into the assessment of children diagnosed with JIA. A sudden reduction in TMJ function and/or orofacial pain should prompt increase attention and appropriate referral of the patient for further examination, and if necessary, initiation of treatment.

Abbreviations

JIA: Juvenile idiopathic arthritis; OHRQOL: Oral health-related quality of life; TMJ: Temporomandibular joint

Acknowledgements

We thank the entire clinical team at the Section of Orthodontics, Aarhus University, Denmark, for their help with the questionnaires. We thank Kasper Dahl Kristensen for his help with the graphical display. We acknowledge the important contribution of Professor Bernd Koos, Tübingen, Germany, in the preparation of the patient questionnaire.

Authors' contributions

PS, MT, TH, TKP and HR designed the study. Questionnaires were prepared by PS, MT, TH, LS and HR HR and PS administred data collection, analyzed data and created a draft for the manuscript. The data was available to all authors throughout the study. All authors revised the results and the manuscript and approved of the final version before submission.

Competing interests

The authors declare that they have no competing interests.

Author details

[1]Department of Pediatrics, Aarhus University Hospital, Palle Juul-Jensens Boulevard 121, 8200 Aarhus N, Denmark. [2]Department of Pediatrics, Division of Rheumatology, Alberta Children's Hospital, 2888 Shaganappi Trail NW, Calgary, AB, Canada. [3]Division of Rheumatology, The Hospital for Sick Children, 555 University Avenue, Toronto, ON, Canada. [4]Department of Oral and Maxillofacial Surgery, Aarhus University Hospital, Nørrebrogade 44, 8000 Aarhus C, Denmark. [5]Section of Orthodontics, Department of Dentistry and Oral Health, Aarhus University, Vennelyst Boulevard 9-11, 8000 Aarhus C, Denmark.

References

1. Kuseler A, Pedersen TK, Gelineck J, Herlin T. A 2 year followup study of enhanced magnetic resonance imaging and clinical examination of the temporomandibular joint in children with juvenile idiopathic arthritis. J Rheumatol. 2005;32:162–9.
2. Weiss PF, Arabshahi B, Johnson A, Bilaniuk LT, Zarnow D, Cahill AM, et al. High prevalence of temporomandibular joint arthritis at disease onset in children with juvenile idiopathic arthritis, as detected by magnetic resonance imaging but not by ultrasound. Arthritis Rheum. 2008;58:1189–96.
3. Cannizzaro E, Schroeder S, Muller LM, Kellenberger CJ, Saurenmann RK. Temporomandibular joint involvement in children with juvenile idiopathic arthritis. J Rheumatol. 2011;38:510–5.
4. Kristensen KD, Stoustrup P, Kuseler A, Pedersen TK, Twilt M, Herlin T. Clinical predictors of temporomandibular joint arthritis in juvenile idiopathic arthritis: a systematic literature review. Semin Arthritis Rheum. 2016;45:717–32.
5. Stoll ML, Sharpe T, Beukelman T, Good J, Young D, Cron RQ. Risk factors for temporomandibular joint arthritis in children with juvenile idiopathic arthritis. J Rheumatol. 2012;39:1880–7.
6. Stoustrup P, Kristensen KD, Verna C, Kuseler A, Herlin T, Pedersen TK. Orofacial symptoms related to temporomandibular joint arthritis in juvenile idiopathic arthritis: smallest detectable difference in self-reported pain intensity. J Rheumatol. 2012;39:2352–8.
7. Stoustrup P, Twilt M, Spiegel L, Kristensen KD, Koos B, Pedersen TK, et al. Clinical orofacial examination in juvenile idiopathic arthritis: international consensus-based recommendations for monitoring patients in clinical practice and research studies. J Rheumatol. 2017;44:326–33.
8. Cedstromer AL, Andlin-Sobocki A, Berntson L, Hedenberg-Magnusson B, Dahlstrom L. Temporomandibular signs, symptoms, joint alterations and disease activity in juvenile idiopathic arthritis – an observational study. Ped Rheumatol Online J. 2013;11:37.
9. Frid P, Nordal E, Bovis F, Giancane G, Larheim TA, Rygg M, et al. Temporomandibular joint involvement in association with quality of life, disability, and high disease activity in juvenile idiopathic arthritis. Arthritis Care Res. 2017;69:677–86.
10. Bakke M, Zak M, Jensen BL, Pedersen FK, Kreiborg S. Orofacial pain, jaw function, and temporomandibular disorders in women with a history of juvenile chronic arthritis or persistent juvenile chronic arthritis. Oral Surg Oral Med Oral Pathol Oral Radiol Endo. 2001;92:406–14.
11. Engstrom AL, Wanman A, Johansson A, Keshishian P, Forsberg M. Juvenile arthritis and development of symptoms of temporomandibular disorders: a 15-year prospective cohort study. J Orofac Pain. 2007;21:120–6.
12. Beukelman T, Patkar NM, Saag KG, Tolleson-Rinehart S, Cron RQ, DeWitt EM, et al. 2011 American College of Rheumatology recommendations for the treatment of juvenile idiopathic arthritis: initiation and safety monitoring of therapeutic agents for the treatment of arthritis and systemic features. Arthritis Care Res. 2011;63:465–82.
13. Twilt M, Schulten AJ, Verschure F, Wisse L, Prahl-Andersen B, Suijlekom-Smit LW. Long-term followup of temporomandibular joint involvement in juvenile idiopathic arthritis. Arthritis Rheum. 2008;59:546–52.
14. Zwir LM, Terreri MT, Sousa SA, Fernandes AR, Guimaraes AS, Hilario MO. Are temporomandibular joint signs and symptoms associated with magnetic resonance imaging findings in juvenile idiopathic arthritis patients? A longitudinal study. Clin Rheumatol. 2015;34:2057–63.
15. Leksell E, Ernberg M, Magnusson B, Hedenberg-Magnusson B. Orofacial pain and dysfunction in children with juvenile idiopathic arthritis: a case-control study. Scand J Rheumatol. 2012;41:375–8.
16. Ruperto N, Ravelli A, Pistorio A, Malattia C, Cavuto S, Gado-West L, et al. Cross-cultural adaptation and psychometric evaluation of the childhood health assessment questionnaire (CHAQ) and the child health questionnaire (CHQ) in 32 countries. Review of the general methodology Clin Exp Rheumatol. 2001;19:S1–9.
17. Petty RE, Southwood TR, Baum J, Bhettay E, Glass DN, Manners P, et al. Revision of the proposed classification criteria for juvenile idiopathic arthritis: Durban, 1997. J Rheumatol. 1998;25:1991–4.
18. Jokovic A, Locker D, Stephens M, Kenny D, Tompson B, Guyatt G. Validity and reliability of a questionnaire for measuring child oral-health-related quality of life. J Dent Res. 2002;81:459–63.
19. Bland JM, Altman DG. Statistical methods for assessing agreement between two methods of clinical measurement. Lancet. 1986;1:307–10.

7

Circulating adipokines are associated with Kawasaki disease

Xin-yan Zhang[1], Ting-ting Yang[1], Xiu-fen Hu[1], Yu Wen[1], Feng Fang[1] and Hui-ling Lu[1,2*]

Abstract

Background: The pathogenesis of Kawasaki disease are still not well understood. It was designed to investigate the relationship between adipokines including chemerin, omentin-1, adiponectin and acute Kawasaki disease.

Methods: Enzyme-linked immunosorbent (ELISA) was used to detect serum levels of chemerin, omentin-1, adiponectin, and inflammatory cytokines IL-1β and TNF-α in 80 cases of patients diagnosed with Kawasaki disease (KD). In addition, 20 cases of children with fever and 20 cases of healthy children were selected as febrile and normal controls.

Results: (1) Serum levels of chemerin in KD group (87.736 ± 56.310) are higher than that of both the healthy (41.746 ± 10.824) and the febrile controls (59.683 ± 18.282) ($P < 0.01$). (2) Circulating omentin-1 levels in Kawasaki disease group (389.773 ± 238.611) are significantly lower than that of febrile control (542.075 ± 177.995) ($P < 0.01$), also serum adiponectin levels in Kawasaki disease group (16.400 ± 12.243) reduced obviously compared with the febrile control group (35.074 ± 12.486). (3)Serum cytokine levels of IL-1β in Kawasaki disease group (13.656 ± 31.151) are higher than those of normal controls (2.415 ± 6.313) ($P < 0.05$). (4) Correlation analysis indicates that serum levels of chemerin are positively correlated with omentin-1 ($r = 0.224$, 95% CI 0.06–0.529, $P < 0.05$). Further, serum omentin-1 levels and total cholesterol (TC) are positively correlated ($r = 0.358$, 95% CI 0.169–0.518, $P < 0.01$).

Conclusions: Circulating chemerin increased significantly in the acute stage of Kawasaki disease, while omentin-1 and adiponectin levels are decreased. These adipokines are closely associated with the early inflammation and lipid metabolism disorders of acute Kawasaki disease.

Keywords: Adiponectin, Chemerin, Kawasaki disease, Omentin-1

Background

Kawasaki disease(KD) is an acute febrile illness, known as mucocutaneous lymph node syndrome, which mainly occurs in boys under 5 years old [1]. Cardiovascular manifestations are the main complications of KD such as coronary artery abnormalities, myocarditis, pericarditis, pericardial effusion, valvular dysfunction, left ventricular dysfunction, and arrhythmias [2]. And KD is the most common cause of coronary artery aneurysms (CAA) in children or young adults and the leading cause of acquired heart disease [3]. However, treatment of intravenous immunoglobulin (IVIG) plus acetylsalicylic acid (ASA) reduces the prevalence of coronary artery abnormalities from 32 to 50% to approximately 4% [4]. Although the pathogenesis of KD is still not fully understood, innate and specific immunity are always fully activated during the acute stage of KD, in which neutrophils, CD8 + T cells, dendritic cells, and macrophages are also activated successively in infiltration of artery walls [5, 6], then leading to the activation of the nuclear transcription factor NF-κB in monocytes macrophages [7]. This promotes the production of inflammatory cytokines such as IL-6 and TNF-α [8], further infiltrating vascular endothelium and causing immune activation.

Adipose tissue is not only a simple energy metabolism organ but also an important endocrine organ that could secrete numerous of proinflammatory cytokines such as TNF, IL-6, MCP1, leptin, and others [9, 10]. Also, it can secrete a series of anti-inflammatory adipokines including the CTRP family and Sfrp5, which play crucial protective roles in the inflammation and atherosclerosis [11, 12].

* Correspondence: huilinglu25@aliyun.com
[1]Tongji Hospital, Tongji Medical College, Huazhong University of Science and Technology, Wuhan 430000, Hubei, China
[2]Department of Pediatrics, Tongji Hospital, No.1095. Jiefang Road, Qiaokou District, Wuhan City 430000, Hubei Province, China

Adipokines are these pleiotropic molecules mainly secreted by adipocytes. It demonstrated that classical adipokines leptin, adiponectin and resistin play a major role in energy metabolism, inflammation, obesity, diabetes, cardiovascular disease and autoimmune diseases [13–16]. Recently, it has been conducted that adipokines including adiponectin, leptin, resistin, and visfatin were involved in the acute stage of KD and may participate in its progress of coronary artery lesions [17–19]. Therefore, it interests us that whether the more recently identified chemerin, and omentin, play roles in Kawasaki disease and whether they are associated with lipid metabolism disorders and coronary artery abnormalities of KD. In this study, we focus on the anti-inflammatory and pro-inflammatory effects of chemerin,omentin-1, and adiponectin on the acute phase of KD. Fortunately, it showed that adipokines including chemerin, omentin-1 and adiponectin involved in inflammation of acute KD and might be associated with its lipid metabolism disorders in this study.

Methods

Patients and groups

Eighty children diagnosed with Kawasaki disease (49 boys and 31 girls) in hospital from August 2015 to March 2017 and exclude other severe diseases were selected as KD group. This study was completed in April 2017. Inclusion criteria: (1) KD was accurately diagnosed according to the diagnose criteria of KD; (2) KD with coronary artery abnormalities and without coronary artery abnormalities of untreated KD cases were confirmed by heart echocardiography; (3) Clinical and laboratory examination data are completed. Exclusion criteria: (1) Sepsis cases with positive blood culture; (2) Accompanied by other cardiovascular or hypertension diseases, and primary disease associated with tumors, hematological diseases, congenital malformations, genetic metabolic diseases, primary myocarditis, primary diseases of major organs; (3) Relapsed patients have been treated; (4) Clinical and laboratory examination data are incomplete. A classification of coronary artery abnormalities based solely on Z score has been proposed in the new guidelines of 2017 [4]. Z-score classification has been adapted and recommended as follows: (1) No involvement: Always < 2; (2) Dilation only: 2 to < 2.5; or if initially< 2, a decrease in Z score during follow-up ≥1; (3) Small aneurysm: ≥2.5 to 5; (4) Medium aneurysm: ≥5 to ≤10, and absolute dimension < 8 mm; (5) Large or giant aneurysm: ≥10, or absolute dimension ≥8 mm. In this study, there were 24 cases of KD patients with coronary artery abnormalities who were enrolled in the CAL group and other fifty-six children were NCAL group. It must be emphasized that all children with coronary artery abnormalities in this study showed coronary dilatation. In addition, twenty children with general fever and respiratory infections children who were admitted to our hospital at the same time (11cases of pneumonia and 9 cases of bronchitis) were selected as the febrile control group. In addition, 20 children in the healthy group who had a physical examination in our hospital were selected as normal control. It should be noted that these children are all about to enter kindergarten before which they have to conduct a physical examination. And in China, only 3 years old can attend kindergarten. This is the reason why the average age of these healthy children is 3 years old. All patients diagnosed with KD treated with intravenous immunoglobulin (IVIG) (2 g/kg given as a single intravenous infusion) and acetylsalicylic acid (ASA, 30 $mg{\cdot}kg^{-1}{\cdot}d^{-1}$) within the first 10 days of illness. IVIG resistance means that patients with KD have the persistent or recurrent fever after primary therapy with IVIG plus ASA [4]. The diagnosis of typical Kawasaki disease met the diagnostic criteria proposed in the 2017 AHA guidelines [4], in which children with a history of more than 4 days of fever have at least the following four major clinical manifestations, including skin rash, lymphadenectasis, bilateral conjunctival congestion, oral changes, hard swollen and molting of fingertips. Incomplete Kawasaki disease means fever for 5 days or more than 5 days plus only two or three major clinical manifestations, and excludes a diagnosis of scarlet fever, drug hypersensitive syndrome, Stevens-Jonson syndrome, toxic shock syndrome, adenovirus infections, Epstein-Barr febrile illness (BB) and virus infection febrile illness. According to this, there were fourteen incomplete KD and sixty-six complete KD patients in this study.

Methods

Serum adipocytokines chemerin, omentin-1, adiponectin, and cytokines TNF-α and IL-1β detection

Peripheral blood of 2 mL in heparin anticoagulation tube was collected in the acute stage of KD (usually 1-11 days during the course of the disease) prior to receiving IVIG treatment. Blood was also obtained from children in the febrile group prior to receiving treatment and in the healthy group. Blood was centrifuged and serum immediately saved in − 80 °C for later analysis. Enzyme-linked immunosorbent (ELISA) was used to detect serum levels of chemerin, omentin, adiponectin and the inflammatory cytokines IL-1β and TNF-α. Chemerin ELISA kit was supplied by RND operation (DCMHOO), omentin-1 ELISA kit was supplied by Biovender operation (RD191100200R), TNF-α (557966) and IL-1β (550610) ELISA kit were supplied by BD operation and adiponectin ELISA kit was supplied by Ebioscience operation (BMs2032/2). A Siemens automatic enzyme table analyzer(9659) was used for analysis. Serum levels of adipokines including chemerin, omentin, and adiponectin were detected at the same time, as well as cytokines TNF-α and IL-1β. All assays were performed in accordance with the kit instructions, with detection at 450 nm wavelength using the standard curve to calculate the concentrations.

Biochemical indicators, echocardiography, and electrocardiogram

Levels of serum IL-6, high sensitivity c-reactive protein (CRP), erythrocyte sedimentation rate (ESR), Procalcitonin (PCT), NT-proBNP, blood lipid and other parameters in KD patients prior to receiving treatment were performed using an automated biochemical analyzer in the hospital Clinical Biochemistry Laboratory. Heart echocardiography and electrocardiogram were performed by the cardiac function department and the pediatric cardiovascular laboratory respectively.

Statistics analysis

SPASS 20.0 software was used for to statistical processing. Normally distributed continuous data were expressed as the mean ± standard deviation. Comparisons of frequencies between groups were analyzed by t-tests or one-way ANOVA analysis and differences among groups were assessed using chi-square tests. Correlation between different adipokines and other biochemical indicators were analyzed by Pearson or Spearman analysis. The significance of difference was calculated by Scheffe's test and a P value less than 0.05 was considered statistically significant.

Results

Clinical characteristic of patients with KD

Among eighty patients with KD, there are forty-nine boys and thirty-one girls, whose average age is (2.994 ± 2.267) years. There are no significant differences between KD and the febrile and healthy controls ($P > 0.05$). All children in KD group have treated with IVIG within 10 days of hospital admittance. The CAL group, composed of KD patients with coronary artery dilatation, including 24 cases (30%) and accordingly the NCAL group consists of 56 cases (70%). Of eighty cases of KD, a total of fourteen children (17.5%) are diagnosed with incomplete KD and sixty-six patients (82.5%) for typical KD. It's noteworthy that this percentage doesn't represent the prevalence of coronary artery abnormalities and incomplete KD in KD. It just reflects the ratio of CAL or incomplete and KD. The inflammatory markers in the acute stage of KD including CRP, ESR, and PCT are higher than the febrile group ($P < 0.05$). Also, it shows that blood cholesterol and high-density lipoprotein (HDL) is lower than febrile controls ($P < 0.05$) in the acute phase of KD. Notably, NT-proBNP clearly increased (1326.462 ± 2185.425) and then reduced after treating with IVIG 175.156 ± 115.665) ($P < 0.05$). KD patients with CAL (1831.676 ± 2048.909) has higher levels of NT-proBNP compared with NCAl group (1083.960 ± 2247.476), though there are no significant differences ($P > 0.05$), which might due to limited cases of KD in this study. Similarly, patients with typical KD have relative higher NT-proBNP levels compared with patients with incomplete KD. But there's no significant statistical difference ($P > 0.05$), which remains to be further confirmed by larger samples (Tables 1, 2, and 3).

The serum levels of adipokines including chemerin, omentin-1 and adiponectin in the acute stage of KD, general fever and healthy controls

Circulating chemerin in KD group (87.736 ± 56.310) is higher than that of febrile (59.683 ± 18.282, $P < 0.01$) and normal controls (41.75 ± 10.833, $P < 0.01$). It doesn't show any significant differences between KD with CAL (82.584 ± 48.745) and NCAL (89.944 ± 59.534) in the serum levels of chemerin ($P > 0.05$). By contrast, the levels of omentin-1 in acute KD (389.773 ± 238.611) is lower than general febrile control (542.08 ± 177.995, $P < 0.01$). There are no significant differences between KD and healthy control (385.65 ± 105.535, $P > 0.05$), which might because of limited samples and individual variation. In the acute stage of KD, adiponectin levels (16.400 ± 12.243) decreass compared with the general febrile patients (35.074 ± 12.486, $P < 0.05$). There are no significant differences compared with the healthy children (16.959 ± 7.576) ($P > 0.05$). In addition, we didn't find serum levels of both omentin-1 and adiponectin show any significant differences between KD with CAL and NCAL ($P > 0.05$) (Tables 4 and 5).

Levels of cytokines IL-1β and TNF-α in the acute stage of KD, general fever and healthy controls

Circulating TNF-α in acute KD (11.015 ± 8.626) is higher than that of healthy control (7.261 ± 4.056, $P < 0.05$). Similarly, IL-1β levels in patients with KD (13.656 ± 31. 151) are significantly increased compared with healthy children (2.415 ± 6.313, $P < 0.05$), but there are no significant differences between KD group and febrile control ($P > 0.05$, Fig. 1).

Correlation analysis of adipokines and other parameters

Through correlation analysis, it shows chemerin is positively correlated with omentin-1 ($r = 0.224$, 95% CI 0.06–0.529, $P < 0.05$). Further, total cholesterol (TC) is positively correlated with omentin-1 ($r = 0.358$, 95% CI 0.169–0.518, $P < 0.05$), which implied that adipokines especially omentin-1 are associated with disorders of lipid metabolism (Figs. 2 and 3).

Discussion

As recently discovered adipokines, chemerin, omentin-1, and adiponectin play crucial roles in inflammatory response and are closely involved in cardiovascular diseases. Takeshida et al. [20] reported that adiponectin

Table 1 General characteristics of patients with Kawasaki disease

	Gender (M/F)	Age	BMI	Fever time (day)
KD (*n* = 80)	49/31	2.994 ± 2.267	15.0923 ± 1.358	6.788 ± 3.393
Febrile controls (*n* = 20)	12/8	3.278 ± 3.656	16.303 ± 2.413	2.650 ± 2.277
Healthy controls (*n* = 20)	9/11	3.00 ± 0.0	15.153 ± 2.993	0.000
F	–	0. 118	1.837	5.161
P	–	0.889	0.168	< 0.001*

*represents a significant difference between groups, which is $P < 0.05$

levels were significantly higher in KD patients; Nozue et al. [21] also found resistin levels elevated in KD but its concentrations were unlikely to predict the prognosis of the disease in the acute stage; Liu et al. [22] published data suggesting that leptin participates in the systemic inflammatory response but with controversial results; Kim et al. [18] found that resistin is significantly higher in KD patients, although it has no prognostic value to predict coronary anomalies in the acute stage.

This study aimed to evaluate the levels of these three adipokines in the acute phase of KD and to investigate the associations between adipokines and coronary artery abnormalities or lipid metabolism disorders of KD. Our research demonstrated that (1) circulating chemerin levels are increased in the acute stage of KD. (2)By contrast, omentin-1 and adiponectin levels are decreased compared with general fever patients in the acute stage of KD. (3) Furthermore, cytokine IL-1β is elevated in patients with acute KD, which is similar to inflammatory cytokines such as TNF-α. On the other hand, IL-1β has a decreasing trend in CAL compared with the NCAL group, which might imply that IL-1β involved in the process of inflammatory infiltration and immune vasculitis in the acute phase of KD. Moreover, (4) we find that circulating omentin-1 is positively correlated with both chemerin and total cholesterol, which suggests that chemerin and omentin-1 are involved in the lipid metabolism disorders in the acute stage of KD.

Chemerin was identified as a cDNA sequence called TIG2 (Tazarotene-induced gene 2) in 1997 firstly [23], whose expression was up-regulated during the treatment of psoriatic lesion by tazarotene, which is a kind of retinoic acid receptors (RARs). It has been demonstrated that the chemerin as a type of adipokine, whose gene expression and its receptor, chemerin-like receptor1 (CMKLR1), was significantly higher in adipose tissue of obese models through a signal sequence trap in 2007 in the first place [24].Our study firstly indicated that circulating chemerin levels increased significantly in the acute stage of KD, which were associated with its effects on the early phase of immune response and inflammatory reaction. Chemerin could modulate immune responses through its chemotactic effects and accumulation of antigen-presenting cells including macrophages and dendritic cells at the sites of damage areas [25, 26]. Several studies have reported that chemerin was closely associated with the inflammatory response related to obesity, metabolic syndrome, rheumatoid arthritis and cancer [27–30]. Chemerin receptor CMKRL1 expressed in human vascular endothelial cells could bind to chemerin, which induces inflammation and angiogenesis processes [31, 32]. In addition, chemerin was involved in the development of inflammation in cardiovascular disease and atherosclerosis [33–35], and circulating chemerin were associated with soluble ICAM-1 and E-selectin [36], which provide the greatest evidence regarding endothelial-cell activation that could trigger vascular inflammation. We didn't find a direct relationship between circulating chemerin and KD with coronary artery abnormalities, or incomplete KD. This may be explained that chemerin was mainly involved in the process of immune regulation and inflammatory activation in acute KD, also might be associated with the inflammatory infiltration of vascular endothelial cells. However, the pathogenesis of chemerin in coronary

Table 2 General characteristics and biochemical indicators of patients with Kawasaki disease

	KD group (*n* = 80)	Febrile controls (*n* = 20)	t	*P*
CRP mg/L	76.465 ± 52.761	17.100 ± 27.852	−6.601	< 0.001*
ESR mm/H	53.877 ± 26.773	11.583 ± 7.914	−10.493	< 0.001*
IL-6 pg/mL	153.578 ± 331.333	5.900 ± 6.494	−3.803	< 0.001*
PCT ng/L	1.359 ± 3.364	0.135 ± 0.165	−3.153	0.002*
HB g/L	106.526 ± 10.517	117.588 ± 12.430	3.790	< 0.001*
PLT *10^3/L	350.434 ± 125.649	327.588 ± 128.848	−0.675	0.502
TG mmol/L	1.208 ± 0.641	1.287 ± 0.601	0.400	0.690
TC mmol/L	3.129 ± 0.619	3.562 ± 0.591	2.639	0.010*
HDL mmol/L	0.613 ± 0.240	1.146 ± 0.309	−6.269	< 0.000*
LDL mmol/L	1.974 ± 0.562	1.994 ± 0.565	−0.103	0.918

*represents a significant difference between groups, which is $P < 0.05$

Table 3 Biochemical indicators of patients with Kawasaki disease prior treatment and posttreatment of IVIG

	Prior treatment of IVIG	Posttreatment of IVIG	t	*P*
CRPmg/L	81.726 ± 56.671	4.014 ± 4.678	8.424	< 0.001*
ESR mm/H	54.290 ± 26.752	41.207 ± 29.089	1.815	0.075
IL-6 pg/mL	157.145 ± 298.991	3.876 ± 3.032	2.989	0.005*
PCT ng/L	1.982 ± 4.540	0.121 ± 0.131	2.493	0.017*
HB g/L	105.486 ± 8.688	108.841 ± 10.696	−1.473	0.145
PLT *10^3/L	330.432 ± 128.981	497.694 ± 141.631	−5.278	< 0.001*
NF-proBNP pg/mL	1326.462 ± 2185.425	175.156 ± 115.665	3.199	0.003*
TG mmol/L	1.296 ± 0.844	1.565 ± 0.606	−1.239	0.220
TC mmol/L	3.057 ± 0.623	3.571 ± 1.109	−2.526	0.014*
HDL mmol/L	0.613 ± 0.240	0.740 ± 0.215	−1.841	0.071
LDL mmol/L	1.973 ± 0.562	2.343 ± 0.480	−2.177	0.035*
Apo-A1 g/L	0.655 ± 0.249	0.943 ± 0.253	−3.311	0.002*
Apo-B g/L	0.697 ± 0.202	0.681 ± 0.094	0.341	0.753

*represents a significant difference between groups, which is $P < 0.05$

artery lesions of patients with KD still need to be confirmed further.

Omentin-1 or interlectin-1, a new cDNA expressed specifically in omental adipose tissue, was a new adipocytokine identified by Schäffler et al. [37]. Omentin has been reported to enhance insulin-mediated glucose-uptake in adipocytes and to activate protein kinase Akt/PKB, which was also named insulin sensitizer [38, 39]. It is well known that immune vasculitis is the most characteristic pathologic change in KD patients, especially targeting coronary arteries among small and medium vessels. It has been conducted that the omentin-1 levels in synovial joints of patients with rheumatoid arthritis(RA) were lower than those of patients with osteoarthritis(OA) [38]. Patients with obesity showed decreased omentin-1 levels compared with thin patients and they suggested that omentin-1 levels may be predictive of the metabolic consequences or co-morbidities associated with obesity [39, 40]. In this study, we found that serum levels of omentin-1 as a kind of anti-inflammatory adipokine decreased in the acute stage of patients with KD, which could be explained that omentin-1 as a protective factor might play vital roles in anti-inflammation and inhibition the activation of endothelial cells at lower levels. What's more interesting is that we found circulating omentin-1 levels are positively correlated with total cholesterol, which is a crucial biomarker of lipid metabolism. Lower omentin-1 may be beneficial to correct the disorders of lipid metabolism through inhibiting oxLDL-induced foam cell formation and protecting vascular endothelial cells from inflammatory lesions and alleviating vascular injuries of KD [41]. However, Antonella et al. [19] reported that serum omentin levels were higher in KD patients than healthy controls. This result is just inconsistent with our results. This difference may be explained through the following three possible reasons. Firstly, omentin has two different subtypes, which might play different roles in the development of KD. In this study, we focus on the correlation between omentin-1 and acute KD. But it is not clear Antonella and his or her colleague studied which subtype or total in their article. Secondly, we found that omentin-1 in the KD group was lower than febrile controls but not than healthy controls. However, Antonella et al. reported that serum omentin levels were significantly higher in KD patients versus healthy controls. Lastly, we have to take individual differences from different regions into account. In short, these controversial results need to be further confirmed by numerous studies.

Adiponectin is the most abundant adipokine secreted by adipocytes, which exhibits multiple physiological functions through combined to its receptors. In vitro and vivo experiments showed that adiponectin treatment

Table 4 Serum levels of adipokines in the acute phase of KD and control subjects

Groups	Chemerin (ng/mL)	Omentin-1 (ng/mL)	Adiponectin (ug/mL)
Healthy controls($n = 20$)	41.746 ± 10.824	385.662 ± 105.547	16.959 ± 7.576
Febrile controls($n = 20$)	59.683 ± 18.282	542.075 ± 177.995	35.074 ± 12.486
KD group($n = 80$)	87.736 ± 56.310	389.773 ± 238.611	16.400 ± 12.243
P	< 0.001*	0.016*	< 0.001*

*represents a significant difference between groups, which is $P < 0.05$

Table 5 Comparison of serum adipokines levels between CAL and NCAL group in KD patients

Groups	CAL ($n = 24$)	NCAL ($n = 56$)	t	P
Chemerin (ng/mL)	82.584 ± 48.745	89.944 ± 59.534	−0.533	0.595
Omentin-1(ng/mL)	410.312 ± 258.103	407.651 ± 267.921	0.041	0.967
Adiponectin(ug/mL)	20.483 ± 17.349	16.891 ± 14.820	0.943	0.348
TNF-α (pg/ml)	14.678 ± 12.402	9.445 ± 6.024	1.393	0.187
IL-1β (pg/ml)	9.299 ± 20.718	15.523 ± 34.677	−0.817	0.416

*represents a significant difference between groups, which is $P < 0.05$

attenuates lipopolysaccharide (LPS)-induced expression of TNF-a in cultured macrophages through inhibition of NF-κB signaling and overexpression of adiponectin alleviates progression of atherosclerotic lesions in apolipoprotein E knockout (KO) mice, with an accompanying decrease in TNF-a and SR-A expression [42, 43]. Here, this research indicates that adiponectin levels reduced significantly in the acute phase of KD, as with omentin-1 levels. The possible pathogenesis might be that adiponectin plays anti-inflammatory roles through blockade of NF-κB signaling and further inhibits the production of proinflammatory cytokines such as TNF-α and MMP-12 [44, 45]. It is worth noting that TNF-α is still overexpressed in the acute phase of KD might because that it has exceeded the inhibition properties of adiponectin though this still needs to be explored through in vitro and vivo experiments. In addition, we didn't discover any pieces of evidence to support the correlation between adiponectin and coronary artery abnormalities of KD.

Recently, there were some case reports and a clinical trial reported that IL-1 receptor inhibitors (IL-1RA) improve the pathogenetic condition of KD with the restoration of dilation coronary artery [46–49]. We found that a low level of IL-1β in KD patients accompanied coronary artery lesions(CAL). This suggests that IL-1β is involved in the progress of coronary artery lesions, which implied that IL-1βbecome a new target in the treatment of KD or KD accompanied CAL in the future. This study provides evidence for this conclusion.

Ishwarlal et al. reported that lower levels of omentin-1 and higher levels of chemerin in nascent metabolic syndrome were risk factors for diabetes and cardiovascular disease [50]. In this study, disorders of lipid metabolism are present in patients with acute KD, which is consistent with the results reported previously [51]. We also found that serum levels of omentin-1 were positively correlated with both chemerin and total cholesterol, which suggests that chemerin and omentin-1 are directly or indirectly closely related to disorders of lipid metabolism in the acute phase of KD. Adipokines were involved in lipid metabolism in autocrine or paracrine manners and these disorders of lipids metabolism may be associated with inappropriate secretion of omentin-1 and chemerin which suggests that low levels of omentin-1 and chemerin may predict disorders of lipid metabolism, although this still needs to be supported by a larger data sample. Interestingly, it showed that hemoglobin in acute KD was higher than febrile control, which implied that hemoglobin was related to inflammation state in acute KD. Kim et al. [18]. described that resistin and serum IL-6 were significantly elevated and hemoglobin significantly lower in KD patients with coronary anomalies. Hemoglobin levels were negatively correlated with resistin levels in KD patients. However, it's a pity that we didn't find the correlation

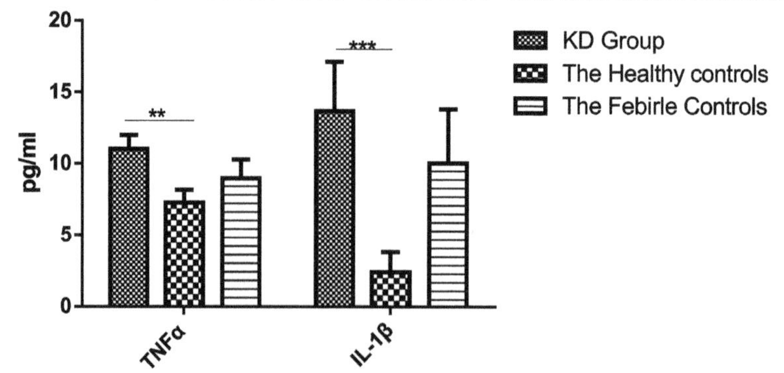

Fig. 1 Serum levels of cytokines in the acute phase of KD and control subjects. This figure shows that the levels of TNF-α in KD group were obviously higher than that of the healthy group ($P < 0.05$). Also, IL-1β levels in KD group were significantly increased compared with healthy group ($P < 0.05$). **Represents a significant difference between groups, which is $P < 0.05$. ***Represents a significant difference between groups, which is $P < 0.01$.

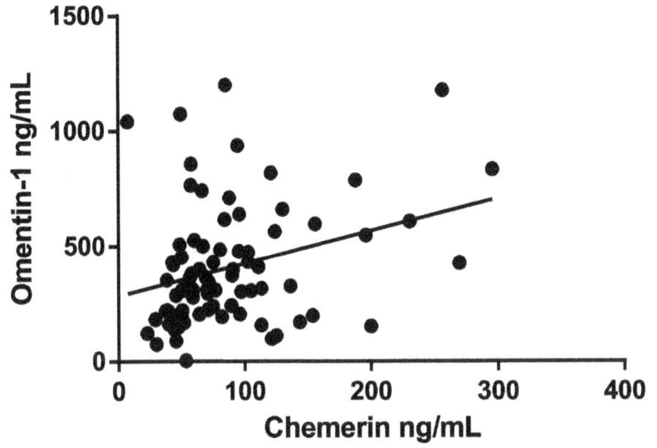

Fig. 2 Chemerin is positively correlated with omentin ($r = 0.224$, $P < 0.05$)

between hemoglobin and adipokines including chemerin, omentin-1, and adiponectin.

However, our study has several limitations. Firstly, we concentrated on the influences of each adipokine on KD respectively but cannot evaluate the interrelationship among different adipokines. Moreover, we only analyzed levels of adipokines including chemerin, omentin-1 and adiponectin in the acute stage without tracking the changing process of adipokines during the full development of KD and without further studying mechanism of action. Finally, our data are confined to a limited number of samples and concentricity of the region, thus further research with a larger sample and covering multi-centers will be more persuasive.

Conclusions

Overall, we demonstrated that high chemerin, low omentin-1 and adiponectin levels are present in the acute stage of KD, suggesting that adipokines chemerin, omentin-1, and adiponectin are involved in acute KD. Furthermore, though the mechanism is unknown, chemerin might play pro-inflammatory, while omentin-1 and adiponectin may play an anti-inflammatory role in inflammation of acute KD. Although it didn't show any relationship between there adipokines and coronary artery abnormalities of KD, we found that chemerin and omentin-1directly or indirectly related to lipid metabolism disorders. This provides new ideas for exploring the pathogenesis and treatment of refractory KD. It will be more interesting and meaningful to study how different isoforms of these adipokines work in inflammation and the relationship between hemoglobin and other adipokines in the acute phase of KD.

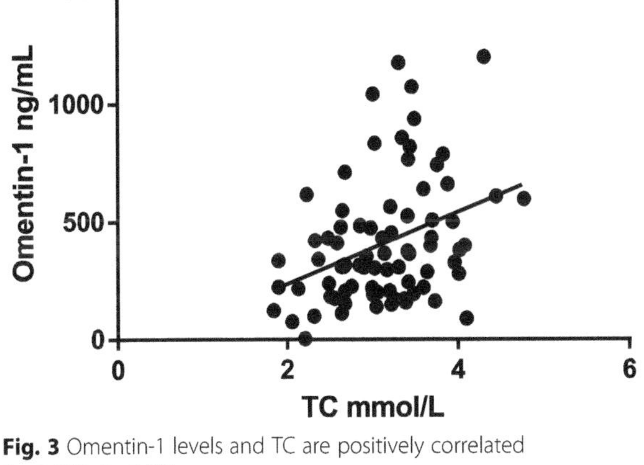

Fig. 3 Omentin-1 levels and TC are positively correlated ($r = 0.358$, $P < 0.05$)

Abbreviations

AOA: Aortic ring diameter; CAL: Coronary artery lesions; CRP: High sensitivity c-reactive protein; ESR: Erythrocyte sedimentation rate; HB: Hemoglobin; HDL: High-density lipoprotein; IVIG: Intravenous immunoglobulin; KD: Kawasaki disease; LCA: Left coronary artery; LDL: Low-density lipoprotein; NCAL: No coronary artery lesion group; PCT: Procalcitonin; PLT: Platelet; RCA: Right coronary artery; TC: Total cholesterol; TG: Triglyceride

Acknowledgments

This study was supported by Natural Science Foundation of China (81270949). And the abstract of this study has been selected as the oral presentation in the 6th congress of Asia-pacific pediatric cardiac society and a poster display in the 13th Congress of Asian Society for Pediatric Research.

Funding

Natural Science Foundation of China (81270949).

Authors' contributions

XyZ participated in the design of the study, carried out the detection of the serum levels of adipokines and cytokines by ELISA and finished the manuscript. HIL carried out the design of the study, performed the statistical analysis and helped to modify the manuscript. TtY conceived of the study and participated in the process of the experiments. XfH, YW, and FF participated in the sample collection, data analysis and helped to modify the manuscript. All authors read and approved the final manuscript.

Competing interests

The authors declare that they have no competing interests.

References

1. Newburger JW, Takahashi M, Burns JC. Kawasaki Disease. J Am Coll Cardiol. 2016;67(14):1738–49.
2. Denby KJ, Clark DE, Markham LW. Management of Kawasaki disease in adults. Heart. 2017;103(22):1760–9.
3. Son MBF. Kawasaki Disease. Pediatr Rev/Am Acad Pediatr. 2018;39(2):78–90.

4. McCrindle BW, Rowley AH, Newburger JW, Burns JC, Bolger AF, Gewitz M, et al. Diagnosis, treatment, and long-term Management of Kawasaki Disease: a scientific statement for health professionals from the American Heart Association. Circulation. 2017;135(17):e927–99.
5. Takahashi K, Oharaseki T, Naoe S, Wakayama M, Yokouchi Y. Neutrophilic involvement in the damage to coronary arteries in acute stage of Kawasaki disease. Pediatr Int. 2005;47(3):305–10.
6. Brown TJ, Crawford SE, Cornwall ML, Garcia F, Shulman ST, Rowley AH. CD8 T lymphocytes and macrophages infiltrate coronary artery aneurysms in acute Kawasaki disease. J Infect Dis. 2001;184(7):940–3.
7. Tian J, An X, Niu L. Correlation between NF-kappaB signal pathway-mediated caspase-4 activation and Kawasaki disease. Exp Ther Med. 2017;13(6):3333–6.
8. Collart MA, Baeuerle P, Vassalli P. Regulation of tumor necrosis factor alpha transcription in macrophages: involvement of four kappa B-like motifs and of constitutive and inducible forms of NF-kappa B. Mol Cell Biol. 1990;10(4): 1498–506.
9. Ouchi N, Parker JL, Lugus JJ, Walsh K. Adipokines in inflammation and metabolic disease. Nat Rev Immunol. 2011;11(2):85–97.
10. Cao H. Adipocytokines in obesity and metabolic disease. J Endocrinol. 2014; 220(2):T47–59.
11. Carbone F, Mach F, Montecucco F. The role of adipocytokines in atherogenesis and atheroprogression. Curr Drug Targets. 2015;16(4):295–320.
12. Ouchi N, Higuchi A, Ohashi K, Oshima Y, Gokce N, Shibata R, et al. Sfrp5 is an anti-inflammatory adipokine that modulates metabolic dysfunction in obesity. Science. 2010;329(5990):454–7.
13. Fruhbeck G, Catalan V, Rodriguez A, Ramirez B, Becerril S, Salvador J, et al. Involvement of the leptin-adiponectin axis in inflammation and oxidative stress in the metabolic syndrome. Sci Rep. 2017;7(1):6619.
14. Freitas LL, Braga VA, Do SDFS, Cruz JC, Sousa Santos SH, de Oliveira Monteiro MM, et al. Adipokines, diabetes and atherosclerosis: an inflammatory association. Front Physiol. 2015;6:304.
15. Hui X, Lam KS, Vanhoutte PM, Xu A. Adiponectin and cardiovascular health: an update. Br J Pharmacol. 2012;165(3):574–90.
16. Bednarska-Makaruk M, Graban A, Wisniewska A, Lojkowska W, Bochynska A, Gugala-Iwaniuk M, et al. Association of adiponectin, leptin and resistin with inflammatory markers and obesity in dementia. Biogerontology. 2017;18(4):561–80.
17. Kemmotsu Y, Saji T, Kusunoki N, Tanaka N, Nishimura C, Ishiguro A, et al. Serum adipokine profiles in Kawasaki disease. Mod Rheumatol. 2012;22(1):66–72.
18. Kim HJ, Choi EH, Kil HR. Association between adipokines and coronary artery lesions in children with Kawasaki disease. J Korean Med Sci. 2014; 29(10):1385–90.
19. Fioravanti A, Simonini G, Cantarini L, Generoso M, Galeazzi M, Bacarelli MR, et al. Circulating levels of the adipocytokines vaspin and omentin in patients with Kawasaki disease. Rheumatol Int. 2012;32(5):1481–2.
20. Takeshita S, Takabayashi H, Yoshida N. Circulating adiponectin levels in Kawasaki disease. Acta Paediatr. 2006;95(10):1312–4.
21. Nozue H, Imai H, Saitoh H, Aoki T, Ichikawa K, Kamoda T. Serum resistin concentrations in children with Kawasaki disease. Inflamm Res. 2010;59(11):915–20.
22. Liu R, He B, Gao F, Qian L, Qijian Y. Relationship between adipokines and coronary artery aneurysm in children with Kawasaki disease. Transl Res. 2012;160(2):131–6.
23. Nagpal S, Patel S, Jacobe H, DiSepio D, Ghosn C, Malhotra M, et al. Tazarotene-induced gene 2 (TIG2), a novel retinoid-responsive gene in skin. J Invest Dermatol. 1997;109(1):91–5.
24. Bozaoglu K, Bolton K, McMillan J, Zimmet P, Jowett J, Collier G, et al. Chemerin is a novel adipokine associated with obesity and metabolic syndrome. Endocrinology. 2007;148(10):4687–94.
25. Zabel BA, Zuniga L, Ohyama T, Allen SJ, Cichy J, Handel TM, et al. Chemoattractants, extracellular proteases, and the integrated host defense response. Exp Hematol. 2006;34(8):1021–32.
26. Parolini S, Santoro A, Marcenaro E, Luini W, Massardi L, Facchetti F, et al. The role of chemerin in the colocalization of NK and dendritic cell subsets into inflamed tissues. Blood. 2007;109(9):3625–32.
27. Landgraf K, Friebe D, Ullrich T, Kratzsch J, Dittrich K, Herberth G, et al. Chemerin as a mediator between obesity and vascular inflammation in children. J Clin Endocrinol Metab. 2012;97(4):E556–64.
28. Lehrke M, Becker A, Greif M, Stark R, Laubender RP, von Ziegler F, et al. Chemerin is associated with markers of inflammation and components of the metabolic syndrome but does not predict coronary atherosclerosis. Eur J Endocrinol. 2009;161(2):339–44.
29. Erdogan S, Yilmaz FM, Yazici O, Yozgat A, Sezer S, Ozdemir N, et al. Inflammation and chemerin in colorectal cancer. Tumour Biol. 2016;37(5):6337–42.
30. Dessein PH, Tsang L, Woodiwiss AJ, Norton GR, Solomon A. Circulating concentrations of the novel adipokine chemerin are associated with cardiovascular disease risk in rheumatoid arthritis. J Rheumatol. 2014;41(9):1746–54.
31. Kaur J, Adya R, Tan BK, Chen J, Randeva HS. Identification of chemerin receptor (ChemR23) in human endothelial cells: chemerin-induced endothelial angiogenesis. Biochem Biophys Res Commun. 2010;391(4):1762–8.
32. Bozaoglu K, Curran JE, Stocker CJ, Zaibi MS, Segal D, Konstantopoulos N, et al. Chemerin, a novel adipokine in the regulation of angiogenesis. J Clin Endocrinol Metab. 2010;95(5):2476–85.
33. Gu P, Cheng M, Hui X, Lu B, Jiang W, Shi Z. Elevating circulation chemerin level is associated with endothelial dysfunction and early atherosclerotic changes in essential hypertensive patients. J Hypertens. 2015;33(8):1624–32.
34. Yan Q, Zhang Y, Hong J, Gu W, Dai M, Shi J, et al. The association of serum chemerin level with risk of coronary artery disease in Chinese adults. Endocrine. 2012;41(2):281–8.
35. Lachine NA, Elnekiedy AA, Megallaa MH, Khalil GI, Sadaka MA, Rohoma KH, et al. Serum chemerin and high-sensitivity C reactive protein as markers of subclinical atherosclerosis in Egyptian patients with type 2 diabetes. Ther Adv Endocrinol Metab. 2016;7(2):47–56.
36. Glowinska B, Urban M, Peczynska J, Florys B. Soluble adhesion molecules (sICAM-1, sVCAM-1) and selectins (sE selectin, sP selectin, sL selectin) levels in children and adolescents with obesity, hypertension, and diabetes. Metabolism. 2005;54(8):1020–6.
37. Schaffler A, Neumeier M, Herfarth H, Fürst A, Schölmerich J, Büchler C. Genomic structure of human omentin, a new adipocytokine expressed in omental adipose tissue. Biochimica et Biophysica Acta (BBA) - Gene Struct Expr. 2005;1732(1–3):96–102.
38. Senolt L, Polanska M, Filkova M, Cerezo LA, Pavelka K, Gay S, et al. Vaspin and omentin: new adipokines differentially regulated at the site of inflammation in rheumatoid arthritis. Ann Rheum Dis. 2010;69(7):1410–1.
39. Menzel J, di Giuseppe R, Biemann R, Wittenbecher C, Aleksandrova K, Eichelmann F, et al. Association between chemerin, omentin-1 and risk of heart failure in the population-based EPIC-Potsdam study. Sci Rep. 2017;7(1):14171.
40. de Souza BC, Yang RZ, Lee MJ, Glynn NM, Yu DZ, Pray J, et al. Omentin plasma levels and gene expression are decreased in obesity. Diabetes. 2007; 56(6):1655–61.
41. Watanabe K, Watanabe R, Konii H, Shirai R, Sato K, Matsuyama TA, et al. Counteractive effects of omentin-1 against atherogenesisdagger. Cardiovasc Res. 2016;110(1):118–28.
42. Ohashi K, Shibata R, Murohara T, Ouchi N. Role of anti-inflammatory adipokines in obesity-related diseases. Trends Endocrinol Metab. 2014;25(7):348–55.
43. Nigro E, Scudiero O, Monaco ML, Palmieri A, Mazzarella G, Costagliola C, et al. New insight into adiponectin role in obesity and obesity-related diseases. Biomed Res Int. 2014;2014:658913.
44. Shibata S, Tada Y, Hau C, Tatsuta A, Yamamoto M, Kamata M, et al. Adiponectin as an anti-inflammatory factor in the pathogenesis of psoriasis: induction of elevated serum adiponectin levels following therapy. Br J Dermatol. 2011;164(3):667–70.
45. Ouchi N, Walsh K. Adiponectin as an anti-inflammatory factor. Clin Chim Acta. 2007;380(1–2):24–30.
46. Lee Y, Schulte DJ, Shimada K, Chen S, Crother TR, Chiba N, et al. Interleukin-1beta is crucial for the induction of coronary artery inflammation in a mouse model of Kawasaki disease. Circulation. 2012;125(12):1542–50.
47. Tremoulet AH, Jain S, Kim S, Newburger J, Arditi M, Franco A, et al. Rationale and study design for a phase I/IIa trial of anakinra in children with Kawasaki disease and early coronary artery abnormalities (the ANAKID trial). Contemp Clin Trials. 2016;48:70–5.
48. Sanchez-Manubens J, Gelman A, Franch N, Teodoro S, Palacios JR, Rudi N, et al. A child with resistant Kawasaki disease successfully treated with anakinra: a case report. BMC Pediatr. 2017;17(1):102.
49. Cohen S, Tacke CE, Straver B, Meijer N, Kuipers IM, Kuijpers TW. A child with severe relapsing Kawasaki disease rescued by IL-1 receptor blockade and extracorporeal membrane oxygenation. Ann Rheum Dis. 2012;71(12):2059–61.
50. Jialal I, Devaraj S, Kaur H, Adams-Huet B, Bremer AA. Increased chemerin and decreased omentin-1 in both adipose tissue and plasma in nascent metabolic syndrome[J]. J Clin Endocrinol Metab. 2013;98(3):E514–7.
51. Fukunaga H, Kishiro M, Akimoto K, Ohtsuka Y, Nagata S, Shimizu T. Imbalance of peroxisome proliferator-activated receptor gamma and adiponectin predisposes Kawasaki disease patients to developing atherosclerosis. Pediatr Int. 2010;52(5):795–800.

8

Pediatric rheumatology infusion center: report on therapeutic protocols and infusions given over 4 Years with focus on adverse events over 1 Year

Surabhi S. Vinod[1], Annelle B. Reed[2], Jamelle Maxwell[2], Randy Q. Cron[1,2] and Matthew L. Stoll[1,2*]

Abstract

Background: Children with chronic rheumatic disease often require intravenous (IV) therapy. Our center has instituted standardized protocols for use of IV medications in rheumatology patients. Herein, we introduce the therapeutic protocols and report on their short-term safety.

Methods: This was an institutional review board (IRB) approved retrospective chart review of all patients who had received IV infusions between the years 2012 and 2015 at a single center, prescribed by a pediatric rheumatologist. Infusion medications included abatacept, belimumab, cyclophosphamide, immune globulin, infliximab, methylprednisolone, N-acetylcysteine, pamidronate disodium, rituximab, and tocilizumab. For calendar year 2015, all adverse infusions reactions were recorded along with treatment strategies used to manage them, and outcomes. Rates of adverse events were calculated per infusion medication.

Results: During calendar years 2012–2015, 7585 IV infusions were administered to 398 unique patients. In the year 2015, 2187 infusions were administered to 224 patients, with 34 patients experiencing 41 infusion reactions (1.9% of all infusions). Rituximab had the highest rate of adverse drug reactions with 10 patients experiencing reactions during 106 infusions (9.4%). None of the reactions were life-threatening, and only 6 resulted in discontinuation of therapy.

Conclusions: In a recent 4-year span, the UAB Pediatric Rheumatology Infusion Center has given thousands of IV infusions with minimal adverse reactions over a one-year reporting period. The combination of standard infusion protocols, experience of and communication between physicians and nurses who staff the center, and safety of the medications themselves, allows for safe IV administration of a variety of therapies for pediatric rheumatology patients.

Keywords: Infusion center, Adverse reaction, Therapeutic protocols, Infliximab, Methylprednisolone, Rituximab

Background

Intravenous (IV) infusion therapy is now critical for the treatment and maintenance of many pediatric rheumatic diseases, such as juvenile idiopathic arthritis (JIA), systemic lupus erythematosus (SLE), and inflammatory bowel disease (IBD) associated arthritis. Prior to biologic infusion therapy, non-steroidal anti-inflammatory drugs (NSAIDs), corticosteroids (CS), and non-biologic disease modifying anti-rheumatic drugs (DMARDs) were a mainstay of treatment [1, 2]. However, due to the strong adverse event (AE) profile of CS and the limited benefit to side effect ratio of NSAIDs, these drugs are often now used as a means of bridging therapy until better alternatives are used [2]. In this era, biologic therapies have become increasingly used treatment approaches, and have made lasting changes in the quality of life of patients affected by diseases such as JIA [3]. Many of these novel

* Correspondence: mstoll@peds.uab.edu
[1]Department of Pediatrics, University of Alabama School of Medicine, Birmingham, AL, USA
[2]Division of Pediatric Rheumatology, Children's of Alabama, Birmingham, AL 35233-1711, USA

biologic therapies require or at least may be administered as IV infusions. While some patients receive such therapies at home via home health or through local infusion centers, which have advantages of decreased travel burden and in some cases more flexible hours, the majority of families prefer to receive them in a well-equipped infusion center associated with a tertiary hospital, and certain medications (e.g., rituximab) are never administered via home health agencies. Although receipt of the infusions at the tertiary hospital poses some inconvenience for the family, this is mitigated to some extent by scheduling visits on the same day as the infusion, which can take place in the infusion center or in the adjacent rheumatology clinic.

In order to cope with the increased demand for providing IV infusion therapies for children with rheumatic diseases, there has been a need for expanding existing, or creating new, infusion facilities. With the creation of new pediatric rheumatology program at the University of Alabama at Birmingham (UAB) in 2007, a novel pediatric rheumatology infusion clinic (7 beds) was constructed. Protocols were created and modified to provide safe and effective IV infusions for this pediatric rheumatology population. Herein, the breadth of clinical diagnoses treated, the variety of IV therapies provided (from 2012 to 2015), and the associated AEs (2015) are reported. This information can be used to assist current and future pediatric rheumatology infusion centers in the care of pediatric rheumatology patients requiring a variety of repeated IV infusion therapies.

Methods

Overview of study

This is an IRB approved retrospective chart review of all patients given infusions as ordered by UAB pediatric rheumatology providers (6 physicians and 3 nurse practitioners) in the Pediatric Rheumatology Infusion Center from 2012 to 2015, including medications used off-label for the given indications. The Pediatric Rheumatology Infusion Center at UAB operates Monday-Friday from 8:00 am to 4:30 pm with infusions, depending on the medication and dose, lasting between two and 8 h (Table 1). The medications infused include abatacept, belimumab, cyclophosphamide, immune globulin, infliximab, methylprednisolone, N-acetylcysteine, pamidronate disodium, rituximab, and tocilizumab, which were given as outlined by developed standardized protocols (see Additional file 1). The protocols include pre-medications to prevent allergic reactions as well as rescue medicines should allergic-type reactions occur.

Data collection

Clinical data about the infusion patients was collected directly from the electronic medical record (EMR). This data included diagnosis, gender, infusion medications given, age at first and last infusions, and number of infusions given per patient. For calendar year 2015, a hand-search of each infusion was performed to identify any AEs that occurred during the infusions, as well as management of the reactions. All infusions are documented in the EMR. Every 15 min during the first hour of the infusion, every 30 min during the second hour of the infusion, and every 60 min thereafter, the nursing staff responsible for the infusion documents the patient's vital signs, response to therapy, rate changes, and IV site condition. Adverse drug events, as well as phone calls made and actions taken, are documented in the EMR as well. Safety events that occurred outside of the infusions (e.g., infections) were not collected as part of this report.

Table 1 Duration of infusions

Medications by Generic Name	Duration of Infusion
Abatacept	2 h
Belimumab	2 h
Cyclophosphamide	6–8 h
Immune Globulin-IVIG	2–8 h
Infliximab	2–6 h
Methylprednisolone	2 h
N-acetyl cysteine	5 h
Pamidronate	4–6 h
Rituximab	6-8 h
Tocilizumab	2–4 h

Statistical analysis

Comparisons of dichotomous variables were performed with the Chi-squared or Fisher exact tests, as appropriate; comparisons of continuous variables were performed with the Student's t-test. Microsoft Excel and SPSS (Version 25) were used for analyses of the data.

Results

From 2012 through 2015, a total of 7585 IV infusions were given to 398 patients in the UAB Pediatric Rheumatology Infusion Center. During the calendar year 2015 alone, a total of 2187 infusions were given to 224 patients. Demographic and clinical data on the patients are shown in Table 2, and a summary of the medications administered by diagnosis is included in Table 3. Among those, thirty-four patients experienced 41 infusion reactions, for a rate of infusion reactions of 1.9% of all infusions (Table 4.) The most common infusion reactions, occurring in 17 patients in total, were nausea/vomiting and throat discomfort, including tightness, itching, or pain. Medications with infusion reactions were abatacept, infliximab, immune globulin, methylprednisolone, rituximab, and tocilizumab. Rituximab had the highest rate of adverse

Table 2 Demographic and clinical features of the patient population

Feature	*n* (224)
DIAGNOSIS	
Juvenile idiopathic arthritis	100
RF-negative polyarticular	35
Enthesitis-related arthritis	24
Oligoarticular	17
Psoriatic	12
Systemic	7
RF+ polyarticular	5
Systemic lupus erythematosus	40
Inflammatory bowel disease-associated arthritis	18
Juvenile dermatomyositis	12
Idiopathic uveitis	10
Sjogren syndrome	8
Mixed connective tissue disease	7
Henoch-Schonlein purpura	5
Sarcoidosis	4
Chronic recurrent multifocal osteomyelitis	3
Other[1]	14
DEMOGRAPHICS	
Female sex	161 (72%)
Age at initiation of infusion (years: mean ± SD)	11.5 ± 4.2
Age in 2015[2] (years: mean ± SD)	13.3 ± 4.0
THERAPY	
Therapy duration (start – September 30, 2017); years: mean ± SD	2.8 ± 2.4
Use of antimetabolites[3]	183 (82%)
Outcome of infusions used in 2015	
Continued into 2016	139[4]
Patient transferred care	19
Changed to home/local infusions or subcutaneous administration	11
Stopped due to disease control	33
Stopped due to inefficacy	21[4]
Stopped due to adverse events	6
Stopped as per parental choice	5

[1]The following diagnoses had 1 patient each: Behcet Syndrome, *CREST* (Calcinosis, Raynaud, Esophageal dysmotility, Sclerodactyly, Telangiectasia) syndrome, cutis laxa with restrictive lung disease, eosinophilic granulomatosis with polyangiitis, hyper IgD syndrome, idiopathic pulmonary hemosiderosis, immune-mediated glomerulonephritis, idiopathic thrombocytopenic purpura, mucolipidosis type IV, orbital pseudotumor, pemphigoid, primary angiitis of the central nervous system, polymyositis, relapsing polychondritis. [2]Calculated as age mid-year (June 30, 2015). [3]azathioprine, cyclophosphamide, leflunomide, methotrexate, mycophenolate mofetil. [4]Ten patients were counted in both rows, due to switching from one infusion to another in 2015

drug reactions with 10 events over 106 infusions (9.4%), while belimumab, cyclophosphamide, and pamidronate were not associated with any. All but one of these reactions terminated with conservative therapy (e.g., non-steroidal anti-inflammatory drugs, diphenhydramine, IV fluids); flushing (rash) following infusion with abatacept was treated with subcutaneous epinephrine. All of the drug-specific protocols have nursing instructions in the event of any infusion reaction (see Additional file 1). Following those protocols, all reactions were managed by placing the infusion on hold and giving established treatments. Specifically, pain was treated with ibuprofen or acetaminophen; rashes, itching, and flushing were managed with diphenhydramine; and nausea with or without emesis were treated were ondansetron or promethazine. As per protocol, if the symptoms were deemed non-life threatening and resolved with conservative therapy as above, re-starting of the infusion was permitted. Infliximab and rituximab were often re-started at slower rates, which were gradually increased as tolerated. Only six of these infusion reactions required discontinuation of therapy (infliximab, $n = 3$; methylprednisolone, $n = 2$; rituximab, $n = 1$); the patient who received epinephrine for suspected anaphylactic reaction to abatacept successfully tolerated additional doses. Overall, of the 224 patients who received infusions in 2015, 139 continued to receive infusions at our center in 2016, 19 transferred care due to moving out of state or graduating to adult care, 11 switched to a more convenient location or method of delivery, and 33 discontinued due to disease control. Only 6 discontinued due to adverse events, 5 due to parental choice, and 21 due to inefficacy, of whom 10 successfully switched to a different infusion.

Of the 224 patients receiving IV infusions, 183 (82%) received one or more anti-metabolites (azathioprine, cyclophosphamide, leflunomide, methotrexate, mycophenolate mofetil). Among the medications as a whole, there was no obvious association between development of infusion reactions and use of an anti-metabolite. Infusion reactions were observed in 9/41 (22%) of patients not taking an anti-metabolite versus 25/183 (14%) of patients on one ($p = 0.181$). However, among patients taking infliximab, there was a trend towards an association, with infusion reactions observed in 3/12 (25%) of patients not taking an anti-metabolite versus 6 / 82 (7.3%, $p = 0.087$, Fisher's exact test) among patients who were taking an anti-metabolite. Interestingly, among those taking infliximab, patients with an infusion reaction were younger (10 ± 3.8 versus 14 ± 3.8 years, $p = 0.008$, Student's t-test) than those who did not; this association did not hold for the group as a whole (data not shown). Female patients (29/161, 18%) may have been more likely to develop infusion reactions than males (5/63, 7.9%, $p = 0.059$).

Table 3 List of infusions by diagnosis

Disease	ABT	Belimumab	CYT	IVIg	INX	MP	Pamidronate	RTX	TCZ
JIA	29		1	1	57	32	1	1	12
SLE		2	14	8		35		22	
IBD-a					17	5			
JDM				11		11			
Uveitis					9	2		1	
Sjogren						8		7	
MCTD	2			1	1	6		3	
HSP			1	3		5		3	
Sarcoidosis					4	3			
CRMO					2	1	1		
GPA						3		3	
Other			1	6	4	9	1	5	
Total patients	31	2	17	30	94	120	3	45	12
Total infusions	237	26	76	266	816	513	7	106	140

Abbreviations: *ABT* Abatacept, *CRMO* Chronic recurrent multifocal osteomyelitis, *GPA* Granulomatosis with polyangiitis, *HSP* Henoch-Schonlein purpura, *IBD-a* Inflammatory bowel disease-associated arthritis; *INX* Infliximab, *IVIg* Intravenous immunoglobulin, *JDM* Juvenile dermatomyositis, *JIA* Juvenile idiopathic arthritis, *MCTD* Mixed connective tissue disease, *MP* Methylprednisolone, *RTX* Rituximab, *SLE* Systemic lupus erythematosus, *TCZ* Tocilizumab

Discussion

Modern therapeutics have dramatically altered the landscape for children with a variety of rheumatic diseases, including JIA and lupus [3, 4]. Although many biologics have the convenience of injectable delivery that the patient or family can self-administer, still others require IV infusions. In addition to the well-known risks associated with immunosuppressive therapy, in general [5], IV medications have their attendant risks of infusion reactions, that while unusual, can in very rare cases prove life-threatening [6]. With medications such as rituximab and infliximab, it is estimated that up to 10% of adults have an infusion reaction severe enough to warrant permanent discontinuation of therapy [7–9]. There is mixed data as to the risk of infusion reactions in the pediatric population. Aeschlimann et al. [10] reported infusion reactions in only 46/2446 (2%) of infliximab infusions, of which only six resulted in discontinuation. However, Al-Mayouf et al. [11] reported 10 suspected anaphylaxis reactions, 8 of which were associated with infliximab among 52 patients taking infusions. Likewise, Lahdenne et al. [12] reported 12 infusion reactions, 8 of which were deemed severe, among 64 patients taking infliximab despite 100% use of anti-metabolites. In contrast to these experiences, our experience has been

Table 4 Number of infusion reactions in 2015

Reaction	ABT (237)	IVIG (266)	INX (816)	MP (513)	RTX (106)	TCZ (140)	Total Infusion Reactions
Rash	1	2			1		4
Nausea/Vomiting		2	1	5		1	9
Cough			1		2		3
Throat Tightness/Itching/Pain	1	2			5		8
Chest Pain/Tightness		1	1				2
Headache	3	2	3				8
Swelling			2		1		3
Wheezing				1			1
Hives					1		1
Blurry Vision				1			1
Abdominal Pain			1				1
Total Events	5	9	9	7	10	1	41

Medications not associated with any infusion reactions are not included in the table
Abbreviations: *ABT* Abatacept, *INX* Infliximab, *IVIG* Intravenous immunoglobulin, *MP* Methylprednisolone, *RTX* Rituximab, *TCZ* Tocilizumab

largely positive. As a whole, we administered 7585 IV infusions to 398 unique patients from 2012 to 2015. In 2015 alone, 2187 infusions were given to 224 patients. Of those, 41 (1.9%) were associated with an infusion reaction of any sort. However, only 1 reaction was treated with an emergency medication, and only 6 of those 2187 infusion reactions (0.27%) resulted in discontinuation of therapy. All of the reactions that did occur in 2015 would fall under the heading of mild adverse reactions, as defined by the Rheumatology Common Toxicity criteria (RCTC) [13].

Several factors may be responsible for our success with the administration of IV therapy. First, we have a skilled team of medical professionals overseeing the delivery of the infusions. All nurses working in the Infusion Center graduated from an accredited school of nursing with an RN license, possess at least one year of recent nursing experience upon hiring, are certificated in Basic Life Support, and are certificated for the administration of chemotherapy within six months of securing employment. Second, the infusion clinic shares space with the rheumatology clinic, and by policy, at least one pediatric rheumatology physician or nurse practitioner must be present on campus at all times during operation of the infusion clinic. This facilitates rapid telephone or in person assessment of the patient. Consequently, symptoms such as flushing or chest pain that could fall anywhere on the spectrum from anxiety to anaphylaxis are rapidly and efficiently assessed by skilled providers. Third, the detailed infusion protocols (see Additional file 1) provide for pre-medications, call for availability of emergency bedside medications, and specify actions taken during both mild as well as potentially life-threatening infusion reactions. For patients receiving rituximab, data from a randomized trial indicated that pre-treatment with 100 mg of methylprednisolone resulted in decreased risk of infusion reactions [14]. With respect to infliximab, the role of pre-medication is less clear. A randomized trial indicated that pre-medication with betamethasone provided no benefit [15], while observational studies have yield mixed evidence with respect to benefits of anti-histamines [10, 12, 16, 17]. Arguably, however, the rarity (9/816) and mild nature of the infusion reactions among patients taking infliximab provide scant impetus to adjust the protocols. Finally, our positive experiences also speak to the general safety of the medications used. Additional factors that may promote the safety of the medications described herein are high doses accompanied by frequent administration of drugs such as infliximab [18] and frequent use of concomitant DMARDs. Eighty-two percent of patients taking any infusion and 88% of our patients on infliximab used an anti-metabolite. With respect to dose, the mean infliximab dose was 13.8 mg/Kg, with none of our patients receiving doses < 6 mg/Kg. This appears to reflect a strong difference between our patients and those reported by Lahdenne et al. [12] , in whom the average total dose was 243 mg ; the article by Al-Mayouf et al. [11] did not discuss medication doses or pre-medications. These factors appear to result in decreased incidence of development of anti-drug antibodies and of infusion reactions in general [19, 20], and use of anti-metabolites appeared to be protective against the development of infusion reactions among patients taking infliximab in our study; levels of anti-drug antibodies were not routinely available in our patients. It is possible that the safety profile described herein is due to the fact that many of the patients had been on therapy for several years (Table 2) and thus, those patients who were prone to infusion reactions may have already discontinued the therapy. However, infusion reactions were no more likely among those patients newly started on therapy in 2015 (11/80, 14%) as compared to those who had started prior to 2015 (23/144, 16%, p = 0.657); similar trends were observed among the sub-group taking infliximab (data not shown). Ultimately, the precise factors responsible for the safety of the infusions reported herein cannot be determined, however.

Some of the symptoms reported in the infusion reactions (Table 4) overlap with those that would be seen during life-threatening anaphylactic events, e.g. itching and swelling of the throat and face, hives, rash, and cough, with one episode of nausea/vomiting. The most frequent culprit in our study was rituximab, in which 10 such reactions were observed over 106 infusions (9.4%) given over 2015. A similar experience was reported by Moss et al. [21], in their report of 10 infusions reactions over 185 infusions. In their study, as in ours, all reactions resolved with conservative management, and patients were able to receive subsequent infusions. Similarly, Lequerre et al. [22] reported that instituting a protocol in which similar infusion reactions were treated with slowing the rate of the infusion permitted continuation of therapy in patients who in the past would have had to discontinue treatment with the offending agent. True anaphylactic reactions do not resolve with diphenhydramine, nor would slowing the rate of infusion provide any safety benefit, and repeat infusions would not be tolerated. Therefore, although tryptase levels were not obtained, such events likely represented anaphylactoid reactions. The overlapping symptoms between these reactions and true anaphylaxis underscore the benefits of having an experienced nursing staff as well as immediate availability of trained clinicians. While delays in the treatment of anaphylaxis can be fatal, there are also substantial risks associated with falsely labeling a reaction as anaphylactic, thus permanently depriving the patient of use of a potentially life-saving medication.

Conclusions

In recent years, the UAB Pediatric Rheumatology Infusion Center has treated a wide variety of diagnoses and given thousands of IV infusions with very few adverse reactions. These reactions were mild and transient, and resolved after using protocol derived management strategies. Together, the use of standardized infusion protocols, the combined experience of physicians and nurses who manage the treatment, effective communication between the nurses providing the infusions and the rheumatology-trained clinicians, and the safety profile of the medications themselves, combine to allow for safe IV infusions for pediatric rheumatology patients, and can serve as a model for the development of future infusion centers.

Abbreviations

AE: Adverse event; CS: Corticosteroids; DMARD: Disease modifying anti-rheumatic drug; EMR: Electronic medical record; IBD: Inflammatory bowel disease; IRB: Institutional review board; IV: Intravenous; JIA: Juvenile idiopathic arthritis; NSAID: Non-steroidal anti-inflammatory drug; OMERACT: Outcome measures in rheumatology; RF: Rheumatoid factor; SLE: Systemic lupus erythematosus; TNF: Tumor necrosis factor; UAB: University of Alabama at Birmingham

Acknowledgments

The authors wish to thank the infusion staff at CoA for all their tremendous work.

Funding

Not applicable

Authors' contributions

ABR, JM, and RQC designed the study. ABR generated the individual therapeutic protocols. SV collected and MLS analyzed the patient data. SV, MLS, and RQC performed the bulk of the writing of the manuscript. All authors read and approved the final manuscript.

Competing interest

The authors declare that they have no competing interests.

References

1. Cron RQ. Treatment for JRA in the new millennium. J Clin Rheumatol. 2001; 7:283–5.
2. Stoll ML, Cron RQ. Treatment of juvenile idiopathic arthritis in the biologic age. Rheum Dis Clin N Am. 2013;39:751–66.
3. Stoll ML, Cron RQ. Treatment of juvenile idiopathic arthritis: a revolution in care. Pediatr Rheumatol Online J. 2014;12:13.
4. Mahmoud I, Jellouli M, Boukhris I, Charfi R, Ben Tekaya A, Saidane O, et al. Efficacy and safety of rituximab in the Management of Pediatric Systemic Lupus Erythematosus: a systematic review. J Pediatr. 2017;187:213–9. e2
5. Horneff G. Safety of biologic therapies for the treatment of juvenile idiopathic arthritis. Expert Opin Drug Saf. 2015;14:1111–26.
6. Hastings D, Patel B, Torloni AS, Mookadam F, Betcher J, Moss A, et al. Plasmapheresis therapy for rare but potentially fatal reaction to rituximab. J Clin Apher. 2009;24:28–31.
7. Salmon JH, Perotin JM, Morel J, Drame M, Cantagrel A, Ziegler LE, et al. Serious infusion-related reaction after rituximab, abatacept and tocilizumab in rheumatoid arthritis: prospective registry data. Rheumatology (Oxford). 2018;57:134–9.
8. Krintel SB, Grunert VP, Hetland ML, Johansen JS, Rothfuss M, Palermo G, et al. The frequency of anti-infliximab antibodies in patients with rheumatoid arthritis treated in routine care and the associations with adverse drug reactions and treatment failure. Rheumatology (Oxford). 2013;52:1245–53.
9. Levin AS, Otani IM, Lax T, Hochberg E, Banerji A. Reactions to rituximab in an outpatient infusion center: a 5-year review. J Allergy Clin Immunol Pract. 2017;5:107–13. e1
10. Aeschlimann FA, Hofer KD, Cannizzaro Schneider E, Schroeder S, Lauener R, Saurenmann RK. Infliximab in pediatric rheumatology patients: a retrospective analysis of infusion reactions and severe adverse events during 2246 infusions over 12 years. J Rheumatol. 2014;41:1409–15.
11. Al-Mayouf SM, Alenazi A, AlJasser H. Biologic agents therapy for Saudi children with rheumatic diseases: indications and safety. Int J Rheum Dis. 2016;19:600–5.
12. Lahdenne P, Wikstrom AM, Aalto K, Kolho KL. Prevention of acute adverse events related to infliximab infusions in pediatric patients. Arthritis Care Res (Hoboken). 2010;62:785–90.
13. Woodworth T, Furst DE, Alten R, Bingham CO 3rd, Yocum D, Sloan V, et al. Standardizing assessment and reporting of adverse effects in rheumatology clinical trials II: the rheumatology common toxicity criteria v.2.0. J Rheumatol. 2007;34:1401–14.
14. Emery P, Fleischmann R, Filipowicz-Sosnowska A, Schechtman J, Szczepanski L, Kavanaugh A, et al. The efficacy and safety of rituximab in patients with active rheumatoid arthritis despite methotrexate treatment: results of a phase IIB randomized, double-blind, placebo-controlled, dose-ranging trial. Arthritis Rheum. 2006;54:1390–400.
15. Sany J, Kaiser MJ, Jorgensen C, Trape G. Study of the tolerance of infliximab infusions with or without betamethasone premedication in patients with active rheumatoid arthritis. Ann Rheum Dis. 2005;64:1647–9.
16. Hutsell SQ, Wu M, Park KT. Frequency of severe infusion reactions associated with outpatient infusion of infliximab without Premedications. J Pediatr Gastroenterol Nutr. 2017;65:430–1.
17. Gold SL, Cohen-Mekelburg S, Schneider Y, Shen N, Faggen A, Rupert A, et al. Premedication use in preventing acute infliximab infusion reactions in patients with inflammatory bowel disease: a single center cohort study. Inflamm Bowel Dis. 2017;23:1882–9.
18. Tambralli A, Beukelman T, Weiser P, Atkinson TP, Cron RQ, Stoll ML. High doses of infliximab in the management of juvenile idiopathic arthritis. J Rheumatol. 2013;40:1749–55.
19. Wee JS, Petrof G, Jackson K, Barker JN, Smith CH. Infliximab for the treatment of psoriasis in the U.K.: 9 years' experience of infusion reactions at a single Centre. Br J Dermatol. 2012;167:411–6.
20. Thomas SS, Borazan N, Barroso N, Duan L, Taroumian S, Kretzmann B, et al. Comparative immunogenicity of TNF inhibitors: impact on clinical efficacy and tolerability in the Management of Autoimmune Diseases. A Systematic Review and Meta-Analysis. BioDrugs. 2015;29:241–58.
21. Moss IB, Moss MB, dos Reis DS, Coelho RM. Immediate infusional reactions to intravenous immunobiological agents for the treatment of autoimmune diseases: experience of 2126 procedures in a non-oncologic infusion Centre. Rev Bras Reumatol. 2014;54:102–9.
22. Lequerre T, Vittecoq O, Klemmer N, Goeb V, Pouplin S, Menard JF, et al. Management of infusion reactions to infliximab in patients with rheumatoid arthritis or spondyloarthritis: experience from an immunotherapy unit of rheumatology. J Rheumatol. 2006;33:1307–14.

9

Temporomandibular joint arthritis in juvenile idiopathic arthritis, now what?

Matthew L. Stoll[1*], Chung H. Kau[2], Peter D. Waite[3] and Randy Q. Cron[1]

Abstract

Background: Arthritis involving the temporomandibular joint (TMJ) complicates 40 - 96% of cases of juvenile idiopathic arthritis (JIA), potentially leading to devastating changes to form and function. Optimal evaluation and management of this joint remains a matter of ongoing discussion.

Methods: We performed a PubMed search for all articles with keywords "temporomandibular" and "arthritis", covering the dates 2002 through February 28, 2018. A separate PubMed search was performed for all articles with keywords "temporomandibular joint", "arthritis", and "treatment" covering the same dates.

Findings: The TMJ is a particularly challenging joint to assess, both clinically and with imaging studies. Clinical assessment of the TMJ is hampered by the low sensitivity of joint pain as well as the absence of physical exam findings early in the disease process. As with all joints, plain radiography and computed tomography only detect arthritic sequelae. Additionally, there is mixed data on the sensitivity of ultrasound, leaving magnetic resonance imaging (MRI) as the optimal diagnostic modality. However, several recent studies have shown that non-arthritic children can have subtle findings on MRI consistent with TMJ arthritis, such as joint effusion and contrast enhancement. Consequently, there has been an intense effort to identify features that can be used to differentiate mild TMJ arthritis from normal TMJs, such as the ratio of the enhancement within the TMJ itself compared to the enhancement in surrounding musculature. With respect to treatment of TMJ arthritis, there is minimal prospective data on medical therapy of this complicated joint. Retrospective studies have suggested that the response to medical therapy of the TMJ may lag behind that of other joints, prompting use of intraarticular (IA) therapy. Although most studies have shown short-term effectiveness of corticosteroids, the long-term safety of this therapy on local growth as well as on the development of IA heterotopic bone have prompted recommendations to limit use of IA corticosteroids. Severe TMJ disease from JIA can also be managed non-operatively with splints in a growing child, as well as with surgery.

Conclusion: In this review, we summarize literature on the diagnosis and management of TMJ arthritis in JIA and suggest a diagnostic and therapeutic algorithm for children with refractory TMJ arthritis.

Keywords: Intraarticular corticosteroids, Juvenile idiopathic arthritis, Magnetic resonance imaging, Temporomandibular joint, Treatment

Background

Forty to ninety-six percent of children with juvenile idiopathic arthritis (JIA) develop arthritis of the temporomandibular joint (TMJ) [1–6]; all JIA categories are at risk [7]. There are several features of this joint that warrant particular attention, including its importance for everyday function, potential cosmetic implications of altered dentofacial growth, and the challenges in the evaluation and management of TMJ arthritis. Detailed discussion of the functional implications of TMJ arthritis are available [8, 9], but briefly include pain with talking, difficulty eating, and obvious and potentially embarrassing alterations to the normal facial appearance. This review will focus on the diagnosis and management of TMJ arthritis in children with JIA.

* Correspondence: mstoll@peds.uab.edu
[1]Department of Pediatrics, University of Alabama at Birmingham (UAB), 1600 7th Avenue South, Children's Park Place North Suite G10, Birmingham 35233, AL, USA
Full list of author information is available at the end of the article

Methods

This was not a systematic review. However, one of the authors (RQC) performed a PubMed search for all articles with keywords "temporomandibular" and "arthritis", covering the dates 2002 to the present. For the review of the studies on intraarticular therapy to the TMJ, a different author (MLS) performed a PubMed search for "temporomandibular joint", "arthritis", and "treatment" covering the same dates.

Anatomy and function

The TMJ is a synovial joint composed of 4 articulating surfaces: glenoid fossa of the temporal bone, the upper and lower surfaces of the articular disc, and the mandibular condyle [10]. The disc divides the joint into the superior and inferior compartments. As it can move independently of the condyle, there is a potential for disc displacement, which results in pain, joint noises, and limited range of motion [11]. The TMJ is a complex joint termed ginglymoarthrodial, meaning that it has both hinge and sliding motion. Specifically, motion at the inferior compartment consists of rotation (ginglymoid joint) and manifests as moving the chin, while motion at the superior compartment consists of sliding or translation and manifests as protrusion of the mandible. Both movements are very important for maximum mouth opening and function [12]. A unique aspect of the joint is that both right and left must work in synchrony with partial dislocation. Additionally, the jaw works to maximize intercuspation of the teeth, so any dental anomalies can alter TMJ function and consequently result in condylar or disc abnormalities [11]. The fact that teeth create an abrupt stop and that malocclusion causes complex neuromuscular feedback with altered proprioception leads to a variety of symptoms, presenting as articular and myofascial pain and dysfunction.

Evaluation of TMJ arthritis

History

The TMJ is among the more challenging joints to evaluate clinically, due to the absence of visible joint swelling and lack of symptomatology early during arthritis. Historical findings indicative of damaging TMJ arthritis include the usual symptoms of pain and stiffness, as well as TMJ-specific symptoms of clicking and popping. The former indicates irregularities of the disc with movement, while the latter indicates a sudden prominent movement or dislocation of the disc during translation [13]. A loud pop may indicate abnormal movement of the disc such as anterior dislocation with or without recapture, limiting the range of motion. Joint noise is obvious due to close proximity to the ear cartilage and is commonly asymptomatic. The predictive power of such historical findings has been evaluated in studies of children with JIA, with findings that their sensitivities are low. For example, Weiss et al. (2008) prospectively evaluated 32 newly diagnosed subjects with JIA, finding that symptoms of TMJ pain and dysfunction were only 26% sensitive, albeit 100% specific, for identification of TMJ arthritis, as assessed by MRI [14]. Thus, while certain abnormal physical exam findings are strongly suggestive of TMJ arthritis, their absence is not reassuring. The Weiss study, as well as similar studies evaluating physician examination maneuvers (below), used the MRI with contrast as a gold standard, the limitations of which will be discussed below.

Physical examination

TMJ arthritis does not typically manifest with joint swelling. Moreover, physical exam findings are late in the disease process where the bone growth has been altered by the arthritis. Thus, physical examination consists at the very least of evaluation for joint tenderness, clicking upon mouth opening, asymmetric mouth opening (present only in unilateral or unequal disease, with the jaw deviating towards the more affected side) [15], and assessment of opening. Recently, published recommendations also encouraged palpation of masticatory muscles and an evaluation of TMJ morphology and symmetry [16]. As with the historical signs, no single one of these markers is highly sensitive for arthritis. For example, Koos et al. (2014) prospectively evaluated five physical exam maneuvers (asymmetric mouth opening, pain on palpation of masticatory muscles, pain on palpation of the TMJ, TMJ clicking and reduced maximal incisal opening (MIO)) as predictors of TMJ arthritis, using MRI as the gold standard [17]. The sensitivity of each individual item ranged from a low of 21% (MIO) to a high of 65% (asymmetric opening). Combining the items, the presence of any one of them had a sensitivity of 85%, which will still not only miss a substantial number of cases but is also associated with a low specificity of 54%. Similarly, the studies by Weiss et al. (2008) and Muller et al. (2009) both reported that physical examination maneuvers had low sensitivity as well as low specificity for the detection of MRI-suggested TMJ arthritis in new-onset patients [14, 18]. In contrast, Abramowicz et al. (2013) reported that a combination of abnormal MIO for age and jaw deviation had a positive predictive value of 100% in patients with long-standing JIA, indicating that patients with both had a 100% likelihood of TMJ arthritis. However, in support of the previous work, the negative predictive value was only 46%, meaning that the majority of patients lacking one or both of these findings still had arthritis [19]. Kristensen et al. [19] performed a systematic literature review, concluding that while studies were not directly comparable, no single physical exam finding could accurately predict MRI findings of TMJ arthritis [20].

Plain radiography and computed tomography

As with any joint, radiography of the TMJ provides information only on arthritic sequelae, not active arthritis. The TMJ is difficult to image due to the overlay of the skull base especially by traditional films. Even standard panoramic tomograms contain artifact and are of little value compared to MRI and CT. Computed tomography (CT) provides greater anatomic detail as compared to plain radiography, and is thus of benefit primarily in identifying surgical candidates [21]. A form of CT, known as cone beam CT (CBCT), provides greater focus on the TMJ, thereby minimizing radiation of the surrounding brain and face. Features such as condylar flattening and erosion, as well as osteophyte formation, were readily distinguished between JIA patients and controls who underwent CBCT for unspecified reasons [22].

Ultrasound

Compared to MRI, ultrasound (US) has advantages with respect to cost and lack of requirement for sedation, but it is unclear as to whether it can identify active inflammation and arthritic sequelae as accurately as MRI with contrast. Weiss et al. (2008) compared US and MRI in the same cohort of 32 children studied above, finding that MRI detected both more active (24/32 vs 0/32) and chronic (22/32 vs 9/32) changes [14]. Likewise, Muller et al. reported that MRI and even physical examination were both more sensitive at the detection of active inflammatory changes and arthritic sequelae as compared to US [18]. More recently, Kirkhus et al. compared the correlation between ultrasonography-assessed capsular width and MRI assessment of synovitis (T1 weighted [T1W] signal increase at the synovium following administration of contrast), finding a correlation of 0.483 ($p < 0.001$) at the subcondylar level, concluding in contrast to the previous studies that US may in fact be a useful screening tool for arthritis of the TMJ [23]. In support, several other studies that did not constitute direct comparisons with MRI did show that US frequently detected findings of active arthritis in children with JIA [24–26]. The reason for the variation in these findings is not clear, although they may relate to the operator-dependence of US, as well as challenges to US due to the small anatomy of the TMJ of young children. A review of the literature concluded that US has low sensitivity for detecting joint effusion and may be more valuable to monitor established TMJ arthritis than for its initial detection [27].

Magnetic resonance imaging

Most studies use MRI with contrast as the gold standard for the evaluation of TMJ arthritis [28], as it can identify both active arthritis changes as well as arthritic sequelae. Findings suggestive of active arthritis include joint fluid, bone marrow edema, and contrast enhancement (CE) (Fig. 1); those representing arthritic sequelae include changes to the shape of the condyle or disk, pannus, and osteophytes (Fig. 2). Short of performing biopsies or direct visualization (Fig. 3) of the joint in children with suspected TMJ arthritis, there would be no way to assess the sensitivity of the MRI in a human population. However, its specificity can be assessed by evaluating MRI of the TMJ in children who do not have arthritis. Although, ideally, such studies would be performed in completely healthy children, the requirement for CE, and in many cases sedation, preclude such a study for ethical reasons.

Nevertheless, several studies have evaluated findings at the TMJ in children without known or suspected JIA undergoing brain MRI. The first of these was conducted by Tzaribachev et al. in 2009; this retrospective study found that arthritic changes are very rare in non-arthritic children, with only three of 96 healthy children showing effusions and another three showing CE [29]. Unfortunately, multiple subsequent studies have shown

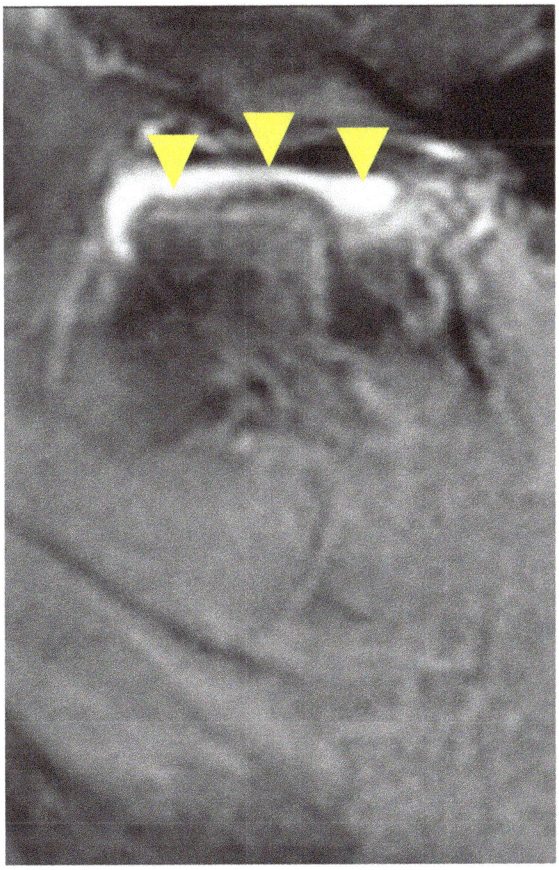

Fig. 1 Active arthritis. Thickened synovium and contrast enhancement seen in the sagittal image of the left TMJ of a 13-year-old female with poly-articular JIA (arrowheads)

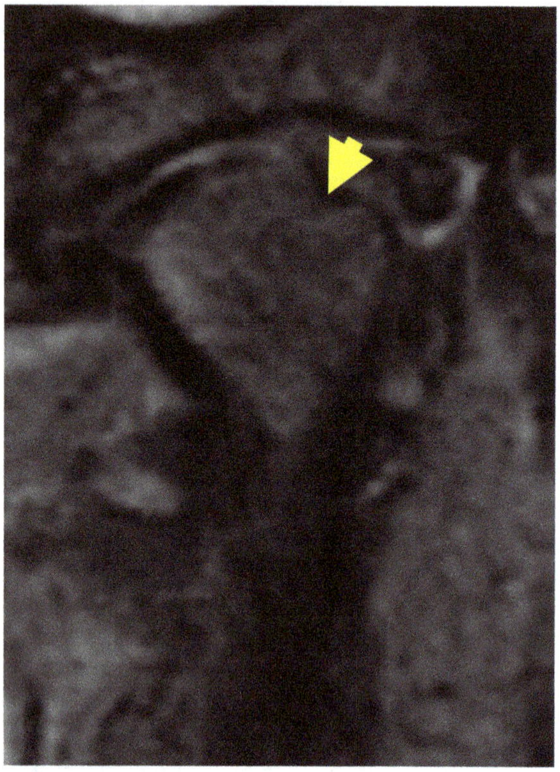

Fig. 2 Arthritic sequelae. Large condylar erosion noted in the sagittal image of the right TMJ of an 11-year-old male with ERA/JIA (arrowhead)

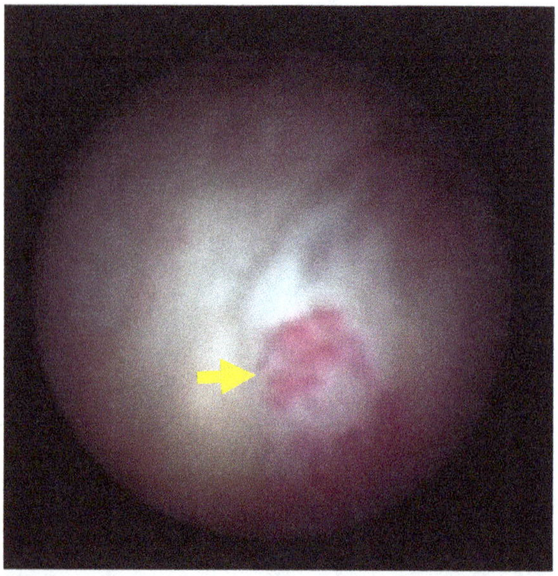

Fig. 3 Arthroscopic images of the inside of a temporomandibular joint in a 17-year-old female with poly-articular JIA. A TMJ image using a mini arthroscope (1.2 mm) reveals clear regions of inflammation (arrow)

contradictory findings. In an uncontrolled study, von Kalle et al. reported that 14 joints from 46 non-arthritic children undergoing MRI of the brain had some degree of CE; additionally, the intensity of CE in the joint tissue post-contrast was 73% higher than pre-contrast, while the intensity of the CE in the joint tissue was a more modest 20% higher than that of the surrounding musculature [30]. An even higher frequency of CE was reported by Kottke et al. in their study of 27 non-arthritic children [31]. Fifty-two of 54 TMJs (96%) demonstrated CE, and 43 of 54 (83%) had effusions. Likewise, Angenete et al. reported CE in 35 of 36 (97%) subjects, as well as mild flattening of the condyle in 20/101 [32]. Finally, Stoll et al. [33] reported CE in 120/122 (98%) non-arthritic controls, with the average size of the enhancement actually larger as compared to that in 35 newly-diagnosed JIA patients (1.1 ± 0.24 vs 0.88 ± 0.27 mm, $p < 0.001$).

In addition to identifying the presence of joint fluid or enhancement in non-arthritic subjects, several recent studies have also sought to determine the optimal method of assessing the presence and extent of enhancement. As CE will increase in any tissue with passage of time following contrast administration [34], comparison of CE in the TMJ with that of a control site present within the field of the view, most commonly the longus capitus muscle, is one approach. This ratio of the signal intensity (SI) in the area of interest divided by the SI in a control location is generally referred to as the enhancement ratio (ER). This method was studied by Peacock et al. in their study of 158 non-arthritic children who underwent MRI of the head. They reported ERs of 1.52 and 1.68 for the inferior and superior joint spaces, respectively [35]. The same group also performed a retrospective controlled study of 72 children with JIA and 71 non-arthritic controls. In this study, both JIA patients and controls had an ER greater than 1, while the JIA patients had a significantly higher ER as compared to the controls (2.52 ± 0.79 versus 1.28 ± 0.16), with ROC analysis identifying 1.55 as the best cutoff value [36].

Similarly, Caruso et al. evaluated three different ratios in a cohort of subjects that included JIA patients with symptoms suggestive of TMJ arthritis, JIA patients without such symptoms, and non-arthritic controls. These ratios were (postGadolinium SI in the TMJ – preGadolinium SI in the TMJ)/(postGadolinium SI in the longus capitus – preGadolinium SI in the longus capitus); (postGadolinium SI in the TMJ – preGadolinium SI in the TMJ)/(postGadolinium of longus capitus); and (postGadolinium SI of TMJ)/(postGadolinium SI of longus capitus). Of those three, they concluded that the most favorable measure was the second (postGadolinium SI in the TMJ – preGadolinium SI in the TMJ)/(postGadolinium of longus capitus), due to optimal discrimination among the three groups and a lack of a substantial increase over time [37]. Likewise, Ma et al. [38] compared a metric that evaluated only the change in SI pre- versus post-administration of gadolinium with a metric that measured a signal to noise ratio based upon enhancement in surrounding tissue, studying 67 children with JIA and 24 non-arthritic controls. Consistent with the study by Caruso et al. [37], Ma et al. concluded that the ER, which incorporated the extent of enhancement in the surrounding tissue, was better able to discriminate JIA patients with mild disease from controls [38]. While the optimal method of assessing the extent of TMJ joint fluid or enhancement in controls may not be entirely clear, it is evident that small amounts of joint fluid and CE in non-arthritic subjects are common. Lastly, there also remain questions as to the optimal protocols, and magnet strengths versus imaging coils in evaluating the TMJ by MRI in children with JIA [39, 40].

Findings of mild degrees of CE in non-arthritic children should not undermine the body of literature indicating a very high frequency of TMJ arthritis in children with JIA. Healthy children do not typically demonstrate retrognathia, micrognathia, and jaw deviation on exam, findings that were once the norm in children with JIA [41–43]. Finally, all of these recent studies of the MRI in non-arthritic children reported fairly mild active arthritic changes, and essentially absent arthritic sequelae, a clear distinction from that seen in children with JIA [14, 41].

Medical treatment of TMJ arthritis

There is minimal prospective data evaluating the effectiveness of systemic immunosuppressive therapy on TMJ arthritis. Randomized clinical trials of conventional and biologic disease-modifying anti-rheumatic drugs generally have not included the TMJ as an outcome. The only prospective study that did evaluate the effectiveness of systemic medications on the TMJ was published over 30 years ago and included two medications that are no longer used (gold and penicillamine) in the management of children with JIA or related disorders [44]. Evidence that the TMJ might not respond as well to current therapies as compared to other joints is observational, e.g., a retrospective study showing that of 73 patients with no evidence of arthritis on physical exam; 36 (49%) nevertheless had TMJ arthritis detectable by MRI [6]. Many of these patients were taking traditional and biologic disease-modifying anti-rheumatic drugs (DMARDs). It is unclear why the TMJ would respond less robustly to systemic medications, as compared to other joints. The joint space is physically close to the growth zone of the condylar head, and evolutionarily it is a distinct synovial joint with a unique biochemical makeup. Moreover, there is precedent for the observation of relative responsiveness to therapy with other joints, e.g., the inability of traditional DMARDs to treat axial spondyloarthritis despite some effectiveness with these medications in the management of peripheral disease [45]. There may also be differences in the biology of arthritis in that joint; as an illustration, one study showed different epigenetic changes of fibroblast-like synoviocytes in the knee as compared to the hip of patients with rheumatoid arthritis [46].

Despite these observations, there is indirect evidence that the TMJ does in fact respond to systemic immunosuppressive therapy. As discussed above, progressive radiographically evident destructive changes were once the norm in children with JIA, while this no longer appears to be the case. Anecdotally, our clinics are no longer heavily populated with children with visually evident facial deformities. Data supporting these observations came from a study by Twilt et al., who performed baseline and 5-year radiographs in 70 children treated with systemic but not local immunosuppressive therapy, finding decreased evidence of TMJ changes on exam as well as by radiography [47]. The findings are all the more impressive given the minimal usage of biologics in this cohort (6/70; Twilt, personal communication). Likewise, Ince et al. reported decreased radiographic evidence of TMJ arthritis among 18 patients with JIA who were taking methotrexate, compared with nine who were not [48]; this was not a controlled study, so it is likely that the children on methotrexate were perceived to have had more severe disease overall than the children not taking any therapies, thus potentially biasing the findings towards the opposite direction. Finally, Stoll et al. (2012) reported that disease duration was protective against the likelihood of having TMJ arthritis in a population of 187 children with JIA, a finding which they took to indicate that therapy itself was protective [6]. These findings are clearly in stark contrast to the older literature, in which disease duration was associated with progressive radiographically evident deterioration [42].

Intraarticular therapy for TMJ arthritis

The safety and effectiveness of intraarticular corticosteroid injections (IACI) for TMJ arthritis has been reviewed twice, with somewhat different conclusions despite inclusion of the same studies [49, 50]. Included studies, as well as studies published since these reviews, are summarized in Tables 1 and 2. These studies have generally reported short-term improvement in markers of TMJ arthritis, including pain, physical examination findings, and MRI findings. Moreover, results were more robust in some studies versus others. In addition, no short-term serious adverse events were reported therein. As Stoustrup (2013) reported, these studies, however, generally lack methodologic rigor, as they are retrospective, uncontrolled, and unblinded in the outcome

Table 1 Overview of studies evaluating local therapy for TMJ arthritis

Study	*n*	Therapy	Injections/TMJ	Localization of IACI	Duration of follow-up
Arabshahi et al. [122]	23	TA 40 mg; TH 20 mg	1	CT	6–12 months
Ringold et al. [106]	25	TA 20–40 mg; TH 10–20 mg	1–5	Anatomic	26 months (5–52)
Weiss et al. [14]	21	TH 10 mg	1	CT	6 months
Parra et al. [123]	83	TH 5–10 mg TA 5–10 mg	1–6	US	6 weeks
Mina et al. [67]	28	DIP 6 mg	8–10	Anatomic	Completion of course
Habibi et al. [124]	39	TH 10–20 mg	1	US	6–8 weeks
Stoll et al. [125]	63	TH 5–10 mg	1–2	Anatomic	5 months
Stoll et al. [56]	24	INX 5–10 mg	ND	Anatomic	7.8 months
Olsen-Bergem et al. [64]	21	Arthrocentesis plus Triamcinolone	1	US	8 months
Olsen-Bergem et al. [64]	17	Arthrocentesis alone	1	US	8 months
Lochbuhler et al. [51]	33	TH 6–20 mg	1–7	Anatomic	5 years
Stoll et al. [55][1]	33	INX	1–7	Anatomic	9 months (2–27)
Stoustrup et al. [126]	13	TH 20 mg	1	Anatomic	333 days (190–600)
Kinard et al. [65]	3	Arthrocentesis alone	1	Anatomic	1 month
Resnick et al. [127]	29	TH 10 mg	1	Anatomic	22.9 months
Resnick et al. [128]	45	TH 10 mg	1	Anatomic or imaging[2]	21–22 months
Antonarakis et al. [66][3]	21 (IACS), 8 (lavage)	TA 20 mg	1	Anatomic	6 months

[1]There is overlap in patients with Stoll et al. [56]; however, patients present in both studied had undergone additional injections in the intervening period. [2]This study compared patients who had received injections via anatomic guidance versus those who had received imaging guidance. For the latter, multiple modalities (CT, US, fluoroscopy) were used. [3]This study compared TMJ lavage alone with lavage plus IACI. *Abbreviations*: *DIP* demamethasone iontophoresis, *INX* infliximab, *TA* triamcinolone acetonide, *TH* triamcinolide hexacetonide

assessments, among other limitations [50]. In addition, the studies may not have captured one recently identified potential safety event: alterations in the growth potential at the TMJ. Lochbuhler et al. performed IACI in 33 children with JIA, finding impaired mandibular growth following this therapy [51]. A unique aspect of this study was that the investigators performed MRI at the time of the injection to evaluate whether the corticosteroid was administered within or immediately outside the joint space. Those subjects who received successful IA placement of the drug demonstrated decreased grade of inflammation yet more impairment of mandibular growth as compared to those subjects in whom MRI demonstrated extra-articular placement of the corticosteroid. Additionally, 21% of the subjects developed heterotopic bone formation (HBF) in the TMJ, which the authors speculated might have resulted from the CS injections themselves, and higher cumulative corticosteroid doses were associated with increased risk of condylar damage, although the issue of confounding by indication was not addressed. Nevertheless, the possibility that IA therapy could promote HBF was subsequently corroborated by Stoll et al. in their study of 238 subjects who had received IACS therapy, of whom 33 developed this outcome; in this study, multivariable analysis revealed that the total number of injections was associated with increased risk of HBF, while delay from diagnosis of JIA to initial injection was protective [52]. Finally, one additional limitation of the studies evaluating the effectiveness and safety of IACI into the TMJ is that as they were all relatively small, they may not have captured rare but potentially serious short-term SAEs, such as rapid TMJ destruction and ankylosis [53, 54].

Another form of IA therapy that has been proposed is IA infliximab [55, 56]. IA therapy with tumor necrosis factor inhibitors into large joints has shown some effectiveness, e.g. [57, 58], even among patients who have failed IACI [59], and may be equivalent to if not superior than some forms of IA corticosteroids [60–62]. There is a single case report of 8 IA injections of infliximab administered to the TMJ over 36 weeks in an adult patient with psoriatic arthritis who had previously failed therapy with systemic infliximab as well as local IACI [63]. This patient had clinical improvement without radiographic deterioration; MRI was not used as an outcome measure. Unfortunately, studies in children with JIA have not been able to replicate this success [55]. The dose that can be administered into the TMJ of a child may be a limiting factor; the study by Carubbi et al. (2016) demonstrated superiority of TNFi over CS only in large joints [62]. Additionally, the subject selection of

Table 2 Outcome of studies evaluating local therapy for TMJ arthritis

Study	Subjective change	Physical exam change	Imaging change	Safety
Arabshahi et al. [122]	Resolution of pain in 10/13 subjects	MIO increase of 4.8 mm	Improved active findings on MRI in > 67% of TMJs (14 subjects)	Transient Cushing syndrome in 2 subjects
Ringold et al. [106]	Decreased incidence of one or more TMJ symptoms (60% to 28%)	MIO increase of 6.6 mm; decreased incidence of jaw deviation (40% to 16%)	CT: worsening changes in 10, no change in 3, and improvement in 2 subjects	Subcutaneous atrophy in 1 subject, IA calcification in two subjects
Weiss et al. [14]	ND	Improved MIO in 9/16 abnormal at baseline	Decreased MRI findings of active arthritis in 5/6	ND
Parra et al. [123][1]	"Good" response in 80/99 encounters, "Partial" response in 10, and "Poor" response in 9	ND	ND	Skin atrophy in 1 subject
Mino et al. [67]	Resolution of pain in 11/15 (73%) with pain at baseline	Improved MIO of 5 mm among the 18 patients with decreased MIO at baseline	ND	Transient painless erythema in 24/28 (86%); metallic taste in one subject
Habibi et al. [124]	Improved pain in 17/17 subjects and improved chewing dysfunction in 5/7 subjects	Improved jaw deviation in 13/14 subjects	ND	Scar in one subject
Stoll et al. [125]	ND	Increased MIO by 2.7 mm	Of 62 TMJs: 24 improved, 30 stable, 8 worse	One subject each with localized swelling, fever x two weeks, and hypopigmentation
Stoll et al. [56]	ND	No change in MIO	No improvement overall by MRI; resolution of inflammation in six TMJs	No AEs
Olsen-Bergem et al. [64]	Improved pain at rest and with palpation	Increased lateral excursion of 3.7 mm (Triamcinolone group)	ND	ND
Olsen-Bergem et al. [64]	Improved pain at rest and with palpation	Increased lateral excursion of 4.6 mm (arthrocentesis alone group)	ND	ND
Lochbuhler et al. [52][2]	ND	ND	Improved inflammatory grade of MRI	Decreased growth of mandibular ramus
Stoll et al. [55]	ND	No change in MIO	Worsening of active and chronic MRI findings	ND
Stoustrup et al. [126]	Improved short-term pain frequency and intensity	No significant changes in MIO, laterotrusion, or protrusion	ND	ND
Kinard et al. [65]	Decreased pain	Improved MIO	ND	Transient subcutaneous atrophy
Resnick et al. [127]	Decreased pain	Improved MIO of 5.8 mm	Decreased ER of 1.06	ND
Resnick et al. [128]	Resolution of pain in 34/37 (92%)	Improved MIO of 5.0 mm (anatomic) or 5.1 mm (image)	Decreased ER of 1.16 (anatomic) or 0.96 (image)	ND
Antonarakis et al. [66]	TA: Decreased VAS 2.6 L: Decreased VAS 1	TA: Improved MIO of 2.3 mm L: Improved MIO of 1.4 mm	TA: Improved in 18 / 42 TMJs L: Improved in 5/16	ND

[1]Some of the reports reflect children who had more than one round of injections. [2]Intra-articular placement was evaluated with MRI. Those with IA placement demonstrated more robust improvement but more impairment of mandibular growth. *Abbreviations*: *ER* enhancement ratio, *L* lavage alone, *MIO* maximal incisal opening, *ND* not documented, *TA* triamcinolone acetonide, *TMJ* temporomandibular joint

JIA patients refractory to traditional and biologic DMARDs plus IA CS is one that is not ideal for the assessment of the effectiveness of IA infliximab. As subsets of TMJ arthritis patients anecdotally appear to benefit from IA corticosteroids and IA infliximab, both in the short and long terms, it will be valuable to identify the factors associated with likelihood of response to these therapies.

Finally, arthrocentesis and lavage without injection of any therapies may also have anti-inflammatory effects. Olsen-Bergem et al. randomized 17 JIA patients with bilateral TMJ arthritis to receive arthrocentesis alone in one joint, versus arthrocentesis accompanied by triamcinolone hexacetonide (TH) in the other; an additional four subjects presumably with unilateral involvement received TH plus arthrocentesis unilaterally, somewhat compromising the analysis of the study [64]. The authors reported improvement in subjective parameters and objective physical examination findings in both groups compared to baseline, without any evident differences between the two treatment groups. Likewise, Kinard et al. published a case series of three children with JIA who underwent arthroscopy with lavage alone, reporting decreased pain at one-month follow-up in all three [65]. Improvements in MIO of 2 and 5 mm were reported in two subjects; a third had unspecified improvement. Most recently, Antonarakis et al. compared outcomes of children receiving IACI with lavage, lavage alone, and no therapy [66]. There appears to have been non-random assignment to all three groups, and they indicated that some of the children who received IACI to one TMJ may have received lavage in the contralateral joint, thus compromising assessment of change in MIO. They reported improvements in both treatment groups, perhaps more so in the group that also received IACI, but few differences that were statistically significant as compared to the no-treatment group. Thus, the benefit of lavage alone remains an open question. Additionally, despite short-term success of IA therapy in general, long-term benefit of IA therapy remains in question.

Iontophoresis

An alternative method of delivering CS to the TMJ was introduced by Mina et al. [67]. This procedure consists of transdermal application of the drug, which is forced into deeper tissues through application of an electrical current. It has been used sporadically in arthritis [68, 69]. Their results were promising, with improved MIO observed in 19/28 and decreased pain observed in 11/15 with pain at baseline. Factors that may limit widespread application of this technique are that this requires a trained physical therapist to perform, as well as multiple visits to their office. No additional studies of this approach in treating TMJ arthritis have been reported.

Orthodontic (functional) devices

In order to preserve normal facial and jaw growth, mechanical (non-anti-inflammatory) approaches have been used in children with JIA. Functional orthodontic appliances (FOA) are splints that can alter mandibular position by stretching local musculature [70], basically braces for the jaw. Two types of FOA are available,: active treatment and distraction (stabilization) splints [70]. Occlusal stabilization splints are used to help support and balance both TMJs and to prevent further pain and discomfort to the TMJ complex. They can be used in growing as well as in skeletally mature patients. They allow the patient to have even contacts when the teeth occlude in all ranges of motion including biting and side to side jaw movements, which can result in decreased pain [71]. In contrast, active treatment splints are only used in the growing phases of a child, typically ages 8–16 years of age, and are intended to add incremental height to the splint platform on the affected side of the arthritic joint, thus potentially reducing asymmetry and need for surgical correction of skeletal deformity [72]. They can also result in more even distribution of muscular forces within the jaw. Both forms of FOA are fairly unobtrusive cosmetically but effective therapy often requires many years of compliance. The general consensus is that they are optimally used when the disease is well-controlled medically [70], although studies evaluating outcomes of JIA patients with versus without active TMJ arthritis who are treated with FOA have not been performed. As reviewed [7], there are no high-quality prospective studies on their effectiveness. Instead, data are generally limited to one large study of children with impaired jaw shape for a variety of reasons [73] and smaller studies limited to children with JIA [74–76], all of which appear to show modest benefit. A recently published retrospective study of 54 children with JIA who were treated with a FOA for two years demonstrated decreased pain and increased MIO, although there was no comparator group. Data in a rabbit model of induced TMJ arthritis demonstrated that stabilization splints significantly reduced the condylar destruction and bone loss compared to untreated rabbits with TMJ arthritis [77], providing rationale for prospective studies in children with TMJ arthritis. No major safety issues have been raised with these devices [70].

Surgery

Once a child has reached skeletal maturity, surgery is the only means of correcting anatomic abnormalities. The consensus is that surgery is not optimally performed in clinically active TMJs, and is generally postponed until growth is complete [78]. However, if TMJ ankyloses develops, surgical intervention such as arthroplasty, or total prosthetic joint replacement is indicated sooner. Surgical options were reviewed in depth by Norholt et al. [78]. Briefly, two options are available: distraction osteogenesis and orthognathic surgery. The former is a procedure, in which a partial osteotomy is performed in the cortex of the ramus, and slow mechanical forces are created daily increasing the desired length. New bone is slowly generated similar to growth. This technique is commonly used in craniofacial deformities such as Pierre Robin Sequence with airway obstruction [79]. Orthognathic surgery is a common procedure to reconstruct the dento-skeletal deformity with precise masticatory function, and TMJ articulation, usually performed in young adults. This may involve a bilateral sagittal osteotomy of the ramus and/or Lefort 1 of the maxilla for alignment of the masticatory system with proper plane of occlusion to the TMJ [80].

Experimental/future therapies

Several IA therapies have been attempted in animal models of TMJ arthritis, whose future applications to human disease remain uncertain. Most of these studies use a model in which disease is introduced in rats or rabbits through intra-TMJ injection of a compound called Complete Freund's Adjuvant, which consists of heat-killed *Mycobacterium tuberculosis* and induces a robust immunologic response. Two groups evaluated low-level laser therapy (LLLT), showing improved histologic features of inflammation [81, 82]. Human studies of LLLT show that it may have a modest analgesic effect [83]; however, its potential mechanism in arthritis is uncertain, and its clinical effects in patients with rheumatoid arthritis appear modest [84]. Another potential therapy is local injection of hyaluronic acid (HA), which reduced histologic and bony morphometric measures of TMJ inflammation in one rat study [85]. There is extensive clinical experience with HA as a therapeutic agent for osteoarthritis OA, for which there is an FDA-approved indication [86]. There is also limited, although positive, experience with HA therapy in RA [87] and isolated enthesopathies [88]. Finally, one group treated juvenile rabbits with induced TMJ arthritis with IA simvastatin, reporting improved bone surface density, although the extent of inflammation was not assessed [89]. In addition to its cholesterol-lowering effects, statins may also have immunomodulatory properties, as evidenced by in vitro studies showing direct effects on the induction of regulatory T cells [90] and in vivo studies demonstrating modest but statistically significant improved disease scores in a randomized trial of atorvastatin versus placebo in adults with RA [91], and decreased risk of RA among long-term users of statins [92]. The potential role of any of these therapies in the management of TMJ arthritis in children with JIA remains unknown and speculative.

Our approach to refractory or isolated TMJ arthritis in children with JIA

In a child presenting with possible isolated TMJ arthritis, the first step is to distinguish JIA limited to the TMJs from its mimic, idiopathic condylar resorption, alternatively called internal condylar resorption (ICR) [93]. A discussion of the surgical treatment of ICR is beyond the scope of this review, but is available elsewhere [94]. Like any other joint, the TMJ can be the initial or sole manifestation of JIA. Indeed, some children presenting with isolated TMJ arthritis will go on to develop arthritis in other joints or uveitis [95]. Differentiating isolated TMJ arthritis from ICR can be challenging, particularly in light of the data summarized above showing that non-arthritic children can have some degree of joint fluid or enhancement, so the presence of these findings, if mild, is not necessarily diagnostic of arthritis. Marked inflammatory changes, such as synovial thickening, appear to be rare in ICR [96], so when present, may suggest JIA. Erosive condylar changes may also help distinguish between the presence of ICR and JIA [22, 97]. In addition, while disc displacement in common in ICR, significant damage to the disc is rare [98]. Finally, unilateral involvement may also suggest JIA over ICR [99, 100], although this has not been established.

A vexing scenario for the pediatric rheumatologist is a child with isolated TMJ arthritis, either at onset or following successful systemic therapy of the remainder of the joints [7]. The management will depend on a variety of factors, including extent of active arthritis and arthritic sequelae on imaging, presence of symptoms or exam findings associated with TMJ arthritis, and availability of corticosteroid preparations. (At the time of this writing, TH, which is the optimal corticosteroid preparation for IA therapy in JIA [101], is not available anywhere in the United States). A flow diagram is shown in Fig. 4.

Children with JIA and completely normal findings on the MRI of the TMJ generally do not warrant further investigations unless signs or symptoms of TMJ arthritis develop. In children with JIA who are old enough to cooperate with the exam, we will typically follow MIO measurements (measured with disposable TheraBite scales, Atos Medical, New Berlin, WI), longitudinally. Unless very low, a single measurement has little prognostic value due to the wide range of measurements in healthy children [102]. However, decreased MIO is likely to indicate TMJ arthritis, as is development of facial asymmetry and other signs or symptoms discussed above. Importantly, the smallest detectable difference in MIO was reported to be just under 0.5 cm [103], so changes of a lesser magnitude may not be clinically

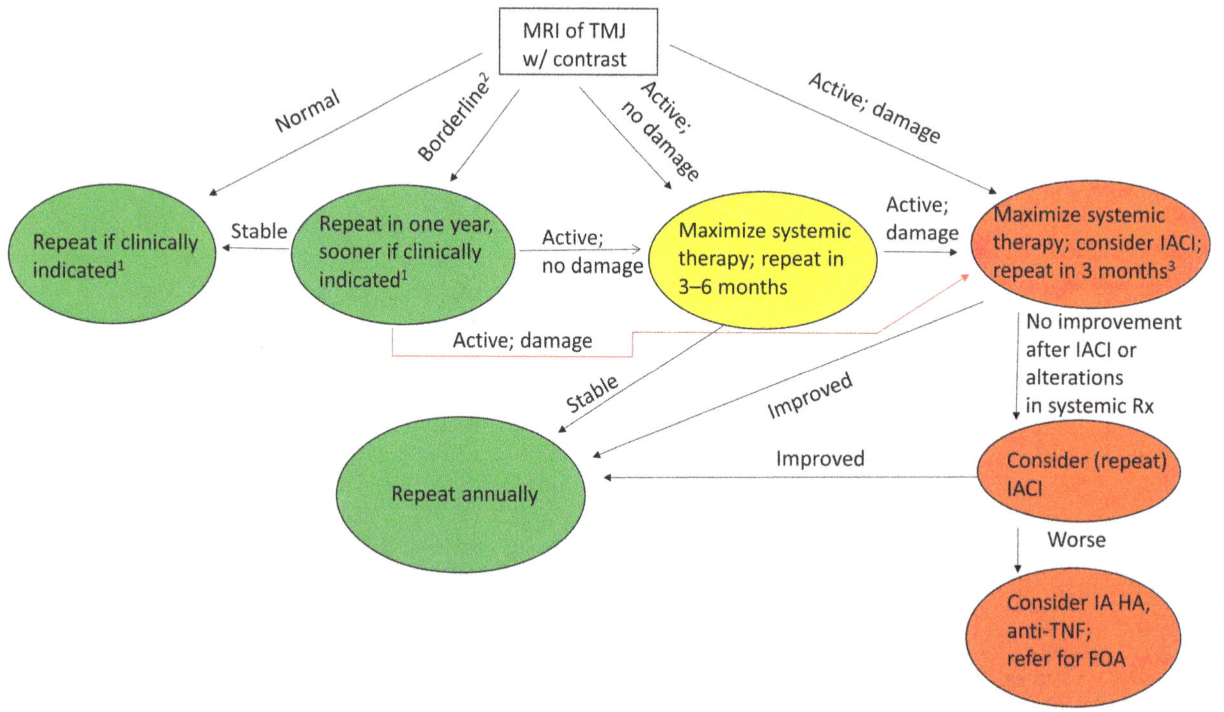

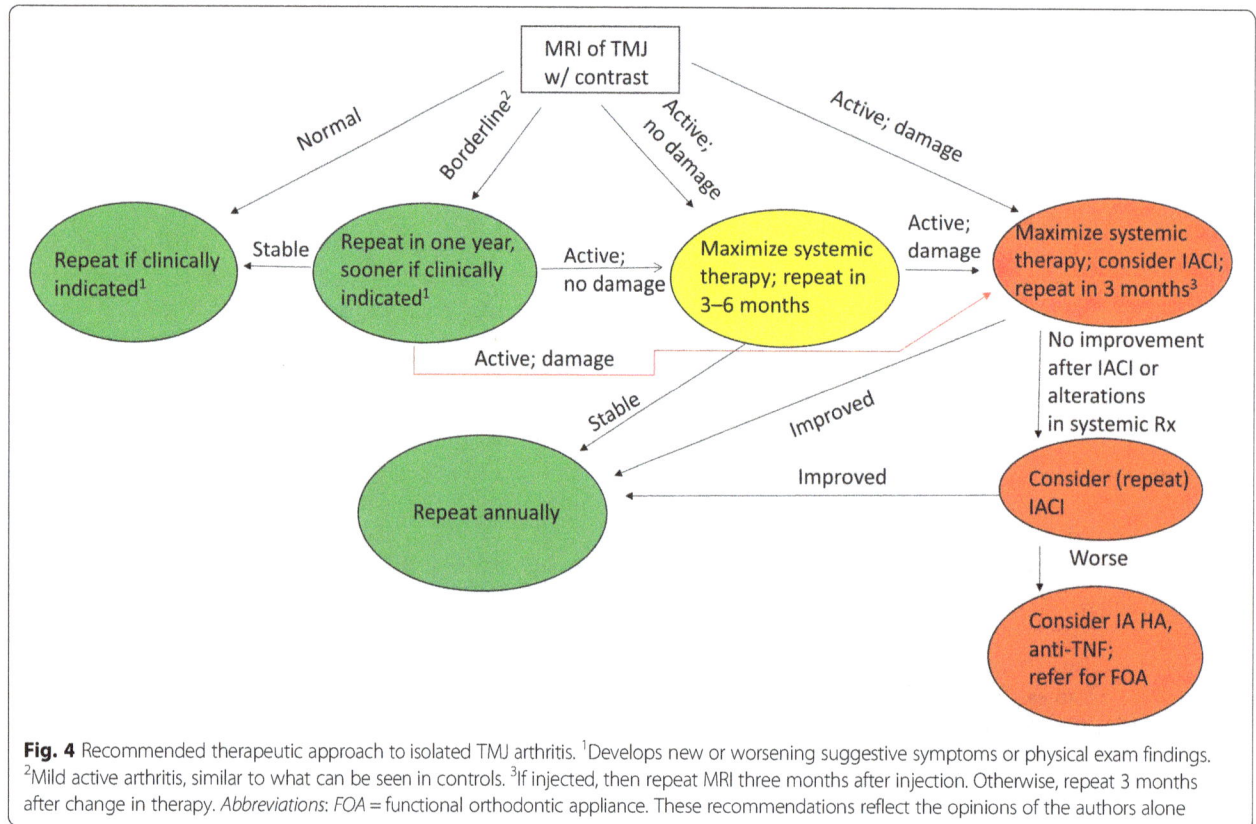

Fig. 4 Recommended therapeutic approach to isolated TMJ arthritis. [1]Develops new or worsening suggestive symptoms or physical exam findings. [2]Mild active arthritis, similar to what can be seen in controls. [3]If injected, then repeat MRI three months after injection. Otherwise, repeat 3 months after change in therapy. *Abbreviations*: *FOA* = functional orthodontic appliance. These recommendations reflect the opinions of the authors alone

significant. Recently, recommendations for monitoring TMJ involvement in JIA were published [16].

In children with mild findings of active arthritis, e.g. effusions or areas of enhancement < 1.5 mm with or without mild bone marrow edema, we recommend repeating the MRI within one year, as these can be normal findings. These mild changes can be observed in non-arthritic pediatric subjects [33], but this does not necessarily mean that it is a negative study. As discussed above, cross-sectional studies using plain radiography clearly demonstrate TMJ changes in at least 40% of JIA patients [42], so the pre-test probability of TMJ arthritis is considerably higher in a JIA patient than in a non-arthritic control. If the findings do not progress over one year, then subsequent imaging studies may not be required.

Children with fairly extensive active findings clearly have TMJ arthritis associated with JIA. However, in light of the recently recognized risks associated with IACI in the TMJ on long-term growth of the joint, as well as risks of HBF, optimal management is uncertain. Such children should have their systemic therapy optimized, e.g., addition of a conventional or biologic DMARD or change in dose; specifically, uses of weekly adalimumab or infliximab at doses upwards of 10 mg/kg/dose have been reported as safe and effective in children with JIA [104, 105], and it may be reasonable to consider to consider switching biologics in some cases. Furthermore, these children should be followed closely for development of TMJ damage as evidenced by MRI and MIO, as well as assessments of dentofacial growth and development of asymmetry. If the arthritis is asymptomatic and is not damaging the joint, then adjustment of the systemic therapies and careful monitoring may be all that is required. However, if the TMJ arthritis is causing significant damage to the joint, e.g., bony erosions or disk displacement, then local therapy in addition to adjustment of systemic therapies may be recommended. It bears emphasis that while mild active changes can be seen in non-arthritic children, significant arthritic sequelae continue to be specific for arthritis, and the presence of such in the context of large areas of enhancement or thickened synovium therefore represent unopposed arthritis and undoubtedly place the child at risk of structural and functional damage. If these steps are not successful, we would not recommend performing more than two IACI into the same TMJ, as children who do not respond to an initial injection generally do not respond well to subsequent injections either [106]. If the arthritis is progressing despite these measures, then alternative albeit somewhat experimental approaches such as injection with a TNFi or HA, or even lavage alone, may be warranted. In addition, orthodontic approaches may be of value in maintaining appropriate jaw growth [71, 74, 107].

For management of TMJ arthritis, as with management of JIA as a whole, there is no clear guidance from the literature as to when therapies may be discontinued. Use of S100 proteins have been studied as a predictive tool among children discontinuing TNFi therapy [108], but these markers are not available for clinical purposes in the United States, nor is there any specific data with respect to their use in the TMJ. We would recommend that all other aspects of the disease (arthritis in other joints, uveitis, systemic symptoms, etc) should be in remission [109] for at least 12–24 months [110], although there is mixed data as to whether prolonged periods of remission increase success of drug withdrawal [111–114]. Then, if MRI with contrast reveals no active findings in the TMJ, one may consider tapering systemic therapy.

Finally, monitoring TMJ arthritis by contrast MRI has been questioned in terms of safety. In 2017, the Food and Drug Administration issued a statement calling into question the safety of gadolinium-based contrast agents (GBCAs; https://www.fda.gov/Safety/MedWatch/SafetyInformation/SafetyAlertsforHumanMedicalProducts/ucm559709.htm). This recommendation is based upon findings of retention of GBCAs in the brain and possibly other tissues following repeat studies [115]. It bears emphasis, however, that there no clear clinical symptoms associated with this deposition, and GBCAs have been safely used in millions of patients with normal renal function [116], and a revised statement released by the FDA in December of 2017 concluded that while we should minimize closely-spaced repeat contrast MRIs, we should not avoid or defer necessary scans (https://www.fda.gov/Safety/MedWatch/SafetyInformation/SafetyAlertsforHumanMedicalProducts/ucm589580.htm). It is advisable when possible to use macrocyclic rather than linear GBCAs, as the former result in decreased deposition [117, 118].

The issue of retention of GBCAs is unrelated to long-recognized safety issue with GBCAs: the risk of nephrogenic systemic fibrosis in patients with renal insufficiency [119]. In these patients, the risks and benefits of a contrast MRI must be weighed very carefully, and our general recommendations above do not apply to them.

Conclusion

Once dubbed the "forgotten joint" [120], there has been an explosion of scholarship in recent years focusing on the diagnosis and management of TMJ arthritis. Yet, the more we learn about this joint, the less we really know about it. There is no doubt that TMJ arthritis is a frequent complication of JIA, and that if untreated, can have devastating effects on the form and function of the joint, jaw, and midface. While distinguishing between normal findings and mild arthritis can be challenging, significant TMJ arthritis resulting in joint damage can still occur, even early in the disease course [14]. Modern therapies have revolutionized the treatment of JIA as a whole [121], but the TMJ appears to have lagged behind [6]. Thus, IA therapy may remain the best option for some children. While we do not discount recent scholarship indicating the IACI may adversely impact the growth of the jaw [51], nor do we discount four decades of scholarship indicating that unopposed arthritis is harmful [42], and to date, corticosteroids are the only local therapy that have clearly shown to be of benefit in the management of TMJ arthritis. Future prospective research is indicated to evaluate alternative local approaches, as well as to understand the natural course among children with active inflammation, so that we can predict which children are likely to develop significant damage among those with active disease.

Abbreviations

CBCT: Cone beam computed tomography; CE: Contrast enhancement; CT: Computed tomography; ER: Enhancement ratio; FOA: Functional orthodontic appliance; GBCA: Gadolinium-based contrast agent; HA: Hyaluronic acid; HBF: Heterotopic bone formation; IACI: Intraarticular corticosteroid injection; ICR: Internal condylar resorption; JIA: Juvenile idiopathic arthritis; LLLT: Low-level laser therapy; MIO: Maximal incisal opening; SI: Signal intensity; TH: Triamcinolone hexacetonide; TMJ: Temporomandibular joint; US: Ultrasound

Authors' contributions

All authors contributed to the writing of this manuscript and approved the final version.

Competing interests

The authors declare that they have no competing interests.

Author details

[1]Department of Pediatrics, University of Alabama at Birmingham (UAB), 1600 7th Avenue South, Children's Park Place North Suite G10, Birmingham 35233, AL, USA. [2]Department of Orthodontics, UAB, 1720 2nd Avenue South, School of Dentistry Building 305, Birmingham 35294, AL, USA. [3]Department of Oral and Maxillofacial Surgery, UAB, 1720 2nd Avenue South, School of Dentistry Building 419, Birmingham 35294, AL, USA.

References

1. Abdul-Aziez OA, et al. Serum S100A12 and temporomandibular joint magnetic resonance imaging in juvenile idiopathic arthritis Egyptian patients: a case control study. Pak J Biol Sci. 2010;13(3):101–13.
2. Abramowicz S, et al. Magnetic resonance imaging of temporomandibular joints in children with arthritis. J Oral Maxillofac Surg. 2011;69(9):2321–8.
3. Argyropoulou MI, et al. Temporomandibular joint involvement in juvenile idiopathic arthritis: clinical predictors of magnetic resonance imaging signs. Eur Radiol. 2009;19(3):693–700.
4. Cannizzaro E, et al. Temporomandibular joint involvement in children with juvenile idiopathic arthritis. J Rheumatol. 2011;38(3):510–5.
5. Cedstromer AL, et al. Temporomandibular condylar alterations in juvenile idiopathic arthritis most common in longitudinally severe disease despite medical treatment. Pediatr Rheumatol Online J. 2014;12:43.

6. Stoll ML, et al. Risk factors for temporomandibular joint arthritis in children with juvenile idiopathic arthritis. J Rheumatol. 2012;39(9):1880–7.
7. Stoll ML, Cron RQ. Temporomandibular joint arthritis in juvenile idiopathic arthritis: the last frontier. Int J Clin Rheumatol. 2015;10:273–86.
8. Hsieh YJ, et al. Facial morphology in children and adolescents with juvenile idiopathic arthritis and moderate to severe temporomandibular joint involvement. Am J Orthod Dentofac Orthop. 2016;149(2):182–91.
9. Ringold S, Cron RQ. The temporomandibular joint in juvenile idiopathic arthritis: frequently used and frequently arthritic. Pediatr Rheumatol Online J. 2009;7:11.
10. Hammer MR, Kanaan Y. Imaging of the pediatric temporomandibular joint. Oral Maxillofac Surg Clin North Am. 2018;30(1):25–34.
11. Niibo P, et al. Contemporary management of TMJ involvement in JIA patients and its orofacial consequences. EPMA J. 2016;7:12.
12. Park JT, et al. Realization of masticatory movement by 3-dimensional simulation of the temporomandibular joint and the masticatory muscles. J Craniofac Surg. 2013;24(4):e347–51.
13. Okeson JP. Critical commentary 1: evaluation of the research diagnostic criteria for temporomandibular disorders for the recognition of an anterior disc displacement with reduction. J Orofac Pain. 2009;23(4):312–5. author reply 323-4
14. Weiss PF, et al. High prevalence of temporomandibular joint arthritis at disease onset in children with juvenile idiopathic arthritis, as detected by magnetic resonance imaging but not by ultrasound. Arthritis Rheum. 2008;58(4):1189–96.
15. Demant S, et al. 3D analysis of facial asymmetry in subjects with juvenile idiopathic arthritis. Rheumatology (Oxford). 2011;50(3):586–92.
16. Stoustrup P, et al. Clinical orofacial examination in juvenile idiopathic arthritis: international consensus-based recommendations for monitoring patients in clinical practice and research studies. J Rheumatol. 2017;44(3):326–33.
17. Koos B, et al. Reliability of clinical symptoms in diagnosing temporomandibular joint arthritis in juvenile idiopathic arthritis. J Rheumatol. 2014;41(9):1871–7.
18. Muller L, et al. Early diagnosis of temporomandibular joint involvement in juvenile idiopathic arthritis: a pilot study comparing clinical examination and ultrasound to magnetic resonance imaging. Rheumatology (Oxford). 2009;48(6):680–5.
19. Abramowicz S, et al. Physical findings associated with active temporomandibular joint inflammation in children with juvenile idiopathic arthritis. J Oral Maxillofac Surg. 2013;71(10):1683–7.
20. Kristensen KD, et al. Clinical predictors of temporomandibular joint arthritis in juvenile idiopathic arthritis: a systematic literature review. Semin Arthritis Rheum. 2016;45(6):717–32.
21. da Motta AT, et al. Superimposition of 3D cone-beam CT models in orthognathic surgery. Dental Press J Orthod. 2010;15(2):39–41.
22. Al-Shwaikh H, et al. Radiologic features of temporomandibular joint osseous structures in children with juvenile idiopathic arthritis. Cone beam computed tomography study. Stomatologija. 2016;18(2):51–60.
23. Kirkhus E, et al. Temporomandibular joint involvement in childhood arthritis: comparison of ultrasonography-assessed capsular width and MRI-assessed synovitis. Dentomaxillofac Radiol. 2016;45(8):20160195.
24. Assaf AT, et al. Is high-resolution ultrasonography suitable for the detection of temporomandibular joint involvement in children with juvenile idiopathic arthritis? Dentomaxillofac Radiol. 2013;42(3):20110379.
25. Jank S, et al. Sonographic investigation of the temporomandibular joint in patients with juvenile idiopathic arthritis: a pilot study. Arthritis Rheum. 2007;57(2):213–8.
26. Melchiorre D, et al. Sonographic evaluation of the temporomandibular joints in juvenile idiopathic arthritis(). J Ultrasound. 2010;13(1):34–7.
27. Hechler BL, et al. Ultrasound versus magnetic resonance imaging of the temporomandibular joint in juvenile idiopathic arthritis: a systematic review. Int J Oral Maxillofac Surg. 2018;47(1):83–9.
28. Kellenberger CJ, Arvidsson LZ, Larheim TA. Magnetic resonance imaging of temporomandibular joints in juvenile idiopathic arthritis. Semin Orthod. 2015;21(2):111–20.
29. Tzaribachev N, Fritz J, Horger M. Spectrum of magnetic resonance imaging appearances of juvenile temporomandibular joints (TMJ) in non-rheumatic children. Acta Radiol. 2009;50(10):1182–6.
30. von Kalle T, Winkler P, Stuber T. Contrast-enhanced MRI of normal temporomandibular joints in children–is there enhancement or not? Rheumatology (Oxford). 2013;52(2):363–7.
31. Kottke R, et al. Contrast-enhanced MRI of the temporomandibular joint: findings in children without juvenile idiopathic arthritis. Acta Radiol. 2015;56(9):1145–52.
32. Angenete OW, et al. Normal magnetic resonance appearances of the temporomandibular joints in children and young adults aged 2-18 years. Pediatr Radiol. 2017;
33. Stoll ML, et al. Defining the normal appearance of the temporomandibular joints by magnetic resonance imaging with contrast: a comparative study of children with and without juvenile idiopathic arthritis. Pediatr Rheumatol Online J. 2018;16(1):8.
34. Kellenberger CJ, et al. Temporomandibular joint atlas for detection and grading of juvenile idiopathic arthritis involvement by magnetic resonance imaging. Pediatr Radiol. 2017;
35. Peacock ZS, et al. Quantifying synovial enhancement of the pediatric temporomandibular joint. J Oral Maxillofac Surg. 2016;74(10):1937–45.
36. Resnick CM, et al. Quantifying temporomandibular joint synovitis in children with juvenile idiopathic arthritis. Arthritis Care Res (Hoboken). 2016;68(12):1795–802.
37. Caruso P, et al. Optimization of quantitative dynamic Postgadolinium MRI technique using normalized ratios for the evaluation of temporomandibular joint synovitis in patients with juvenile idiopathic arthritis. AJNR Am J Neuroradiol. 2017;38(12):2344–50.
38. Ma GM, et al. MRI thresholds for discrimination between normal and mild temporomandibular joint involvement in juvenile idiopathic arthritis. Pediatr Rheumatol Online J. 2015;13:53.
39. Inarejos Clemente EJ, et al. Qualitative and semi-quantitative assessment of temporomandibular joint MRI protocols for juvenile idiopathic arthritis at 1.5 and 3.0T. Eur J Radiol. 2018;98:90–9.
40. Tolend MA, et al. Towards establishing a standardized magnetic resonance imaging scoring system for temporomandibular joints in juvenile idiopathic arthritis. Arthritis Care Res (Hoboken). 2017;
41. Arvidsson LZ, Flato B, Larheim TA. Radiographic TMJ abnormalities in patients with juvenile idiopathic arthritis followed for 27 years. Oral Surg Oral Med Oral Pathol Oral Radiol Endod. 2009;108(1):114–23.
42. Larheim TA, et al. The temporomandibular joint in juvenile rheumatoid arthritis. Radiographic changes related to clinical and laboratory parameters in 100 children. Scand J Rheumatol. 1982;11(1):5–12.
43. Bakke M, et al. Orofacial pain, jaw function, and temporomandibular disorders in women with a history of juvenile chronic arthritis or persistent juvenile chronic arthritis. Oral Surg Oral Med Oral Pathol Oral Radiol Endod. 2001;92(4):406–14.
44. Kvien TK, et al. Radiographic temporomandibular joint abnormalities in patients with juvenile chronic arthritis during a controlled study of sodium aurothiomalate and D-penicillamine. Br J Rheumatol. 1986;25(1):59–66.
45. Caso F, et al. Pharmacological treatment of spondyloarthritis: exploring the effectiveness of nonsteroidal anti-inflammatory drugs, traditional disease-modifying antirheumatic drugs and biological therapies. Ther Adv Chronic Dis. 2015;6(6):328–38.
46. Ai R, et al. Joint-specific DNA methylation and transcriptome signatures in rheumatoid arthritis identify distinct pathogenic processes. Nat Commun. 2016;7:11849.
47. Twilt M, et al. Long-term followup of temporomandibular joint involvement in juvenile idiopathic arthritis. Arthritis Rheum. 2008;59(4):546–52.
48. Ince DO, Ince A, Moore TL. Effect of methotrexate on the temporomandibular joint and facial morphology in juvenile rheumatoid arthritis patients. Am J Orthod Dentofac Orthop. 2000;118(1):75–83.
49. Stoll ML, Cron RQ, Saurenmann RK. Systemic and intra-articular anti-inflammatory therapy of temporomandibular joint arthritis in children with juvenile idiopathic arthritis. Semin Orthod. 2015;21(2):125–33.
50. Stoustrup P, et al. Intra-articular steroid injection for temporomandibular joint arthritis in juvenile idiopathic arthritis: a systematic review on efficacy and safety. Semin Arthritis Rheum. 2013;43(1):63–70.
51. Lochbuhler N, et al. Magnetic resonance imaging assessment of temporomandibular joint involvement and mandibular growth following corticosteroid injection in juvenile idiopathic arthritis. J Rheumatol. 2015;42(8):1514–22.
52. Stoll ML, Amin D, Poholek CH, Harvey RJ, Young D, Cron RQ, and Waite PD. Risk factors for heterotopic bone of the temporomandibular joint in children with chronic arthritis treated with intraarticular therapy. J Rheumatology. https://doi.org/10.3899/jrheum.171306.

53. Schindler C, et al. Severe temporomandibular dysfunction and joint destruction after intra-articular injection of triamcinolone. J Oral Pathol Med. 2005;34(3):184–6.
54. Aggarwal S, Kumar A. A cortisone-wrecked and bony ankylosed temporomandibular joint. Plast Reconstr Surg. 1989;83(6):1084–5.
55. Stoll ML, et al. Magnetic resonance imaging findings following intraarticular infliximab therapy for refractory temporomandibular joint arthritis among children with juvenile idiopathic arthritis. J Rheumatol. 2015;42(11):2155–9.
56. Stoll ML, et al. Safety and efficacy of intra-articular infliximab therapy for treatment-resistant temporomandibular joint arthritis in children: a retrospective study. Rheumatology (Oxford). 2013;52(3):554–9.
57. Nikas SN, et al. Treatment of resistant rheumatoid arthritis by intra-articular infliximab injections: a pilot study. Ann Rheum Dis. 2004;63(1):102–3.
58. Fiocco U, et al. Synovial effusion and synovial fluid biomarkers in psoriatic arthritis to assess intraarticular tumor necrosis factor-alpha blockade in the knee joint. Arthritis Res Ther. 2010;12(4):R148.
59. Conti F, et al. Intra-articular infliximab in patients with rheumatoid arthritis and psoriatic arthritis with monoarthritis resistant to local glucocorticoids. Clinical efficacy extended to patients on systemic anti-tumour necrosis factor. alpha Ann Rheum Dis. 2008;67(12):1787–90.
60. Liang. D.F., et al., *[A randomized, single-blind, parallel, controlled clinical study on single intra-articular injection of etanercept in treatment of inflammatory knee arthritis]*. Zhonghua Nei Ke Za Zhi. 2010;49(11):930–4.
61. Bliddal H, et al. A randomized, controlled study of a single intra-articular injection of etanercept or glucocorticosteroids in patients with rheumatoid arthritis. Scand J Rheumatol. 2006;35(5):341–5.
62. Carubbi F, et al. Safety and efficacy of intra-articular anti-tumor necrosis factor alpha agents compared to corticosteroids in a treat-to-target strategy in patients with inflammatory arthritis and monoarthritis flare. Int J Immunopathol Pharmacol. 2016;29(2):252–66.
63. Alstergren P, Larsson PT, Kopp S. Successful treatment with multiple intra-articular injections of infliximab in a patient with psoriatic arthritis. Scand J Rheumatol. 2008;37(2):155–7.
64. Olsen-Bergem H, Bjornland T. A cohort study of patients with juvenile idiopathic arthritis and arthritis of the temporomandibular joint: outcome of arthrocentesis with and without the use of steroids. Int J Oral Maxillofac Surg. 2014;43(8):990–5.
65. Kinard BE, et al. Arthroscopy of the temporomandibular joint in patients with juvenile idiopathic arthritis. J Oral Maxillofac Surg. 2016;74(7):1330–5.
66. Antonarakis GS, et al. Benefit of temporomandibular joint lavage with intra-articular steroids versus lavage alone in the Management of Temporomandibular Joint Involvement in juvenile idiopathic arthritis. J Oral Maxillofac Surg. 2018; in press.
67. Mina R, et al. Effectiveness of dexamethasone iontophoresis for temporomandibular joint involvement in juvenile idiopathic arthritis. Arthritis Care Res (Hoboken). 2011;63(11):1511–6.
68. Li LC, et al. The efficacy of dexamethasone iontophoresis for the treatment of rheumatoid arthritic knees: a pilot study. Arthritis Care Res. 1996;9(2):126–32.
69. Ozgocmen S, et al. Glucocorticoid iontophoresis for Achilles tendon enthesitis in ankylosing spondylitis: significant response documented by power Doppler ultrasound. Rheumatol Int. 2005;25(2):158–60.
70. Pedersen TK, Carlaberta B. Functional and orthopedic treatment in developing dentofacial growth deviation in juvenile idiopathic arthritis. Semin Orthod. 2015;21(2):134–9.
71. Stoustrup P, et al. Management of temporomandibular joint arthritis-related orofacial symptoms in juvenile idiopathic arthritis by the use of a stabilization splint. Scand J Rheumatol. 2014;43(2):137–45.
72. Stoustrup P, et al. Orthopaedic splint treatment can reduce mandibular asymmetry caused by unilateral temporomandibular involvement in juvenile idiopathic arthritis. Eur J Orthod. 2013;35(2):191–8.
73. Tulloch JF, et al. The effect of early intervention on skeletal pattern in class II malocclusion: a randomized clinical trial. Am J Orthod Dentofac Orthop. 1997;111(4):391–400.
74. Portelli M, et al. Temporomandibular joint involvement in a cohort of patients with juvenile Idiopatic arthritis and evaluation of the effect induced by functional orthodontic appliance: clinical and radiographic investigation. Eur J Paediatr Dent. 2014;15(1):63–6.
75. Kjellberg H, Kiliaridis S, Thilander B. Dentofacial growth in orthodontically treated and untreated children with juvenile chronic arthritis (JCA). A comparison with angle class II division 1 subjects. Eur J Orthod. 1995;17(5):357–73.
76. Farronato G, et al. Craniofacial growth in children affected by juvenile idiopathic arthritis involving the temporomandibular joint: functional therapy management. J Clin Pediatr Dent. 2009;33(4):351–7.
77. von Bremen J, et al. Histologic effects of mandibular protrusion splints in antigen-induced TMJ arthritis in rabbits. Pediatr Rheumatol Online J. 2017;15(1):27.
78. Norholt SE, Bjornland E, Pedersen TK. Jaw surgery for correction of dentofacial anomalies caused by JIA. Semin Orthod. 2015;21(2):140–7.
79. Sahoo NK, et al. Distraction osteogenesis for Management of Severe OSA in Pierre Robin sequence: an approach to elude tracheostomy in infants. J Maxillofac Oral Surg. 2016;15(4):501–5.
80. Resnick CM. Temporomandibular joint reconstruction in the growing child. Oral Maxillofac Surg Clin North Am. 2018;30(1):109–21.
81. Khozeimeh F, et al. Comparative evaluation of low-level laser and systemic steroid therapy in adjuvant-enhanced arthritis of rat temporomandibular joint: a histological study. Dent Res J (Isfahan). 2015;12(3):215–23.
82. Lemos GA, et al. Low-level laser therapy stimulates tissue repair and reduces the extracellular matrix degradation in rats with induced arthritis in the temporomandibular joint. Lasers Med Sci. 2016;31(6):1051–9.
83. Cotler HB, et al. The use of low level laser therapy (LLLT) for musculoskeletal pain. MOJ Orthop Rheumatol. 2015;2(5)
84. Meireles SM, et al. Assessment of the effectiveness of low-level laser therapy on the hands of patients with rheumatoid arthritis: a randomized double-blind controlled trial. Clin Rheumatol. 2010;29(5):501–9.
85. Lemos GA, et al. Effects of high molecular weight hyaluronic acid on induced arthritis of the temporomandibular joint in rats. Acta Histochem. 2015;117(6):566–75.
86. Strand V, Lim S, Takamura J. Evidence for safety of retreatment with a single intra-articular injection of Gel-200 for treatment of osteoarthritis of the knee from the double-blind pivotal and open-label retreatment clinical trials. BMC Musculoskelet Disord. 2016;17:240.
87. Goto M, et al. Intra-articular injection of hyaluronate (SI-6601D) improves joint pain and synovial fluid prostaglandin E2 levels in rheumatoid arthritis: a multicenter clinical trial. Clin Exp Rheumatol. 2001;19(4):377–83.
88. Kumai T, et al. The short-term effect after a single injection of high-molecular-weight hyaluronic acid in patients with enthesopathies (lateral epicondylitis, patellar tendinopathy, insertional Achilles tendinopathy, and plantar fasciitis): a preliminary study. J Orthop Sci. 2014;19(4):603–11.
89. Holwegner C, et al. Impact of local steroid or statin treatment of experimental temporomandibular joint arthritis on bone growth in young rats. Am J Orthod Dentofac Orthop. 2015;147(1):80–8.
90. Forero-Pena DA, Gutierrez FR. Statins as modulators of regulatory T-cell biology. Mediat Inflamm. 2013;2013:167086.
91. McCarey DW, et al. Trial of atorvastatin in rheumatoid arthritis (TARA): double-blind, randomised placebo-controlled trial. Lancet. 2004;363(9426): 2015–21.
92. Tascilar K, et al. Statins and risk of rheumatoid arthritis - a nested case-control study. Arthritis Rheumatol. 2016;
93. Sarver DM, Janyavula S, Cron RQ. Condylar degeneration and diseases – local and systemic etiologies. Semin Orthod. 2013;19:89–96.
94. Bodine TP, et al. Surgical treatment of adolescent internal condylar resorption (AICR) with articular disc repositioning and orthognathic surgery in the growing patient–a pilot study. Prog Orthod. 2016;17:2.
95. Hugle B, et al. Isolated arthritis of the temporomandibular joint as the initial manifestation of juvenile idiopathic arthritis. J Rheumatol. 2017; 44(11):1632–5.
96. Young A. Idiopathic condylar resorption: the current understanding in diagnosis and treatment. J Indian Prosthodont Soc. 2017;17(2):128–35.
97. Sansare K, et al. Management-related outcomes and radiographic findings of idiopathic condylar resorption: a systematic review. Int J Oral Maxillofac Surg. 2015;44(2):209–16.
98. Wolford LM, Goncalves JR. Condylar resorption of the temporomandibular joint: how do we treat it? Oral Maxillofac Surg Clin North Am. 2015;27(1):47–67.
99. Abramowicz S, et al. Juvenile arthritis: current concepts in terminology, etiopathogenesis, diagnosis, and management. Int J Oral Maxillofac Surg. 2016;45(7):801–12.
100. Wolford LM, Galiano A. Adolescent internal condylar resorption (AICR) of the temporomandibular joint, part 1: a review for diagnosis and treatment considerations. Cranio. 2017:1–10.

101. Zulian F, et al. Triamcinolone acetonide and hexacetonide intra-articular treatment of symmetrical joints in juvenile idiopathic arthritis: a double-blind trial. Rheumatology (Oxford). 2004;43(10):1288–91.
102. Muller L, et al. Maximal mouth opening capacity: percentiles for healthy children 4-17 years of age. Pediatr Rheumatol Online J. 2013;11:17.
103. Stoustrup P, et al. Smallest detectable differences in clinical functional temporomandibular joint examination variables in juvenile idiopathic arthritis. Orthod Craniofac Res. 2013;16(3):137–45.
104. Trachana M, et al. Safety and efficacy of adalimumab treatment in Greek children with juvenile idiopathic arthritis. Scand J Rheumatol. 2011;40(2):101–7.
105. Tambralli A, et al. High doses of infliximab in the management of juvenile idiopathic arthritis. J Rheumatol. 2013;40(10):1749–55.
106. Ringold S, et al. Intraarticular corticosteroid injections of the temporomandibular joint in juvenile idiopathic arthritis. J Rheumatol. 2008;35(6):1157–64.
107. Isola G, et al. The effect of a functional appliance in the management of temporomandibular joint disorders in patients with juvenile idiopathic arthritis. Minerva Stomatol. 2017;66(1):1–8.
108. Gerss J, et al. Phagocyte-specific S100 proteins and high-sensitivity C reactive protein as biomarkers for a risk-adapted treatment to maintain remission in juvenile idiopathic arthritis: a comparative study. Ann Rheum Dis. 2012;71(12):1991–7.
109. Wallace CA, Ruperto N, Giannini E. Preliminary criteria for clinical remission for select categories of juvenile idiopathic arthritis. J Rheumatol. 2004;31(11):2290–4.
110. Broughton T, Armon K. Defining juvenile idiopathic arthritis remission and optimum time for disease-modifying anti-rheumatic drug withdrawal: why we need a consensus. Paediatr Drugs. 2012;14(1):7–12.
111. Chang CY, Meyer RM, Reiff AO. Impact of medication withdrawal method on flare-free survival in patients with juvenile idiopathic arthritis on combination therapy. Arthritis Care Res (Hoboken). 2015;67(5):658–66.
112. Foell D, et al. Methotrexate withdrawal at 6 vs 12 months in juvenile idiopathic arthritis in remission: a randomized clinical trial. JAMA. 2010;303(13):1266–73.
113. Baszis K, et al. Clinical outcomes after withdrawal of anti-tumor necrosis factor alpha therapy in patients with juvenile idiopathic arthritis: a twelve-year experience. Arthritis Rheum. 2011;63(10):3163–8.
114. Simonini G, et al. Flares after withdrawal of biologic therapies in juvenile idiopathic arthritis: clinical and laboratory correlates of remission duration. Arthritis Care Res (Hoboken). 2017;
115. Kahn J, et al. Is there long-term signal intensity increase in the central nervous system on T1-weighted images after MR imaging with the Hepatospecific contrast agent Gadoxetic acid? A cross-sectional study in 91 patients. Radiology. 2017;282(3):708–16.
116. Tedeschi E, et al. Gadolinium retention in the body: what we know and what we can do. Radiol Med. 2017;122(8):589–600.
117. Wang YX, et al. Total gadolinium tissue deposition and skin structural findings following the administration of structurally different gadolinium chelates in healthy and ovariectomized female rats. Quant Imaging Med Surg. 2015;5(4):534–45.
118. Frenzel T, et al. Quantification and assessment of the chemical form of residual gadolinium in the brain after repeated Administration of Gadolinium-Based Contrast Agents: comparative study in rats. Investig Radiol. 2017;52(7):396–404.
119. Schlaudecker JD, Bernheisel CR. Gadolinium-associated nephrogenic systemic fibrosis. Am Fam Physician. 2009;80(7):711–4.
120. Arabshahi B, Cron RQ. Temporomandibular joint arthritis in juvenile idiopathic arthritis: the forgotten joint. Curr Opin Rheumatol. 2006;18(5):490–5.
121. Stoll ML, Cron RQ. Treatment of juvenile idiopathic arthritis: a revolution in care. Pediatr Rheumatol Online J. 2014;12:13.
122. Arabshahi B, et al. Utility of corticosteroid injection for temporomandibular arthritis in children with juvenile idiopathic arthritis. Arthritis Rheum. 2005;52(11):3563–9.
123. Parra DA, et al. Use and accuracy of US guidance for image-guided injections of the temporomandibular joints in children with arthritis. Pediatr Radiol. 2010;40(9):1498–504.
124. Habibi S, et al. Safety and efficacy of US-guided CS injection into temporomandibular joints in children with active JIA. Rheumatology (Oxford). 2012;51(5):874–7.
125. Stoll ML, et al. Intra-articular corticosteroid injections to the temporomandibular joints are safe and appear to be effective therapy in children with juvenile idiopathic arthritis. J Oral Maxillofac Surg. 2012;70(8):1802–7.
126. Stoustrup P, et al. Temporomandibular joint steroid injections in patients with juvenile idiopathic arthritis: an observational pilot study on the long-term effect on signs and symptoms. Pediatr Rheumatol Online J. 2015;13:62.
127. Resnick CM, et al. Quantifying the effect of temporomandibular joint intra-articular steroid injection on synovial enhancement in juvenile idiopathic arthritis. J Oral Maxillofac Surg. 2016;74(12):2363–9.
128. Resnick CM, et al. Is intra-articular steroid injection to the temporomandibular joint for juvenile idiopathic arthritis more effective and efficient when performed with image guidance? J Oral Maxillofac Surg. 2017;75(4):694–700.

10

Coexistent sickle-cell anemia and autoimmune disease in eight children: pitfalls and challenges

Valerie Li-Thiao-Te[1*], Florence Uettwiller[2], Pierre Quartier[2,3,4], Florence Lacaille[5], Brigitte Bader-Meunier[2,3,4], Valentine Brousse[6] and Mariane de Montalembert[6]

Abstract

Background: Patients with sickle cell disease (SCD) present a defective activation of the alternate complement pathway that increases the risk of infection and is thought to predispose to autoimmune disease (AID). However, coexisting AID and SCD is rarely reported, suggesting possible underdiagnosis due to an overlapping of the symptoms.

Study design: Among 603 patients with SCD followed between 1999 and June 2016, we retrospectively searched for patients with coexisting SCD and AID.

Results: We identified 8 patients aged from 7 to 17 years diagnosed with AID; juvenile idiopathic arthritis ($n = 3$), systemic lupus erythematosus ($n = 2$), Sjögren's syndrome ($n = 1$) and autoimmune hepatitis (n = 2). The diagnosis of AID was often delayed due to similarities of the symptoms with those of SCD. Patients treated with steroids experienced multiple vaso-occlusive crises and received prophylactic chronic blood transfusions when it was possible. Tolerance to other immunosuppressive and biological treatments, such as anti-TNF agents, was good. A remission of AID was achieved in 4 patients, without worsening the course of the SCD. One patient underwent a geno-identical hematopoietic stem cell transplantation that cured both diseases. Another one underwent a successful liver transplantation.

Conclusion: Coexistence of AID and SCD generates diagnostic and therapeutic challenges. Early diagnosis of AID is important to define the best treatment, which may include targeted biological therapy.

Keywords: Sickle cell disease, Autoimmune disease, Juvenile idiopathic arthritis, Systemic lupus erythematosus, Children, Biological therapy

Background

Sickle cell disease (SCD) is a common inherited condition in African, Caribbean, and Mediterranean countries. Production of abnormal hemoglobin S is responsible for the sickling of red blood cells in deoxygenated conditions. SCD manifests itself as chronic intravascular hemolysis, vaso-occlusion and painful crises. Over time, multiple organ damage can develop. Patients with SCD display a defective activation of the alternate complement pathway, leading to an increased risk of infection with encapsulated bacteria (pneumococci, *Haemophilus influenzae*) [1–3]. It was suggested that complement abnormalities could predispose to autoimmune disease (AID) [4]. However, the frequency of coexisting SCD and AID has not been evaluated, and most data come from case reports [5–14]. Manifestations of AID, such as fever, polyarthritis, and multiorgan involvement, can also be caused by SCD, leading to a delay in diagnosing the AID [11]. Furthermore, antiinflammatory drugs such as steroids and immunosuppressive therapy used to treat AID can induce severe SCD complications.

Study design

Between 1999 and June 2016, 603 patients with SCD aged under 18 years were seen at the hemoglobinopathy reference center of the Necker Hospital, Paris, France.

* Correspondence: lithiaote.valerie@chu-amiens.fr
[1]Onco-Hématologie Pédiatrique, Centre Hospitalier Universitaire Amiens, Amiens, France
Full list of author information is available at the end of the article

Among them, we searched for patients with coexisting SCD and AID.

We retrospectively collected data from the medical records of SCD patients followed in our institution, the largest Pediatric University-Hospital in France, which has a national reference center for SCD and a national reference center for pediatric rheumatology diseases. Started in 2007, data from the patients referred to the pediatric rheumatology team were registered in the CEMARA database, a nationwide web-based information for rare diseases [15] approved by the French patients Data Protection Authority (*Commission Nationale de l'Informatique et Libertés*, CNIL), after patients'/parents' information and verification of their non-opposition. In accordance with the French legislation, no ethics committee agreement was requested for such a retrospective survey.

Results

Among the 603 children with SCD followed between 1999 and June 2016, we identified 8 patients aged from 7 to 17 years, who developed an AID. All patients were Afro-Caribbean homozygous SCD (Hb SS) children either diagnosed by neonatal screening (patient 1, 6, 7 and #8) or during infancy (patient 2, 3, 4 and #5). The diagnoses were juvenile idiopathic arthritis (JIA, $n = 3$), systemic lupus erythematosus (SLE, $n = 2$), Sjögren's syndrome ($n = 1$) and autoimmune hepatitis (n = 2). These 8 patients received joint follow-up by hematologists, rheumatologists and an hepatologist. Table 1 reports the medical history before the diagnosis of the AID and the clinical and laboratory findings that led to the diagnosis of AID.

In one patient, SLE was diagnosed within a few weeks of the onset of the symptoms because of fingers swelling, not a common site of vaso-occlusion in adolescents with SCD. In another patient, alopecia and aphthous stomatitis helped diagnose the SLE several months after the first neurologic symptoms and polyarthritis had appeared. In some patients, the diagnosis was delayed for several years (Table 1). Before the diagnosis of JIA, patients #2 and #4 had had a long history of joint pain and ankle and knee swelling, first ascribed to SCD and treated as SCD complications (analgesics, hyperhydratation, hydroxyurea for patient #2 and exchange transfusion for patient #4). Patients 5 and #8 displayed biological signs of liver dysfunction (elevation of AST and ALT, cholestasis). Liver biopsy showed lymphoplasmocytic infiltrates and mild fibrosis compatible with autoimmune hepatitis. For patient #7 diagnosed with SLE, cerebral MRI was performed in response to the worsening of neurologic symptoms and showed periventricular hyperintensity and cortico-subcortical atrophy compatible with lupus lesions. The tolerance to AID treatment was good. Among the 4 patients treated with steroids, 3 had a concomitant exchange transfusion program in order to prevent vaso-occlusive crises and 1 received hydroxyurea. Red blood cell alloimmunisation in 1 patient required a switch from transfusion to hydroxyurea. Complete remission of the AID was obtained for 4 patients with a classical immunosuppressive treatment ($n = 1$), biological treatment ($n = 2$) or genoidentical hematopoietic stem cell transplantation (n = 1), although 1 patient (patient #4) had arthritis sequelae. Despite being associated with AID, the SCD course was stable for 5 patients. The patient who underwent stem cell transplantation was cured of both AID and SCD. Patient #4 who did not receive hydroxyurea or transfusion experienced several vaso-occlusive crises during the follow up. Patient #8 who underwent liver transplantation due to chronic infectious cholangitis, presented multiple post-transplant complications (rejection, biliary stenosis, high blood pressure, posterior reversible encephalopathy), but had a normal liver function and a much improved quality of life at the last follow up. Table 2 reports the treatments and last follow-up data.

Discussion

We report 8 cases of coexisting SCD and AID including polyarticular JIA and juvenile SLE in a cohort of 603 patients with SCD. The incidence of AID in France in an ethnic matched population is not known, as it is not allowed to compare diseases according to patients' ethnicity. These cases highlight the diagnostic difficulties raised by the symptom overlapping between AID and SCD (e.g., polyarthritis, anemia, and fever) and the therapeutic challenges. Nevertheless, the use of immunosuppressive drugs (except steroids), including new drugs such as TNFα antagonist was well tolerated and provided durable AID remissions, without worsening the course of the SCD when associated to specific SCD treatments.

AID such as SLE [16] and polyarticular JIA [17, 18] are more common in Blacks than in other ethnic groups. In addition to genetics, patients with SCD present functional asplenia and defective activation of the alternate complement pathway [1–4]. Although published data focused on functional complement abnormalities, it would be interesting to assess the impact of functional asplenia itself in the occurrence of AID [19]. However, the coexistence of AID and SCD seems to be rare, potentially underdiagnosed, and its prevalence is unknown. In a study of 30 patients with SCD and connective tissue disease, 15 patients (50%) had rheumatoid arthritis, 13 (44%) had SLE, 1 (3%) had Sjögren's syndrome, and 1 (3%) had sclerodermia [20]. Most data on coexistent AID and SCD come from anecdotal case-reports [5–14] describing patients SLE [2, 8–11], or far less often, JIA [5–7] or autoimmune hepatitis [12–14].

Our patients reflect the diagnostic challenges of JIA in children with SCD. We report diagnostic delays from 1 to 8 years, as could be found in previous reports [5–7].

Table 1 Medical history, clinical and biological findings at presentation in our patients

Patient	1	2	3	4	5	6	7	8
Sex	M	M	F	M	M	F	F	F
Medical history related to SCD	ACS (3 episodes) Recurrent VOC	Recurrent polyarthralgia[a]	Recurrent VOC	Recurrent VOC Osteomyelitis right femur Chronic hepatitis B	Recurrent VOC Acute cholecystitis, *Salmonella* septicemia Bilateral avascular necrosis of femoral heads	Recurrent VOC	Recurrent VOC ACS (3 episodes)	Recurrent VOC ACS Acute splenic sequestration Recurrent cholangitis
Type of AID	SLE	JIA	JIA	JIA	AIH	Sjogrën'syndrome	SLE	AIH
Age at onset of AID (years)	13	4	7	4	17	11	15	3
Age at diagnosis of AID (years)	13	13	7	6	17	13 (11 for initial diagnosis of JIA)	15	3
Symptoms	Asthenia, denutrition polyarthritis fingers and toes hepatomegaly pericarditis	Polyarthritis left knee and right ankle severe arthropathy at 10 y uveitis	Polyarthritis (temporo-mandibular arthritis and sacroiliitis)	Polyarthralgia bilateral knee arthritis Asthenia, weight loss	Polyarthralgia	Polyarthralgia (spine); knee arthritis; Secondary recurrent parotiditis; xerostomia at 13 y	Polyarthritis; pleuritis, pericarditis, aphthous stomatitis, alopecia; pulmonary hypertension; behavior disorder	Hepatomegaly; jaundice
ESR (mm/h)	74	95	34	86	67	14	84	88
IgG (g/l)	38	26	–	–	35	23	30	26
ANA pattern	1/1280 homogeneous	1/160 speckled	Negative	1/80 homogeneous	1/80	1/1280	1/80 speckled	1/160
Others immunological features	Anti-DNA antibodies + (43 UI/ml) Coombs +	RF negative	RF positive		Anti-U1RNP + Farr test 29%	Anti-SSA, SSB + Anti-U1RNP + Antiβ2GP1 + Antiphospholipid antibodies +	Anti-DNA antibodies + (44 U/l) pANCA Coombs + Antiplatelets antibodies + AntiB2GP1 + anticardiolipin + Neutropenia	c-ANCA + Smooth muscle antibodies + (1/50)

VOC vaso-occlusive crises, *ACS* acute chest syndrome, *AID* autoimmune disease, *SLE* systemic lupus erythematosus, *JIA* juvenile idiopathic arthritis, *AIH* autoimmune hepatitis, *M* male, *F* female, *ESR* erythrocyte sedimentation rate, *ANA* antinuclear antibodies, *RF* rheumatoid factor
[a]first ascribed to SCD but probably related to JIA

Features arguing against SCD as the cause included bilateral symmetric pain limited to the joints, failure of hydroxyurea, persistent high erythrocyte sedimentation rate. In most previously reported cases, the recognition of SLE was delayed because of similar clinical features, regardless of involved organs [8–10]. The liver involvement is often misdiagnosed because jaundice is ascribed to hemolysis and not cholestasis.

An autoantibody production is traditionally a manifestation of autoimmunity. Nearly all our patients had detectable antinuclear antibodies. Whether early autoantibody detection might have helped to diagnose AID is discussed. The prevalence of antinuclear antibodies varies from 12 to 30% in healthy individuals overall [21, 22] and from 7 to 39% in Africans [23, 24]. Moreover, high autoantibody titers have been reported in SCD in the absence of autoimmunity [25, 26]. Consequently, routine screening for autoantibodies in the absence of suggestive symptoms is not recommended, because it may be confusing and lead to inadequate diagnosis and therapy. The mechanisms underlying the production of autoantibodies in SCD are unknown but may involve impaired spleen function. Significant autoantibody titers have been found after splenectomy, in the absence of AID [27]. Other hypotheses include immune system overstimulation by multiple transfusions [28] and chronic inflammation [29]. This has not been confirmed in clinical studies [25, 26].

The treatment of coexisting AID and SCD is difficult [30]. Our patients experienced recurrent vaso-occlusive crises while on steroids [7, 10, 13, 30]. Concomitant red blood cell transfusion or exchange transfusion program may help prevent vaso-occlusive crises but increase the risk of anti-erythrocyte alloimmunization. Half of our patients received hydroxyurea in the first line or after chronic blood

Table 2 Treatment and last follow-up in the 8 patients

Patient	1	2	3	4	5	6	7	8
Treatment related to SCD before the diagnosis of AID	None	Hydroxyurea started at 13 y	Hydroxyurea started at 7 y	None	None	Hydroxyurea started at 9 y	Hydroxyurea started at 14 y	Chronic exchange transfusion programme started at 3 y splenectomy
AID	SLE	JIA	JIA	JIA	AIH	Sjogrën's syndrome	SLE	AIH
Treatment of AID First line	NSAIDs Hydroxychloroquine	NSAIDs	NSAIDs for 3 years	Etanercept (No methotrexate because of chronic hepatitis B)	Steroids Chronic blood transfusions then Hydroxyurea[a]	NSAIDs (from age 11 to 13 y)	Steroids Chronic exchange transfusions[a] Hydroxychloroquine Aspirin	Steroids 6-mercaptopurine Chronic exchange transfusions[a]
2nd line	Genoidentical hematopoietic stem cell transplantation at 18 y	Etanercept	Steroids Intra-articular steroids		Azathioprine NSAIDs	Methotrexate Hydroxychloroquine Aspirin	Mycophenolate mofetil Steroids	Azathioprine Steroids Chronic exchange transfusions[a]
3rd line and more			Etanercept for 5 years; (Failure of abatacept, infliximab, adalimumab) Current treatment: Tolicizumab + methotrexate			Mycophenolate mofetil		Liver transplantation at 10 y Ciclosporin and steroids
Last follow-up	CR	PR	Persistant activity	CR	CR	CR	PR	Normal liver function Controlled blood pressure

AID autoimmune disease, *SLE* systemic lupus erythematosus, *JIA* juvenile idiopathic arthritis, *AIH* autoimmune hepatitis, *NSAIDs* non steroidal antiinflammatory drugs, *CR* complete remission, *PR* partial remission

Patient 2: relapse after 3 years, then lost in transition to adult care, patient 7: persistent periventricular hyperintensity on cerebral MRI

[a]in order to prevent occurrence of vasoocclusive crises

transfusion and experienced fewer vaso- occlusive crises. Hydroxyurea seems to be well tolerated by patients taking antiinflammatory drugs [8–10]. TNFα antagonist therapy (etanercept) was promptly effective in our patients with JIA, as reported in patients with polyarticular onsets of JIA and no SCD [31, 32]. No severe etanercept-related complications were recorded. The few available data suggest good effectiveness and tolerance in patients with SCD [5, 20]. The use of others biological therapies as anti-interleukine 1 and 6 has not been reported yet in patients with SCD. Azathioprine was frequently used either for patients with SLE or autoimmune hepatitis and was well tolerated [10, 12–14]. For hydroxychloroquine, ocular toxicity may worsen retinopathy due to SCD and has to be regularly controlled. Finally, immunosuppressive and antiinflammatory drugs can induce renal and hepatic toxicity that may be worsened by SCD-related complications. They may further increase the risk of infection [20], despite the lack of published data concerning infections in patients with both AID and SCD. The initiation of immunosuppressive and/or antiinflammatory therapy should be discussed in reference centers and require close monitoring. Biological treatments, including anti-TNF targeted treatments, might be beneficial to SCD-associated AID / inflammation and in some cases to SCD itself and deserve further evaluation [33]. Hematopoietic stem cell transplantation seems to be a good therapeutic option. Liver transplantation can be discussed in very selected cases.

Conclusion

SCD and AID share many clinical and biological features, and diagnosing AID in patients with SCD can be challenging. Diagnostic delay increases the morbidity and mortality related to both the AID and SCD. Whilst the use of steroids to treat AIDs induced potential severe SCD-related complications, which justified associated chronic red blood cell transfusions, other treatments such as anti-TNF agents were well tolerated. Further studies are needed to determine the prevalence of AID in patients with SCD, to look for pathophysiological links, to earlier diagnose AID, and to define the best therapeutic options.

Abbreviations

ACS: Acute chest syndrome; AID: Autoimmune disease; AIH: Autoimmune hepatitis; CNIL: Commission Nationale Informatique et Libertés; JIA: Juvenile idiopathic arthritis; SCD: sickle cell disease; SLE: Systemic lupus erythematosus; VOC: Vaso-occlusive crises

Acknowledgements

Not applicable.

Funding

The authors declare that they have no funding.

Authors' contributions

VL and FU collected data and wrote the manuscript; MM, VB, FL, BB and PQ were involved in the clinical care of the patients and provided data for the study. MM, FL and PQ helped with data management, edited and reviewed the manuscript. All authors read and approved the manuscript.

Competing interests

The authors declare that they have no competing interests.

Author details

[1]Onco-Hématologie Pédiatrique, Centre Hospitalier Universitaire Amiens, Amiens, France. [2]Unité d'Immunologie-Hématologie et Rhumatologie Pédiatrique, Centre de référence pour la Rhumatologie et les maladies Auto-immunes Systémiques de l'Enfant, Hôpital Necker-Enfants Malades, Assistance Publique Hôpitaux de Paris, Paris, France. [3]Université Paris-Descartes, Paris, France. [4]IMAGINE Institute, Paris, France. [5]Hépatologie-Gastroentérologie-Nutrition Pédiatrique, Hôpital Necker-Enfants Malades, Assistance Publique Hôpitaux de Paris, Paris, France. [6]Pédiatrie Générale, Centre de Référence des Hémoglobinopathies, Hôpital Necker-Enfants Malades, Assistance Publique Hôpitaux de Paris Labex-GR-Ex, Paris, France.

References

1. Johnston RB Jr, Newman SL, Struth AG. An abnormality of the alternate pathway of complement activation in sickle-cell disease. N Engl J Med. 1973;288:803–8.
2. Wilson WA, Nicholson GD, Hughes GR, Amin S, Alleyne G, Serjeant GR. Systemic lupus erythematosus and sickle-cell anaemia. Br Med J. 1976;1:813.
3. Koethe SM, Casper JT, Rodey GE. Alternative complement pathway activity in sera from patients with sickle cell disease. Clin Exp Immunol. 1976;23:56–60.
4. Wilson WA, De Ceulaer K, Morgan AG. Sickle cell anemia, complement, and systemic lupus erythematosus. Arthritis Rheum. 1979;22:803.
5. Adelowo O, Edunjobi AS. Juvenile idiopathic arthritis coexisting with sickle cell disease: two case reports. BMJ. 2011; doi: https://doi.org/10.1136/bcr.2011.4889.
6. Eberhard BA. Coexistent sickle cell disease and juvenile rheumatoid arthritis: 2 cases with delayed diagnosis and severe destructive arthropathy. J Rheumatol. 2002;29:1802. author reply 1802-3
7. Nistala K, Murray KJ. Co-existent sickle cell disease and juvenile rheumatoid arthritis. Two cases with delayed diagnosis and severe destructive arthropathy. J Rheumatol. 2001;28:2125–8.
8. Appenzeller S, Fattori A, Saad ST, Costallat LT. Systemic lupus erythematosus in patients with sickle cell disease. Clin Rheumatol. 2008;27:359–64.
9. Khalidi NA, Ajmani H, Varga J. Coexisting systemic lupus erythematosus and sickle cell disease: a diagnostic and therapeutic challenge. J Clin Rheumatol. 2005;11:86–92.
10. Saxena VR, Mina R, Moallem HJ, Rao SP, Miller ST. Systemic lupus erythematosus in children with sickle cell disease. J Pediatr Hematol Oncol. 2003;25:668–71.
11. Maamar M, Tazi-Mezalek Z, Harmouche H, Mounfaloti W, Adnaoui M, Aouni M. Systemic lupus erythematosus associated with sickle-cell disease: a case report and literature review. J Med Case Rep. 2012;6:366.
12. Chuang E, Ruchelli E, Mulberg AE. Autoimmune liver disease and sickle cell anemia in children: a report of three cases. J Pediatr Hematol Oncol. 1997;19:159–62.
13. Lykavieris P, Benichou JJ, Benkerrou M, Feriot JP, Bernard O, Debray D. Autoimmune liver disease in three children with sickle cell disease. J Pediatr Gastroenterol Nutr. 2006;42:104–8.
14. El Younis CM, Min AD, Fiel MI, Klion FM, Thung SN, Faire B, Miller CM, Bodenheimer HC Jr. Autoimmune hepatitis in a patient with sickle cell disease. Am J Gastroenterol. 1996;91:1016–8.
15. Landais P, Messiaen C, Rath A, Le Mignot L, Dufour E, Ben Said M, Jais JP, Toubiana L, Baujat G, Bourdon-Lanoy E, Gérard-Blanluet M, Bodemer C, Salomon R, Aymé S, Le Merrer M, Verloes A, CEMARA task force.

CEMARA an information system for rare diseases. Stud Health Technol Inform. 2010;160:481–5.
16. Hopkinson ND, Doherty M, Powell RJ. Clinical features and race-specific incidence/prevalence rates of systemic lupus erythematosus in a geographically complete cohort of patients. Ann Rheum Dis. 1994;53:675–80.
17. Saurenmann RK, Rose JB, Tyrrell P, Feldman BM, Laxer RM, Schneider R, Silverman ED. Epidemiology of juvenile idiopathic arthritis in a multiethnic cohort: ethnicity as a risk factor. Arthritis Rheum. 2007;56:1974–84.
18. Haffejee IE, Raga J, Coovadia HM. Juvenile chronic arthritis in black and Indian south African children. S Afr Med J. 1984;65:510–4.
19. Vaiopoulos G, Konstantopolous K, Osterland CK. Asplenia in systemic lupus erythematosus: a simple coincidence? Clin Exp Rheumatol. 1995;13:513–5.
20. Michel M, Habibi A, Godeau B, Bachir D, Lahary A, Galacteros F, Fifi-Mah A, Arfi S. Characteristics and outcome of connective tissue diseases in patients with sickle-cell disease: report of 30 cases. Semin Arthritis Rheum. 2008;38:228–40.
21. de Vlam K, De Keyser F, Verbruggen G, Vandenbossche M, Vanneuville B, D'Haese D, Veys EM. Detection and identification of antinuclear autoantibodies in the serum of normal blood donors. Clin Exp Rheumatol. 1993;11:393–7.
22. Hilário MO, Len CA, Roja SC, Terreri MT, Almeida G, Andrade LE. Frequency of antinuclear antibodies in healthy children and adolescents. Clin Pediatr. 2004;43:637–42.
23. Adebajo AO, Charles P, Maini RN, Hazleman BL. Autoantibodies in malaria, tuberculosis and hepatitis B in a west African population. Clin Exp Immunol. 1993;92:73–6.
24. Greenwood BM, Herrick EM, Holborow EJ. Speckled antinuclear factor in African sera. Clin Exp Immunol. 1970;7:75–83.
25. Baethge BA, Bordelon TR, Mills GM, Bowen LM, Wolf RE, Bairnsfather L. Antinuclear antibodies in sickle cell disease. Acta Haematol. 1990;84:186–9.
26. Toly-Ndour C, Rouquette AM, Obadia S, M'bappe P, Lionnet F, Hagege I, Boussa-Khettab F, Tshilolo L, Girot R. High titers of autoantibodies in patients with sickle cell disease. J Rheumatol. 2011;38:302–9.
27. Balsalobre B, Hernández-Godoy J, Planelles D. Autoantibodies in splenectomized patients as a consequence of abdominal trauma. J Investig Allergol Clin Immunol. 1992;2:91–5.
28. Aygun B, Padmanabhan S, Paley C, Chandrasekaran V. Clinical significance of RBC alloantibodies and autoantibodies in sickle cell patients who received transfusions. Transfusion. 2002;42:37–43.
29. Allen RC, Dewez P, Stuart L, Gatenby PA, Sturgess A. Antinuclear antibodies using HEp-2 cells in normal children and in children with common infections. J Paediatr Child Health. 1991;27:39–42.
30. Couillard S, Benkerrou M, Girot R, Brousse V, Ferster A, Bader-Meunier B. Steroid treatment in children with sickle-cell disease. Haematologica. 2007;92:425–6.
31. Quartier P, Taupin P, Bourdeaut F, Lemelle I, Pillet P, Bost M, Sibilia J, Koné-Paut I, Gandon-Laloum S, LeBideau M, Bader-Meunier B, Mouy R, Debré M, Landais P, Prieur AM. Efficacy of etanercept for the treatment of juvenile idiopathic arthritis according to the onset type. Arthritis Rheum. 2003;48:1093–101.
32. Horneff G, Schmeling H, Biedermann T, Foeldvari I, Ganser G, Girschick HJ, Hospach T, Huppertz HI, Keitzer R, Küster RM, Michels H, Moebius D, Rogalski B, Thon A, Paediatric Rheumatology Collaborative Group. The German etanercept registry for treatment of juvenile idiopathic arthritis. Ann Rheum Dis. 2004;63:1638–44.
33. Solovey A, Somani A, Chen C, et al. Interference with TNFα using long-term etanercept in $S^{+}S^{Antilles}$ sickle transgenic mice ameliorates abnormal endothelial activation, vasoocclusion, and pulmonary hypertension including its pulmonary arterial wall remodeling. Blood. 2013;122:728.

The transcription factor CREM drives an inflammatory phenotype of T cells in oligoarticular juvenile idiopathic arthritis

Kim Ohl[1], Helge Nickel[1], Halima Moncrieffe[2,3], Patricia Klemm[1], Anja Scheufen[1], Dirk Föll[4], Viktor Wixler[5], Angela Schippers[1], Norbert Wagner[1], Lucy R. Wedderburn[6,7,8] and Klaus Tenbrock[1*]

Abstract

Background: Inflammatory effector T cells trigger inflammation despite increased numbers of Treg cells in the synovial joint of patients suffering from juvenile idiopathic arthritis (JIA). The cAMP response element (CREM)α is known to play a major role in regulation of T cells in SLE, colitis, and EAE. However, its role in regulation of effector T cells within the inflammatory joint is unknown.

Methods: CREM expression was analyzed in synovial fluid cells from oligoarticular JIA patients by flow cytometry. Peripheral blood mononuclear cells were incubated with synovial fluid and analyzed in the presence and absence of CREM using siRNA experiments for T cell phenotypes. To validate the role of CREM in vivo, ovalbumin-induced T cell dependent arthritis experiments were performed.

Results: CREM is highly expressed in synovial fluid T cells and its expression can be induced by treating healthy control PBMCs with synovial fluid. Specifically, CREM is more abundant in $CD161^+$ subsets, than $CD161^-$ subsets, of T cells and contributes to cytokine expression by these cells. Finally, development of ovalbumin-induced experimental arthritis is ameliorated in mice with adoptively transferred $CREM^{-/-}$ T cells.

Conclusion: In conclusion, our study reveals that beyond its role in SLE T cells CREM also drives an inflammatory phenotype of T cells in JIA.

Keywords: CREM, JIA, Effector T cells

Background

Juvenile idiopathic arthritis (JIA) is the most common inflammatory rheumatic disease in children and is an autoimmune disease of unknown origin. Apart from cells of the innate immune system like neutrophils and monocytes, which trigger inflammation, T cells play a dominant role in the inflammatory reaction of the joint. Recent investigations indicate an accumulation of highly inflammatory $CD4^+CD161^+$ cells in the joints [1–3]. Although the functional relevance of CD161 ligation on T cell function is less clear, CD161 expression is a useful indicator of inflammatory T cells. They belong to either Th1, Th17 or Th1/Th17, so called non-classical Th1, cells and their proportions in synovial fluid (SF) correlate positively with parameters of disease activity [1, 4, 5]. The inflammatory potential of these effector T cells within the joint is controlled by regulatory T cells (Tregs). The control, however, is inefficient despite the high presence of Tregs in arthritic joints. Tregs typically are not pro-inflammatory, but recent reports showed that some Tregs also may share functional capabilities with conventional T cells, like production of inflammatory cytokines in the context of autoimmunity or chronic inflammation [6–8]. These Tregs are part of the CD161 population and also enriched in joints of JIA and rheumatoid arthritis (RA) patients [2, 9].

The cAMP response element modulator (CREM) α binds to promoters of genes with cAMP response elements (CRE) and regulates transcription via a chromatin-dependent mechanism. Under physiological

* Correspondence: ktenbrock@ukaachen.de
[1]Department of Pediatrics, Medical Faculty, RWTH Aachen, Pauwelsstr. 30, D-52074 Aachen, Germany
Full list of author information is available at the end of the article

conditions, the production of CREM is tightly regulated and involves the differential use of alternate promoters and splicing processes, resulting in cell- and tissue-specific expression patterns [10, 11]. Quite interesting is that in T cells of SLE patients CREMα mRNA and protein expression is increased and this significantly alters the expression of various T lymphocyte-specific target genes, including IL-2 and IL-17 family cytokines [12–15]. Notably, the observed effects of CREMα on IL-2 and IL-17a cytokine production in humans are also observed in transgenic mice with T cell-specific CREMα overexpression [16]. These mice have decreased IL-2 and increased IL-17a levels and are more prone to develop signs of autoimmunity (including lymphadenopathy and higher autoantibody titers against double-stranded DNA) when an additional genetic deletion of the *cd95* gene (Fas) is present [16, 17]. Beyond its role in SLE CREMα also contributes to T cell dysregulations in asthma, LPS-induced lung injury, colitis, and EAE [18–21]. Although it is known that T cells contribute to pathogenesis in JIA, the role of CREM here has not been addressed so far.The aim of this study was to evaluate the role CREM expressing T cells in oligoarticular JIA. Our findings indicate that beyond its role in SLE CREMα also contributes to T cell pathophysiology in oligoarticular JIA by modulating inflammatory and regulatory T cells.

Methods

Flow cytometry

For surface staining, single cell suspensions were stained with anti-CD3 (UCHT1), anti-CD4 (RPA-T4), anti-CD161 (HP-3G10) antibodies (all from eBioscience, Germany). To analyze Foxp3 and CREM expression, cells were fixed and permeabilized with a FOXP3 staining buffer set (eBioscience, Germany) following the manufacturer's instructions and stained with anti-Foxp3 (PCH101) antibodies (eBioscience, Germany), monoclonal anti-CREM (Abcam, Great Britain) or IgG isotype control antibodies for 30 min. Monoclonal anti-CREM antibodies and IgG isotype control antibodies were labeled with Alexa Fluor Antibody Labeling Kits (Thermo Fisher Scientific, USA) according to manufactures instructions. For measurement of intracellular cytokines, cells were treated with propidium iodide (P/I) and GolgiPlug (BD Bisciences, Germany) for 5 h and fixed and permeabilized with FoxP3 staining buffer set (eBioscience, Germany) following the manufacturers' instructions. Intracellular cytokines were stained with anti-IFN-γ (4S.B3) APC and anti-IL-17 PE (64DEC17) (both eBioscience, Germany) antibodies.

Patients and healthy donors

All patients were diagnosed as having oligoarticular JIA and were receiving nonsteroidal anti-inflammatory drugs before therapeutic aspiration of SF and administration of corticosteroids. JIA patients were diagnosed according to internationally agreed criteria.Cells were pelleted by centrifugation and supernatants were individually stored at – 20 °C, with this more than twenty different SFs and HC sera were collected and are included in different experiment in this study. Ethical approval for all experiments was obtained from the local ethics committee. All patients provided fully informed consent or age-appropriate assent where applicable. Sera from healthy controls (HC) were obtained from peripheral blood. For co-incubation wit HC Sera and SF, cells from healthy donors were isolated from buffy coats provided by the local blood bank, Transfusionsmedizin, UniversitätsklinikumAachen, Germany).

Cell isolation

Human mononuclear cells from patients with JIA were isolated onto a Ficoll (PAN Biotech, Germany) gradient either from peripheral blood (PB) or synovial fluid (SF). Erythrocytes were lysed and cells were washed twice. Peripheral blood mononuclear cells (PBMC) were isolated from healthy donors by the same procedure.

Cell culture

PBMCs from healthy donors were incubated with 10% allogenic SF or serum from allogenic healthy controls (HC) in RPMI (Gibco, Germany) with 10% FCS (Biochrom, Germany). When indicated, cells were stimulated with plate-bound anti-CD3 and anti-CD28 antibodies (both at 3 μg/ml; BD Bioscience, Germany) in individual wells of 96-well round-bottom microtiter plates. To knock-down CREM expression, PBMCs and SFMCs were transfected with 5 nM CREM-specific siRNA or irrelevant control siRNA (Origene, USA) using the Amaxa transfection system (Lonza, Switzerland). After four hours cells were transferred in fresh media and either left unstimulated and analyzed after 24 h or stimulated and anyalzed as indicated.

RNA isolation, complementary DNA (cDNA) synthesis, and quantitative real-time polymerase chain reaction (PCR)

Total RNA was extracted from cells using an RNeasy Mini Kit (Qiagen, Germany) and transcribed to cDNA using a First Strand cDNA Synthesis Kit (Thermo Fisher Scintific, USA) according to the manufacturer's instructions. Standard quantitative real-time PCR was carried out on a TaqMan 7900 (Applied Biosystems, USA) using the DNA intercalating dye SYBR Green.

Ovalbumin (OVA)-induced arthritis model

OVA-induced arthritis was induced in mice, as described previously [22]. Briefly, 2×10^6 OVA-specific $CD4^+CD25^-$ T cells from either wild-type (WT) or $CREM^{-/-}$ OT-II mice were injected intraperitoneally into C57BL/6 $RAG^{-/-}$ mice. Two independent experiments were performed and overall 6 mice per group were analyzed. One day later recipients were immunized with 100 μg cationized OVA (Sigma-Aldrich, Germany) in PBS at the base of the tail. On day 7 mice were rechallenged with 60 μg cationized OVA injected intra-articularly into the left knee joint. Knee swelling was assessed using calipers at definite time points as the difference between the right (arthritic) before and after OVA-injection.

Mice

Experiments were performed withage-matched $RAG^{-/-}$, WT OT-II and $CREM^{-/-}$ OT-II mice (all C57BL/6). $CREM^{-/-}$ animals were originally cloned and provided by Prof. G. Schütz (Deutsches Krebsforschungszentrum, Heidelberg, Germany) [23]. $CREM^{-/-}$ OT-II mice were generated by crossing $CREM^{-/-}$ mice with OT-II mice. All mice were bred in our animal facility and kept under standardized conditions. The study was approved by the regional government authorities and animal procedures were performed according to German legislation for animal protection.

Histology

Knee joints from mice were fixed in 4% neutral buffered formalin solution for 24 h. Afterwards they were placed in an EDTA-decalcifying solution (20% EDTA) for 20 days, dehydrated, and embedded in paraffin blocks. Sections were cut along a longitudinal axis at 6 μm and stained with hematoxylin and eosin. Hematoxylin and eosin stained slides were evaluated and scored blindly for exudates, granulocyte infiltration, hyperplasia, fibroblast proliferation/mononuclear cell infiltration, periarticular mononuclear cell infiltration (each scoring 0–3), bone/cartilage destruction (scoring 0–4), and an additional score of 1 for visible fibrin deposition and periarticular granulocyte infiltration, resulting in a maximum score of 21.

Statistical analysis

All data are presented as mean ± standard error (SEM). Differences between two groups were evaluated using two-tailed unpaired or paired (if indicated), Student's t-test if data were normally distributed. Otherwise, a non-parametric Mann-Whitney test or Wilcoxon matched-pairs signed rank test were performed. All statistical analysis and subsequent graphics generation were performed using GraphPad Prism version 7.0 (GraphPad Software, USA). A p-value < 0.05 was considered to be statistically significant.

Results

CREMα is overexpressed in synovial fluid T cells of juvenile arthritis patients

T cells from SLE patients have previously been shown to display enhanced CREMα levels, thus pointing to the relevance of CREMα in human disease. Based on these findings we asked if expression of CREMα is also upregulated during another autoimmune disease in which T cells are involved in pathogenesis. We therefore investigated expression of CREMα in synovial fluid T cells from JIA patients. As shown in Fig. 1, percentages of $CREM^{high}$ cells within $CD3^+$ T cells were indeed more abundant in the synovial fluid of JIA patients than in the peripheral blood of healthy controls (Fig. 1a and b).

Incubation of control PBMCs with synovial fluid upregulates FoxP3 and IL-17 expression and involves upregulation of CREM

Synovial fluid of JIA patients contains high amounts of $FoxP3^+$ and $IL\text{-}17^+$ cells [24, 25]. Hence, we asked whether SF of JIA patients contains factors responsible for differentiation of these type of immune cells and whether this went along with increased expression of CREM. Thus we mimicked the inflammatory setting in the joint in vitro by incubating PBMCs from healthy controls with 10% allogenic synovial fluid from individual patients for 24 h. As a control we incubated PBMCs from the same healthy controls with 10% allogenic serum from individual healthy controls for 24 h. We observed increased percentages of FoxP3 positive cells in particular (Fig. 1c and d) and an increase in FoxP3 mRNA in general (Fig. 1e) when PBMC were incubated in the presence of synovial fluid for 24 h. In addition, when restimulated with P/I in the presence of Brefeldin A, percentages of $IL\text{-}17^+$ T cells (Fig. 1f and g) and IL-17 mRNA (Fig. 1h) were also increased in SF-stimulated PBMC. Moreover, incubation with SF also upregulated CREM mRNA expression in PBMC (Fig. 1j) and CREM protein expression specifically in T cells (Fig. 1i). Hence, incubation of control PBMCs with SF not only upregulates FoxP3 and IL17 expression but also CREM expression in T cells. Therefore, we hypothesize that soluble factors within the synovial fluid induce CREM transcription in SF T cells which leads to enhanced expression of CREM in SF T cells.

SF-induced expression of IFN-γ, IL-17, and FoxP3 in T cells can be reversed by CREM knock down with CREM-specific siRNA

We next asked if expression of CREM directly influences activation of T cells and therefore analyzed T cell activation in the absence of CREM. We isolated $CD4^+CD25^-$ cells from healthy donors, transfected them with CREM-specific siRNA or control siRNA. Flow cytometric

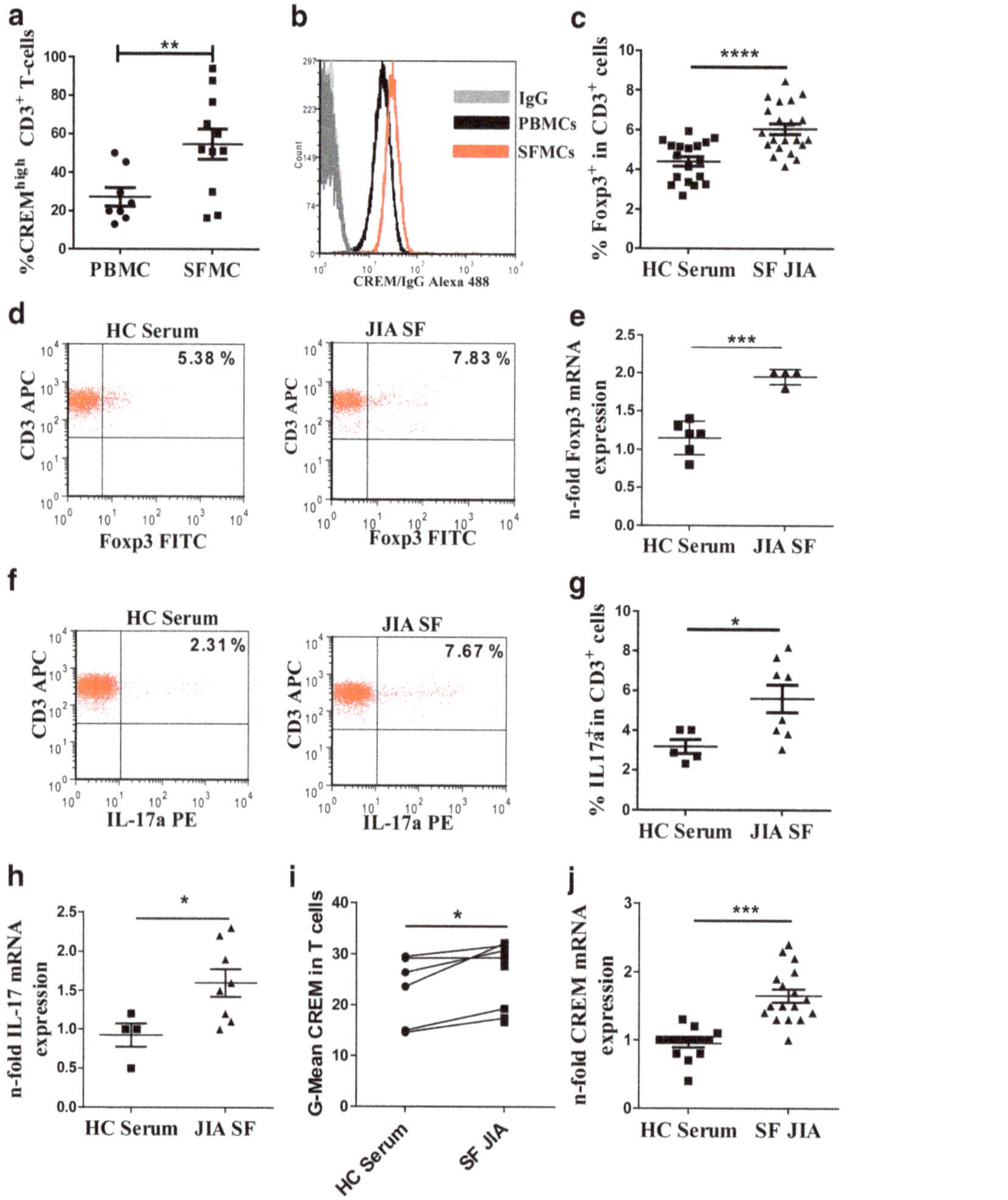

Fig. 1 CREM is overexpressed in JIA T cells. **a** Percentages of CREM high expressing T cells of 8 healthy control PBMCs and of 11 oligoarticular JIA SFMCs as assessed by flow cytometry. **b** Representative histogram showing mean fluorescent intensity of CREM expression in CD3+ T cells. **c-j** HC PBMCs were treated with 10% SF or HC Serum in RPMI for 24 h. **c** Percentages of Foxp3+ cells within CD3+ T cells. **d** Representative dot plot of Foxp3 expressing T cells. **e** Foxp3 mRNA expression. **f** Representative dot plot of IL-17+ expressing T cells after restimulation with P/I in the presence of Brefeldin A. **g** Percentages of IL-17+ cells within CD3+ T cells after restimulation with P/I in the presence of Brefeldin A. **h** IL-17 mRNA expression. **i** Geometric (G)-Mean of CREM expression, paired, two tailed t-test. **j** CREM mRNA expression, two-tailed Mann Whitney test. Symbols present individual patients, SFs or HC sera and horizontal bars show SEM. A two-tailed unpaired t-test was used to calculate *p*-values in **a, b, e, g** and **h**

analysis revealed that siRNA knockdown results in reduced protein expression of CREM (Fig. 2a and b). We next incubated the cells with anti-CD3/CD28 antibodies. Our analysis showed that percentages of IL-17a$^+$, IFN-γ$^+$ and FoxP3$^+$ cells were significantly reduced in CREM siRNA transfected cells (Fig. 2c, d and e). To further analyze if CREM is required for IL-17a and FoxP3 expression under the inflammatory environment we stimulated CD4$^+$ T cells with knocked down CREM by incubation in SF from JIA patients. Stimulation of CD4$^+$ T cells with

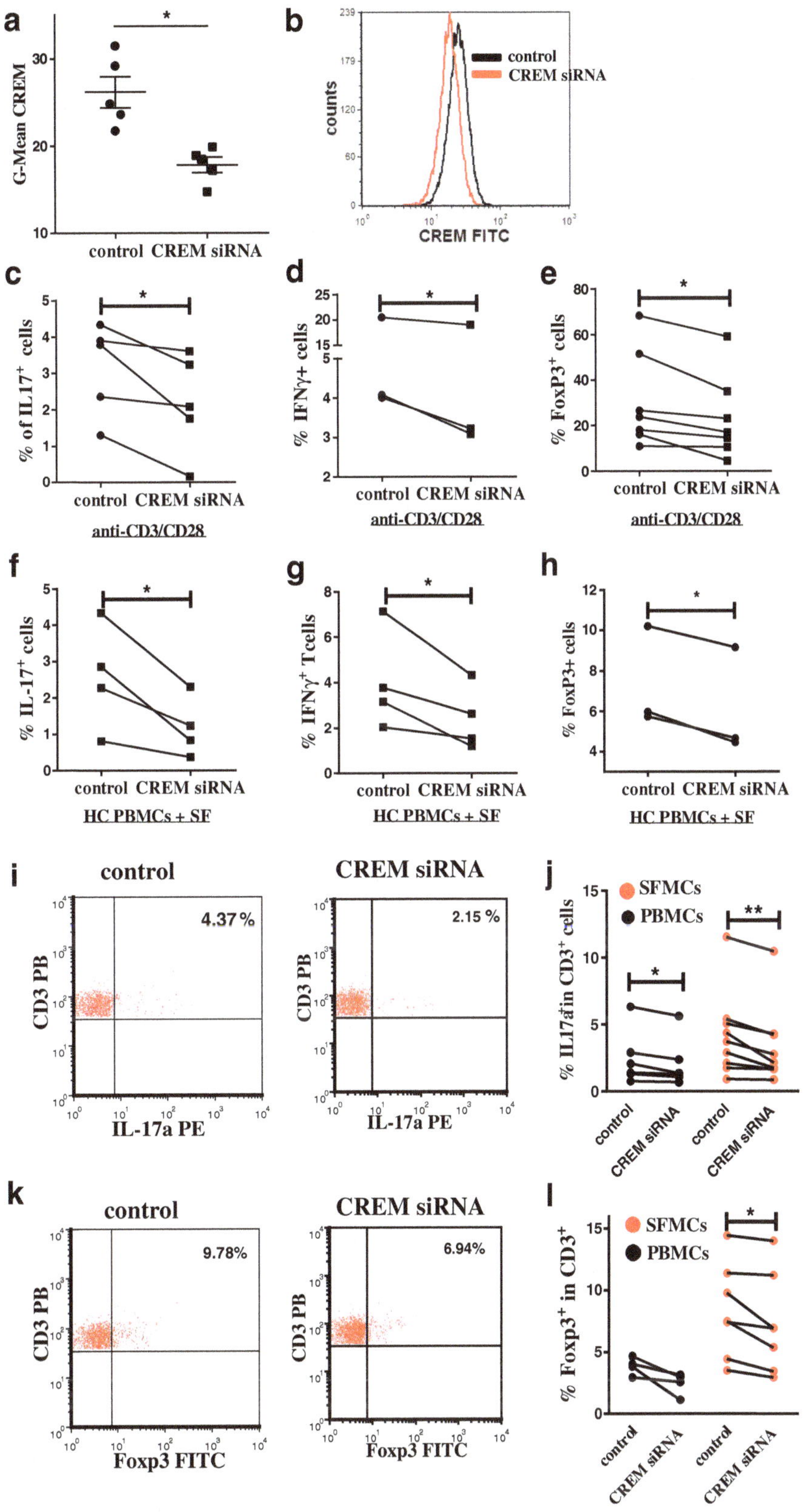

Fig. 2 (See legend on next page.)

(See figure on previous page.)

Fig. 2 CREM contributes to T cell dysregulations in JIA. **a** Healthy control PBMCs were transfected with control siRNA or with CREM siRNA and G-Mean of CREM expression was analyzed by flow cytometry, two-tailed paired t-test. **b** Representative histogram of CREM expression after transfection with control siRNA (black) or CREM siRNA (red). **c-e** Healthy control PBMCs were transfected with control siRNA or with CREM siRNA and stimulated with anti-CD3 and anti CD28 antibodies for 3 days, symbols present individual healthy controls incubated with different allogenic HC sera or SFs, two-tailed paired t-tests. **c** Percentages of IL-17$^+$ cells within CD3$^+$ T cells after restimulation with P/I in the presence of Brefeldin A. **d** Percentages of IFN-γ$^+$ cells within CD3$^+$ T cells after restimulation with P/I in the presence of Brefeldin. **e** Percentages of Foxp3$^+$ cells within CD3$^+$ T cells. F-H) Healthy control PBMCs were transfected with control siRNA or with CREM siRNA and incubated with 10% SF in RPMI for 24 h, two-tailed, paired t-tests were used to calculate *p*-values. **f** Percentages of IL-17$^+$ cells within CD3$^+$ T cells **g** Percentages of IFN-γ$^+$ cells within CD3$^+$ T cells. **h** Percentages of Foxp3$^+$ cells within CD3$^+$ T cells after restimulation with P/I in the presence of Brefeldin A. **i-l** PBMCs and SFMCs from JIA patients were transfected with control siRNA or with CREM siRNA and **i-h**) percentages of IL-17$^+$ cells after restimulation with P/I in the presence of Brefeldin A, Wilcoxon matched-pairs signed rank test was used to calculate p-values and of **k-l**) Foxp3$^+$ cells were assessed by flow cytometry after 24 h, two-tailed paired t-tests were used to calculate p-values

healthy control serum served as control. Similar to anti-CD3/CD28 antibody mediated stimulation of CD4$^+$ T cells, also the SF-induced expression of IFN-γ, IL-17a and FoxP3 could be reversed in CD4$^+$ T cells by expression of CREM-specific siRNA (Fig. 2f, g, and h). To establish the involvement of CREMα in the regulation of IL-17a, FoxP3 and IFN-γ expression in JIA we transfected ex vivo isolated SFMC with either unrelated control siRNA or siRNA directed against CREM. SFMC transfected with CREM-specific siRNA expressed significantly lower percentages of FoxP3$^+$ and IL17a$^+$ cells (Fig. 2i-l). Hence, these experiments provide evidence for the involvement of CREMα in the regulation of IL-17 and FoxP3 expression in juvenile arthritic joints.

CREM regulates inflammatory CD161$^+$ T cells and determines the outcome in inflammatory arthritis

Among CD4$^+$ cells the subset of CD161$^+$ T cells are the most important in maintaining the inflammatory process and exactly this cell population is increased in the SF of JIA patients [1, 5]. We thus analyzed the role of CREMα within this population of CD4$^+$ cells. We found enhanced expression of CREMα in CD161$^+$CD4$^+$ PBMC and of SFMC from JIA patients compared to their CD161$^-$ counterparts (Fig. 3a). Treatment of HC PBMCs with SF upregulated CD161$^+$CD4$^+$IL-17$^+$ cells in the presence of CREM, while knock down of CREM inhibited the SF induced expression of this inflammatory subset (Fig. 3b). Unfortunately, in contrast to humans, mice do not express CD161 in cytokine-producing T cells and therefore we could not validate these data in vivo. Nevertheless, we performed a T cell dependent arthritis model in mice to analyze how CREM signaling in T cells influences the fate of an inflammatory arthritis.

To this end, we transferred CD4$^+$CD25$^-$ T cells from either OTII-CREM$^{-/-}$ or control OTII-wild-type (WT) mice into RAG$^{-/-}$ mice and immunized the mice with OVA to expand the T cells (Fig. 3c). On day 7 we induced arthritis by injecting cationic OVA-peptide into the right knee. As seen in Fig. 3d, transfer of CREM$^{-/-}$ T cells resulted in a faster remission of arthritis and significantly lower histological scores for inflammation and tissue destruction (Fig. 3d-f).

Discussion

For the first time we provide evidence that CREM plays a role in T cell dysregulation in oligoarticular JIA patients. Our conclusion is based on several levels of evidence. First, we observed enhanced expression of CREM in SF T cells from JIA patients. Enhanced expression of CREM could also be induced after ex vivo culture of PBMCs from healthy donors with SF from JIA patients. CREM expression is also enhanced in SLE T cells and as well as SF Sera from SLE patients also induces CREM expression [26]. However, expression of CREM is regulated by complex mechanism and by at least two different promoter regions that are differentially activated in SLE and normal T cells [10]. Further studies will show which promoter regions are activated by SF. Second, we found enhanced expression of CREM in CD4$^+$CD161$^+$ cells, which are known producers of inflammatory cytokines. Third, incubation with SF induced expression of IFN-γ, IL-17 and FoxP3 in T cells, which could be reversed by knock down of CREM. Finally deficiency of CREM in T cells ameliorated OVA induced arthritis in vivo.

There are some limitations to our study. While our data suggest that CREM directly regulates CD4$^+$CD161$^+$ T cells in human JIA, we cannot fully transfer this observation to our in vivo arthritis model as the murine analog of CD161 has not yet been identified. Furthermore, we could only analyze a small number of patients and further work is required to confirm our data.

Regarding the pathophysiology of JIA, the inflammatory reaction within the joint is initiated by cells of the innate immune system like neutrophils and macrophages, but cells of the adaptive immune system like B cells and T cells play a dominant role in perpetuating the disease. Pathogenic T cells within the joint display a mixed Th17/Th1 phenotype characterized by the production of IL-17 as well as IFN-γ and expression of both lineage transcription factors T-bet and RORγT [2].

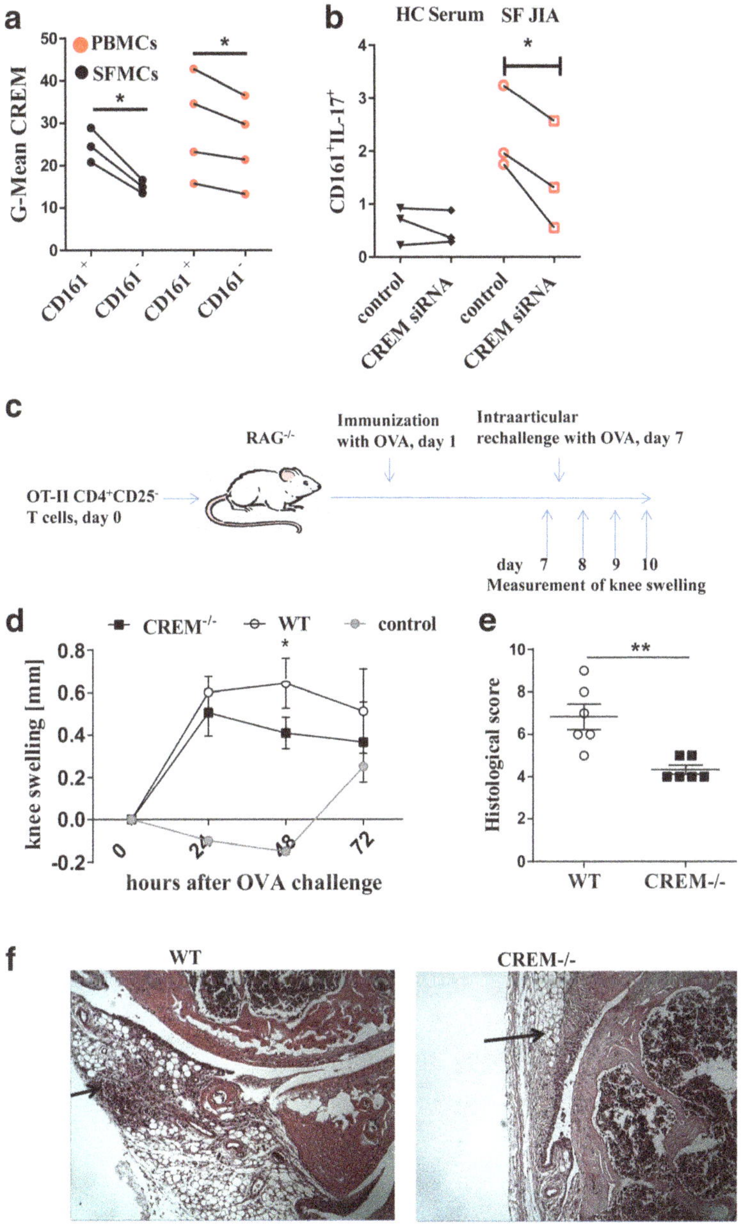

Fig. 3 CREM regulates T cell inflammation in arthritis. **a** Geometric (G)-Mean of CREM expression in PBMCs and SFMCs from JIA patients, two-tailed paired t-tests were used to calculate p-values. **b** PBMCs and SFMCs from JIA patients were transfected with control siRNA or with CREM siRNA and cultivated in RPMI for 24 h and percentages of $CD161^{+}IL\text{-}17^{+}$ in $CD3^{+}$ T cells after restimulation with P/I in the presence of Brefeldin were determined, two-tailed paired t-tests were used to calculate p-values. **c** Graphic showing T cell mediated arthritis model. **d** Knee swelling of $RAG^{-/-}$ mice after adoptive transfer of OT-II cells either from WT or from $CREM^{-/-}$ mice, immunization with OVA and subsequent intraarticular injection of cationic ovalbumin. **e** Histological scores of arthritis-induced knee joints, Mann Whitney test were used to calculate *p*-values. **f** Hematoxylin and eosin staining of knee joint sections (arrow on the loft shows cellular infiltration, arrow on the right shows thickening of the synovial membrane)

Furthermore, in humans, these cells display a high expression of CD161, low expression of the TCR ζ chain (CD247) and low expression of IL-2 as well as low response to stimulation with IL-2 [27]. In addition, the TCR ζ chain has been established recently as an independent risk factor for JIA in linkage analysis studies [28]. The same is true for the IL2- receptor [29]. Interestingly, despite abundance of pathogenic T cells within the inflamed joint, the expression of detectable IL-2 within the joint is negligible [30]. This could be the result of decreased expression of IL-2 by the Th17 cells [27] or of consumption by the abundant regulatory T cells, which are dependent on IL-2. CREMα has been shown before to downregulate the TCR ζ chain and the

IL-2 expression in SLE while enhancing secretion of IL-17 and IL-21 [12, 13, 16, 20, 31] and as shown here also dysregulates T cell responses in JIA as shown by our siRNA and in vivo studies. We therefore suggest that CREM regulates T cells in JIA by several mechanisms, which similarly to consequences of CREM overexpression in SLE contributes to an aberrant cytokine-expression profile and an enhanced occurrence of Th17 cells. How exactly CREM is activated in the synovium remains to be elucidated.

Recent studies underline the importance of a balance between inflammatory T cells and Tregs within inflamed joints [32] and CREM mediated mechanism might have potential as a therapeutic strategy for Th17-driven autoimmune diseases. It is therefore noticeable that genetic or pharmacologic inhibition of calcium/calmodulin-dependent protein kinase IV (CaMK4) reduced Il-17 transcription through decreased activation of CREMα [21]. Furthermore a recent clinical trial demonstrated the safety and efficacy of low-dose IL-2 treatment on SLE [33]. This shows that there are already advances to re-establish CREM-mediated dysregulations in T cells in autoimmune diseases and our study suggests that it would be valuable to further analyze the therapeutic potential of these mechanisms in JIA as well.

Conclusion

T cell dysregulations critically contribute to ongoing inflammation in juvenile arthritis joints. By identifying CREM as a transcriptional activator that contributes to increased occurrence of inflammatory effector T cells within the joints; our study puts CREMα in a central role within JIA and makes it a possible attractive target for pharmacological intervention.

Abbreviations

CREM: cAMP responsive element modulator; HC: Healthy control; JIA: Juvenile idiopathic arthritis,; OVA: Ovalbumin; PB: Peripheral blood; PBMC: Peripheral blood mononuclear cells; SF: Synovial fluid

Funding

HM was supported in part by National Institutes of Health Grant Award Numbers: National Institute of Arthritis and Musculoskeletal and Skin Diseases P30 AR070549, Eunice Kennedy Shriver National Institute of Child Health and Human Development R01 HD089928, National Institute of Allergy and Infectious Diseases (NIAID) U01 AI130830. The content is solely the responsibility of the authors and does not necessarily represent the official views of the National Institutes of Health. LW is supported by the NIHR Biomedical Research Centre at Great Ormond Street Hospital for Children NHS Foundation Trust; HM and LW were supported by grants from SPARKS UK reference 08ICH09.

The study was supported by a grant of the Novartis foundation.

Authors' contributions

All authors were involved in drafting the article or revising it critically for important intellectual content, and all authors approved the final version to be published. Dr. T had full access to all of the data in the study and takes responsibility for the integrity of the data and the accuracy of the data analysis. KO, HN, HM, PK and AS contributed to the acquisition of data, analysis and interpretation of data. VW, DF and LW contributed to the acquisition of samples, contributed to study design and provided critical feedback on intellectual content. KT conceived the study and wrote the paper.

Competing interests

The authors declare that they have no competing interests.

Author details

[1]Department of Pediatrics, Medical Faculty, RWTH Aachen, Pauwelsstr. 30, D-52074 Aachen, Germany. [2]Center for Autoimmune Genomics & Etiology, Cincinnati Children's Hospital Medical Center, Cincinnati, OH, USA. [3]Department of Pediatrics, University of Cincinnati, College of Medicine, Cincinnati, OH, USA. [4]Department of Pediatric Rheumatology and Immunology, University Hospital Muenster, Muenster, Germany. [5]Institute of Virology, Westfaelische Wilhelms University, 48149 Muenster, Germany. [6]Arthritis Research UK Centre for Adolescent Rheumatology at UCL UCLH and GOSH, London, UK. [7]UCL GOS Institute of Child Health, University College London, London, UK. [8]NIHR- Great Ormond Street Hospital Biomedical Research Centre (BRC), London, UK.

References

1. Nistala K, Adams S, Cambrook H, Ursu S, Olivito B, de Jager W, et al. Th17 plasticity in human autoimmune arthritis is driven by the inflammatory environment. Proc Natl Acad Sci U S A. 2010;107(33):14751–6.
2. Pesenacker AM, Bending D, Ursu S, Wu Q, Nistala K, Wedderburn LR. CD161 defines the subset of FoxP3+ T cells capable of producing proinflammatory cytokines. Blood. 2013;121(14):2647–58.
3. Duurland CL, Brown CC, O'Shaughnessy RF, Wedderburn LR. CD161(+) Tconv and CD161(+) Treg share a transcriptional and functional phenotype despite limited overlap in TCRbeta repertoire. Front Immunol. 2017;8:103.
4. Cosmi L, De Palma R, Santarlasci V, Maggi L, Capone M, Frosali F, et al. Human interleukin 17-producing cells originate from a CD161+CD4+ T cell precursor. J Exp Med. 2008;205(8):1903–16.
5. Cosmi L, Cimaz R, Maggi L, Santarlasci V, Capone M, Borriello F, et al. Evidence of the transient nature of the Th17 phenotype of CD4+CD161+ T cells in the synovial fluid of patients with juvenile idiopathic arthritis. Arthritis Rheum. 2011;63(8):2504–15.
6. Kryczek I, Wu K, Zhao E, Wei S, Vatan L, Szeliga W, et al. IL-17+ regulatory T cells in the microenvironments of chronic inflammation and cancer. J Immunol. 2011;186(7):4388–95.
7. Dominguez-Villar M, Baecher-Allan CM, Hafler DA. Identification of T helper type 1-like, Foxp3+ regulatory T cells in human autoimmune disease. Nat Med. 2011;17(6):673–5.
8. Beriou G, Costantino CM, Ashley CW, Yang L, Kuchroo VK, Baecher-Allan C, et al. IL-17-producing human peripheral regulatory T cells retain suppressive function. Blood. 2009;113(18):4240–9.
9. Afzali B, Mitchell PJ, Edozie FC, Povoleri GA, Dowson SE, Demandt L, et al. CD161 expression characterizes a subpopulation of human regulatory T cells that produces IL-17 in a STAT3-dependent manner. Eur J Immunol. 2013;43(8):2043–54.
10. Rauen T, Benedyk K, Juang YT, Kerkhoff C, Kyttaris VC, Roth J, et al. A novel intronic cAMP response element modulator (CREM) promoter is regulated by activator protein-1 (AP-1) and accounts for altered activation-induced CREM expression in T cells from patients with systemic lupus erythematosus. J Biol Chem. 2011;286(37):32366–72.
11. Rauen T, Hedrich CM, Tenbrock K, Tsokos GC. cAMP responsive element modulator: a critical regulator of cytokine production. Trends Mol Med. 2013;19(4):262–9.
12. Tenbrock K, Juang YT, Tolnay M, Tsokos GC. The cyclic adenosine 5'-monophosphate response element modulator suppresses IL-2 production in stimulated T cells by a chromatin-dependent mechanism. J Immunol. 2003;170(6):2971–6.

13. Tenbrock K, Kyttaris VC, Ahlmann M, Ehrchen JM, Tolnay M, Melkonyan H, et al. The cyclic AMP response element modulator regulates transcription of the TCR zeta-chain. J Immunol. 2005;175(9):5975–80.
14. Tenbrock K, Juang YT, Gourley MF, Nambiar MP, Tsokos GC. Antisense cyclic adenosine 5'-monophosphate response element modulator up-regulates IL-2 in T cells from patients with systemic lupus erythematosus. J Immunol. 2002;169(8):4147–52.
15. Rauen T, Hedrich CM, Juang YT, Tenbrock K, Tsokos GC. cAMP-responsive element modulator (CREM)alpha protein induces interleukin 17A expression and mediates epigenetic alterations at the interleukin-17A gene locus in patients with systemic lupus erythematosus. J Biol Chem. 2011;286(50): 43437–46.
16. Lippe R, Ohl K, Varga G, Rauen T, Crispin JC, Juang YT, et al. CREMalpha overexpression decreases IL-2 production, induces a T(H)17 phenotype and accelerates autoimmunity. J Mol Cell Biol. 2012;4(2):121–3.
17. Ohl K, Wiener A, Schippers A, Wagner N, Tenbrock K. IL-2 treatment reverses effects of CREMalpha-overexpressing T cells in autoimmune-prone mice. Clin Exp Immunol. 2015;181(1):76–86.
18. Verjans E, Ohl K, Yu Y, Lippe R, Schippers A, Wiener A, et al. Overexpression of CREMalpha in T cells aggravates lipopolysaccharide-induced acute lung injury. J Immunol. 2013;191(3):1316–23.
19. Verjans E, Ohl K, Reiss LK, van Wijk F, Toncheva AA, Wiener A, et al. The cAMP response element modulator (CREM) regulates TH2 mediated inflammation. Oncotarget. 2015;6(36):38538–51.
20. Ohl K, Wiener A, Lippe R, Schippers A, Zorn C, Roth J, et al. CREM alpha enhances IL-21 production in T cells in vivo and in vitro. Front Immunol. 2016;7:618.
21. Koga T, Hedrich CM, Mizui M, Yoshida N, Otomo K, Lieberman LA, et al. CaMK4-dependent activation of AKT/mTOR and CREM-alpha underlies autoimmunity-associated Th17 imbalance. J Clin Invest. 2014;124(5):2234–45.
22. Stittrich AB, Haftmann C, Sgouroudis E, Kuhl AA, Hegazy AN, Panse I, et al. The microRNA miR-182 is induced by IL-2 and promotes clonal expansion of activated helper T lymphocytes. Nat Immunol. 2010;11(11):1057–62.
23. Blendy JA, Kaestner KH, Weinbauer GF, Nieschlag E, Schutz G. Severe impairment of spermatogenesis in mice lacking the CREM gene. Nature. 1996;380(6570):162–5.
24. Nistala K, Moncrieffe H, Newton KR, Varsani H, Hunter P, Wedderburn LR. Interleukin-17-producing T cells are enriched in the joints of children with arthritis, but have a reciprocal relationship to regulatory T cell numbers. Arthritis Rheum. 2008;58(3):875–87.
25. de Kleer IM, Wedderburn LR, Taams LS, Patel A, Varsani H, Klein M, et al. CD4+CD25bright regulatory T cells actively regulate inflammation in the joints of patients with the remitting form of juvenile idiopathic arthritis. J Immunol. 2004;172(10):6435–43.
26. Juang YT, Wang Y, Solomou EE, Li Y, Mawrin C, Tenbrock K, et al. Systemic lupus erythematosus serum IgG increases CREM binding to the IL-2 promoter and suppresses IL-2 production through CaMKIV. J Clin Invest. 2005;115(4):996–1005.
27. Santarlasci V, Maggi L, Capone M, Querci V, Beltrame L, Cavalieri D, et al. Rarity of human T helper 17 cells is due to retinoic acid orphan receptor-dependent mechanisms that limit their expansion. Immunity. 2012;36(2):201–14.
28. Hinks A, Cobb J, Sudman M, Eyre S, Martin P, Flynn E, et al. Investigation of rheumatoid arthritis susceptibility loci in juvenile idiopathic arthritis confirms high degree of overlap. Ann Rheum Dis. 2012;71(7):1117–21.
29. Hinks A, Ke X, Barton A, Eyre S, Bowes J, Worthington J, et al. Association of the IL2RA/CD25 gene with juvenile idiopathic arthritis. Arthritis Rheum. 2009;60(1):251–7.
30. Lepore L, Pennesi M, Saletta S, Perticarari S, Presani G, Prodan M. Study of IL-2, IL-6, TNF alpha, IFN gamma and beta in the serum and synovial fluid of patients with juvenile chronic arthritis. Clin Exp Rheumatol. 1994;12(5):561–5.
31. Ohl K, Wiener A, Schippers A, Wagner N, Tenbrock K. Interleukin-2 treatment reverses effects of cAMP-responsive element modulator alpha-over-expressing T cells in autoimmune-prone mice. Clin Exp Immunol. 2015; 181(1):76–86.
32. Maggi L, Cosmi L, Simonini G, Annunziato F, Cimaz R. T cell subpopulations in juvenile idiopathic arthritis and their modifications after biotherapies. Autoimmun Rev. 2016;15(12):1141–4.
33. von Spee-Mayer C, Siegert E, Abdirama D, Rose A, Klaus A, Alexander T, et al. Low-dose interleukin-2 selectively corrects regulatory T cell defects in patients with systemic lupus erythematosus. Ann Rheum Dis. 2016;75(7): 1407–15.

12

MBL2 gene polymorphism rs1800450 and rheumatic fever with and without rheumatic heart disease: an Egyptian pilot study

Maher Hassan Gomaa[1*], Shawkey Sadik Ali[1], Aya Mohamed Fattouh[2], Hala Salah Hamza[2] and Mohamed Mohamed Badr[1]

Abstract

Background: Rheumatic fever (RF) is the result of an autoimmune response to pharyngitis caused by infection with *Streptococcus pyogenes*. RF is most prevalent in Africa and the Middle East. Rheumatic heart disease (RHD) is the most serious complication of RF. Mannose-binding lectin 2 gene (MBL2) has been reported to be correlated with different cardiac conditions. In Egyptian patients as a new studied ethnic population, it is the first time to evaluate the association between MBL2 gene polymorphism rs1800450 and RF with and without RHD.

Methods: One hundred and sixty RF patients (80 with RHD and 80 without RHD) and eighty healthy ethnically matched controls were studied. MBL2 (rs1800450) was genotyped by real-time PCR using TaqMan® allele discrimination assay. The MBL level was measured by ELISA. Westergren erythrocytes sedimentation rate (ESR), anti-streptolysin O titer (ASOT), C-reactive protein (CRP) and complements (C3 and C4) were determined.

Results: The AA genotype with high production of MBL was associated with increased risk of RHD more than the B allele carrying subjects. However, MBL2 genotype related to the low production of MBL was more frequently observed in those patients without RHD.

Conclusions: Our results suggested the involvement of MBL2 (rs1800450) polymorphism and its protein in RHD pathogenesis. Also, it might be a promising future strategy to utilize this polymorphism to help differentiate patients with RHD from those without RHD.

Keywords: Rheumatic fever, Rheumatic heart disease, MBL2 gene polymorphism

Background

Globally, rheumatic heart disease (RHD) is still the leading cause of acquired heart disease among the young [1]. Many echocardiographic screening studies put the prevalence of RHD at 8–57 out of 1000 children meaning that the prevalence may rest closer to 62–78 million individuals worldwide with up to 1.4 million deaths each year [2, 3]. A large African study indicated that RHD prevails as the most frequent cause of heart failure (HF) among children and young adults [4].

Despite being preventable and imminently treatable disease, sadly, RHD can go undetected until patients' presentation with debilitating HF. At this stage, surgery is the only possible treatment option [5]. Patients living in poor countries have limited or no access to expensive heart surgery. To prevent these serious complications, it is very important to find out the most patients vulnerable to RHD to receive their further medical follow-up.

The main hypothesis for RF development is an autoimmune reaction resulting from molecular mimicry between streptococcal antigen and cardiac, articular and central nervous system proteins [6].

The innate immune response provides the first line of defense against *Streptococcus pyogenes* infections, in the

* Correspondence: mahergomaa30@yahoo.com
[1]Biochemistry Department-Faculty of Pharmacy (Boys), Al-Azhar University, Almokhayam Aldaem Street, 6th Province - 13465 Nasr City, Cairo, Egypt
Full list of author information is available at the end of the article

case of RF, with complement cascade activation. Mannose-binding lectin (MBL) is an acute phase inflammatory protein and functions as a soluble pathogen recognition receptor. It binds to a wide variety of sugars on the surface of pathogens and plays a major role in innate immunity due to its ability to opsonize pathogens, enhancing their phagocytosis and activating the complement cascade via the lectin pathway [7]. N-acetylglucosamine, one of the main constituents of the streptococci cell wall [8] and of human heart valves [9] is a strong ligand for MBL.

Upon binding of the MBL's higher-order oligomers to the identified carbohydrates moieties, they form complexes with MBL-associated serine proteases (MASPs), which help in activation of the complement system through the lectin pathway and generation of multiple opsonic and inflammatory fragments, which ultimately result in phagocytosis and several immune-mediated reactions [7].

The MBL2 gene is located on the chromosome 10 and comprises four exons. Inherited MBL insufficiency, which results in impaired innate immune function and enhanced susceptibility to infection, is essentially caused by three structural variants in exon 1. These three polymorphisms alter significantly the serum concentrations of MBL, with the variant alleles (D, B, C) resulting from mutations in codons 52, 54 and 57, respectively. The variant alleles are collectively named O, and the normal allele, A. The allele D changes CGT to TGT, changing arginine to cysteine (p.Arg52Cys). The B allele changes GGC to GAC and causes an amino acid replacement of glycine to aspartic acid (p.Gly54Asp) while the allele C changes GGA to GAA substituting glycine to glutamic acid (p.Gly57Glu) [7, 10].

Single nucleotide polymorphism (SNP) B, as it designates an exchange of the glycine in the glycine-rich motif, is associated with a decreased stability of the collagenous region of the protein. Although this MBL2 variant is indeed able to form multimers [11], they are more rapidly degraded and exist primarily as lower order oligomers. Functionally, they have a lower binding capacity to N-acetylglucosamine and do not activate complement [12], presumably due to lacking the capability of binding to MASPs [13].

The information surrounding the role of MBL2 polymorphism in RF pathogenesis remains insufficient. Few previous studies on limited ethnic population showed a direct variation about the MBL2 genotypes associated with the risk of RF and RHD [10]. Based on these findings, the current study was the 1st to demonstrate the association between MBL2 gene polymorphism and RF in Egyptians of different ethnic groups than the most of the studies and as a part of North Africa and the Middle East. And to find if there is a clinical value for this SNP to be predictive for RF complications.

Methods

Patients and control

This study was conducted on 160 patients with a history of RF chosen from outpatient RF Clinic, Abol-Reich Hospital, Kasr Al-Aini School of Medicine; Cairo University at the period between January 2015 and June 2015. RF patients were divided into 80 patients with RHD and 80 patients without RHD. Our patients were cases diagnosed, 4 to 12 months before enrolled in the study and not acute RF. All included patients were on monthly intramuscular injection of long-acting penicillin (benzathine penicillin) since their first diagnosis. No one required valvular heart surgery as no one was in HF. The control group included eighty healthy subjects matched with the patients for the ethnic, geographic and socioeconomic background. The study was approved by ethical committee of Abol-Reich Hospital. A written informed consent was obtained from all study subjects or their parents. The diagnosis of RF was made using the modified Jones criteria [14]. Patients presenting infective endocarditis, congenital heart diseases or other inflammatory or immunological disorders were excluded from this study. All the patients were subjected to complete history taking, thorough clinical examination as well as revision of their pre-registered data which included their laboratory investigations. Echocardiography was performed in all patients to assess the valve affection and all patients with RHD had a history of mild to moderate mitral valve regurge. The diagnosis of RHD was based on World Heart Federation criteria [15]. Overnight fasting blood samples from control and all patients were obtained. Each blood sample was distributed into three tubes; the first tube contained citrate, used for determination of 1st-hour erythrocytes sedimentation rate (ESR) using Westergren method [16]. The second tube was allowed to clot for 30 min and then centrifuged at 4000 rpm for 10 min. The obtained sera were used for determination of anti-streptolysin O titer (ASOT), C-reactive protein (CRP), complements (C3 and C4) by turbidimetric immunoassay method using commercially available kits (BioSystems S.A., Costa Brava, Barcelona, Spain). Serum MBL concentration was measured by enzyme-linked immunosorbent assay (ELISA) using commercial kits (Boster Biological Technology Co., Ltd., Pleasanton, USA) according to manufacturer's instructions and recommendations.

Genetic analysis

The third tube contained EDTA, used for genomic DNA (gDNA) extraction and purification using Gene JET™ Whole Blood DNA Purification Mini Kit (Thermo Fisher Scientific Inc., USA) and then stored at − 80 °C until analyzed. The gDNA concentration and purity (A260/280) for each sample was determined using NANODROP™ 2000 spectrophotometer (Thermo Fisher Scientific Inc., USA). The extracted DNA was genotyped for MBL2 (AB; codon 54, rs1800450) exon 1 polymorphism by StepOne™ (Applied Biosystems, CA, USA) real-time polymerase chain reaction (PCR) using TaqMan® allele discrimination assay (Applied Biosystems, CA, USA). Probes and primers were designed by Applied Biosystems (ID: C_2336609_20), context sequence TGGTTCCCCCTTTTCTCCCTTGGTG[**C**/**T**]C ATCACGCCCATCTTTGCCTGGGAA. Further details are restricted to Applied Biosystems and cannot be provided. TaqMan PCR was performed in a total volume of 20 μl (20 ng of DNA, 10 μl TaqMan master mix and 0.5 μl TaqMan® allele discrimination assay) placed in 48-well plates. Thermal cycling conditions were initiated by AmpliTaq Gold® polymerase activation at 95 °C for 10 min, followed by 45 cycles (denaturation at 95 °C for 15 s, then annealing/extension at 60 °C for 1 min). After PCR amplification, an endpoint plate read was carried out using the Applied Biosystems real-time PCR system. The fluorescence measurements that made during the plate read used by the sequence detection system software to plot the fluorescence values based on the signals from each well. The plotted fluorescence signals indicated which alleles are in each sample.

Statistical analysis

GraphPad Prism 6.0 (GraphPad software 2010, San Diego, USA) was used for analysis. Data of the groups were analyzed by D'Agostino and Pearson omnibus normality test to determine the normal distribution pattern. Normally distributed variables are presented as mean ± SE. Skewed distributed variables are presented as median (inter-quartile range). All results were compared by Kruskal-Wallis test (with multiple comparisons using Dunn's test). Correlations between variables were tested using the Spearman's correlation coefficients. The genotypes distribution for polymorphism was analyzed for deviation from the Hardy–Weinberg equilibrium (HWE) and any deviation between the observed and expected frequencies was tested for significance using the χ^2 test. Differences in genotype and allele frequencies between groups were analyzed using the Fisher's exact tests. In addition, we calculated the odds ratios (ORs) and 95% confidence intervals (CIs) regarding the presence RHD with respect to the existence of the polymorphism. All statistical tests were two-sided. A *p*-value < 0.05 was considered to be statistically significant. The receiver operator characteristic (ROC) curve was constructed to obtain the diagnostic accuracy, cutoff values, sensitivity and specificity for MBL. As an accuracy indicator, the area under the curve (AUC) was used for assessment of the diagnostic performance.

Results

Regarding ASOT, 1st-h ESR, CRP and C3, significantly increased values were obtained in RF patients without RHD as compared to control. Also, RF patients with RHD showed significantly increased values concerning to 1st-h ESR, CRP, C3 and MBL as compared to controls. In addition, MBL showed significantly increased values in RF patients with RHD as compared to both patients without RHD and controls. However, a significant decrease of CRP was obtained in RF patients with RHD as compared to those without RHD as shown in Table 1.

Using ROC curve analysis, we found that the critical serum level of MBL associated with the risk of RHD was 1383 ng/ml (AUC = 0.74, SE = 0.037, 95% CI = 0.67 to 0.82, p = < 0.0001, 73.3% sensitivity and 80% specificity).

The RF patients showed negative significant correlations between (MBL) against ASOT (r – 0.22, p 0.013), 1st-hr ESR (r – 0.2, p 0.026), and CRP (r – 0.25, p 0.005). However, MBL showed negative insignificant correlations with C3 (r – 0.03, p 0.757) and C4 (r 0.016, p 0.86).

The genotype distribution for the studied SNP (AB; codon 54, rs1800450) showed no deviation from HWE. Higher frequency of the AA genotype was present in patients with RHD when compared to controls. However, a lower frequency of AB and BB genotypes was observed in RHD

Table 1 Characteristics of the 240 study subjects

Characteristics		Controls (*n* = 80)	RF (*n* = 160)	
			Without RHD (*n* = 80)	With RHD (*n* = 80)
Gender	Female n (%)	48 (60.0)	46 (57.5)	48 (60.0)
	Male n (%)	32 (40.0)	34 (42.5)	32 (40.0)
Age (years)		15.2 ± 0.29	14.5 ± 0.43	14.3 ± 0.33
ASOT (IU/ml)		29.0 (11.3–97.0)	116 (26.3–172) [a]	63.0 (19.0–127)
1st-h ESR (mm/h)		6.00 (5.00–8.00)	21.5 (13.25–31.50) [a]	16.5 (11.00–25.0) [a]
CRP (mg/l)		2.90 (1.70–3.87)	6.55 (5.75–7.37) [a]	4.30 (3.10–6.25) [a, b]
C3 (mg/dl)		108.0 (98.0–122)	122.5 (111–136) [a]	127.5 (113–139) [a]
C4 (mg/dl)		30.5 (21.0–36.8)	31.5 (27.3–37.8)	32.0 (26.0–36.0)
MBL (ng/ml)		450.6 (290.2–563.1)	591.2 (478.0–1005)	1614 (1419–1945) [a, b]

Data are presented as n (%), mean ± SE or median (inter-quartile range)
[a] significant from control group, [b] significant from RF without RHD group

patients as compared to healthy controls. In addition, a lower frequency of the B allele was observed in RF patients with RHD when compared to the controls. Patients without RHD showed insignificant differences in the frequency of all genotypes and B allele when compared to controls, as illustrated in Tables 2 and 3.

In this study, RF group was classified according to the MBL2 gene (rs1800450) genotypes into subjects carrying AA genotype and subjects carrying AB+BB genotypes. As shown in Table 4, regarding C4, a significant difference was found between AA of RF group as compared to AB+BB. Looking at the MBL level, the genotype AA in RF group was associated with highly significant concentrations of MBL in serum as compared to individuals carrying the B allele (AB+BB) in the same group. In genotype AB+BB individuals, the MBL levels were reduced 4 times than AA genotype.

Discussion

Despite the vital role of the lectin pathway in complement activation and host defense against infection and autoimmunity, studies on the significance of components of this pathway in RF and RHD are still scarce [17, 18].

In the current study, regarding ASOT, significantly increased values were found in RF group without RHD as compared to control, which was confirmed by Sainani and Sainani, [19] who reported that the significant increase of ASOT in RF group as compared to control may be explained by recent streptococcal infection in RF patients.

In agreement with Kumar [20] and Farghaly et al., [21], concerning the 1st-h ESR and CRP, there were significantly increased values in RF group as compared to control. These elevations may be explained by the ongoing inflammatory nature of the disease as suggested by Gölbasi et al., [22], Veasy and Tani, [23] and Chiu-Braga et al., [24].

Given the level of C3, it was significantly increased in RF group than the control subjects which is in agreement with Schafranski et al., [25, 26] who suggested the presence of continuous inflammation with probable complement activation. The C3 is an acute phase protein which significantly increases in response to infections or to an inflammatory reaction.

However, the involvement of complement system in RF and RHD has been shown in different studies. Antibodies found in RF patients' sera that show molecular mimicry between streptococcal and human antigens were able to cause human fibroblasts lyses in vitro in the presence of complement [25].

These results confirmed the involvement of complement system components in the pathogenesis of RF as described by Schafranski et al., [26].

As the best to our knowledge, this is the 1st study in Egypt evaluating MBL levels and MBL2 genotype (A/B; codon 54, rs1800450) in the development of RF.

In the current study, the level of MBL was significantly higher in patients with RHD than both controls and patients without RHD, indicating the high MBL levels could be a cause of undesirable complement activation in carditis patients, contributing to the pathogenesis of rheumatic cardiomyopathy [25]. This result may encourage further studies on anti-MBL as an interesting alternative therapy for patients with this disease.

The negative significant correlation between serum MBL and ASOT in this study could be explained by the subsequent triggering of MBL to the complement system that may be responsible for either a direct complement-dependent killing of the bacteria or increased phagocytosis through the opsonization [27].

Table 2 Distribution of MBL2 genotypes (rs1800450) in patients with history of RF and controls

	Controls (n = 80)	RF (n = 160)		p	OR	95% CI
		Without RHD (n = 80)	With RHD (n = 80)			
Genotypes						
AA n (%)	44 (55)	42 (52.5)	69 (86.25)	1.00 [a]	0.90	0.37–2.17
				0.0003 [b]	5.13*	2.10–12.5
AB n (%)	24 (30)	34 (42.5)	11 (13.75)	0.50 [a]	1.48	0.57–3.84
				0.02 [b]	0.29*	0.11–75.0
BB n (%)	12 (15)	4 (5)	0 (0)	0.26 [a]	0.29	0.06–1.58
				0.001 [b]	0.03*	0.002–0.60
HWE	$\chi^2 = 3.3, p > 0.05$	$\chi^2 = 0.38, p > 0.05$	$\chi^2 = 0.44, p > 0.05$			

OR of AA: by comparison between AA versus (AB+BB) (dominant model)
OR of AB: by comparison between AB versus AA (co-dominant model)
OR of BB: by comparison between BB versus (AA+AB) (recessive model)
[a] RF without RHD versus controls. [b] RF with RHD versus controls
* significant difference at $p < 0.05$

Table 3 Distribution of MBL2 alleles (rs1800450) in patients with history of RF and controls

	Controls (n = 80)	RF (n = 160)		p	OR	95% CI
		Without RHD (n = 80)	With RHD (n = 80)			
Allele						
A n (%)	112 (70)	118 (73.8)	149 (93.1)			
B n (%)	48 (30)	42 (26.2)	11 (6.9)	0.720 [a]	0.83	0.42–1.65
				0.0001[b]	0.17*	0.08–0.37

a RF without RHD versus controls. [b] RF with RHD versus controls
* significant difference at $p < 0.05$

These findings confirmed the positive impact of MBL in streptococcal innate immune defense.

The current study showed a significant negative correlation between MBL and ESR that may be explained by either the expression of functional MBL protein is largely genetically determined by polymorphisms found in the first exon of the structural gene [28] or by the characteristic pattern of ESR in rheumatic disease [29].

Our results disclosed a negative significant correlation between MBL and CRP levels that may be related to the following two different functional mechanisms: 1) MBL is involved in the lectin pathway while CRP is involved in the classical complement activation pathway. 2) Although, both MBL and CRP have a common terminal pathway, MBL mainly plays a role in the early responses of the host innate immune system, while CRP mainly plays a role in the late stage of adaptive immune responses [30].

However, in the current study, there were insignificant correlations between C3, C4 and MBL levels, indicating that elevated MBL concentration might be an independent event [31].

In the present study, the homozygous wild genotype AA was more prevalent in patients with RHD than healthy controls. In addition, the frequency of variant allele B was significantly lower in patients with RHD than controls. These findings were in accordance with

Table 4 Biochemical and demographic characteristics of RF patients according to MBL2 gene (rs1800450) genotypes

	RF patients	
	AA	AB+BB
Age (years)	14.44 ± 0.30	14.35 ± 0.55
ASOT (IU/ml)	64.5 (19–139.5)	113 (28–189)
1st-h ESR (mm/h)	17 (11–25)	23.5 (14–42.25)
CRP (mg/l)	5.1 (3.5–6.8)	6.2 (5.1–7.9)
C3 (mg/dl)	122.5 (112.8–135.0)	134 (110.8–146)
C4 (mg/dl)	32 (26–36)	25 (19.75–30.25) [a]
MBL (ng/ml)	1544 (1328–1906)	412.9 (338–501.2) [a]

Data are presented in mean ± SE or median (inter-quartile range)
[a] significant difference between AB+BB and AA at $p < 0.05$

Schafranski et al., [26] and Reason et al., [32], who concluded that the AA genotype could be involved in the development of cardiac manifestation in RF and the relationship was due to genetic effect of MBL2 polymorphisms rather than to an acute phase reaction. They also suggested a role for AA MBL2 genotype in the susceptibility to rheumatic carditis.

Many previous studies reported the association between MBL deficiency and risk of recurrent different infections [33]. While RF is a result of untreated streptococcal pharyngeal infection [6], previous studies [26, 32] and our results suggested an association between high MBL levels and RF that could be explained by the auto immune nature of RF and RHD [34]. Moreover, the role of MBL in the pathogenesis of rheumatic carditis could be related to the stressful conditions and the inflammatory processes of this carditis which could result in glycosylation of the self-cell surfaces [35]. In the heart valves of RF patients, there is a lot of myxomatous tissue which rich in hyaluronic acid. The N-acetylglucosamine is a major constituent of this hyaluronic acid. So, it can act as a ligand for the high levels of MBL that argue the chronic inflammatory activity present in the RHD individuals and contribute to valve injury through complement activation [9]. In addition, MBL may act as an immunomodulatory molecule, inducing a higher secretion of cytokines by macrophages [36].

Thus, the high blood concentrations of MBL could be considered as a double-edged sword molecule in the physiopathology of RF and rheumatic carditis, on one hand conferring protection against the initial infection by rheumatogenic *Streptococci* which is good, but on the other hand eliciting inflammation and complement dependent tissue damage in the chronic stage of the disease [10].

In contrast to the previous results, in an initial study in Chinese patients, there was no association between the B allele and RHD [37]. However, they suggested an assumed role for MBL deficiency in the progression of RHD, by considering their patient's age of onset of heart disease. The mean age of onset of cardiac symptoms of patients with the deficient B allele was significantly lower compared with patients with MBL2 genotype AA. These findings supported the hypothesis that MBL deficiency caused by the B allele could facilitate the development and accelerate the progression of RHD in younger people. In addition, higher levels of serum MBL in control group as compared to RHD patients were reported by Scalzi et al. [38] in Yemen population.

Also, in another study on patients from São Paulo, Brazil who suffered from chronic severe rheumatic aortic regurgitation (AR), Ramasawmy et al., [39] observed that B allele had similar frequencies in both AR patients and controls. They postulated that continuous exposure to

Table 5 Studies on MBL2 gene polymorphism in RHD

Polymorphism	Population	Polymorphism association	Refs
– 221 XY A (52C, 54G, 57G), O (52T, 54A, 57A)	Brazilian	RHD patients with mitral valve lesion showed an association with the A allele	[26, 32]
A (52C, 54G, 57G), O (52T, 54A, 57A)	Chinese	RHD displayed no association with the B allele	[37]
A (52C, 54G, 57G), O (52T, 54A, 57A)	Brazilian	RHD patients with AR displayed an association with the O allele	[39]

Streptococcus antigens in MBL-deficient individuals would lead to the subsequent abnormal immune response against heart proteins, leading to rheumatic AR. Studies done on MBL2 gene polymorphisms in RHD could be summarized in Table 5.

The contradiction between these results could be attributed to the difference in ethnicity, clinical manifestations of the studied subjects or due to the difference in the sample size.

In the present study, it was found that the AA genotype of RF patients was associated with high levels of MBL as compared to subjects carrying AB+BB in the same group indicating the suppressive effect of the mutant B allele on the levels of serum MBL that was in agreement with Reason et al., [32] and Schafranski et al., [26].

Some limitations should be considered when interpreting this study results. First, the sample size of the selected patients is not large enough to give a bigger picture about the distribution of MBL2 genotypes. So, further larger sample studies are recommended to verify these findings in Egyptians and other Mediterranean ethnics. Second, the selected SNP was based on the scientific literature, other SNPs may be more prominently implicated in our study included ethnics. Third, this study was independent on patients' follow-up while the long-term follow-up of patients with RF without valve consequence is necessary in order to identify which patients actually progress to RHD and the risk factors associated with it. Fourth, the age of our studied population may not allow a homogeneous representation of the population with RF.

Conclusions

The AA genotype associated with a higher production of MBL seems to represent a risk factor for the development of RHD. In addition, the highly significant frequencies of B allele in both controls and patients without RHD when compared to patients with RHD may indicate that the presence of B allele would be a protective factor against rheumatic carditis. In addition, this polymorphism could be suggested in the differentiation between RF patients with and without RHD.

Abbreviations

AR: Aortic regurgitation; ASOT: anti-streptolysine O titer; C3: complement 3; C4: complement 4; CRP: C-reactive protein; ESR: erythrocyte sedimentation rate; HF: heart failure; MASPs: MBL-associated serine proteases; MBL: mannose-binding lectin; RF: rheumatic fever; RHD: rheumatic heart disease; SNP: Single nucleotide polymorphism

Acknowledgements

We gratefully acknowledge the cooperation of the patients and their families and normal control individuals involved in this study.

Authors' contributions

MHG acquired the data. MHG and MMB carried out the molecular genetic studies. MHG did the literature search and the statistical analysis, and wrote the paper. SSA and HSH participated in study design and coordination and helped to draft the manuscript. MHG and AMF interpreted the data and were responsible for the manuscript preparation. All authors read and approved the final manuscript.

Competing interests

The authors declare that the research was conducted in the absence of any commercial or financial relationships that could be construed as a potential conflict of interest.

Author details

[1]Biochemistry Department-Faculty of Pharmacy (Boys), Al-Azhar University, Almokhayam Aldaem Street, 6th Province - 13465 Nasr City, Cairo, Egypt. [2]Department of Pediatrics, Kasr Al-Aini School of Medicine, Cairo University, P.O. Box 99, Manial El-Roda, Cairo 11553, Egypt.

References

1. Zuhlke L, Mirabel M, Marijon E. Congenital heart disease and rheumatic heart disease in Africa: recent advances and current priorities. Heart. 2013; 99(21):1554–61.
2. Zuhlke L, Mayosi BM. Echocardiographic screening for subclinical rheumatic heart disease remains a research tool pending studies of impact on prognosis. Curr Cardiol Rep. 2013;15(3):343.
3. Zuhlke L, Engel ME, Karthikeyan G, Rangarajan S, Mackie P, Cupido B, Mauff K, Islam S, Joachim A, Daniels R, et al. Characteristics, complications, and gaps in evidence-based interventions in rheumatic heart disease: the global rheumatic heart disease registry (the REMEDY study). Eur Heart J. 2015; 36(18):1115–1122a.
4. Damasceno A, Mayosi BM, Sani M, Ogah OS, Mondo C, Ojji D, Dzudie A, Kouam CK, Suliman A, Schrueder N. The causes, treatment, and outcome of acute heart failure in 1006 Africans from 9 countries: results of the sub-Saharan Africa survey of heart failure. Arch Intern Med. 2012;172(18):1386–94.
5. Nishimura RA, Otto CM, Bonow RO, Carabello BA, Erwin JP, Guyton RA, O'Gara PT, Ruiz CE, Skubas NJ, Sorajja P. 2014 AHA/ACC guideline for the management of patients with valvular heart disease. Circulation. 2014; 129(23):2440–92.
6. Carapetis JR, Beaton A, Cunningham MW, Guilherme L, Karthikeyan G, Mayosi BM, Sable C, Steer A, Wilson N, Wyber R: PRIMER. 2016.
7. Takahashi K, Ip WE, Michelow IC, Ezekowitz RA. The mannose-binding lectin: a prototypic pattern recognition molecule. Curr Opin Immunol. 2006;18(1):16–23.
8. Guilherme L, Ramasawmy R, Kalil J. Rheumatic fever and rheumatic heart disease: genetics and pathogenesis. Scand J Immunol. 2007;66(2-3):199–207.
9. Nayar S, Nayar PG, Cherian KM. Heart valve structure: a predisposing factor for rheumatic heart disease. Heart. 2006;92(8):1151–2.

10. Beltrame MH, Catarino SJ, Goeldner I, Boldt AB, de Messias-Reason IJ. The lectin pathway of complement and rheumatic heart disease. Front Pediatr. 2014;2(148):148.
11. Super M, Gillies SD, Foley S, Sastry K, Schweinle JE, Silverman VJ, Ezekowitz RA. Distinct and overlapping functions of allelic forms of human mannose binding protein. Nat Genet. 1992;2(1):50–5.
12. Garred P, Larsen F, Madsen HO, Koch C. Mannose-binding lectin deficiency–revisited. Mol Immunol. 2003;40(2–4):73–84.
13. Matsushita M, Ezekowitz RA, Fujita T. The Gly-54->Asp allelic form of human mannose-binding protein (MBP) fails to bind MBP-associated serine protease. *Biochem J.* 1995;311 (Pt 3)(3):1021–3.
14. Gewitz MH, Baltimore RS, Tani LY, Sable CA, Shulman ST, Carapetis J, Remenyi B, Taubert KA, Bolger AF, Beerman L, et al. Revision of the Jones criteria for the diagnosis of acute rheumatic fever in the era of Doppler echocardiography: a scientific statement from the American Heart Association. Circulation. 2015;131(20):1806–18.
15. Remenyi B, Wilson N, Steer A, Ferreira B, Kado J, Kumar K, Lawrenson J, Maguire G, Marijon E, Mirabel M, et al. World heart federation criteria for echocardiographic diagnosis of rheumatic heart disease–an evidence-based guideline. Nat Rev Cardiol. 2012;9(5):297–309.
16. Gilmour D, Sykes AJ. Westergren and Wintrobe methods of estimating ESR compared. Br Med J. 1951;2(4746):1496–7.
17. Neth O, Jack DL, Dodds AW, Holzel H, Klein NJ, Turner MW. Mannose-binding lectin binds to a range of clinically relevant microorganisms and promotes complement deposition. Infect Immun. 2000;68(2):688–93.
18. Boldt AB, Goeldner I, de Messias-Reason IJ. Relevance of the lectin pathway of complement in rheumatic diseases. Adv Clin Chem. 2012;56:105–53.
19. Sainani G, Sainani AR. Rheumatic fever-how relevant in India today? J Assoc Physicians India. 2006;54(N):42–7.
20. Kumar R. Spectrum of clinical presentation of rheumatic fever and rheumatic heart disease patients. Annals of International Medical and Dental Research. 2016;2(3):49–51.
21. Farghaly HS, Gad EF, Hassan A-EA, MAA A. Evaluation of Adrenomedullin levels in children with acute rheumatic Feverand its correlation to left ventricular function. American Journal of Medicine and Medical Sciences. 2017;7(2):74–8.
22. Gölbasi Z, Uçar Ö, Keles T, Sahin A, Çagli K, Çamsari A, Diker E, Aydogdu S. Increased levels of high sensitive C-reactive protein in patients with chronic rheumatic valve disease: evidence of ongoing inflammation. Eur J Heart Fail. 2002;4(5):593–5.
23. Veasy LG, Tani LY. A new look at acute rheumatic mitral regurgitation. Cardiol Young. 2005;15(6):568–77.
24. Chiu-Braga Y, Hayashi S, Schafranski M, Messias-Reason I. Further evidence of inflammation in chronic rheumatic valve disease (CRVD): high levels of advanced oxidation protein products (AOPP) and high sensitive C-reactive protein (hs-CRP). Int J Cardiol. 2006;109(2):275–6.
25. Schafranski M, Stier A, Nisihara R, MESSIAS-REASON I. Significantly increased levels of mannose-binding lectin (MBL) in rheumatic heart disease: a beneficial role for MBL deficiency. Clin Exp Immunol. 2004;138(3):521–5.
26. Schafranski MD, Pereira Ferrari L, Scherner D, Torres R, Jensenius JC, de Messias-Reason IJ. High-producing MBL2 genotypes increase the risk of acute and chronic carditis in patients with history of rheumatic fever. Mol Immunol. 2008;45(14):3827–31.
27. Yaroslavskyy O. The association of mannose-binding lectin with parameters of metabolic syndrome and early atherosclerosis markers. PhD, Universitat Regensburg. 2013;
28. Eddie Ip W, Takahashi K, Alan Ezekowitz R, Stuart LM. Mannose-binding lectin and innate immunity. Immunol Rev. 2009;230(1):9–21.
29. Neto R, Salles N, JFd C. The use of inflammatory laboratory tests in rheumatology. Rev Bras Reumatol. 2009;49(4):413–30.
30. Liu XH, Li Q, Zhang P, Su Y, Zhang XR, Sun Q. Serum mannose-binding lectin and C-reactive protein are potential biomarkers for patients with community-acquired pneumonia. Genet Test Mol Biomarkers. 2014;18(9):630–5.
31. Lappegård KT, Garred P, Jonasson L, Espevik T, Aukrust P, Yndestad A, Mollnes TE, Hovland A. A vital role for complement in heart disease. Mol Immunol. 2014;61(2):126–34.
32. Reason IJM, Schafranski MD, Jensenius JC, Steffensen R. The association between mannose-binding lectin gene polymorphism and rheumatic heart disease. Hum Immunol. 2006;67(12):991–8.
33. Heitzeneder S, Seidel M, Förster-Waldl E, Heitger A. Mannan-binding lectin deficiency—good news, bad news, doesn't matter? Clin Immunol. 2012; 143(1):22–38.
34. Guilherme L, Kalil J. Rheumatic fever and rheumatic heart disease: cellular mechanisms leading autoimmune reactivity and disease. J Clin Immunol. 2010;30(1):17–23.
35. Collard CD, Vakeva A, Morrissey MA, Agah A, Rollins SA, Reenstra WR, Buras JA, Meri S, Stahl GL. Complement activation after oxidative stress: role of the lectin complement pathway. Am J Pathol. 2000;156(5):1549–56.
36. Turner MW. The role of mannose-binding lectin in health and disease. Mol Immunol. 2003;40(7):423–9.
37. Jin Z, Ji Z, Hu J. Mannose-binding lectin gene site mutations and the susceptibility of rheumatic heart disease. Zhonghua Yi Xue Za Zhi. 2001; 81(21):1284–6.
38. Scalzi V, Hadi HA, Alessandri C, Croia C, Conti V, Agati L, Angelici A, Riccieri V, Meschini C, Al-Motarreb A, et al. Anti-endothelial cell antibodies in rheumatic heart disease. Clin Exp Immunol. 2010;161(3):570–5.
39. Ramasawmy R, Spina GS, Fae KC, Pereira AC, Nisihara R, Reason IJM, Grinberg M, Tarasoutchi F, Kalil J, Guilherme L. Association of mannose-binding lectin gene polymorphism but not of mannose-binding serine protease 2 with chronic severe aortic regurgitation of rheumatic etiology. Clinic Vaccine Immunol. 2008;15(6):932–6.

13

Defining the normal appearance of the temporomandibular joints by magnetic resonance imaging with contrast: a comparative study of children with and without juvenile idiopathic arthritis

Matthew L. Stoll[1*], Saurabh Guleria[2,3], Melissa L. Mannion[1], Daniel W. Young[2], Stuart A. Royal[2], Randy Q. Cron[1] and Yoginder N. Vaid[2]

Abstract

Background: Up to 80% of children with juvenile idiopathic arthritis (JIA) develop arthritis involving their temporomandibular joint (TMJ). Recent studies have questioned the sensitivity of an abnormal MRI in the diagnosis of active arthritis.

Methods: 122 children without arthritis undergoing contrast MRI of the head were prospectively consented to undergo a simultaneous contrast MRI of their TMJs. As a comparison point, the initial MRI of the TMJ of 35 newly diagnosed children with JIA were retrospectively scored. The presence and size of effusion and contrast enhancement were measured in the left TMJ in all subjects.

Results: 62/122 (51%) controls compared to only 10/35 JIA (29%) patients had an effusion ($p = 0.022$). Contrast enhancement was present in ≥97% of both groups, although the size of the enhancement was, on average, 0. 2 mm larger in controls (1.1 ± 0.24 vs 0.88 ± 0.27 mm, $p <$ 0.001). Among JIA patients, the size of the enhancement correlated inversely with disease duration ($r = -0.475$, $p = 0.005$). Chronic changes were present in none of the controls versus 2/35 (5.5%) of the JIA patients ($p = 0.049$).

Conclusion: Findings consistent with minimally active TMJ arthritis appear to be equally likely in children with JIA as compared to non-inflamed controls, while this and other studies confirm that chronic changes are specific to JIA. Thus, small amounts of effusion or contrast enhancement, in the absence of chronic changes, should be interpreted with caution.

Keywords: Juvenile idiopathic arthritis, Temporomandibular joint, Magnetic resonance imaging

Background

Juvenile idiopathic arthritis (JIA) is the most common form of chronic arthritis in children, affecting approximately 1 in 1000 children [1]. Forty to 80% of children with JIA develop arthritis of the temporomandibular joint (TMJ) [2–4]. TMJ arthritis can occur even in the absence of typical symptoms of pain, stiffness, or swelling, and in the presence of a normal physical exam [2, 5]. Thus, diagnosis is typically made with imaging studies. As radiographs only capture late stages of TMJ arthritis, advanced imaging modalities are typically used, with several studies indicating that magnetic resonance imaging (MRI) may have improved ability to detect TMJ arthritis as compared to ultrasound [5, 6].

A limitation of studies evaluating the use of advanced imaging tools for the diagnosis of TMJ arthritis is the absence of a gold standard, as it would clearly be unethical to subject children to biopsy in order to test the

* Correspondence: mstoll@peds.uab.edu
[1]Department of Pediatrics, University of Alabama at Birmingham, CPP N G10 / 1600 7th Avenue South, Birmingham, AL 35233, USA
Full list of author information is available at the end of the article

performance characteristics of MRI. In particular, in light of recent evidence indicating that local therapy of TMJ arthritis may impair TMJ growth in children [7], interest in the specificity of an abnormal TMJ MRI has arisen. A retrospective study by Tzaribachev et al. [8] indicated that abnormal MRIs of the pediatric TMJ are rare in those without arthritis elsewhere, with effusions observed in only 3 of 96 children TMJs and enhancement observed in another three children. In contrast, von Kalle et al. [9] retrospectively evaluated the TMJs of 46 children who underwent MRI of the head, finding contrast enhancement in all TMJs with a mean signal intensity of 75% higher than pre-contrast [9]. A subsequent study from the group showed similar contrast signal intensity between patients and controls, with the major difference being in the extent of synovial hypertrophy [10]. Likewise, Ma et al. [11] found that the signal to noise ratio of 24 healthy controls was higher post-contrast as compared to pre-contrast. A similar approach was taken by Resnick et al. [12], who retrospectively evaluated the TMJs of 72 children with JIA and 71 non-inflamed controls. They calculated the enhancement ratio (ER), defined as the intensity of contrast enhancement in the superior TMJ space divided by that of a nearby muscle. They reported significantly higher ER in the JIA patients (2.52 ± 0.79) versus the controls (1.28 ± 0.16), with ROC analysis showing that a cutoff of 1.55 was optimal for distinguishing the two groups. Thus, MRI findings of synovial fluid or mild synovial enhancement in the TMJ may be within normal limits.

A limitation of these studies is that they were retrospective in design, and they were limited to children who underwent contrast MRI of the brain, in whom the TMJ was visualized after the fact. This limitation is potentially problematic, due to lack of use of TMJ coils and other technical issues that may restrict visualization of the joint, although the Resnick study was limited to children with head coils and appropriate visualization of both the TMJ and the surrounding musculature [12]. While the ideal study would be a prospective study of healthy children, such a study would be ethnically challenging due to the requirement for contrast as well as the need for sedation in many young children. Kottke et al. [13] performed a prospective study of children undergoing MRI of the head to evaluate for intracranial pathology, finding joint fluid and contrast enhancement in 83% and 97% of TMJs, respectively, among 27 children studied. To avoid both the limitations of retrospective studies as well as the risks of exposing healthy children to unnecessary contrast MRI studies, we conducted a prospective study of children who underwent contrast MRI of the brain for diagnostic purposes, who agreed to allow us to obtain an MRI of the TMJs simultaneously. We also compared our findings in these controls to findings in children with newly diagnosed JIA undergoing initial MRI screening of the TMJ for arthritis.

Methods

Study design

This was a study of children undergoing MRI of the brain/TMJ. Two groups of subjects were included in this study: controls undergoing MRI of the brain were studied prospectively, and children with newly diagnosed JIA undergoing routine MRI of the TMJ were studied retrospectively. This study was approved by the local IRB. Informed consent was obtained from the legal guardians of all individual participants included in the prospective study, as well as participants age 14 or older. Waiver of informed consent was obtained for the retrospective component to the study, as the MRIs of the TMJ were obtained as per standard of care.

Controls

Children age 1–18 who were undergoing MRI of the brain as per standard of care were considered for the study. Exclusion criteria included (1) active infections; (2) immunodeficiency; (3) known rheumatic disease; (4) sickle cell disease; (5) radiation to the TMJ; (6) TMJ pain; (7) failure to receive contrast enhancement; and (8) excessive motion artifact precluding interpretation of the images. To assess for undiagnosed rheumatic disease, subjects were screened via questionnaire (Additional file 1); anyone who answered affirmatively to any of the questions was excluded.

Cases

Children age 1–18 newly diagnosed with JIA (symptom onset under 16 years of age) who underwent initial MRI of the TMJ during the same time period during which controls were recruited were identified retrospectively. Their MRIs were reviewed by the same radiologists who reviewed the control studies. Clinical and demographic data were abstracted from their electronic medical records. Maximal incisal opening (MIO) was routinely measured using the Therabite Measuring Scale (Atos Medical, Hörby, Sweden).

MRI sequences

For the controls, two additional study sequences were obtained in addition to the clinically indicated MRI. All MRIs were performed with an Ingenia 1.5 Tesla (T), Ingenia 3.0 T, or an Avanto 1.5 T scanner (Philips Medical Systems, and Seimens Healthcare, respectively). Both sequences were obtained after all of the clinically indicated sequences and were therefore both post-contrast. These were a fast spin echo T2 and a spin echo T1-weighted fat-saturated sequence of the left TMJ in the sagittal plane. In-plane resolution (pixel size) varied from 0.5–0.8, and slice thickness was 2 mm with no gap.

MRIs of the patients were performed as previously described [14]. For this study, the only images that were retrospectively reviewed were T2-weighted fat-saturated pre-contrast and T1-weighted post-contrast sagittal images of the left TMJ.

Interpretation

Interpretation of the MRIs was performed by two board certified pediatric radiologists; one has s 26 years of experience post-training, and the other has 10 years of experience; additionally, the Radiology Department at our hospital interprets approximately 500 pediatric MRIs of the TMJ annually. In both controls and newly diagnosed JIA cohorts, the left TMJ was assessed for the presence or absence of joint fluid (Fig. 1) and synovial enhancement (Fig. 2). Any amount of fluid or synovial enhancement was measured in maximal thickness (in mm), regardless of location (anterior/posterior, inferior/superior joint recesses). The thickness of enhanced synovial lining was measured taking particular care to exclude diffusion of contrast within joint fluid. In addition, chronic changes (pannus formation, condylar flattening, bony erosions, disc deformities, and bony destruction) were assessed in all subjects with the pre-contrast images [14].

Statistical analysis

Continuous data are presented as means (± SD), and dichotomous data are presented as proportions. The concordance correlation coefficient (CCC) was calculated to quantify the agreement between raters for both the effusion measurement and the enhancement measurement. The CCC measures the degree that matched pairs fall on the concordance line and thus contains the measurements of accuracy and precision. While Cohen's kappa is often reported as a measure of inter-rater reliability, it is optimally used for categorical or ordinal variables and is less appropriate than the CCC in this case. The CCC was developed as a measure of agreement between continuous variables in a dependent sample [15]. Comparisons between JIA patients and controls, as well as between 1.5 T versus 3 T MRI scanners, were performed with the Chi squared or Fisher exact tests as appropriate for proportional data, and the Student's t-test for continuous data. The Pearson correlation coefficient was used to assess correlations between continuous variables. The CCC calculation was performed using SAS software, Version 9.3 (copyright, SAS Institute, Inc., Cary, NC, USA).

Ethical approval

All procedures performed in studies involving human participants were in accordance with the ethical standards of the institutional and/or national research committee, and with the 1964 Helsinki declaration and its later amendments or comparable ethical standards.

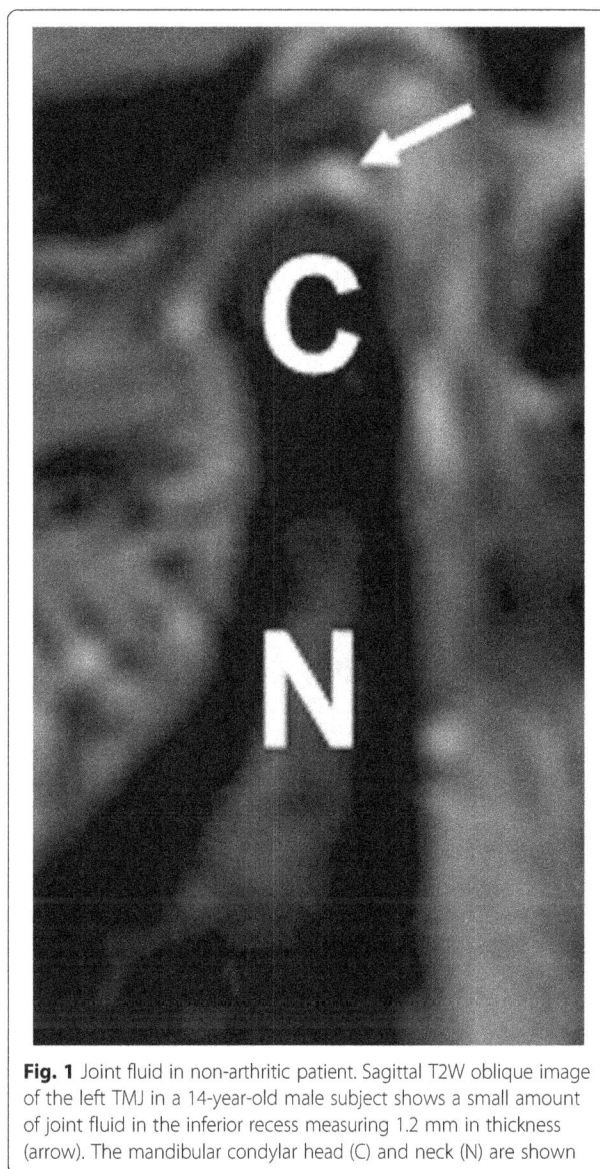

Fig. 1 Joint fluid in non-arthritic patient. Sagittal T2W oblique image of the left TMJ in a 14-year-old male subject shows a small amount of joint fluid in the inferior recess measuring 1.2 mm in thickness (arrow). The mandibular condylar head (C) and neck (N) are shown

Results

Subjects

One-hundred-and-twenty-two arthritis-free control subjects were included in the study. Their demographic features and clinical indications for MRI are summarized in Table 1; 38 (31%) had a history of malignancy, of whom 12 (9.8% of the total population) had received chemotherapy or radiation; the rest of the children with malignancy were presumably enrolled at or near the time of diagnosis. None of the subjects had any historical features suggestive of arthritis, nor had any been evaluated by pediatric rheumatology. As a comparison, 35 children with JIA were included; their demographic and clinical information is summarized in Table 2. Of the 17 children using biologic therapies, 14 were taking tumor

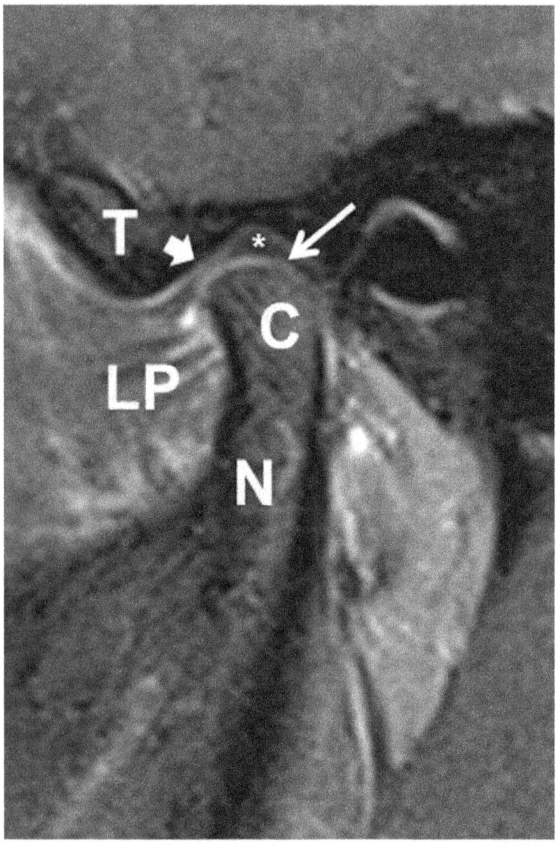

Fig. 2 Joint enhancement in non-arthritic patient. Post-contrast sagittal T1W oblique image of the left TMJ in a 16-year-old male subject shows enhancement of the synovium in both the inferior (arrow) and superior (arrowhead) recesses with maximal thickness measuring 1.2 mm in thickness. The condylar head (C), condylar neck (N), left lateral pterygoid muscle (LP), glenoid tubercle (T), and meniscus (*) are shown

Table 1 Demographic and clinical features of the control population

Feature	Number
n	122
Sex	
Male	67 (55%)
Female	55 (45%)
Race	
Hispanic	2 (1.6%)
Caucasian	101 (83%)
African-American	18 (15%)
Asian	1 (0.8%)
Age (years; mean ± SD)	7.5 ± 4.5
Indication for head MRI	
Evaluation for intracranial malignancy	51 (42%)
Known intracranial malignancy	41 (34%)
Evaluation for pituitary disease	21 (17%)
Evaluation for white matter disease	7 (5.7%)
Trauma	1 (0.8%)
Suspected cerebral vascular accident	1 (0.8%)
Prior chemotherapy	5 (4.1%)
Prior radiation therapy	9 (7.4%)

necrosis factor inhibitors, and 3 (all with systemic JIA) were on the interleukin-1 receptor antagonist, anakinra. The duration from diagnosis to MRI ranged from one day to just under six months, with a mean of 2.2 ± 1.7 months.

MRI findings (Table 3)

Among the controls, 62 (51%) had an effusion in the TMJ; when present, the mean (± SD) diameter was 0.90 ± 0.22 mm. One-hundred-and-twenty (98%) had contrast enhancement; when present, the mean (± SD) diameter was 1.06 ± 0.24 mm. The maximum sizes of the effusions and enhancement were 1.4 and 1.8 mm, respectively. An illustration of a control subject with abnormal MRI findings is shown in Fig. 1. Among JIA patients, only 10/35 (29%) had an effusion, a statistically significant difference ($p = 0.022$) compared to controls. When present, the sizes of the effusions were non-significantly larger in the JIA patients compared to controls (1.5 ± 1.3 versus 0.89 ± 0.23 mm, $p = 0.192$), and effusions larger than 1.5 mm were only seen in JIA patients ($n = 3$); in contrast, the sizes of the enhancement were statistically significantly larger in the controls compared to patients (1.1 ± 0.24 versus 0.88 ± 0.27 mm, $p < 0.001$). The maximum sizes of the effusions in the controls and JIA patients were 1.4 and 4.5 mm respectively; and for enhancements, the maximum sizes were 1.8 mm in both groups. Chronic changes were seen in none of the controls and in two (5.7%) of the JIA patients ($p = 0.049$). One child had condylar flattening, erosive changes, and pannus; and the other had condylar flattening, osteophytes, and pannus. Both 1.5 T and 3 T MRI scanners were used during the course of the study. The MRI field strength was available on 152 / 157 of the subjects; the 3 T device was used in 24 / 117 (21%) of the control subjects for whom this information was obtainable, compared to 15 / 35 (43%) patients with JIA. Among the controls, the 3 T MRI scanner identified an increased frequency of effusions compared to the 1.5 T MRI (22 / 24 [92%] versus 35 / 93 [38%], respectively, $p < 0.001$). A similar trend was observed among the JIA patients (7 / 15 [47%] versus 3 / 20 [15%], $p = 0.062$). MRI field strength did not appear to impact size of the effusion in either group (data not shown), while 3 T scans were associated with larger sizes of enhancement in controls (1.20 ± 0.20

Table 2 Demographic and clinical features of the JIA population. Continuous variables are presented as mean ± sd

Feature	Number
n	35
Sex	
Male	11 (31%)
Female	24 (69%)
Race	
Biracial	1 (2.9%)
Caucasian	28 (80%)
African-American	6 (17%)
Age at MRI (years; mean ± SD)	9.6 ± 4.7
Time from diagnosis to MRI (months; mean ± SD)	2.2 ± 1.8
Time from initial symptom to MRI (months; mean ± SD)	12 ± 17
JIA category	
Oligoarticular	5 (14%)
Systemic	3 (8.6%)
RF- polyarticular	14 (40%)
RF+ polyarticular	3 (8.6%)
Psoriatic	7 (20%)
Enthesitis-related arthritis	3 (8.6%)
Disease activity assessments	
Swollen joint count	8.2 ± 8.3
ESR (n = 32; mm / hr)	32 ± 28
Physician global assessment (0–10)	3.3 ± 1.4
Exam findings of TMJ activity or damage	
Maximal incisal opening (n = 34; mm)	4.5 ± 0.9
Jaw deviation (n = 29)	7 (24%)
Medications	
None	4 (11%)
Prednisone alone	2 (5.7%)
Methotrexate alone	13 (37%)
Biologic alone	3 (8.6%)
Methotrexate plus biologic	13 (37%)

Abbreviations: ESR erythrocyte sedimentation rate, *TMJ* temporomandibular joint

Table 3 MRI findings in controls compared to JIA patients

Feature	Controls	JIA patients	*p*-value
Frequency of effusion	62 (51%)	10 (29%)	0.022
Size of effusion (mm; mean ± sd)	0.89 ± 0.23	1.5 ± 1.3	0.192
Frequency of enhancement	120 (98%)	34 (97%)	0.533
Size of enhancement (mm; mean ± sd)	1.1 ± 0.24	0.88 ± 0.27	< 0.001
Frequency of chronic changes	0	2 (5.7%)	0.049

versus 1.03 ± 0.25 mm, $p = 0.003$) but not patients (data not shown).

To assess the impact of medical therapy on TMJ MRI findings in JIA patients, we tested the correlation of disease duration to the size of effusions and enhancements. While there was no association between effusion size and disease duration from diagnosis to the MRI ($r = -0.231$, $p = 0.188$), there was a robust inverse association between enhancement and disease duration ($r = -0.475$, $p = 0.005$). Neither methotrexate nor TNF inhibitors were associated with the presence or size of effusions or contrast enhancement in children with JIA (data not shown), although these findings are likely influenced by the short duration from diagnosis to MRI in many patients.

Agreement

All of the MRIs of the control subjects were reviewed by both radiologists. When effusions or enhancement were dichotomized to present or absent, agreement between the two radiologists was present in 120 / 122 (98%) for effusion and 122 / 122 (100%) for enhancement. When evaluated on a continuous scale, the two radiologists were within 0.2 mm of each other in 120 / 122 (98%) of subjects with respect to size of the effusion, and in 114 / 122 (93%) subjects with respect to the size of the enhancement. The concordance correlation coefficient indicated inter-reader agreement was 0.98 for effusion and 0.92 for enhancement, representing high levels of agreement for both.

Discussion

One-hundred-and-twenty-two children were prospectively evaluated for TMJ inflammation while undergoing a clinically indicated MRI of their brains for reasons other than TMJ arthritis screening. Of these subjects, 62 had effusions up to 1.4 mm, and 120 had contrast enhancement up to 1.8 mm. The frequency and size of the areas of effusion and enhancement were similar between JIA patients and controls, with effusions surprisingly more common in the latter. This cannot be explained by MRI field strength, as controls were more likely to have been scanned with a 1.5 T device, which detected a lower frequency of effusions among both groups of subjects. However, the largest effusions were present in those children with JIA, and effusions larger than 1.5 mm were seen only in JIA patients. Thus, our data support several previous studies in this field [9–13], with only the study by Tzaribachev et al. [8] yielding contradictory findings.

The reasons for these widely discrepant findings with respect to the frequency of inflammatory changes in the TMJ of non-arthritic subjects are not entirely clear. To some extent, it may pertain to the study methodology, with respect to looking for specific areas of effusion or enhancement as opposed to dynamic contrast studies that compare the overall pattern of signal intensity pre-versus post-contrast. Additionally, as noted above, retrospective studies by definition involve children who did not undergo dedicated MRI of the TMJ. The field strength of the MRI (1.5 T vs 3 T) may also influence sensitivity with 3 T providing higher resolution images, although the use of TMJ coils in the 1.5 T scanners at least in our institution partially compensated for this limitation. Finally, there may be differences pertaining to the interpretation of the images or the patient populations themselves.

The clear message from this and other recent studies is that small amounts of joint effusion and contrast enhancement are not necessarily pathologic. Perhaps the intensity of the enhancement or the extent of synovial hypertrophy are more appropriate indicators of JIA [10–12]; these were not assessed in our study. It must be emphasized, though, that these findings do not detract from the body of literature indicating that children with JIA are at substantial risk of TMJ arthritis [16]. While the size of the effusions and enhancement in our subjects were typically under 1.5 mm, children with JIA can have changes up to 3–4 mm. Furthermore, none of the 96 children in the study by Tzaribachev [8], only 3 of 46 (6.5%) of the subjects in the study by von Kalle [9], 1 of 27 (3.7%) subjects in the study by Kottke [13], and 0 / 122 in the present study had morphological changes suggestive of advanced TMJ arthritis. In contrast, studies of children with JIA, particularly those conducted prior to the biologic era, demonstrated substantial alterations in the morphology of the TMJ [17, 18]. Such changes can lead to devastating alterations in the form and function of the jaw [17]. Only two JIA subjects in this study had chronic changes by MRI; in part, this is due to the short disease duration, although it is unclear why these results differ from those previously reported in newly diagnosed subjects with JIA, in which chronic changes were seen in 69% at baseline (within 2 months of diagnosis) [5]. It may be related to earlier use of systemic biologic therapies or earlier diagnoses.

We acknowledge some limitations of this study. Although control subjects were screened by questionnaire, no rheumatologist was involved in their evaluation. However, given the rarity of JIA (~ 1 in 1000), it is highly unlikely that any of these subjects were in fact affected with TMJ arthritis. Additionally, some of the control children received chemotherapy or radiation, and many of the JIA subjects were on immunosuppressive therapy, which appeared to have had an effect on the size of the enhancement. There may also have been a delay in the attainment of the images in the control population that was not present in the patients, as the former underwent initial dedicated MRIs of the brain; such a delay could result in increased contrast uptake, thus biasing the study towards findings of increased TMJ inflammation in controls [19]. This is nevertheless important information, as in routine practice, there will likely be variations in the rate at which post-contrast images are obtained, and such information will not necessarily be available to the rheumatologist, underscoring the need to interpret small amounts of contrast uptake with caution. There were also differences in the field strength of the MRI used in patients versus controls, although these differences if anything may have attenuated the differences between the two groups of subjects. Strengths of the study include the following: the number of children evaluated (and in a prospective fashion), the precise measurements of the extent of joint fluid and contrast enhancement, the high level of agreement between the two radiologists, and the comparison with the subjects with JIA.

In conclusion, our study confirms previous findings that a small amount of joint fluid or enhancement can be within the range of normal, particularly when 3 T MRI scanners are used. However, even a small effusion of minimal synovial enhancement may reflect ongoing TMJ arthritis in the setting of a child with JIA. Thus, timely follow-up TMJ MRI examination is necessary to evaluate for progression of disease. This information should be taken into account when interpreting the TMJ MRI of a child with JIA.

Conclusion

Findings consistent with minimally active TMJ arthritis appear to be equally likely in children with JIA as compared to non-inflamed controls. However, chronic changes and large areas of effusion appear specific for JIA.

Abbreviations

CCC: Concordance correlation coefficient; ER: Enhancement ratio; JIA: Juvenile idiopathic arthritis; T Tesla: (MRI field strength); TMJ: Temporomandibular joint

Acknowledgements

None.

Funding

This work was not supported by any commercial sources.

Authors' contributions

The radiologists SG, DY, SR, and YV designed and implemented the study, reviewing all of the imaging data. MS abstracted the clinical information and wrote the draft of the manuscript. MM performed the statistical analyses. RC supervised all aspects of this study. All authors read and approved the final manuscript.

Competing interests
The authors declare that they have no competing interests.

Author details
[1]Department of Pediatrics, University of Alabama at Birmingham, CPP N G10 / 1600 7th Avenue South, Birmingham, AL 35233, USA. [2]Department of Radiology at Children's of Alabama, CH 2 FL / 1600 7th Avenue South, Birmingham, AL 35233, USA. [3]Present affiliation: Austin Radiological Associates, Austin, TX, USA.

References
1. Krause ML, Crowson CS, Michet CJ, Mason T, Muskardin TW, Matteson EL. Juvenile idiopathic arthritis in Olmsted County, Minnesota, 1960-2013. Arthritis Rheum. 2016;68:247–54.
2. Stoll ML, Sharpe T, Beukelman T, Good J, Young D, Cron RQ. Risk factors for temporomandibular joint arthritis in children with juvenile idiopathic arthritis. J Rheumatol. 2012;39:1880–7.
3. Cannizzaro E, Schroeder S, Muller LM, Kellenberger CJ, Saurenmann RK. Temporomandibular joint involvement in children with juvenile idiopathic arthritis. J Rheumatol. 2011;38:510–5.
4. Carmody RN, Gerber GK, Luevano JM Jr, et al. Diet dominates host genotype in shaping the murine gut microbiota. Cell Host Microbe. 2015;17:72–84.
5. Weiss PF, Arabshahi B, Johnson A, et al. High prevalence of temporomandibular joint arthritis at disease onset in children with juvenile idiopathic arthritis, as detected by magnetic resonance imaging but not by ultrasound. Arthritis Rheum. 2008;58:1189–96.
6. Muller L, Kellenberger CJ, Cannizzaro E, et al. Early diagnosis of temporomandibular joint involvement in juvenile idiopathic arthritis: a pilot study comparing clinical examination and ultrasound to magnetic resonance imaging. Rheumatology (Oxford). 2009;48:680–5.
7. Lochbuhler N, Saurenmann RK, Muller L, Kellenberger CJ. Magnetic resonance imaging assessment of temporomandibular joint involvement and mandibular growth following corticosteroid injection in juvenile idiopathic arthritis. J Rheumatol. 2015;42:1514–22.
8. Tzaribachev N, Fritz J, Horger M. Spectrum Of magnetic resonance imaging appearances of juvenile temporomandibular joints (TMJ) in non-rheumatic children. Acta Radiol. 2009;50:1182 6.
9. von Kalle T, Winkler P, Stuber T. Contrast-enhanced MRI of normal temporomandibular joints in children–is there enhancement or not? Rheumatology (Oxford). 2013;52:363–7.
10. von Kalle T, Stuber T, Winkler P, Maier J, Hospach T. Early detection of temporomandibular joint arthritis in children with juvenile idiopathic arthritis - the role of contrast-enhanced MRI. Pediatr Radiol. 2015;45:402–10.
11. Ma GM, Amirabadi A, Inarejos E, et al. MRI thresholds for discrimination between normal and mild temporomandibular joint involvement in juvenile idiopathic arthritis. Pediatr Rheumatol Online J. 2015;13:53.
12. Resnick CM, Vakilian PM, Breen M, et al. Quantifying temporomandibular joint synovitis in children with juvenile idiopathic arthritis. Arthritis Care Res (Hoboken). 2016;69:1795–802.
13. Kottke R, Saurenmann RK, Schneider MM, Muller L, Grotzer MA, Kellenberger CJ. Contrast-enhanced MRI of the temporomandibular joint: findings in children without juvenile idiopathic arthritis. Acta Radiol. 2015;56:1145–52.
14. Vaid YN, Dunnavant FD, Royal SA, Beukelman T, Stoll ML, Cron RQ. Imaging of the temporomandibular joint in juvenile idiopathic arthritis. Arthritis Care Res (Hoboken). 2014;66:47–54.
15. Lin LI. A concordance correlation coefficient to evaluate reproducibility. Biometrics. 1989;45:255–68.
16. Stoll ML, Cron RQ. Temporomandibular joint arthritis in juvenile idiopathic arthritis: the last frontier. Int J Clin Rheumatol. 2015;10:273–86.
17. Stabrun AE. Impaired mandibular growth and micrognathic development in children with juvenile rheumatoid arthritis. A longitudinal study of lateral cephalographs. Eur J Orthod. 1991;13:423–34.
18. Larheim TA, Hoyeraal HM, Stabrun AE, Haanaes HR. The temporomandibular joint in juvenile rheumatoid arthritis. Radiographic changes related to clinical and laboratory parameters in 100 children. Scand J Rheumatol. 1982; 11:5–12.
19. Rieter JF, de Horatio LT, Nusman CM, et al. The many shades of enhancement: timing of post-gadolinium images strongly influences the scoring of juvenile idiopathic arthritis wrist involvement on MRI. Pediatr Radiol. 2016;46:1562–7.

14

Anatomy of the sacroiliac joints in children and adolescents by computed tomography

Anna Zejden[1*] and Anne Grethe Jurik[1,2]

Abstract

Background: Diagnosing sacroiliitis by magnetic resonance imaging (MRI) in children/adolescents can be difficult due to the growth-related changes. This study analyzed the normal osseous anatomy of the sacroiliac joints (SIJ) in a juvenile population using computed tomography (CT).

Methods: The anatomy of the SIJ was retrospectively analyzed in 124 trauma patients aged 9 months – <18 years by CT, based on 2 mm slices in axial, semi-axial and semi-coronal planes. The following anatomical features were recorded: intersegmental fusion of the sacral vertebral segments 1–3 (S1-S3), ossified nuclei (antero-superior at S1, lateral to the intervertebral spaces and lateral to S1 and S2) and joint facet defects larger than 3 mm.

Results: Fusion of S1/S2 started at the age of 6 years and was complete after the age of 13 years in most girls and after the age of 14 years in most boys. Fusion of S2/S3 started at the age of 9 years, but could remain incomplete up to 18 years in both genders. Ossified nuclei antero-lateral at S1 and/or in the joint space were observed until the age of 18 years and occurred in 77% of individuals ≥13 years with intraarticular localization in 64% of girls and 60% of boys. Joint facet defects >3 mm occurred in 21 children/adolescents (17%) located to both the iliac and sacral joint facets.

Conclusions: Normal osseous SIJ structures in children and adolescents vary considerably. Attention to these normal anatomical structures during growth may help to avoid false positive findings by MRI.

Keywords: Sacroiliac joints, Computed tomography, Juvenile individuals, Anatomy, Sacroiliitis, Juvenile spondyloarthritis

Background

The sacroiliac joints (SIJ) play an important role in spondyloarthritis as the diagnosis often is confirmed based on sacroiliitis by imaging. In adults the early diagnosis of sacroiliitis is currently based on magnetic resonance imaging (MRI) [1, 2]. Since 2009 bone marrow edema (BME), highly suggestive of sacroiliitis, has been part of the classifications criteria for adult SpA as defined by Assessment of SpondyloArthritis (ASAS) International Society [1]. Inflammatory changes in the sacroiliac joints is also frequent in juvenile spondyloarthritis (JSpA) [3, 4] but the classification or diagnostic criteria used in adults seems not to be applicable in juvenile patients [5]. One of the explanations for somewhat different sacroiliac joints changes in children/adolescents compared with adults is the persistence of growth related edematous changes and lack of a clear delineation of minor osseous structures by MRI; in juvenile patients this is often a big challenge for radiologists [6, 7]. Usually both active and chronic MRI findings are required to establish the diagnosis in children and adolescents and distinct knowledge about the complicated anatomy of SIJ is therefore important [8]. Computed tomography (CT) is superior to MRI for visualizing detailed osseous anatomy in addition to pathological structural lesions [9–11] and can display chronic osseous changes in sacroiliitis, but not signs of inflammatory activity [9, 12, 13]. However, due to exposure to ionizing radiation, CT is not commonly used as the diagnostic method for diagnosing SIJ changes, especially not in children and adolescents.

For both adults and children/adolescents, early and correct diagnosis of inflammatory changes in the SIJ is

* Correspondence: annazejd@rm.dk
[1]Department of Radiology, Aarhus University Hospital, Noerrebrogade 44, 8000 Aarhus C, Denmark
Full list of author information is available at the end of the article

only possible with precise knowledge of the structural anatomy and developmental variation of SIJ. A literature review resulted in a few studies analyzing the anatomy of the SIJ based on CT in adults [10, 13–15]; two of these focused on prevalence and appearance of anatomical variants [14, 15]. In children and adolescents, CT evaluation was performed in one study with the purpose of evaluating developmental features. A total of 25 juvenile individuals were examined by single slice CT resulting in the detection of ossification centers in the SIJ in individuals aged >15 years [16].

The purpose of this study was to analyze the normal osseous anatomy of the SIJ in children and adolescents using current multislice CT technique.

Methods

Study population

The study was designed as a retrospective analysis conducted at the Department of Radiology, Aarhus University Hospital, Denmark.

The study population comprised patients selected from a local trauma database at our hospital between January 2012 and August 2016. A total of 194 juvenile patients met our trauma team activation criteria according to the international ABCDE-system having a score ≥ 2 [17] and the indication for total-body CT used by Treskes et al. in the REACT-2 trial [18]. They all underwent CT scanning encompassing the head, neck, chest, abdomen and pelvis. Inclusion criteria to our study were: Age below 18 years and no CT detectable traumatic changes in the spine, pelvis, abdomen and chest. Exclusion criteria: Traumatic skeletal and/or organ lesions in the chest, abdomen, pelvis and spine, changes in the SIJ suggestive of sacroiliitis, previous spine or pelvic surgery, CT reconstructions in a bony setting not including the whole SIJ (Fig. 1). In total, 124 patients aged 9 months – <18 years (mean age 11 years 8 months), 57 girls and 67 boys, were included in our study. One girl was examined twice: at the age of 13 years and at the age of 15 years.

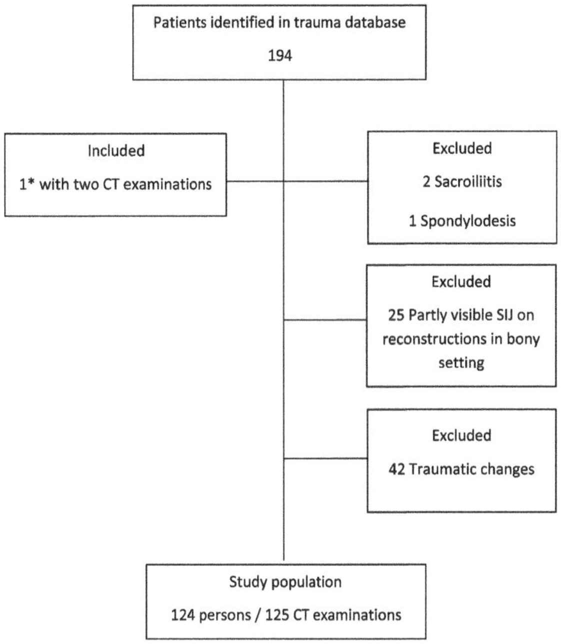

Fig. 1 Flowchart of study population. * 1 girl included with two CT examinations being 13 and 15 years old

CT examination

All patients were examined in supine position using a 64-slice Philips Brilliance CT scanner (USA, Cleveland), according to the standard department guidelines. A post-contrast CT examination of the thorax, abdomen and pelvis was performed using a beam collimation of 0.625 mm, slice thickness of 2 mm, increment 1 mm, kV 100–140 and mAs 100–350 appropriately adjusted for patient size and shape. Axial spine reformats, including the SIJ, with a slice thickness of 1 mm and an increment of 0.5 mm, using a bony reconstruction filter D, were routinely performed and post-processed at a Philips IntelliSpace workstation with software version 6.0.4.02700 for reconstructions of the SIJ. Axial, semi-axial and semi-coronal 2 mm thick contiguous CT slices covering the entire SIJ were used for evaluation of the SIJ.

Evaluation of CT examination

The following anatomical features were recorded: 1) Intersegmental fusion of the sacral vertebral segments 1–3 (S1-S3) (Fig. 2), 2) ossified nuclei antero-superior

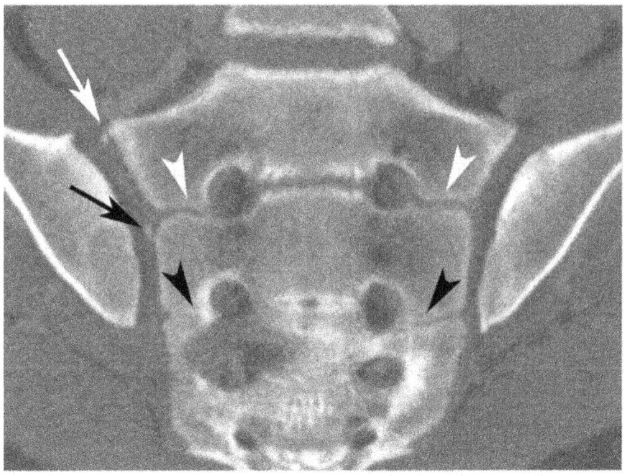

Fig. 2 Fusion between sacral segments S1-S3 in a 14-year-old boy. Semi-coronal slice. Open space (no fusion) at the level S1/S2 – white arrowhead; partial fusion at the level S2/S3 – black arrowhead. Note also ossified nucleus antero-superior at S1 (white arrow) and lateral to the intervertebral space S1/S2 (black arrow) on the right side

at S1 (Fig. 3), 3) ossified nuclei lateral to the intersegmental spaces at S1/S2 and S2/S3 (Fig. 2), 4) ossified nuclei lateral to vertebral segment S1 and S2, respectively (Fig. 4), and 5) joint facet defects larger than 3 mm (Fig. 5).

Intersegmental fusion of sacral vertebrae S1 - S3 was characterized as absent when no osseous bridging was observed in the intersegmental space on all coronal slices. Partial fusion was reported in case of ossification in intersegmental spaces and complete fusion at the time of no detectable space between the sacral segments.

All 125 CT examinations of the SIJ were evaluated by a senior musculoskeletal radiologist (AZ). The reliability of the evaluations was assessed based on an independently evaluation of 48 examinations/96 SIJ by another senior radiologist (AGJ). Inter-observer agreement was based on these results.

Statistical analysis

The frequency of segmental fusion and occurrence of ossified nuclei were analyzed descriptively in relation to age and gender. Gender related developmental differences were analyzed using Pearson's chi-squared test or Fisher exact test. A level of $p < 0.05$ was considered significant.

Inter-observer variation regarding nuclei in the 96 joint spaces was assessed by Bland-Altman analysis using plots, bias and 95% confidence interval, and disagreements were subsequently analyzed to obtain consensus.

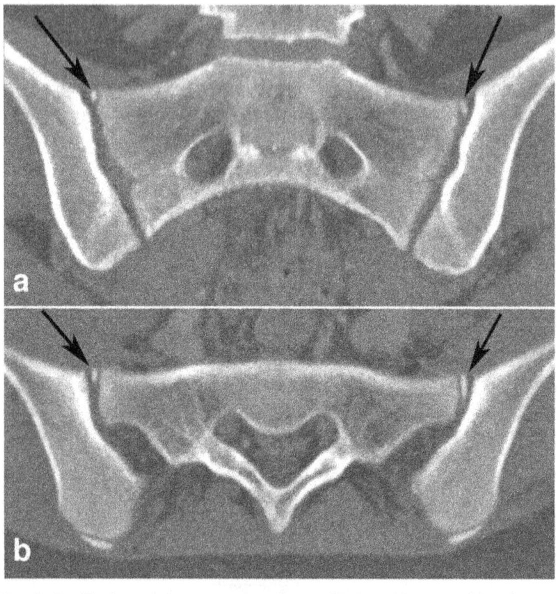

Fig. 3 Ossified nuclei antero-superior at S1 in a 13-year-old girl. Bilateral ossified nuclei antero-superior at S1 - black arrows. **a** - semi-coronal and (**b**) - semi-axial slice

Results

The two radiologists agreed on intersegmental fusion except in two (4%) of the 48 individuals and disagreed on joint facet defects in three of the 192 (1,5%) articular surfaces. They agreed on the number of nuclei in the joint space in 85 of the 96 (88%) joints. The disagreement regarding the number of nuclei was low with a bias of 0.1 and a 95% confidence interval of 0.0–0.2.

Results of the age and gender distribution of intersegmental fusion of S1-S3, occurrence of ossified nuclei antero-superior at S1 and in the SIJ space, and joint facet defects are shown in Table 1.

Fusion of S1/S2 intersegmental space was not seen before the age of 6 years, and the frequency increased with age. Complete fusion was seen in one girl at 7 years and 10 months but predominantly occurred in girls after the age of 13; however, with remnants of space in one girl aged >16 years. Complete fusion was less common in boys occurring significantly less frequently in boys ≥14 years than in girls in the same age range ($X^2 = 6.94$, $p = 0.008$).

Fusion of the intersegmental space S2/S3 started at the age of 9 years, but there were remnants of space in both genders up to the age of 18 years. Complete fusion between S2 and S3 was observed 2 years earlier in girls than in boys, occurring in four of six girls aged 13–14 years and in three of seven boys aged 15–16 years, though not statistically significant.

Nuclei antero-superior at S1 and in the joint space rarely occurred before the age of 13 years, observed in three girls; two of them had both nuclei antero-superior at S1 and in the join space (in a 11-year-old girl lateral to S1 and in a 12-year-old girl lateral to S1 and at the level S1/S2, respectively). In individuals aged ≥13 years ossified nuclei at or in the joint space were frequent, occurring in 21 of 28 girls (75%) and in 26 of 33 boys (79%).

The antero-superior area at S1 was the most frequent location of ossified nuclei in individuals ≥13 years old, observed in 19 of 28 (68%) girls and 21 of 33 (64%) boys. The nuclei often occurred bilaterally and were visualized on both coronal and axial slices (Fig. 3). Nuclei at this location were first observed at the age of 10 years in a girl but were not seen in boys before the age of 13 years. Although they predominantly occurred in the age range 14 - ≤17 years, nuclei at this location were observed in two girls and three boys in the age range 17 - <18 years.

Intraarticular localization of ossified nuclei was seen in 18 of 28 (64%) girls and in 20 of 33 (60%) boys >13 years. In total, 25 of 61 persons (41%) aged ≥13 years had multiple (≥ three) ossified nuclei in the joint space, observed in 11 (39%) girls and 14 (42%) boys, respectively. Persistence of ≥ three nuclei located intraarticularly was observed in one girl and three boys ≥17 years old.

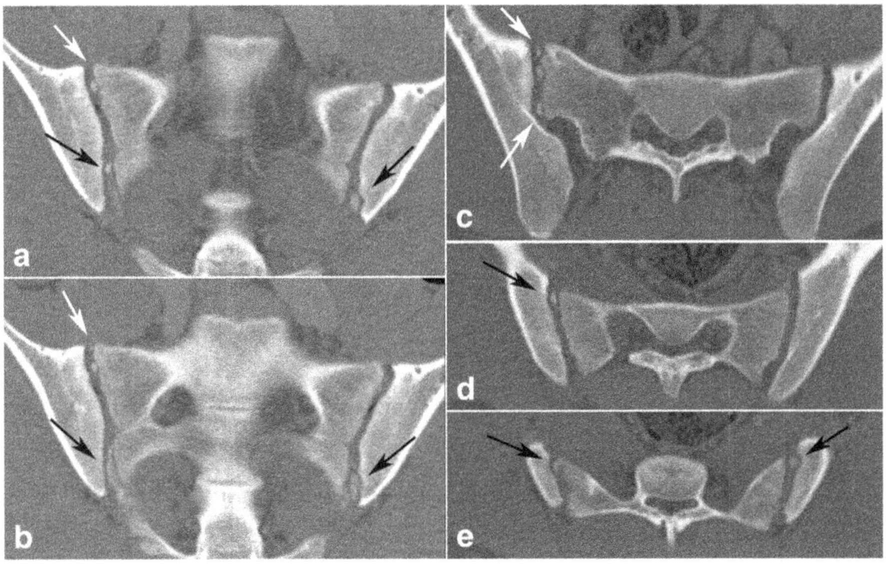

Fig. 4 Multiple (≥ three) ossified nuclei in the joint space in a 16-year-old boy. Left images labeled (**a**), (**b**) – semi-coronal slices; right semi-axial images marked by (**c**) at the level of S1 and (**d**), (**e**) at the level of S2. White arrows – ossified nuclei lateral to the first sacral segment; black arrows – ossified nuclei lateral to the second sacral segment

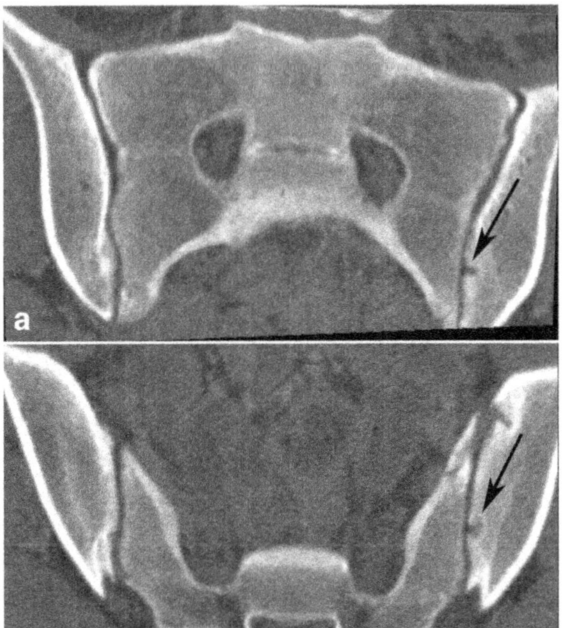

Fig. 5 Joint facets defects ≥3 mm. 14-year-old girl with joint facets defect larger than 3 mm in the left iliac surface - black arrow; (**a**) - semi-coronal and (**b**) - semi-axial slice

Joint facet defects over 3 mm were observed in 21 children (17%), 10 girls and 11 boys, occurring in all age groups. Bilateral defects occurred in one boy who had a total of three lesions (Fig. 5). Thirteen of the defects were localized to the iliac joint facet and ten to the sacral joint facet.

Discussion

The present study highlights the complex osseous anatomy of juvenile SIJs during skeletal growth. There is a frequent occurrence of ossified nuclei antero-lateral to S1 or in the joint space in children and adolescents over 13 years (77% of individuals ≥13 years in current study). The occurrence of joint facet defects over 3 mm was observed in all age groups, but in 21% of individuals ≥13 years. Both ossified nuclei and joint facet defects could be challenging for radiologists or rheumatologists assessing MRI regarding inflammatory changes as growth related changes may simulate inflammatory lesions.

Computed tomography of juvenile SIJs is rarely use in the diagnosis of sacroiliitis due to the exposure to ionizing radiation. Review of the literature resulted in one study where 25 children/adolescents were examined by CT for unknown reasons. A total of seven individuals aged 15–19 years had ossified nuclei in the SIJ, all apparently occurring at the first sacral segment. The age of the remaining individuals in the study was not stated [16]. Another age range than in the present study may have influenced the lower frequency of nuclei compared to our detection of

Table 1 Age and gender distribution of intersegmental fusion S1- S3, ossified nuclei, and joint facet defects

Age, years		<12		12- < 13		13- < 14		14- < 15		15- < 16		16- < 17		17- < 18	
Number of persons		Girls *n* = 27	Boys n = 27	Girls *n* = 3	Boys *n* = 7	Girls *n* = 6	Boys *n* = 7	Girls *n* = 8	Boys *n* = 8	Girls *n* = 4	Boys *n* = 7	Girls *n* = 4	Boys *n* = 3	Girls *n* = 6	Boys *n* = 8
S1/S2 fusion: no		20	17	0	1	0	3	0	1	0	0	0	0	0	0
partial		6[a]	10[b]	3	6	2	4	3	7	2	4	0	1	1	4
complete		1[c]	0	0	0	4	0	5	0	2	3	4	2	5	4
S2/S3 fusion: no		20	24	0	1	1	2	1	2	0	0	0	0	0	1
partial		7[d]	3[e]	3	6	1	5	5	6	1	4	1	1	1	3
complete		0	0	0	0	4	0	2	0	3	3	3	2	5	4
Nuclei															
Ant/sup S1	bilateral	0	0	1	0	3	1	8	5	3	5	2	3	1	3
	unilateral	2[f]	0	0	0	1	1	0	2	0	1	0	0	1	0
Lat ISP S1/S2	bilateral	0	0	1	0	2	1	3	3	0	3	2	1	1	2
	unilateral	0	0	0	0	0	0	1	1	3	2	0	0	0	2
Lat ISP S2/S3	bilateral	0	0	0	0	0	0	4	1	1	0	2	3	1	1
	unilateral	0	0	0	0	0	0	0	1	0	1	0	0	0	0
Lat S1	bilateral	0	0	0	0	2	1	3	3	1	4	1	2	0	2
	unilateral	1[g]	0	1	0	0	0	1	1	2	2	0	0	1	0
Lat S2	bilateral	0	0	0	0	1	0	1	0	0	0	0	1	0	0
	unilateral	0	0	0	0	0	0	0	1	0	0	0	0	0	1
Joint facet defects															
bilateral		0	0	0	0	0	1	0	0	0	0	0	0	0	0
unilateral		1[h]	3[i]	1	3	3	1	2	2	1	1	1	0	1	0

[a]Occurrence at age 9 and 11 years, respectively; [b] Occurrence at age 6, 7, 9, 10 and 11, respectively; [c]Occurrence at age 7 years; [d] Occurrence at age 9, 10 and 11 years, respectively; [e] Occurrence at age 10 and 11, respectively; [f] Occurrence at age 10 and 11 years, respectively; [g] Occurrence at age 11 years; [h]Occurrence at age 11 years; [i]Occurrence at age 7 and 8 years, respectively

ossified nuclei in 50 of 125 (40%) individuals including nuclei in the joint space in 40 (32%) individuals. In the current study, ossified nuclei were observed 5 years earlier than in the study by Götz et al. [16] with the occurrence of ossified nuclei antero-lateral at S1 in one 10-year-old girl. We also detected nuclei more distally located in the joint space. Such nuclei were not detected by Götz et al. at CT, but their histological analyses of three autopsy specimens revealed the presence of nuclei at the level of the second and third sacral segment. It is therefore possible that the different scan techniques may influence results. The present use of 2 mm slices in three different reconstruction planes ought to increase the detectability of nuclei compared to axial 4–8 mm slices used in the study by Götz et al. [16].

The SIJ anatomy has also been evaluated by MRI [6]. Based on 114 individuals aged 8–17 years, findings regarding intersegmental fusion were rather similar to our observations with fusion occurring earlier in girls than in boys. Apophyses/nuclei lateral to S1 or at the intersegmental space S1/S2 were also observed between the age of 9 to 17 years. This is in accordance with the present findings except that Bollow et al. found complete ossification and apparently fusion of the nuclei at S1 in the 25 oldest children, mean age 15.9 ± 1.3 years. In the present study persistence of nuclei was also observed in the age group 17- < 18 years, in both girls and boys. The difference is probably due to a better delineation of minor osseous structures by CT than by MRI.

Growth-related changes can lead to false positive MRI results regarding both activity and structural lesions. Recent findings have revealed a limited specificity of BME alone to define a positive MRI for SpA in both children/adolescents and adults [19, 20]. Subtle non-specific BME at the SIJ suggestive of sacroiliitis was reported in 20% of a juvenile control group as well as in 21% of adult patients with low back pain (LBP) [20, 21]. The causes of subchondral non–inflammatory BME at the SIJ in juvenile subjects have not yet been analyzed. However, the high prevalence of ossified nuclei in the joint space in children and adolescents over 13 years could be the cause of the observed BME in 20% of the juvenile control subjects with a mean age ± SD of 15;1 ± 2;3 years [20]. An increased bone turn-over during ossification of cartilage-preformed bone could be a possible explanation. The ossified nuclei detected in the current study are probably located in the sacral cartilage, as shown histopathologically in three autopsy specimens [16]. The process resulting in fusion of the ossified nuclei to the main ossified sacral segment thus corresponds to the growth process occurring as part of epiphyseal cartilage fusion in tubular bones where the process is accompanied by BME. It has to our knowledge not been evaluated whether or not BME in healthy juvenile persons predominantly occur in the sacrum.

The presence of erosions was found to be a rather specific MRI feature for sacroiliitis in juvenile SpA patients, as it was reported to be present in 58–96% of patients [8, 20]. However, erosions by MRI of the SIJ were reported in 9% of a juvenile control group as well as in 11% of adults with non-inflammatory LBP [20, 21]. Defining erosion by MRI may be difficult due to a poor visualization of cortical bone in the widely used T1-weighted sequences and a high variability of the appearance of erosions. This is supported by moderate inter-observer agreement in juvenile individuals as well as in adults [20, 22]. Several studies evaluating the value of CT in the diagnosis of sacroiliitis in adults have shown higher specificity of CT for detection of erosions and subchondral sclerosis compared to radiography and the commonly used T1-weighted MR-images [11–13, 23–25]. Similar analyses have not been performed in juvenile populations to avoid radiation exposure by CT. Radiation disadvantages by CT have also been a limiting factor for assessing CT morphology in the healthy adult population. However, a study of 45 asymptomatic adults revealed bilateral erosions in only one case, indicating erosions to be rather specific signs of sacroiliitis [26]. In our study, irregularity of the osseous margins of the iliac and/or sacral articular surface with articular defects over 3 mm occurred in 17% and may simulate erosions by MRI.

One of the strengths of the current study is the wide age distribution illustrating the anatomical variety of the juvenile SIJ. Another strength is a uniform study recruitment and the standardized CT technique including reconstructions.

Some limitations need to be considered. The number of persons included in the analysis was rather small, resulting in few representatives among girls and boys in some of the age groups. Thus, our results must be interpreted with some caution. Only one reader evaluated all SIJ examinations, but the inter-observer agreement was good.

Knowledge of osseous anatomy at the SIJ is crucial to make a correct early diagnosis in children/adolescents, especially considering the appearance of structural changes in the early phase of SpA [27–29]. Further studies in a larger population and analyses of the correlation between CT and MRI appearances of structural findings in SIJ would be optimal but probably not feasible. A prospective study with MRI supplementing a CT examination performed on a clinical indication such as suspicious traumatic changes can be a possibility, though difficult to perform. However, the results of the current study could be used to define the anatomy of the SIJ by MRI in clinical practice. The possible presence of subchondral BME in relation to ossified nuclei in the articular cartilage needs to be investigated. An evaluation of SIJ anatomy in healthy juvenile persons using dedicated cartilage sequences and high-resolution 3 T image quality can potentially visualize the complex anatomy and explain BME distribution on concomitant STIR or T2-weighted fat suppressed sequences.

Conclusions

Normal osseous SIJ structures in children and adolescents vary considerably. Intraarticular ossified nuclei are frequent after the age of 13 years and can persist up to the age of 18 years in both genders. Attention to normal anatomical structures during growth may help to avoid false positive MRI findings.

Abbreviations

ASAS: Assessment of SpondyloArthritis International Society; BME: Bone marrow edema; CT: Computed tomography; JSpA: Juvenile Spondyloarthritis; LBP: Low back pain; MRI: Magnetic resonance imaging; SIJ: Sacroiliac joints; SpA: Spondyloarthritis

Acknowledgements

Not applicable.

Funding

There were no grants or financial supports of the study.

Authors' contributions

All authors were involved in drafting the article and revising it critically for important intellectual content, and all authors approved the final version to be published. Study conception and design: AGJ, AZ. Acquisition of data: AZ, AGJ. Analysis and interpretation of data: AZ, AGJ.

Competing interest

The authors declare that they have no competing interests.

Author details

[1]Department of Radiology, Aarhus University Hospital, Noerrebrogade 44, 8000 Aarhus C, Denmark. [2]Department of Clinical Medicine, Aarhus University, Nordre Ringgade 1, 8000 Aarhus C, Denmark.

References

1. Rudwaleit M, Jurik AG, Hermann KG, Landewe R, van der Heijde D, Baraliakos X, et al. Defining active sacroiliitis on magnetic resonance imaging (MRI) for classification of axial spondyloarthritis: a consensual approach by the ASAS/OMERACT MRI group. Ann Rheum Dis. 2009;68: 1520–7.
2. Weber U, Zubler V, Pedersen SJ, Rufibach K, Lambert RG, Chan SM, et al. Development and validation of a magnetic resonance imaging reference criterion for defining a positive sacroiliac joint magnetic resonance imaging finding in spondyloarthritis. Arthritis Care Res (Hoboken). 2013;65:977–85.
3. Hussein A, Abdul-Khaliq H, von der Hardt H. Atypical spondyloarthritis in children: proposed diagnostic criteria. Eur J Pediatr. 1989;148:513–7.
4. Strom H, Lindvall N, Hellstrom B, Rosenthal L. Clinical, HLA, and roentgenological follow up study of patients with juvenile arthritis: comparison between the long term outcome of transient and persistent arthritis in children. Ann Rheum Dis. 1989;48:918–23.
5. Herregods N, Dehoorne J, Van den Bosch F, Jaremko JL, Van Vlaenderen J, Joos R, et al. ASAS definition for sacroiliitis on MRI in SpA: applicable to children? Pediatr Rheumatol Online J. 2017;15:24-017–0159.
6. Bollow M, Braun J, Kannenberg J, Biedermann T, Schauer-Petrowskaja C, Paris S, et al. Normal morphology of sacroiliac joints in children: magnetic resonance studies related to age and sex. Skelet Radiol. 1997;26:697–704.
7. Weiss PF, Xiao R, Biko DM, Chauvin NA. Assessment of Sacroiliitis at diagnosis of juvenile Spondyloarthritis by radiography, magnetic resonance imaging, and clinical examination. Arthritis Care Res (Hoboken). 2016;68: 187–94.
8. Herregods N, Dehoorne J, Joos R, Jaremko JL, Baraliakos X, Leus A, et al. Diagnostic value of MRI features of sacroiliitis in juvenile spondyloarthritis. Clin Radiol. 2015;70:1428–38.
9. Devauchelle-Pensec V, D'Agostino MA, Marion J, Lapierre M, Jousse-Joulin S, Colin D, et al. Computed tomography scanning facilitates the diagnosis of sacroiliitis in patients with suspected spondylarthritis: results of a prospective multicenter French cohort study. Arthritis Rheum. 2012;64:1412–9.
10. Geijer M, Gadeholt Gothlin G, Gothlin JH. The validity of the New York radiological grading criteria in diagnosing sacroiliitis by computed tomography. Acta Radiol. 2009;50:664–73.
11. Puhakka KB, Jurik AG, Egund N, Schiottz-Christensen B, Stengaard-Pedersen K, van Overeem HG, et al. Imaging of sacroiliitis in early seronegative spondylarthropathy. Assessment of abnormalities by MR in comparison with radiography and CT. Acta Radiol. 2003;44:218–29.
12. Hu L, Huang Z, Zhang X, Chan Q, Xu Y, Wang G, et al. The performance of MRI in detecting subarticular bone erosion of sacroiliac joint in patients with spondyloarthropathy: a comparison with X-ray and CT. Eur J Radiol. 2014;83:2058–64.
13. Tuite MJ. Sacroiliac joint imaging. Semin Musculoskelet Radiol. 2008;12(1): 72–82.
14. Demir M, Mavi A, Gumusburun E, Bayram M, Gursoy S, Nishio H. Anatomical variations with joint space measurements on CT. Kobe J Med Sci. 2007;53:209–17.
15. Prassopoulos PK, Faflia CP, Voloudaki AE, Gourtsoyiannis NC. Sacroiliac joints: anatomical variants on CT. J Comput Assist Tomogr. 1999;23:323–7.
16. Gotz W, Funke M, Fischer G, Grabbe E, Herken R. Epiphysial ossification centres in iliosacral joints: anatomy and computed tomography. Surg Radiol Anat. 1993;15:131–7.
17. Kool D, Blickman JG. Advanced trauma life support. ABCDE from a radiological point of view. Emerg Radiol. 2007;14:135–41.
18. Treskes K, Bos SA, Beenen LFM, Sierink JC, Edwards MJR, Beuker BJA, et al. High rates of clinically relevant incidental findings by total-body CT scanning in trauma patients; results of the REACT-2 trial. Eur Radiol. 2017;27: 2451–62.
19. Arnbak B, Jensen TS, Egund N, Zejden A, Horslev-Petersen K, Manniche C, et al. Prevalence of degenerative and spondyloarthritis-related magnetic resonance imaging findings in the spine and sacroiliac joints in patients with persistent low back pain. Eur Radiol. 2016;26:1191–203.
20. Jaremko JL, Liu L, Winn NJ, Ellsworth JE, Lambert RG. Diagnostic utility of magnetic resonance imaging and radiography in juvenile spondyloarthritis: evaluation of the sacroiliac joints in controls and affected subjects. J Rheumatol. 2014;41:963–70.
21. Arnbak B, Grethe Jurik A, Horslev-Petersen K, Hendricks O, Hermansen LT, Loft AG, et al. Associations between Spondyloarthritis features and magnetic resonance imaging findings: a cross-sectional analysis of 1,020 patients with persistent low back pain. Arthritis Rheumatol. 2016;68: 892–900.
22. Arnbak B, Jensen TS, Manniche C, Zejden A, Egund N, Jurik AG. Spondyloarthritis-related and degenerative MRI changes in the axial skeleton–an inter- and intra-observer agreement study. BMC Musculoskelet Disord. 2013;14:274.
23. Kozin F, Carrera GF, Ryan LM, Foley D, Lawson T. Computed tomography in the diagnosis of sacroiliitis. Arthritis Rheum. 1981;24:1479–85.
24. Carrera GF, Foley WD, Kozin F, Ryan L, Lawson TL. CT of sacroiliitis. AJR Am J Roentgenol. 1981;136:41–6.
25. Yu W, Feng F, Dion E, Yang H, Jiang M, Genant HK. Comparison of radiography, computed tomography and magnetic resonance imaging in the detection of sacroiliitis accompanying ankylosing spondylitis. Skelet Radiol. 1998;27:311–20.
26. Vogler JB 3rd, Brown WH, Helms CA, Genant HK. The normal sacroiliac joint: a CT study of asymptomatic patients. Radiology. 1984;151:433–7.
27. Weber U, Jurik AG, Lambert RG, Maksymowych WP. Imaging in Spondyloarthritis: controversies in recognition of early disease. Curr Rheumatol Rep. 2016;18:58.
28. Weber U, Lambert RG, Ostergaard M, Hodler J, Pedersen SJ, Maksymowych WP. The diagnostic utility of magnetic resonance imaging in spondylarthritis: an international multicenter evaluation of one hundred eighty-seven subjects. Arthritis Rheum. 2010;62:3048–58.
29. Althoff CE, Sieper J, Song IH, Haibel H, Weiss A, Diekhoff T, et al. Active inflammation and structural change in early active axial spondyloarthritis as detected by whole-body MRI. Ann Rheum Dis. 2013;72:967–73.

15

Final adult height of patients with childhood-onset systemic lupus erythematosus: a cross sectional analysis

Merav Heshin-Bekenstein[1*], Liat Perl[2], Aimee O. Hersh[3], Emily von Scheven[1], Ed Yelin[4,5], Laura Trupin[4], Jinoos Yazdany[4] and Erica F. Lawson[1]

Abstract

Background: To compare final height to mid-parental target height among adults with childhood-onset systemic lupus erythematosus (cSLE) versus adult-onset SLE (aSLE), and to evaluate the impact of age at SLE onset on final height.

Methods: Data derived from the Lupus Outcomes Study, a longitudinal cohort of adults with SLE, was used for this cross-sectional analysis ($N = 728$). Participants aged 18–63 years with complete height data were included ($N = 566$) and were classified as cSLE if age at diagnosis was < 18 years (N = 72). The Tanner formula was used to calculate mid-parental target height. Multivariate linear regression was used to determine mean difference between final height and target height. Multivariate logistic regression was used to compare odds of substantially reduced final height, defined as > 2 SD below target height. Separate analyses were conducted for females and males to account for differences in timing of the pubertal growth spurt for each sex.

Results: Participants with cSLE were, on average, 2.4 cm shorter than their target height (95% CI -4, − 0.7). The adjusted odds ratio (OR) for substantially reduced final height was 3.9 (95% CI + 2.0, + 7.2, $p < 0.001$) as compared to participants with aSLE. Females diagnosed between 11 and 13 years were at greatest risk for substantially reduced final height, with adjusted OR of 11.2 (95% CI + 3.4, + 36.3) as compared to participants with aSLE ($p < 0.001$).

Conclusions: cSLE is associated with shorter-than-expected final height. Onset of SLE in the pubertal period, near the time of maximum linear growth, may have a particularly significant impact on final height.

Keywords: SLE, Childhood-onset SLE, Adult-onset SLE, Final adult height, Mid-parental target height, Growth hormone

Background

Childhood-onset systemic lupus erythematosus (cSLE) is a multi-system autoimmune disease characterized by autoantibody production. It is estimated to account for 10% to 20% of all cases of systemic lupus erythematosus (SLE), with an average age at onset of 12 years [1].

cSLE is often more severe than adult-onset SLE (aSLE), with higher levels of disease activity, greater likelihood of renal and neurological involvement, lower complement levels and a more frequent need for immunosuppressive therapy [2–5]. Survival in SLE has improved dramatically, from five-year survival rates of 42–72% in the 1960's to 95% today [6–8]. As a result, SLE in adults and children has shifted from being a predominantly fatal disease to a chronic condition [9, 10]. As life expectancy of children with SLE has increased, assessing outcomes of the disease, including the effects of therapy, has become increasingly important.

Impaired linear growth is commonly encountered in children with chronic inflammatory conditions, including SLE. These children may experience delayed onset of puberty and attenuated pubertal growth spurts, especially when the disease presents in late childhood or early adolescence [11, 12]. Poor growth may lead to short stature, and ultimately shorter-than-expected adult

* Correspondence: meravheshin@gmail.com
[1]Division of Pediatric Rheumatology, University of California San Francisco, Benioff Children's Hospital, 550 16th Street, 5th Floor, San Francisco, CA 94143-0632, USA
Full list of author information is available at the end of the article

height, which may impact quality of life [11]. Multiple factors may contribute to the underlying pathophysiology of growth failure in chronic illness, including suboptimal nutrition, prolonged use of glucocorticoids, comorbidities and the chronic inflammatory process itself [11, 13]. Growth failure may result from suppression of the Growth Hormone (GH)-IGF-1 axis or at the level of the growth plate [11].

Significant differences between target and final adult height has been shown in systemic-onset juvenile idiopathic arthritis (sJIA), although these reports do not reflect the more recent outcomes of patients treated with biologics, which may reduce steroid use and subsequent growth impairment [11, 14]. Studies of adults with childhood-onset inflammatory bowel diseases (IBD) also reveal a difference between target and actual height [11], especially in males [15]. In a cohort of 123 patients with pediatric onset Crohn's disease, mean adult height was 2.4 cm less than target height, and 19% of patients were more than 8 cm shorter than their target height [16].

Growth failure was added to the Modified SLICC/ACR SLE Damage Index (M-SDI) by Bandeira et al. [17] and Gutierrez-Suarez et al. [18] as a damage measure for pediatric SLE. Although Bandeira et al. documented growth failure in 15.8% at 3 years of follow up of cSLE, the percentage of participants with growth failure was smaller (7.7%) at 5 years of follow up, demonstrating the potential for catch-up growth in children. As a result, Hiraki et al. proposed final height as a preferred measure of damage in pediatric SDI [12], recognizing that only reduced final height represents an irreversible outcome, since children with cSLE and growth failure may experience significant catch-up growth once the disease is better controlled and steroid dose is tapered.

The purpose of this study was to assess final adult height in an adult cohort of patients with both cSLE and aSLE, comparing final height to target height and evaluating the impact of age of SLE onset on final height. To our knowledge, this work represents the first study of final adult height in cSLE.

Patients and methods

Data sources

Data was derived from the 2007 cycle of Lupus Outcome Study (LOS) (Fig. 1). The LOS is a longitudinal, U.S.-based cohort of over 1200 adults with SLE, 10% of whom had disease onset in childhood (defined as age at diagnosis < 18 years). Details regarding LOS eligibility and enrollment are described elsewhere [19]. Briefly, participants were recruited from community (70%) and clinical (30%) sources, with data collected annually via telephone by trained interviewers. All participants had a confirmed diagnosis of SLE according to chart review supervised by a rheumatologist, using the American College of Rheumatology (ACR) classification criteria for SLE [20]. The survey included validated items pertaining to demographic and socioeconomic characteristics, SLE manifestations, medications, general health, mental health, cognition, employment, and health care utilization. All study data were obtained by participant self-report.

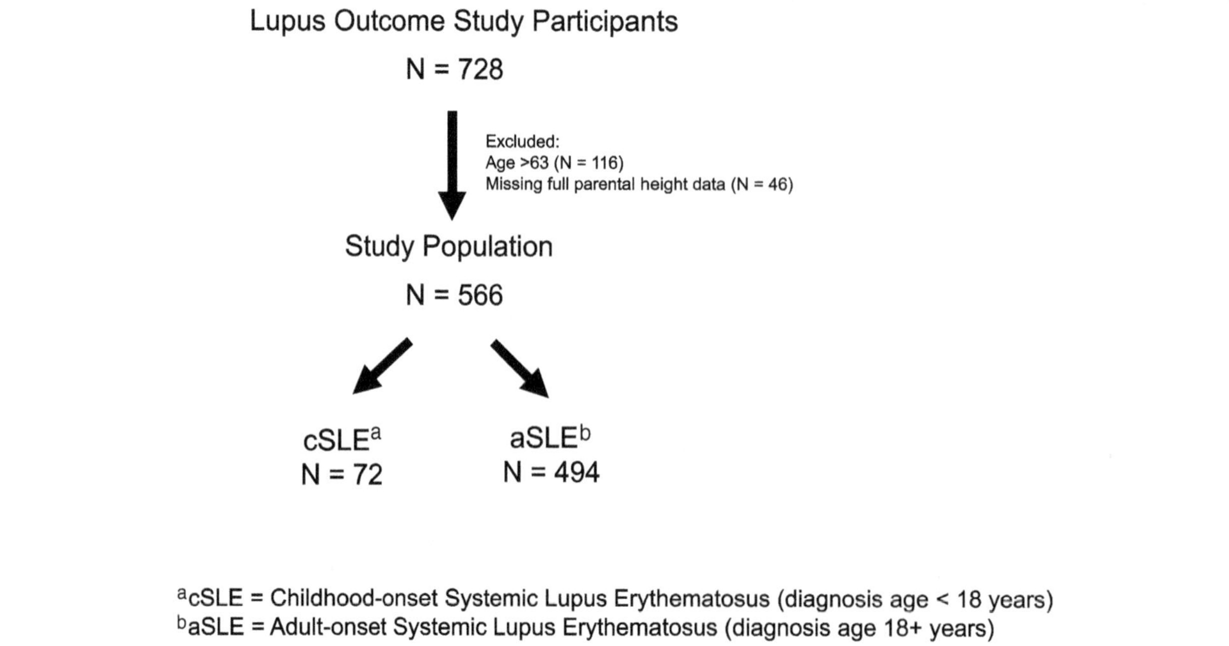

Fig. 1 Study Population of Adults with SLE from the Lupus Outcome Study included in the Analysis

Measures

The primary outcome measures for this analysis were 1) difference between patient-reported final adult height and mid-parental target height, and 2) substantially reduced final height. Target height was calculated from patient-reported biologic-parent heights using the Tanner formula, a validated measure used to estimate genetic height potential: mean parental height plus 6.5 cm for males, and mean parental height minus 6.5 cm for females [21]. Substantially reduced final height was defined as final adult height more than 2 standard deviations (SD) below the mid-parental target height, consistent with the clinical definition of short stature [22]. The SD for the target height in the general population is approximately 2.5 cm [23]; therefore, we identified patients with final adult height more than 5 cm below the target height as having substantially reduced final height.

The primary predictor variable was cSLE, defined as age < 18 years at diagnosis. To further explore the impact of age at SLE onset on final adult height, we subdivided the cSLE cohort into groups based on age at disease onset (< 11, 11–13, 14–15, 16–17 years). Age groups were defined based on timing of pubertal growth spurts in healthy girls and boys. On average, the pubertal growth spurt occurs between the ages of 11 and 13 years in females and 14 to 15 years in males. Demographic predictors included sex and race/ethnicity. Race/ethnicity was categorized as White, Hispanic, African American, Asian and other. SLE-associated predictors included year of diagnosis, disease duration, steroid use ever, cyclophosphamide use ever, and history of end-stage renal disease (defined as history of dialysis or kidney transplant). Year of diagnosis was included in the final model as a predictor to account for the changes in the standard of care for SLE over time. Cyclophosphamide use and end-stage renal disease (ESRD) were included as proxies for disease severity.

Study sample

Data from the 2007 cycle of the LOS were used for this cross-sectional analysis ($N = 728$). All participants age 18–63 years with complete height data were included ($N = 566$). Since the oldest participant with cSLE was 63 years old at time of interview, aSLE patients age > 63 years were excluded ($N = 116$) in order to maximize overlap between groups, as well as to avoid the potential confounding effect of linear height loss among elderly participants.

Statistical analysis

Baseline characteristics of the cSLE and aSLE groups were summarized and compared using bivariate statistics (Student's t-test, rank sum and chi-square test), as appropriate. Multivariate linear regression was used to determine adjusted and unadjusted mean differences between final adult height and target height. Multivariate logistic regression was used to compare unadjusted and adjusted odds of substantially reduced final height between participants with cSLE and aSLE. The final models included cSLE vs. aSLE status, sex, race/ethnicity and predictors of substantially reduced final height with $p < 0.2$ in univariate analysis among participants with cSLE (year of diagnosis, cyclophosphamide use and ESRD).

Among participants with cSLE, one-way ANOVA testing was used to determine whether the difference between final and target height varied according to timing of cSLE onset (age < 11, 11–13, 14–15, 16–17 years). Separate ANOVA analyses were conducted for females and males to account for differences in the average timing of the pubertal growth spurt, and post-hoc Tukey testing was conducted to account for multiple comparisons.

Bivariate and multivariate logistic regression analyses were conducted to determine whether timing of SLE onset is associated with significantly shorter-than-expected final height among female participants with cSLE. Analyses were not conducted for males alone due to the small number of male participants.

Finally, to further explore the impact of disease severity on final height among individuals with cSLE, we examined the association between substantially reduced final height and history of cyclophosphamide treatment in the cSLE cohort, using univariate and multivariate logistic regression. Covariates included sex, race/ethnicity, timing of cSLE onset (age < 11, 11–13, 14–15, 16–17 years), year of diagnosis and history of ESRD. Statistical analyses were performed using STATA 13.0 (StataCorp, College Station, TX.)

Results

Demographics

The study population consisted of 566 participants with SLE, including 72 (13%) with cSLE. The baseline characteristics of the cSLE and aSLE subgroups are described in Table 1. As compared to participants with aSLE, those with cSLE were younger at the time of the interview (mean age 33 ± 9 versus 49 ± 9 years; $p < 0.001$), more likely to be male (12% versus 6%; $p = 0.01$) and less likely to be white (51% versus 70%; $p < 0.001$). Mean age at diagnosis was 14 ± 3 versus 33 ± 10 years ($p < 0.001$), with ranges of age of diagnosis being 2–17 and 18–58 respectively. Respondents with cSLE were more likely to have ever required dialysis (18% versus 7%; $p = 0.001$) and to have undergone kidney transplantation (14% versus 5%; $p = 0.003$). All cSLE participants and nearly all aSLE participants reported a history of steroid use (100% versus 94%; $p = 0.02$). There was no difference between

Table 1 Baseline characteristics of childhood and adult onset SLE patients enrolled in Lupus Outcome Study

Variable	cSLE[a] (*N* = 72)	aSLE[b] (*N* = 494)	*p*-value
Sociodemographics	*N* (%) or Mean ± SD		
Age at diagnosis, years	14 ± 3	33 ± 10	< 0.001
Age at interview, years	33 ± 9	49 ± 9	< 0.001
Sex, female	63 (88%)	465 (94%)	0.01
Race/Ethnicity (%)			< 0.001
White	37 (51%)	347 (70%)	
Hispanic	11 (15%)	39 (8%)	
African American	5 (7%)	35 (7%)	
Asian	11 (15%)	50 (10%)	
Other	8 (11%)	23 (5%)	
SLE Characteristics			
Dialysis ever (A)	13 (18%)	34 (7%)	0.001
Renal transplant ever (B)	10 (14%)	24 (5%)	0.003
End-stage ever (A and/or B)	15 (21%)	37 (7%)	< 0.001
Treated w Steroids ever	72 (100%)	465 (94%)	0.02
Treated w Cyclophosphamide ever	10 (14%)	66 (13%)	0.9

[a]cSLE = Childhood-onset Systemic Lupus Erythematosus (diagnosis age < 18 years)
[b]aSLE = Adult-onset Systemic Lupus Erythematosus (diagnosis age 18+ years)

groups in the likelihood of having received cyclophosphamide (14% versus 13%; $p = 0.9$).

Impact of age at SLE onset on final height

In bivariate analysis, participants with cSLE were, on average, 2.4 cm shorter than their target height (95% CI -4, − 0.7). This differed significantly from aSLE participants ($p < 0.001$), who were a mean of 0.6 cm taller than expected (95% CI 0.03, 1.1). When dividing the groups by sex, females were on average 2.5 cm shorter than their target height (95% CI -4.3, − 0.6), as compared to aSLE ($p < 0.001$). Males were 2 cm shorter than their target height, but the difference was not significant (95% CI -7.5, 3.6, $p = 0.2$) (Fig. 2). In a multivariate linear regression model controlling for sex, race/ethnicity, year of SLE diagnosis, cyclophosphamide use and ESRD, individuals with cSLE were on average 2.8 cm shorter than their target height (95% CI -4.2, − 1.3), and this also differed significantly as compared to aSLE individuals ($p < 0.001$), who were on average 0.6 cm taller than expected (95% CI 0.07, 1.2).

Among cSLE participants, mean difference between actual and target height differed significantly according to age at disease onset ($p < 0.001$, Fig. 3). Females with cSLE diagnosed between 11 and 13 years old were shorter than expected by 6.8 cm (95% CI -11.7, − 1.8), which differed significantly from females with aSLE ($p < 0.001$), who were on average 0.5 cm taller than expected (95% CI -0.0, + 1.1). In a multivariate linear regression model controlling for race/ethnicity, year of SLE diagnosis, cyclophosphamide use and ESRD, females with cSLE diagnosed between 11 and 13 years old were on average 8 cm shorter than their target height (95% CI -11, − 5), $p < 0.001$. Females diagnosed at 14 or 15 years old were shorter than expected by 0.5 cm, which approached statistical significance when compared to females diagnosed at 11–13 years (95% CI -3, + 2, $p = 0.06$). Males diagnosed with SLE at the youngest ages (< 11, 11–13, 14–15) were on average shorter than expected, while males diagnosed at age 16–17 or in adulthood were on average taller than expected. However, these differences did not reach statistical significance.

Finally, we compared the odds of substantially reduced final height, or actual height more than 2 SD (> 5 cm) below target height. A higher proportion of cSLE participants had substantially reduced final height when compared to the adult-onset group (31% vs 14%, $p < 0.001$). In logistic regression analyses, participants with cSLE were more likely to have substantially reduced final height, with an unadjusted OR of 2.8 (95% CI + 1.6, + 4.9, $p < 0.001$). After adjustment for sex, ethnicity/race, year of SLE diagnosis, cyclophosphamide use and ESRD, the odds of short stature in cSLE participants rose to 3.9 (95% CI + 2.0, + 7.2, $p < 0.001$). Females diagnosed between the ages of 11 and 13 years were at greatest risk for substantially reduced final height, with unadjusted odds ratio of 6.3 (95% CI + 2.3, + 17.3, $p < 0.001$) and adjusted odds ratio of 11.2 (95% CI + 3.4, + 36.3; $p < 0.001$) as compared to participants with aSLE (Fig. 4).

Impact of cyclophosphamide on substantially reduced final height

Individuals in the cSLE cohort who received cyclophosphamide were clinically significant shorter in univariate analysis (27% vs 8%, $p = 0.03$). In multivariate logistic regression analysis accounting for sex, race/ethnicity, timing of cSLE onset (age < 11, 11–13, 14–15, 16–17 years), year of diagnosis and history of ESRD, cSLE participants with history of cyclophosphamide use were again much more likely to demonstrate substantially reduced final height, with an adjusted OR of 9.0 (95% CI + 1.5, + 53, $p = 0.01$).

Discussion

In this cohort of adults with SLE, we found that individuals with cSLE were significantly less likely to reach their target height as compared to those with adult-onset SLE. Our results further demonstrate that onset of SLE in the pubertal period, a time of rapid linear growth, may have a particularly significant impact on final adult height.

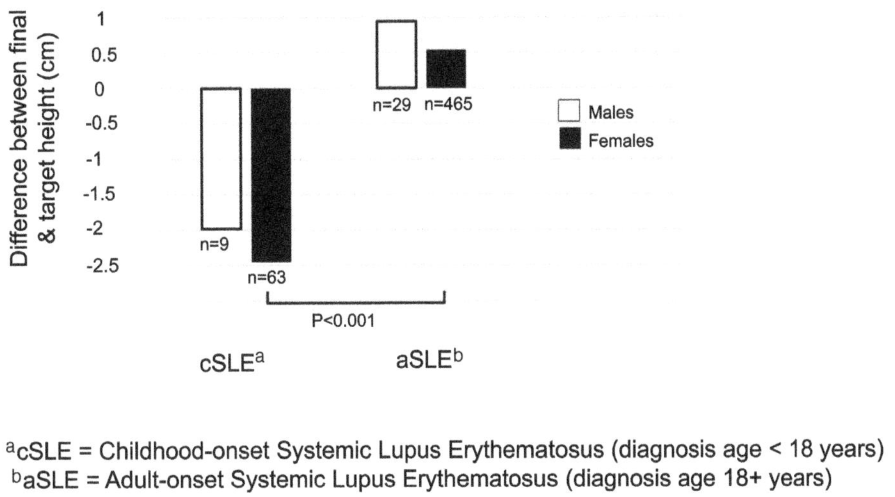

Fig. 2 Mean difference between final height and mid-parental target height among participants with childhood-onset versus adult-onset SLE, by sex ($n = 566$). This graph demonstrates the mean difference between final height and mid-parental target height among males and females with cSLE and aSLE. Females with cSLE were on average 2.5 cm shorter than their target height (95% CI -4.3, – 0.6) which differed significantly from females with aSLE ($p < 0.001$). Males with cSLE were on average 2 cm shorter than target height, but did not differ significantly from males with aSLE (95% CI -7.5, 3.6, $p = 0.2$)

Due to the rarity of cSLE and the lack of longitudinal cohort studies, information regarding growth and final height in cSLE has been limited. In a cross-sectional study of 1015 cSLE patients with a mean age of 15. 9 years, growth failure, defined as height more than 2 standard deviations (SD) below the mean for age, was reported in 15.3% [18]. No information on target height or final adult height was included. Another cross-sectional study of 70 patients with cSLE found that mean height of the cohort was significantly lower than healthy matched controls; however, this cohort consisted of patients aged 9–49 years, and therefore did not reflect the final adult height for all patients, and did not take into account the target height for each individual [24]. In a similar study that examined 32 cSLE patients for a mean period of 4.3 years during the 1980s, short stature (defined as height for age less than the 5th percentile) was present in 38%. This study also did not include final height for all participants [25]. In a longitudinal study, the Paediatric Rheumatology International Trials Organization (PRINTO) examined growth in 331 cSLE patients with a median age of 13.9 years over 26 months, comparing patients' height to mid-parental height [26]. At the end of the study period, growth failure (defined as a parental height z-score < – 1.5) was seen in 15% of the female patients and 25% of the male patients. Furthermore, growth failure was seen in 22.4% of women with disease onset before the age of 12 compared to 3.3% of women with disease onset after 12 years of age. Again, final adult height was not assessed.

Timing of the pubertal growth spurt is different in males and in females. The pubertal growth spurt in females occurs during early adolescence. The peak linear growth velocity corresponds most closely with Tanner stage 2 in females, which occurs in 95% of the girls by the age of 12.1 years. For males, the growth spurt occurs later in puberty, around Tanner stage 3 and age 14 years [23]. The differences between females and males in our analysis can be partially explained by this difference in timing of the pubertal growth spurt. In our analysis, SLE onset in females around the age of peak linear growth (11–13 years old) was associated with significantly shorter than expected adult height, whereas SLE diagnosed later in puberty (age 14–15 years and 16–17 years), after the growth spurt is completed for most females, did not significantly affect final adult height. Males demonstrated similar results, though these findings did not achieve statistical significance, likely due to the very small number of male participants in our study. Males who were diagnosed around the time of peak linear growth (age 14–15 years) were shorter than expected by a mean of 3.6 cm. Disease onset between ages 11 to 13 years in males did affect final height as well, but to a lesser extent than in the female population.

Final height greater than 2 SD below the mid-parental height (> 5 cm) has been previously suggested by Hiraki et al. as a damage measure in cSLE [12]. In our analyses, individuals with cSLE were more than three times more likely to meet this criterion as compared to the aSLE population. Odds of

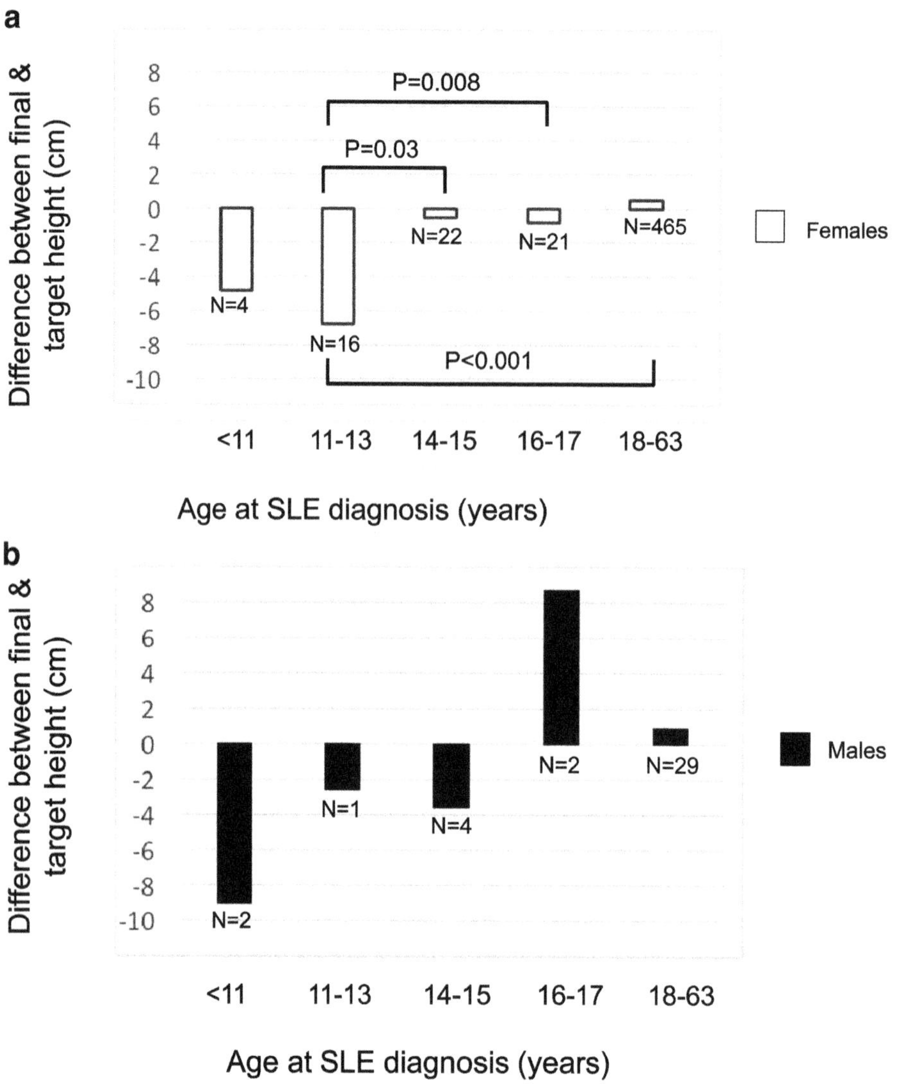

Fig. 3 Mean difference between final height and mid-parental target height among participants by age at SLE diagnosis. **a** Mean difference between final height and mid-parental target height among females with SLE, by age at lupus diagnosis. Females diagnosed between 11 and 13 years of age were shorter than expected by 6.8 cm (95% CI -11.7, −1.8), which differed significantly from females diagnosed later in childhood (14–15, 16–17 years) or during adulthood. **b** Males diagnosed with SLE at the youngest ages (< 11, 11–13, 14–15) were on average shorter than expected, while males diagnosed at age 16–17 or in adulthood were on average taller than expected. However, these differences did not reach statistical significance

short stature were the greatest among females diagnosed between the ages of 11–13 years.

Our analyses demonstrated that childhood-onset lupus patients with a history of cyclophosphamide exposure may be at significantly higher risk for reduced final height. As individuals with cSLE who receive cyclophosphamide typically have severe disease, they are likely to have had higher levels of systemic inflammation and steroid exposure, both of which can inhibit linear growth.

Although to date recombinant GH therapy is not indicated in the treatment of chronic inflammatory disease, cSLE patients with significant short stature may be considered for GH therapy in the future. In other inflammatory diseases like juvenile idiopathic arthritis, randomized controlled trials have confirmed that GH therapy can improve final adult height and also suggest a modest effect on short to medium term catch-up growth [11]. The benefit versus risk from GH therapy should be considered, with the main risks being decrease in insulin sensitivity, skeletal complications like avascular necrosis, increased risk of malignancies and the theoretical risk of worsening the inflammatory disease process itself. In the literature, there are only case reports of GH therapy in cSLE. Gorska et al. reports on GH therapy given to a 17-year-old female patient with

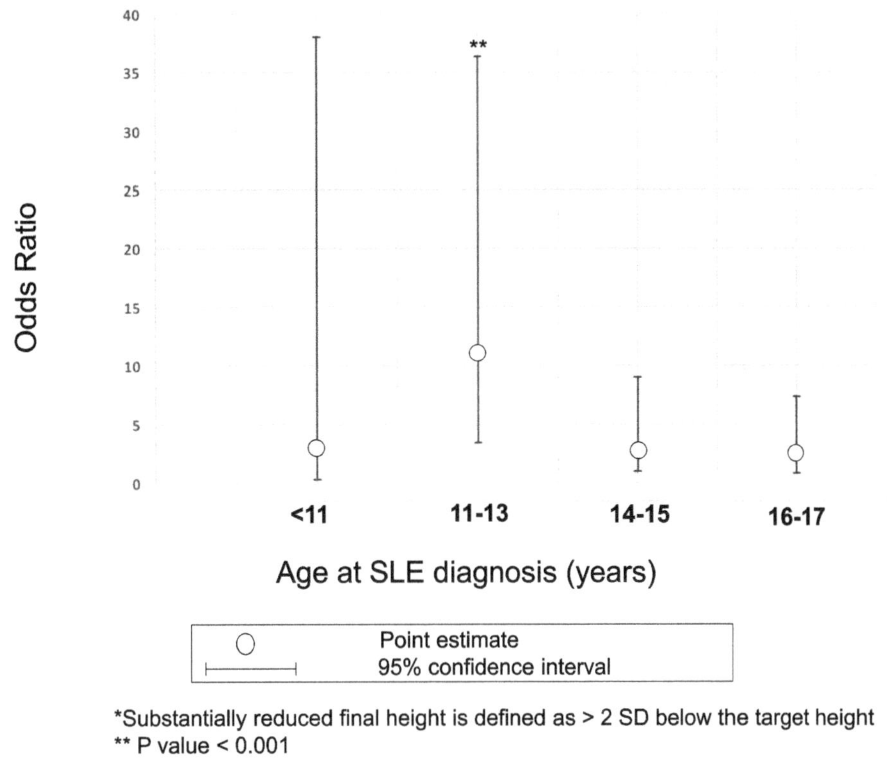

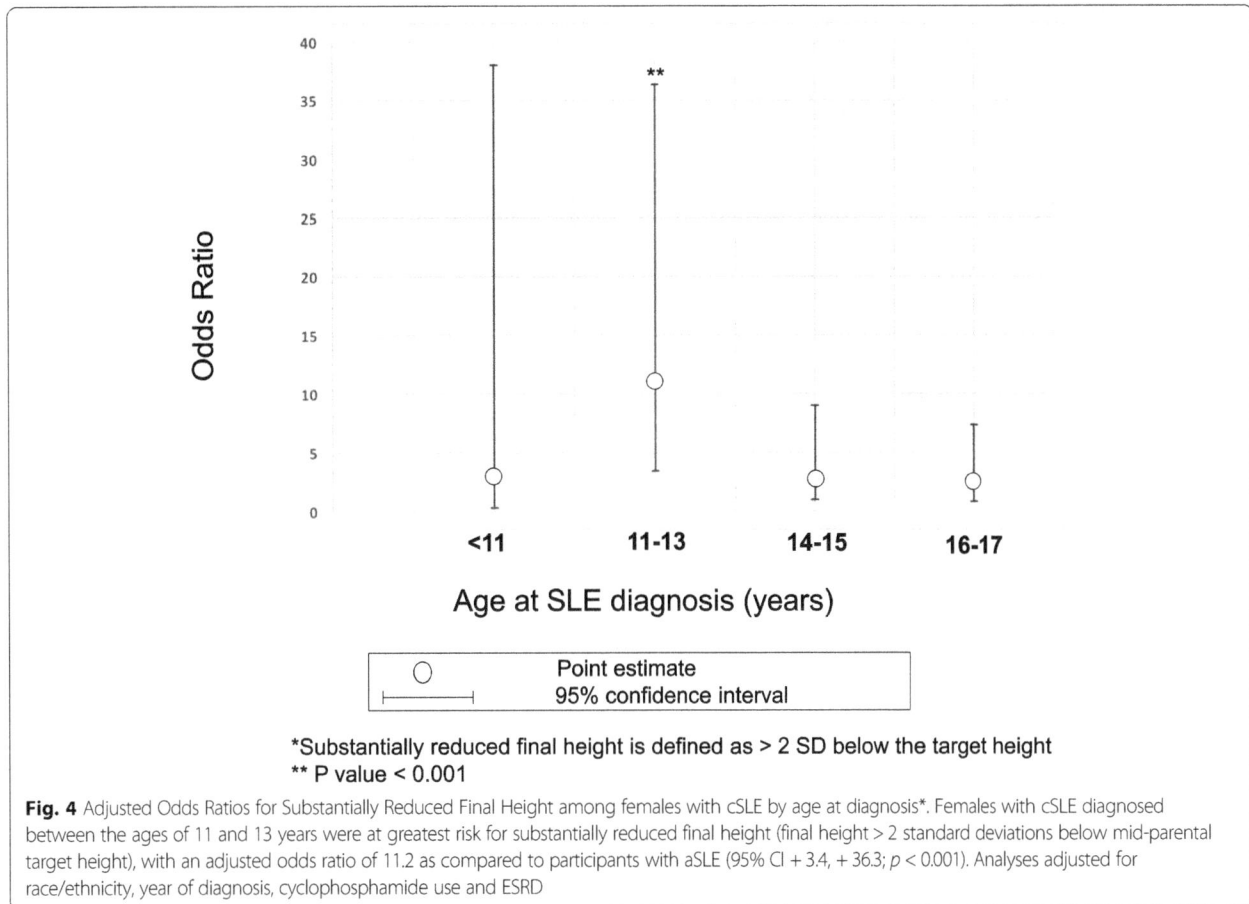

Fig. 4 Adjusted Odds Ratios for Substantially Reduced Final Height among females with cSLE by age at diagnosis*. Females with cSLE diagnosed between the ages of 11 and 13 years were at greatest risk for substantially reduced final height (final height > 2 standard deviations below mid-parental target height), with an adjusted odds ratio of 11.2 as compared to participants with aSLE (95% CI + 3.4, + 36.3; $p < 0.001$). Analyses adjusted for race/ethnicity, year of diagnosis, cyclophosphamide use and ESRD

short stature and bone age of 11 years [27]. Following one-year of GH therapy, the girl achieved catch-up growth, with no significant side effects. Bae et al. reported a case of a 19-year-old man with a history of cSLE, treated with GH and testosterone at the age of 16 for hypogonadism and growth impairment [28]. Nine months after GH initiation, height increased by 10 cm. However, GH therapy was discontinued due to increased disease activity, which improved after cessation of GH therapy. Yap et al. described improved growth velocity after initiation of supra-physiological doses of GH in a 15-year-old male with cSLE, though the patient subsequently developed worsening of lupus nephritis, which improved following cessation of the GH treatment [29].

There are several limitations to our study. First, since the height data in our cohort relies on participant self-report, inaccuracies may occur. However, self- and family member- reporting of heights are widely used in the literature, and have been proven accurate in the adult population [30, 31]. Second, since the LOS collected data from individuals with cSLE in adulthood, we do not have detailed data on exposures or outcomes that occurred during childhood, such as cumulative steroid exposure, disease activity measurements, nutritional status or financial status. Since we lack information on cumulative steroid exposure or steroid dosing during childhood, the present study cannot assess whether the effect of steroids on the final height is dose-dependent, or whether there is a dose that minimizes the risk of shorter-than-expected final height. Despite the absence of disease activity measurements at the time of cSLE diagnosis, it can be assumed that SLE is active at the time of diagnosis. Therefore, if SLE was diagnosed at the time of puberty, lupus activity and treatment may impede the pubertal growth spurt, ultimately limiting adult height. It is important to note that we do not have data on the exact timing of puberty relative to SLE diagnosis, e.g. age at menarche or Tanner stage at diagnosis. Therefore, we used age as a proxy for the timing of the pubertal growth spurt. However, age may not accurately reflect pubertal stage, especially among adolescents with cSLE that may be at risk for delayed puberty. Similarly, we do not have data to specify the timing of other events that occurred in cSLE participants, such as the onset of ESRD during childhood vs. adulthood. Third, the number of male participants is our study was small, which reflects the fact that SLE is much more common in females. This reduced our power to detect statistically significant differences among male participants. Finally, it is important to note that our cSLE cohort is on average younger than the aSLE cohort. Since younger generations have become progressively taller over the past century [32], as reflected by the fact that our aSLE cohort was on average taller than mid-parental target height, the true target height of our cSLE cohort may actually be greater than their mid-parental height. Therefore, the true difference in the odds of clinically significant short stature between our aSLE and cSLE cohorts may be greater than reported here.

This study is the first to assess final adult height in individuals with childhood-onset SLE, which is a more accurate indicator of permanent damage than growth failure. Our study also included data on mid-parental height, which allowed us to account for the impact of genetics in a multi-ethnic cohort.

Our study suggests that disease onset at the period of maximum linear growth may predict shorter-than-expected stature in adulthood. Per our results, clinicians should closely monitor growth in patients with pubertal onset of SLE and consider underlying pubertal development in their determination of future risk for short stature. Treatment strategies that minimize steroid exposure and promote tight disease control, including aggressive use of second-line immunosuppressive agents, should be applied when possible, as minimizing systemic inflammation and steroid exposure may help to prevent short stature in cSLE. Individuals with severe short stature may benefit from GH therapy; however, further data is needed in order to determine risk versus benefit and to identify the sub-groups for whom this treatment is most appropriate. The development of predictive models for future short stature would be informed by prospective studies that assess all potential risk factors for reduced final height, including detailed assessments of disease features, medication exposure and pubertal stage.

Conclusion

In conclusion, our study showed that childhood-onset SLE is associated with shorter-than-expected final adult height. Onset of SLE in the pubertal period, a time of rapid linear growth, may have a particularly significant impact on final adult height.

Abbreviations

aSLE: Adult-onset Systemic Lupus Erythematosus; cSLE: Childhood-onset Systemic Lupus Erythematosus; GH: Growth Hormone; LOS: Lupus Outcome Study; SLE: systemic lupus erythematosus

Acknowledgements

The authors would like to thank Robert Lustig and Nadav Rappoport for their valuable comments to improve the quality of this paper.

Funding

Dr. Heshin-Bekenstein was supported by the NIH NIAMS T32-AR007304 grant, Dr. Ed Yelin and Ms. Laura Trupin were supported by the NIH NIAMS P60 AR-053308 grant and Erica Lawson was supported by NCATS UCSF-CTSI UL1-TR001872 grant and the Hellman Fellows Fund.

Authors' contributions

Study conception: EFL, LT, EY, JY. Study design: LT, EFL, MHB, LP. Analysis and interpretation of data: MHB, EFL, LT. The first and subsequent versions of the manuscript were written by MHB, edited by EFL and revised critically by all remaining co-authors. All authors read and approved the final version of the manuscript.

Competing interests

The authors declare that they have no competing interests in this section.

Author details

[1]Division of Pediatric Rheumatology, University of California San Francisco, Benioff Children's Hospital, 550 16th Street, 5th Floor, San Francisco, CA 94143-0632, USA. [2]Division of Pediatric Endocrinology, University of California San Francisco, San Francisco, CA, USA. [3]Division of Pediatric Rheumatology, University of Utah, Salt Lake City, UT, USA. [4]Division of Rheumatology, University of California San Francisco, San Francisco, CA, USA. [5]Philip R Lee Institute for Health Policy Studies, University of California, San Francisco, CA, USA.

References

1. Klen-Gitelman M, Lane JC. Systemic lupus erythematosus. In: Petty RE, Laxer RM, Lindsley CB, Wedderburn LR, editors. Textbook of pediatric rheumatology. Textb. Pediatr. Rheumatol. Philadelphia: Elsevier; 2016. p. 286.
2. Sousa S, Gonçalves MJ, Inês LS, Eugénio G, Jesus D, Fernandes S, et al. Clinical features and long-term outcomes of systemic lupus erythematosus: comparative data of childhood, adult and late-onset disease in a national register. Rheumatol. 2016;36:955–60.
3. Brunner HI, Gladman DD, Ibañez D, Urowitz MD, Silverman ED. Difference in disease features between childhood-onset and adult-onset systemic lupus erythematosus. Arthritis Rheum. 2008;58:556–62.
4. Tucker LB, Uribe AG, Fernandez M, Vila LM, McGwin G, Apte M, et al. Adolescent onset of lupus results in more aggressive disease and worse outcomes: results of a nested matched case—control study within LUMINA, a multiethnic US cohort (LUMINA LVII). Lupus. 2010;17:314–22.
5. Tucker LB, Menon S, Schaller JG, Isenberg DA. Adult- and childhood-onset systemic lupus erythematosus: a comparison of onset, clinical features, serology, and outcome. Br J Rheumatol. 1995;34:866–72.
6. Meislin AG, Rothfield N. Systemic lupus erythematosus in childhood. Analysis of 42 cases, with comparative data on 200 adult cases followed concurrently. Pediatrics. 1968;42:37–49.
7. Lee P-Y, Yeh K-W, Yao T-C, Lee W-I, Lin Y-J, Huang J-L. The outcome of patients with renal involvement in pediatric-onset systemic lupus erythematosus – a 20-year experience in Asia. Lupus. 2013;22:1534–40.
8. Lerang K, Gilboe I-M, Steinar Thelle D, Gran JT. Mortality and years of potential life loss in systemic lupus erythematosus: a population-based cohort study. Lupus. 2014;23:1546–52.
9. Gladman DD. Prognosis of systemic lupus erythematosus and the factors that affect it. Curr Opin Rheumatol. 1991;3:789–96.
10. Ravelli A, Ruperto N, Martini A. Outcome in juvenile onset systemic lupus erythematosus. Curr Opin Rheumatol. 2005;17:568–73.
11. Wong SC, Dobie R, Altowati MA, Werther GA, Farquharson C, Ahmed SF. Growth and the growth hormone-insulin like growth factor 1 Axis in children with chronic inflammation: current evidence, gaps in knowledge, and future directions. Endocr Rev. 2016;37:62–110.
12. Hiraki LT, Hamilton J, Silverman ED. Measuring permanent damage in pediatric systemic lupus Erythematosus. Lupus. 2007;16:657–62.
13. MacRae VE, Wong SC, Farquharson C, Ahmed SF. Cytokine actions in

growth disorders associated with pediatric chronic inflammatory diseases (review). Int J Mol Med. 2006;18:1011–8.
14. Simon D, Fernando C, Czernichow P, Prieur A-M. Linear growth and final height in patients with systemic juvenile idiopathic arthritis treated with longterm glucocorticoids. J Rheumatol. 2002;29:1296–300.
15. Gupta N, Lustig RH, Kohn MA, McCracken M, Vittinghoff E. Sex differences in statural growth impairment in Crohn's disease: role of IGF-1. Inflamm Bowel Dis. 2011;17:2318–25.
16. Sawczenko A, Ballinger AB, Savage MO, Sanderson IR. Clinical features affecting final adult height in patients with pediatric-onset Crohn's disease. Pediatrics. 2006;118:124–9.
17. Bandeira M, Buratti S, Bartoli M, Gasparini C, Breda L, Pistorio A, et al. Relationship between damage accrual, disease flares and cumulative drug therapies in juvenile-onset systemic lupus Erythematosus. Lupus. 2006;15:515–20.
18. Gutiérrez-Suárez R, Ruperto N, Gastaldi R, Pistorio A, Felici E, Burgos-Vargas R, et al. A proposal for a pediatric version of the systemic lupus international collaborating clinics/American College of Rheumatology Damage Index based on the analysis of 1,015 patients with juvenile-onset systemic lupus erythematosus. Arthritis Rheum. 2006;54:2989–96.
19. Yelin E, Trupin L, Katz P, Criswell L, Yazdany J, Gillis J, et al. Work dynamics among persons with systemic lupus erythematosus. Arthritis Rheum. 2007; 57:56–63.
20. Hochberg MC. Updating the American College of Rheumatology revised criteria for the classification of systemic lupus erythematosus. Arthritis Rheum. 1997;40:1725.
21. Tanner JM. Normal growth and techniques of growth assessment. Clin Endocrinol Metab. 1986;15:411–51.
22. Rosenbloom AL. Idiopathic short stature: conundrums of definition and treatment. Int J Pediatr Endocrinol. 2009;2009:470378.
23. Backelijauw PF, Dattani MT, Cohen P, Rosenfeld RG. Disorders of growth hormone/ I growth factors secretion and action. In: Sperling MA, editor. Pediatric endocrinology. Philadelphia: Elsevier Saunders; 2014. p. 292–404.
24. Lilleby V, Lien G, Frey Frøslie K, Haugen M, Flatø B, Førre Ø. Frequency of osteopenia in children and young adults with childhood-onset systemic lupus erythematosus. Arthritis Rheum. 2005;52:2051–9.
25. Lacks S, White P. Morbidity associated with childhood systemic lupus erythematosus. J Rheumatol. 1990;17:941–5.
26. Rygg M, Pistorio A, Ravelli A, Maghnie M, Di Iorgi N, Bader-Meunier B, et al. A longitudinal PRINTO study on growth and puberty in juvenile systemic lupus erythematosus. Ann Rheum Dis. 2012;71:511–7.
27. Górska A, Gardziejczyk M, Urban M. [growth hormone administration in the treatment of growth retardation in juvenile SLE–case history]. Pediatr. Endocrinol. Diabetes Metab. 2007;13:171–3.
28. Bae Y-S, Bae S-C, Lee S-W, Yoo D-H, Kim T, Kim S. Lupus flare associated with growth hormone. Lupus. 2001;10:448–50.
29. Yap HK, Loke KY, Murugasu B, Lee BW. Subclinical activation of lupus nephritis by recombinant human growth hormone. Pediatr Nephrol. 1998;12:133–5.
30. Reed DR, Price RA. Estimates of the heights and weights of family members: accuracy of informant reports. Int J Obes Relat Metab Disord. 1998;22:827–35.
31. Kuczmarski MF, Kuczmarski RJ, Najjar M. Effects of age on validity of self-reported height, weight, and body mass index: findings from the Third National Health and Nutrition Examination Survey, 1988–1994. J. Am. Diet. Assoc. 2001;101:28–34-6.
32. Stulp G, Barrett L. Evolutionary perspectives on human height variation. Biol Rev. 2016;91:206–34.

16

Mental health care for youth with rheumatologic diseases – bridging the gap

Alaina M. Davis[1*], Tamar B. Rubinstein[2], Martha Rodriguez[3] and Andrea M. Knight[4,5,6]

Abstract

Youth with rheumatologic diseases have a high prevalence of comorbid mental health disorders. Individuals with comorbid mental health disorders are at increased risk for adverse outcomes related to mental health as well as their underlying rheumatologic disease. Early identification and treatment of mental health disorders has been shown to improve outcomes, but current systems of care fall short in providing adequate mental health services to those in need. Pediatric rheumatologists are uniquely positioned to provide mental health screening and intervention for youth with rheumatologic diseases due to the frequency of patient encounters and ongoing therapeutic relationship with patients and families. However, additional training is likely required for pediatric rheumatologists to provide effective mental health care, and focusing efforts on providing trainees with mental health education is key to building competency. Potential opportunities for improved mental health education include development of clinical guidelines regarding mental health screening and management within pediatric rheumatology settings and incorporation of mental health didactics, workshops, and interdisciplinary clinic experiences into pediatric rheumatology fellowship curricula. Additional steps include mental health education for patients and families and focus on system change, targeting integration of medical and mental health care. Research is needed to better define the scope of the problem, determine effective strategies for equipping pediatric rheumatologists with skills in mental health intervention, and develop and implement sustainable systems for delivery of optimal mental health care to youth with rheumatologic diseases.

Keywords: Pediatrics, Rheumatologic diseases, Mental health, Medical education

Background

Beyond the long-established detrimental impact that chronic disease has on an individual's mental health, we now appreciate that the relationship between chronic physical disease and mental illness is bidirectional [1]. As such, providers that care for patients with chronic diseases must consider their patients' mental health as both an outcome of the disease they are treating and a contributor to their patients' overall health. Understanding the relationship between mental and physical health is of utmost importance in pediatric populations, in which both poor physical and mental health outcomes can affect development and lead to long-lasting consequences. Empowering pediatric rheumatologists to effectively address mental health disorders should be seen as an integral part of optimizing the care for youth with rheumatologic diseases. This review article aims to describe the burden and impact of mental health disorders in youth with rheumatologic diseases, assess current practices, and explore opportunities to improve mental health care for this population of vulnerable children.

* Correspondence: alaina.m.davis@vanderbilt.edu
[1]Division of Pediatric Rheumatology, Vanderbilt University Medical Center, Monroe Carell Junior Children's Hospital at Vanderbilt, 2200 Children's Way, Doctor's Office Tower 11240, Nashville, TN 37232, USA
Full list of author information is available at the end of the article

Burden of mental health disorders in youth with rheumatologic diseases

Children with chronic diseases have a higher prevalence of mental illness [2–5], and youth with rheumatologic diseases are no exception. Psychological comorbidity in pediatric rheumatology has been studied most for juvenile idiopathic arthritis (JIA), systemic lupus erythematosus (SLE), and fibromyalgia. Current prevalence estimates for depression and anxiety among patients with these diseases in North America, South America, Europe, and Asia range from 15 to 65% [6–14], with suicidal ideation rates as high as 14–34% [6, 15, 16]. These prevalences are disproportionately higher than those observed in healthy controls [6, 7, 9, 13, 17], and by some measures are higher compared to children with special health care needs other chronic diseases such as diabetes and asthma [18–20]. Moreover, recent studies indicate that individuals with childhood-onset rheumatologic disease may be at higher risk for mental health disorders than individuals with adult-onset disease [21, 22].

Discrepancies in reported prevalence of mental health disorders in this population are potentially due to small sample sizes with limited generalizability and the varying use of symptoms, screeners, or diagnosis codes to define mental health disease. These limitations and the overall paucity of existing data regarding mental health comorbidities across pediatric rheumatologic diseases emphasize the need for further research to describe better the burden of mental health disorders in this patient population. Large collaborative studies that draw on diverse demographics of patients will be important in defining the scope of the problem and understanding risk factors for mental health disorders in youth with rheumatologic diseases.

Impact of mental health disorders in youth with rheumatologic diseases

Preliminary studies show that mental health disorders adversely impact quality of life, development, and disease outcomes in youth with rheumatologic diseases. Understanding these effects can illuminate strategies to optimize overall care. In youth with JIA, depression has been associated with higher disease activity, worse pain, worse general health, greater functional disability, and overall lower health related quality of life (HRQL) scores [8, 23]. In youth with SLE, depression and anxiety have been associated with higher disease activity and increased medical services use across ambulatory and acute care settings [9, 24, 25]. However, it is unclear whether these are causal relationships. Further research to investigate these relationships and other potential adverse outcomes related to mental health disorders in pediatric rheumatologic diseases is needed in order to guide development and assessment of future targeted interventions.

While the scope of the problem of mental illness in youth with rheumatologic diseases has yet to be fully investigated, studies of other pediatric chronic diseases indicate that mental illness can lead to poor outcomes during childhood [10, 26–29] and can affect development and risk of mental illness in adulthood [30–32]. To our knowledge, no studies have assessed long-term consequences of mental illness specifically in youth with rheumatologic diseases, but studies of adults with JIA found worse mental health, lower health-related quality of life scores, and higher levels of unemployment than in healthy controls [33, 34].

The impact of mental health disorders on rheumatologic diseases has been more robustly studied in adults than in children. In adults with SLE, depression is cited as the most significant predictor of poor health-related quality of life [35, 36], and positive depression screens have been associated with elevated disease activity scores in studies from around the globe including South America and Asia [37–40]. Similarly, comorbid mental health disorders in patients with rheumatoid arthritis and psoriatic arthritis have been associated with higher disease activity scores and lower likelihood of achieving remission [41–43]. Furthermore, depression is a risk factor for nonadherence to chronic medical treatment [44, 45]; and poor adherence has been associated with increased disease activity, increased ambulatory and acute care, and overall poor prognosis in adults with SLE [46–49].

Fortunately, early recognition and treatment of mental health disorders improves outcomes. In small, randomized controlled trials cognitive behavioral therapy was found to lower levels of functional disability and reported depressive symptoms in adolescents with fibromyalgia [50] and improve quality of life and adaptive pain cognitions in children with JIA [51]. Recent systematic reviews of psychological interventions for pediatric chronic illness describe programs implemented within various settings (i.e. community, school, and clinical practices) that have resulted in consistent improvement of a variety of clinical outcomes, particularly when subthreshold symptoms are recognized and managed [52–54]. In adults, early identification of depression, including subthreshold symptoms, decreases the risk for major depression and suicide [55, 56], improves social function, increases productivity, and decreases absenteeism [57, 58]. Specifically, cognitive-behavioral intervention in adults with SLE has led to significant reduction in the level of depression and anxiety compared to controls and an overall improvement in quality of life scores [59].

Mental health care gap for youth with rheumatologic diseases

Given the impact of mental health disorders on health outcomes and the effectiveness of psychological interventions, the United States Preventive Services Task Force and the Canadian Network for Mood and Anxiety Treatment recommend screening adolescents for depression [60, 61]. The resulting American Academy of Pediatrics (AAP) Recommendations for Preventive Pediatric Health Care and the Guidelines for Adolescent Depression in Primary Care developed from a collaborate initiative in the United States (US) and Canada encourage annual depression screening for all adolescents in primary care settings [62, 63]. However, less than 1% of clinic visits included depression screening in a sample from ambulatory pediatric settings across the US between 2004 and 2013 [64]. Furthermore, in a recent survey by the AAP nearly 40% of the 512 responding pediatricians reported they lacked confidence in their ability to recognize mental health problems and greater than 50% reported they lacked confidence in their ability to treat them. These factors likely contributed to the responses from 44% of those surveyed who reported they were not interested in treating, managing, or co-managing childhood mental health disorders [65].

This situation might be acceptable if access to pediatric mental health providers were not exceedingly limited. Workforce data from the American Academy of Child and Adolescent Psychiatry indicates that there are approximately 8300 practicing child and adolescent psychiatrists in the US with over 15 million youth in need of one [66]. Additional data describes that 96% of counties in the US have an unmet need for prescribing mental health professionals [67], with an uneven distribution leaving rural and low-income populations underserved [68]. Similar data has been reported by the Child and Adolescent Mental Health in Europe project that summarized collective experiences from 15 countries within the European Union and highlighted specific gaps in provider education and available preventative services [69].

Thus, the current systems of care fall short in terms of meeting the mental health needs for youth with rheumatologic diseases. In a survey by the Childhood Arthritis and Rheumatology Research Alliance (CARRA), which includes pediatric rheumatologists from both US and Canada, 52% of surveyed members reported inadequate symptom identification; and 45% reported inadequate treatment of depression and anxiety in adolescents with SLE, identifying limited staff resources and availability of mental health providers as top barriers to mental health intervention [70]. These barriers are not exclusive to pediatric rheumatology settings and have been cited as barriers to identification and management of psychosocial problems within general pediatrics settings as well [65]. Yet, it is notable that only 31% of the 100 CARRA pediatric rheumatology centers report having an affiliated social worker or psychologist. When these providers were surveyed, 35% reported inadequate connection of patients to mental health services; and 52% reported inadequate follow-up of mental health referrals at their practice [71].

Value of pediatric rheumatologists for identifying and addressing mental health disorders

The increased risk of mental health disorders in youth with rheumatologic diseases and their impact on clinical and psychosocial outcomes, as well as the shortage of mental health providers, underscore the need for pediatric rheumatologists to be proficient in addressing mental health needs for these vulnerable patients. Pediatric rheumatologists are optimally positioned to improve mental health intervention due to the frequency and intensity of their patient-provider interactions. Youth with SLE and MCTD have on average twice the number of rheumatology visits compared to primary care visits, and one study found youth with SLE and depressive symptoms to have fewer primary care visits than youth with SLE and no depressive symptoms [6]. Furthermore, in a qualitative interview study, almost all parents of youth with SLE and MCTD said they would feel comfortable bringing concerns about their child's mental health to the rheumatologist; reasons for this included trust and confidence in the therapeutic relationship with his/her rheumatologist, whom they viewed as the primary doctor for their child [72]. In fact, the majority of patients surveyed in an ongoing mood screening project for youth with SLE believe that emotional health should be addressed by their rheumatologist [Rubinstein, unpublished data]. Additionally, a preliminary study of cognitive-behavioral therapy to improve pain and well-being in children with JIA indicated that this intervention within the pediatric rheumatology setting was acceptable to patients and families [51].

Current state of mental health education for pediatric rheumatologists

To begin closing the mental health care gap for youth with rheumatologic diseases, pediatric rheumatologists must feel adept in the screening and initial management of mental health disorders. Symptoms of mental health disorders are often subtle and can be easily overlooked despite multiple interactions between youth with chronic conditions and the health care system. Thus, pediatric subspecialists need to learn how to implement formal screening methods into routine clinical care, effectively communicate with patients, families, and other providers regarding mental health, and assist with establishing and sustaining appropriate mental health intervention.

Current training program requirements outlined by the Accreditation Council of Graduate Medical Education simply call for adequate resources for an education in mental health and social services [73]. The American Board of Pediatrics (ABP) provides slightly more detailed expectations in subspecialty content outlines used to develop questions for board certification examinations. For pediatric rheumatology, the ABP lists the following three learning objectives relevant to mental health care: recognize the cardinal features of depression, determine when depression requires professional consultation, and recognize suicide warning signs [74]. The Objectives of Training in the Subspecialty of Adult and Pediatric Rheumatology from the Royal College of Physicians and Surgeons of Canada and the European Union of Medical Specialists Training Requirements for the Specialty of Rheumatology do not specifically address training for management of mental health comorbidities [75, 76].

Therefore, current training programs likely insufficiently prepare pediatric rheumatologists to manage mental health comorbidities in youth with rheumatologic disease. In a CARRA survey of 130 pediatric rheumatologists, two-thirds reported formal mental health training only in medical school and nearly 10% reported no training at all. Importantly, the respondents with higher levels of mental health training perceived a lower frequency of barriers to mental health screening, and greater than 90% of respondents expressed interest in further mental health training [70]. These data highlight the potential value that mental health education for pediatric rheumatologists may have on improving care for youth with rheumatologic diseases.

Opportunities for improved mental health education for pediatric rheumatologists

The most basic measure to tackle this educational need might be to provide guidelines for mental health screening to pediatric rheumatologists. The American Diabetes Association and the American College of Gastroenterology both issued 2017 guidelines for standards of medical care in diabetes and preventive care in inflammatory bowel disease, respectively, that include recommendations for routine depression and anxiety screening [77, 78]. Such guidelines, however, do not exist for rheumatology. While 85% of surveyed CARRA-affiliated pediatric rheumatologists support routine screening for depression and anxiety in adolescents with SLE, only 2% of practices report routine screening with a standardized instrument [70]. Several standardized and validated instruments exist for mental health screening in children and adolescents, and many of these instruments are available free of charge and with translations in multiple languages [79, 80]. Setting a standard of pediatric rheumatology care inclusive of routine mental health screening, via guidelines and recommendations from professional associations in rheumatology, may be highly valuable to educate pediatric rheumatologists about mental health screening.

For pediatric rheumatology trainees, mental health education could be delivered in didactics within fellowship core curricula or offered in workshops at academic conferences. However, mastery of the skills to elicit information on the symptoms of a mental health disorder in a patient interview likely requires more intensive instruction from behavioral health specialists. Dedicated rotations in behavioral health clinics could provide this needed education if protected time for trainees and mental health providers is secured. Furthermore, training pediatric rheumatologists in the setting of interdisciplinary clinics, where rheumatology and behavioral health trainees work side by side, may offer the most comprehensive opportunity to educate providers and improve mental health care in pediatric rheumatology. While it potentially involves restructuring the way care is provided to patients, it has been proven to be effective for enhancing pediatric resident education in the management of behavioral health problems and improving collaboration between pediatricians and behavioral health specialists [81]. Accordingly, efforts are ongoing by the ABP to promote longitudinal partnerships between trainees and behavioral health providers within integrated ambulatory and inpatient settings [82]. These types of programs are also viewed by physicians and patients as a valuable strategy to improve access to mental health services and ease care coordination for at risk populations [83], and the approach is endorsed in a 2016 perspectives paper from the National Academy of Medicine [84].

Further research is needed to develop effective education programs that will optimize mental health care for youth with rheumatologic diseases. The National Academy of Medicine has outlined a research agenda to support an integrative mental health training paradigm with attention to the following topics: comparative studies of different structural configurations of the interface of pediatric medical care and behavioral health support; development of quality indicators that assess competencies for integrative team training and that lead to improved health outcomes for children; and study of new integrative training models for children with chronic disorders [84]. Studies investigating these topics will help determine best training practices that lead to the greatest impact on mental health for youth with rheumatologic diseases.

Additional steps for improved mental health care for youth with rheumatologic diseases

Early and ongoing mental health education for patients and families of youth with rheumatologic diseases is essential to help increase mental health awareness and normalize attention to mental health as part of the overall care of youth with rheumatologic diseases. Normalization of mental health care is critical in reducing stigma and fear, both of which have been reported by youth with SLE and their parents as common barriers to seeking mental health treatment [72]. Partnerships with community providers and foundations can enhance dissemination of educational information and normalize mental health issues. For example, the National Resource Center on Lupus sponsored by Lupus Foundation of America publishes online educational information to help patients and families recognize warning signs of mental health disorders and find assistance for management of these disorders [85].

Increasing the availability of peer support groups and networks also has the potential to improve mental health education of youth with rheumatologic diseases. Specifically, the iPeer2Peer Program, a novel online peer mentoring program for adolescents with JIA developed by investigators in Canada, improved participants' perceived ability to manage their disease compared to controls [86]. Similarly, Teens Taking Charge, an internet-based self-management program including disease-specific information and social support for youth with JIA in Canada, led to higher levels of knowledge and lower pain reports [87]. Improving support for families of youth with rheumatologic diseases also may positively impact patient outcomes, as higher caregiver psychological distress has been associated with worse HRQL in patients with JIA [88, 89].

While improved mental health education for both pediatric rheumatologists and patients and their families is necessary, education alone is insufficient. Sustainable systems for the delivery of mental health services must be developed. Dedicated application of implementation science principles and quality improvement methodology has been successfully utilized to improve mental health care for youth with other chronic diseases [90]. Funding is needed to support implementation research and quality improvement initiatives aimed at optimizing mental health care for youth with rheumatologic diseases. Required funding for overall increased mental health resources for this population should not be overlooked either, particularly given reported lack of time and adequate staffing for mental health screening and treatment in pediatric rheumatology settings [70]. The necessity of this funding priority aligns with the goals and expectations of our patients, as indicated in a mixed methods study of youth with SLE showing that research focused on alleviating poor psychological outcomes is viewed as a top priority in this population [91].

Conclusions

The prevalence and burden of mental health disorders in youth with rheumatologic diseases is high. The evidence from pediatric and adult literature of rheumatologic diseases indicates that mental illness has a pervasive impact on multiple areas of health behaviors, disease outcomes, and quality of life. Improved identification and early treatment of mental health disorders may improve outcomes in this population, and pediatric rheumatologists are well situated to provide mental health screening and offer early intervention. Additional training for pediatric rheumatologists is necessary to enable provision of effective mental health care. Potential educational strategies include the development of clinical guidelines for mental health screening within pediatric rheumatology settings and revision of pediatric rheumatology fellowship cuuricula to include mental health didactics, workshops, and clinical experience in behavioral health. Improved education of patients and families is also essential in order to increase awareness of and normalize inclusion of mental health as part of overall care. Future work should focus on developing and implementing sustainable systems for the delivery of mental health care alongside medical care for youth with rheumatologic diseases. Increased advocacy for mental health resources and research funding is needed to support the above initiatives.

Abbreviations

AAP: American Academy of Pediatrics; ABP: American Board of Pediatrics; CARRA: Childhood Arthritis and Rheumatology Research Alliance; HRQL: health related quality of life; JIA: juvenile idiopathic arthritis; MCTD: mixed connective tissue disease; SLE: systemic lupus erythematosus; US: United States

Acknowledgements

Not applicable.

Funding

No specific funding was secured for the development this manuscript.

Authors' Contributions

All authors made substantial contributions to the conception and design of this manuscript including the review of the literature. AMD wrote the original draft of the article. TBR, MR, and AMK contributed to the content and revisions. All authors read and approved the final manuscript and agree to be accountable for all aspects of the work.

Competing interests

The authors declare that they have no competing interests.

Author details

[1]Division of Pediatric Rheumatology, Vanderbilt University Medical Center, Monroe Carell Junior Children's Hospital at Vanderbilt, 2200 Children's Way, Doctor's Office Tower 11240, Nashville, TN 37232, USA. [2]Division of Pediatric Rheumatology, Albert Einstein College of Medicine, Children's Hospital at Montefiore/ Albert Einstein College of Medicine, 3415 Bainbridge Avenue, Bronx, NY 10467, USA. [3]Section of Pediatric Rheumatology, Riley Hospital for Children at Indiana University Health, 705 Riley Hospital Dr, Indianapolis, IN 46202, USA. [4]Division of Rheumatology, The Children's Hospital of Philadelphia, Roberts Center for Pediatric Research, 2716 South St, Ste 10253, Philadelphia, PA 19146, USA. [5]The Children's Hospital of Philadelphia, Roberts Center for Pediatric Research, Center for Pediatric Clinical Effectiveness, 2716 South St, Ste 10253, Philadelphia, PA 19146, USA. [6]The Children's Hospital of Philadelphia, Roberts Center for Pediatric Research, PolicyLab, 2716 South St, Ste 10253, Philadelphia, PA 19146, USA.

References

1. United States Department of Health and Human Services, Office of Disease Prevention and Health Promotion. Healthy People 2020. https://www.healthypeople.gov. Accessed 7 Aug 2017.
2. Suryavanshi MS, Yang Y. Clinical and economic burden of mental disorders among children with chronic physical conditions, United States, 2008–2013. Prev Chronic Dis. 2016;13:E71.

3. Pinquart M, Shen Y. Depressive symptoms in children and adolescents with chronic physical illness: an updated meta-analysis. J Pediatr Psychol. 2011; 36:375–84.
4. Bennett D. Depression among children with chronic medical problems: a meta-analysis. J Pediatr Psychol. 1994;19:149–69.
5. Pao M, Bosk A. Anxiety in medically ill children/adolescents. Depress Anxiety. 2011;28:40–9.
6. Knight A, Weiss P, Morales K, Geredes M, Gustein A, Vickery M, et al. Depression and anxiety and their association with healthcare utilization in pediatric lupus and mixed connective tissue disease patients: a cross-sectional study. Pediatr Rheuamtol Online J. 2014;12:42.
7. Krause M, Zamora-Legoff JA, Crowson CS, Wampler Muskardin T, Mason T, Matteson EL. Population-based study outcomes of patients with juvenile idiopathic arthritis (JIA) compared to non-JIA subjects. Semin Arthritis Rheum. 2017;46:439–43.
8. Shaw KL, Southwood TR, Duffy CM, McDonagh JE. Health-related quality of life in adolescents with juvenile idiopathic arthritis. Arthritis Rheum. 2006;55: 199–207.
9. Knight AM, Xie M, Mandell DS. Disparities in psychiatric diagnosis and treatment for youth with systemic lupus erythematosus: analysis of a national US Medicaid sample. J Rheumatol. 2016;43:1427–33.
10. Jones JT, Cunningham N, Kashikar-Zuck S, Brunner HI. Pain, fatigue, and psychosocial impact on health-related quality of life in childhood-onset lupus. Arthritis Care Res (Hoboken). 2016;68:73–80.
11. Kohut SA, Williams TS, Jayanthikumar J, Landolt-Marticorena C, Lefebvre A, Silverman E, et al. Depressive symptoms are prevalent in childhood-onset systemic lupus erythematosus (cSLE). Lupus. 2013;22:712–20.
12. Kashikar-Zuck S, Parkins IS, Graham TB, Lynch AM, Passo M, Johnston M, et al. Anxiety, mood, and behavioral disorders among pediatric patients with juvenile fibromyalgia syndrome. Clin J Pain. 2008;24:620–6.
13. Makay B, Emiroglu N, Unsal E. Depression and anxiety in children and adolescents with familial Mediterranean fever. Clin Rheumatol. 2010;29:375–9.
14. Nery FG, Borba EF, Viana VS, Hatch JP, Soares JC, Bonfa E, et al. Prevalence of depressive and anxiety disoders in systemic lupus erythematosus and their association with anti-ribosomal P antibodies. Prog Neuro-Psychopharmacol Biol Psychiatry. 2008;32:695–700.
15. Nassi L, Punaro L, Morton A, Fribley C, Baisch J, Xu Z, et al. Suicidal ideation common in childhood-onset systemic lupus erythematosus (cSLE): genetic expression and depressive symptoms in cSLE. Arthritis Rheum. 2009; 60(Suppl 10):1532.
16. Lim LS, Lefebvre A, Benseler S, Peralta M, Silverman ED. Psychiatric illness of systemic lupus erythematosus in childhood: sprectrum of clinically important manifestations. J Rheumatol. 2013;40:506–12.
17. Kashikar-Zuck PIS, Ting TV, Verkamp E, Lynch-Jordan A, Passo M, et al. Controlled follow-up study of physical and psychosocial functioning of adolescents with juvenile primary fibromyalgia syndrome. Rheumatology (Oxford). 2010;49:2204–9.
18. Child and Adolescent Health Measurement Initiative, Data Resource Center on Child and Adolescent Health. National Survey of Children with Special Health Care Needs. 2010. http://www.childhealthdata.org/browse/ata-snapshots/cshcn-profiles/condition-specific?rpt=12&cond=15&geo=1&ind=144. Accessed 21 Sept 2017.
19. Child and Adolescent Health Measurement Initiative, Data Resource Center on Child and Adolescent Health. National Survey of Children with Special Health Care Needs. 2010. http://childhealthdata.org/browse/data-snapshots/cshcn-profiles/condition-specific?rpt=12&cond=7&geo=1&ind=144. Accessed 21 Sept 2017.
20. Child and Adolescent Health Measurement Initiative, Data Resource Center on Child and Adolescent Health. National Survey of Children with Special Health Care Needs. 2010. http://childhealthdata.org/browse/data-snapshots/cshcn-profiles/condition-specific?cond=1&geo=1&rpt=12&ind=144. Accessed 21 Sept 2017.
21. Knight Am, Trupin L, Katz P, Lawson EF. Depression risk in young adults with childhood- and adult-onset lupus: 12 years of follow-up. Arthritis Care Res (Hoboken). 2017 [Epub ahead of print].
22. Shih M, Hootman JM, Strine TW, Chapman DP, Brady TJ. Serious psychological distress in U.S. adults with arthritis. J Gen Intern Med. 2006;21:1160–6.
23. Tarakci E, Yeldan I, Kaya Mutlu E, Baydogan SN, Kasapcopur O. The relationship between physical activity level, anxiety, depression, and functional ability in children and adolescents with juvenile idiopathic arthritis. Clin Rheumatol. 2011;30:1415–20.
24. Knight A, Weiss P, Morales K, Gerdes M, Rearson M, Vickery M, et al. Identifying differences in risk factors for depression and anxiety in pediatric chronic disease: a matched cross-sectional study of youth with lupus/mixed connective tissue disease and their peers with diabetes. J Pediatrics. 2015; 167:1397–403.
25. Knight AM, Davis AM, Klein-Gitelman MS, Cidav Z, Mandell D. The impact of psychiatric comorbidity on health care utilization for youth with systemic lupus erythematosus. Arthritis Rheumatol. 2017;69 Suppl 10 [abstract].
26. Bernstein CM, Stockwell MS, Gallagher MP, Rosenthal SL, Soren K. Mental health issues in adolescents and young adults with type I diabetes: prevalence and impact on glycemic control. Clin Pediatr (Phila). 2013;52:10–5.
27. Bitsko MJ, Everhart RS, Rubin BK. The adolescent with asthma. Paediatr Respir Rev. 2014;15:146–53.
28. Calsbeek H, Rijken M, Bekkers MJ, Dekker J, van Berge Henegouwen GP. School and leisure activites in adolescents and young adults with chronic digestive disorders: impact and burden of disease. Int J Behav Med. 2006;13: 121–30.
29. Reigada LC, Bruzzese JM, Benkov KJ, Levy J, Waxman AR, Petkova E, et al. Illness-specific anxiety: implications for functioning and utilization in systemic lupus erythematosus. J Spec Pediat Nurs. 2011;16:207–15.
30. Harrington R, Fudge H, Rutter M, Pickles A, Hill J. Adult outcomes of childhood and adolescent depression. I. Psychiatric status. Arch Gen Psychiatry. 1990;47:465–73.
31. Kim-Cohen J, Caspi A, Moffitt TE, Harrington H, Milne BJ, Poulton R. Prior Juvenile diagnosis in adults with mental disorder: developmental follow-back of a prospective-longitudinal cohort. Arch Gen Psychiatry. 2003;60:709–17.
32. Fombonne E, Wostear G, Cooper V, Harrington R, Rutter M. The Maudsley long-term follow-up of child and adolescent depression. 1. Psychiatric outcomes in adulthood. Br J Psychiatry. 2001;179:210–7.
33. Foster HE, Marshall N, Myers A, Dunkley P, Griffiths ID. Outcome in adults with juvenile idiopathic arthritis: a quality of life study. Arthritis Rheum. 2003;48:767–75.
34. Barth S, Haas JP, Schlchtiger J, Molz J, Bisdorff B, Michels H, et al. Long-term health-related quality of life in German pateints with juvenile idiopathic arthritis in comparison to German general population. PLoS One. 2016;11:e0153267.
35. Moldovan I, Katsaros E, Carr FN, Coorey D, Torralba K, Shinada S, et al. The patient reported outcomes in lupus (PATROL) study: role of depression in health-related quality of life in Southern California lupus cohort. Lupus. 2011;20:1285–92.
36. Choi ST, Kang JI, Park IH, Lee YW, Song JS, Park YB, et al. Subscale analysis of quality of life in patients with systemic lupus erythematosus: association with depression, fatigue, disease activity, and damage. Clin Exp Rheumatol. 2012;30:665–72.
37. Skare T, da Silva Magalhaes D, Siquiera RE. Systemic lupus erythematosus activity and depression. Rheumatol Int. 2014;34:445–6.
38. Nery FG, Borba EF, Hatch JP, Soares JC, Bonfa E, Neto FL. Major depressive disorder and disease activity in systemic lupus erythematosus. Compr Psychiatry. 2007;48:14–9.
39. Alsowaida N, Alrasheed M, Mayet A, Alsuwaida A, Omair MA. Medication adherence, depression and disease activity among patients with systemic lupus erythematosus. Lupus 2017 [Epub ahead of print].
40. Shen B, Tan W, Feng G, He Y, Liu J, Chen W, et al. The correlations of disease activity, socioeconomic status, quality of life, and depression/anxiety in Chinese patients with systemic lupus erythematosus. Clin Dev Immunol 2013 [Epub ahead of print].
41. Inanc N, Yilmaz-Onar S, Can M, Sokka T, Direskeneli H. The role of depression, anxiety, fatigue, and fibromyalgia on the evaluation of the remission status in patients with rheumatoid arthritis. J Rheumatol. 2014;41:1755–60.
42. Rathbun AM, Reed GW, Harrold LR. The temporal relationship between depression and rheumatoid arthritis disease activity, treatment persistence, and response: a systemic review. Rheumatology (Oxford). 2013;52:1785–94.
43. Michelsen B, Kristianslund EK, Sexton J, Hammer HB, Fagerli KM, Lie E, et al. Do depression and anxiety reduce the likelihood of remission in rheumatoid arthritis and psoriatic arthritis? Data from the prospective multicenter NOR-DMARD study. Ann Rheum Dis. 2017; [Epub ahead of print]
44. DiMatteo MR, Lepper HS, Croghan TW. Depression is a risk factor for noncompliance with medical treatment: meta-analysis of the effects of anxiety and depression on patient adherence. Arch Intern Med. 2000;160:2101–7.
45. Julian LJ, Yelin E, Yazdany J, Panopalis P, Trupin L, Criswell LA, et al. Depression, medication adherence, and service utilization in systemic lupus erythematosus. Arthritis Rheum. 2009;61:240–6.

46. Petri M, Perez-Gutthann S, Longenecker JC, Hochberg M. Morbidity of systemic lupus erythematosus: role of race and socioeconomic status. Am J Med. 1991;91:345–53.
47. Adler M, Chambers S, Edwards C, Neild G, Isenberg D. An assessment of renal failure in an SLE cohort with special reference to ethnicity, over a 25-year period. Rheumatol. 2006;45:1144–7.
48. Rojas-Serrano J, Cardiel MH. Lupus patients in an emergency unit. Causes of consultation, hospitalization, and outcome. A cohort study. Lupus. 2000;9:601–6.
49. Costedoat-Chalumeau N, Pouchot J, Guettrot-Imbert G, Le Guern V, Marra D, Morel N, et al. Adherence to treatment in systemic lupus erythematosus patients. Best Pract Res Clin Rheumatol. 2013;27:329–40.
50. Kashikar-Zuck S, Swain NF, Jones BA, Graham TB. Efficacy of cognitive-behavioral intervention for juvenile pediatric primary fibromyalgia syndrome. J Rheumatol. 2005;32:1594–602.
51. Lomholt JJ, Thastum M, Christensen AE, Leegaard A, Herlin T. Cognitive behavioral group intervention for pain and well-being in children with juvenile idiopathic arthritis: a study of feasibility and preliminary efficacy. Pediatr Rheumatol Online J. 2015;13:35.
52. Beale IL. Scholarly literature review: efficacy of psychological interventions for pediatric chronic illness. J Pediatr Psychol. 2006;31:437–51.
53. Wesselhoeft R, Sorensen MJ, Heiervang ER, Bilenberg N. Subthreshold depression in children and adolescents – a systematic review. J Afffect Disord. 2013;151:7–22.
54. Leslie LK, Mehus CJ, Hawkins JD, et al. Primary health care: potential home for family focused preventative interventions. Am J Prev Med. 2016;51(Suppl 2):106–18.
55. Halfin A. Depression: the benefits of early and appropriate treatment. Am J of. Manag Care. 2007;13(Suppl 4):92–7.
56. Kupfer DJ, Frank E, Perel JM. The advantage of early treatment intervention in recurrent depression. Arch Gen Psychiatry. 1989;46:945–8.
57. Coulehan JL, Schulberg HC, Block MR, Madonia MJ, Rodrigues E. Treating depressed primary care patients improves their physical, mental, and social functioning. Arch Intern Med. 1997;157:1113–20.
58. Rost K, Smith JL, Dickinson M. The effect of improving primary care depression management on employee absenteeism and productivity. A randomized trial. Med Care. 2004;42:1202–10.
59. Navarrete-Navarrete N, Peralta-Ramirez MI, Sabio-Sanchez JM, Coin MA, Robles-Ortega H, Hidalgo-Tenorio C, et al. Efficiency of cognitive behavioral therapy for the treatment of chronic stress in patients with lupus erythematosus: a randomized controlled trial. Psychother Psychosom. 2010;79:107–15.
60. US Preventive Services. Task force. Screening and treatment for major depressive disorder in children and adolescents: US preventive services task force recommendation statement. Pediatrics. 2009;123:1223–8.
61. MacQueen GM, Frey BN, Ismail Z, Jaworska N, Steiner M, Van Lieshout R, et al. Canadian network for mood and anxiety treatments (CANMAT) 2016 clinical guidelines for the management of adults with major depressive disorder. Can J Psychiatr. 2016;61:588–603.
62. American Academy of Pediatrics. Recommendations for preventive pediatric health care. http://www.aap.org/en-us/professional-resources/practice-support/Periodicity/Periodicity%20Schedule_FINAL.pdf. Accessed 3 Aug 2017.
63. Zuckerbrot RA, Cheung AH, Jensen PS, Stein REK, Laraque D. GLAD-PC steering group. Guidelines for adolescent depression in primary care (GLAD-PC): I. Identification, assessment, and initial management. Pediatrics. 2007; 120:e1299–312.
64. Zenlea IS, Milliren CE, Mednick L, Rhodes ET. Depression screening in adolescents in the United States: a national study of ambulatory office-based practice. Acad Pediatr. 2014;133:e981–92.
65. Horwitz SM, Storfer-Isser A, Kerker BD, Szilagyi M, Garner A, O'Connor KG, et al. Barriers to the identification and management of psychosocial problems: changes from 2004 to 2013. Acad Pediatr. 2015;15:613–20.
66. American Academy of Child and Adolescent Psychiatry. Workforce Issues. https://www.aacap.org/aacap/resources_for_primary_care/Workforce_Issues.aspx. Accessed 4 Sept 2017.
67. Konrad TR, Ellis AR, Thomas KC, Holzer CE, Morrissey JP. County-level estimates of need for mental health professionals in the United States. Psychiatr Serv. 2009;60:1307–14.
68. Ricketts TC. Workforce issues in rural areas: a focus on policy equity. Am J Public Health. 2005;95:42–8.
69. Braddick F, Carral V, Jenkins R, Jané-Llopis E. Child and adolescent mental health in Europe: infrastructures, policy and programmes. http://ec.europa.eu/health/ph_determinants/life_style/mental/docs/camhee_infrastructures.pdf. Accessed 25 Nov 2017.
70. Knight AM, Vickery ME, Muscal E, Davis AM, Harris JG, Soybilgic A, et al. Identifying targets for improving mental healthcare for adolescents with systemic lupus erythematosus: perspectives from pediatric rheumatology clinicians in the United States and Canada. J Rheumatol. 2016;43:1136–45.
71. Knight A, Vickery M, Muscal E, Davis A, Harris J, Hersh AO, et al. Mental health care for adolescents with rheumatologic conditions: perspectives from pediatric behavioral health providers in North America. Arthritis Rheumatol. 2016;68 Suppl 10 [abstract].
72. Knight AM, Vickery ME, Fiks AG, Barg FK. Barriers and facilitators for mental healthcare in pediatric lupus and mixed connective tissue disease: a qualitative study of youth and parent perspectives. Pediatr Rheumatol Online J. 2015;13:52.
73. The Accreditation Council of Graduate Medical Education. ACGME Program Requirements for Graduate Medical Education in the Subspecialties of Pediatrics. http://www.acgme.org/Portals/0/PFAssets/ProgramRequirements/320S_pediatric_subs_2016.pdf. Accessed 28 Jun 2016.
74. The American Board of Pediatrics. Content Outline, Pediatric Rheumatology: Subspecialty In-Training, Certification and Maintenance of Certification (MOC) Examinations. https://www.abp.org/sites/abp/files/pdf/pediatric_rheumatology_content_outline.pdf. Accessed 28 June 2016.
75. Royal College of Physicians and Surgeons of Canada. Objectives of Training in the Subspecialty of Adult and Pediatric Rheumatology. http://www.royalcollege.ca/cs/groups/public/documents/document/mdaw/mdg4/~edisp/088807.pdf. Accessed 24 Nov 2017.
76. European Union of Medical Specilaists. Training Requirements for the Specialty of Rheumatology: Euopean Standards of Postgraduate Medical specialist Training. https://www.uems.eu/__data/assets/pdf_file/0005/44438/UEMS-2014.21-European-Training-Requirements-Rheumatology-.pdf. Accessed 24 Nov 2017.
77. American Diabetes Association. Standards of medical care in diabetes – 2017. Diabetes Care. 2017;40 Suppl 1:1–142.
78. Farraye FA, Melmed GY, Lichtenstein GR, Kane SV. Preventive Care in Inflammatory Bowel Disease. Am J Gastroenterol. 2017;112:241–58.
79. Beidas RS, Stewart RE, Walsh L, Lucas S, Downey MM, Jackson K, et al. Free, brief, and validated: standardized instruments for low-resource mental health settings. Cogn Behav Pract. 2015;22:5–19.
80. American Academy of Pediatrics Inc. Mental Health Screening and Assessment Tools for Primary Care. In: Addressing Mental Health Concerns in Primary Care: A Clinician's Toolkit. https://www.aap.org/en-us/advocacy-and-policy/aap-health-initiatives/Mental-Health/Documents/MH_ScreeningChart.pdf. Accessed 8 Aug 2017.
81. Garfunkel LC, Pisani AR, leRoux P, Siegel DM. Educating residents in behavioral health care and collaboration: comparison of conventional and integrated training models. Academic Medicine: Journal of the Association of American Medical Colleges. 2011;86:174–9.
82. McMillan JA, Land M Jr, Leslie LK. Pediatric residency education and the behavioral and mental health crisis: a call to action. Pediatrics 2017;139: e20162141.
83. Khazan O. Therapy for everybody. The Atlantic 22 Jun 2017.
84. Boat TF, Land M, Leslie LK, et al. Workforce development to enhance cognitive, affective and behavioral health of children and youth: opportunities and barriers in child health care training, perspectives paper. National Academy of Medicine https://nam.edu/wp-content/uploads/2016/11/Workforce-Development-to-Enhance-the-Cognitive-Affective-and-Behavioral-Health-of-Children-and-Youth.pdf. Accessed 7 Sept 2017.
85. Knight AM. Mental health issues in children and teens with lupus. In: National Resource Center on lupus. Lupus Foundation of America http://resources.lupus.org/entry/mental-health-in-children. Accessed 8 Aug 2017.
86. Stinson J, Ahola Kohut S, Forgeron P, Amaria K, Bell M, Kaufman M, et al. The iPeer2Peer program: a pilot randomized controlled trial in adolescents with juvenile idiopathic arthritis. Pediatr Rheumatol Online J. 2016;14:48.
87. Stinson JN, McGrath PJ, Hodnett ED, Feldman BM, Duffy CM, Huber AM, et al. An internet-based self-management program with telephone support for adolescents with arthritis: a pilot randomized controlled trial. J Rheumatol. 2010;37:1944–52.
88. Toupin April K, Cavallo S, Ehrmann Feldman D, Ni A. The associations among economic hardship, caregiver psychological distress, disease activity,

and health-related quality of life in children with juvenile idiopathic arthritis. Qual Life Res. 2012;21:1185–91.

89. Seid M, Huang B, Niehaus S, Brunner HI, Lovell DJ. Determinants of heath-related quality of life in children newly diagnosed with juvenile idiopathic arthritis. Arthritis Care Res (Hoboken). 2014;66:263–9.
90. Corathers SD, Kichler J, Jones NH, Houchen A, Jolly M, Morwessell N, et al. Improving depression screening for adolescents with type 1 diabetes. Pediatrics. 2013;132:e1395–402.
91. Tunnicliffe DJ, Singh-Grewal D, Craig JC, Howell M, Tugwell P, Mackie F, et al. Healthcare and research priorities of adolescents and young adults with systemic lupus erythematosus a mixed-methods study. J Rheumatol. 2017; 44:444–51.

17

Incidence and risk factors for recurrent Henoch-Schönlein purpura in children from a 16-year nationwide database

Wei-Te Lei[1], Po-Li Tsai[2], Szu-Hung Chu[1], Yu-Hsuan Kao[1], Chien-Yu Lin[3], Li-Ching Fang[1], Shyh-Dar Shyur[1], Yu-Wen Lin[4] and Shu-I Wu[5,6,7*]

Abstract

Background: The recurrence rate of Henoch-Schönlein purpura (HSP) is 2.7%–30%, with varied average intervals between the first and second episodes. Few studies have explored the incidence and risk factors for recurrent HSP.

Methods: We used a 16-year nationwide database to analyze the incidence of recurrent HSP. Patients with HSP were identified, and risk factors for recurrent HSP were explored. Kaplan-Meier and Cox regression model analyses were performed, and covariates were adjusted in the multivariate model.

Results: From January 1, 1997 to December 31, 2012, among 2,886,836 individuals in the National Health Insurance Research Database, 1002 HSP patients aged < 18 years were identified. Among them, 164 had ≥2 HSP episodes (recurrence rate, 16.4%; incidence of recurrent HSP, 7.05 per 100 person-years); 83.6% patients with one HSP episode remained free of secondary HSP. The average time intervals between the first and second and second and third HSP episodes were 9.2 and 6.4 months, respectively. After adjusting for demographic parameters, comorbidities, and socioeconomic status, recurrent HSP was found to occur more frequently in patients who had renal involvement (adjusted hazard ratio, 2.41; 95% confidence interval [CI], 1.64–3.54; $p < 0.001$), were receiving steroid therapy for > 10 days (adjusted hazard ratio, 8.13; 95%CI, 2.51–26.36; $p < 0.001$), and had allergic rhinitis (adjusted hazard ratio, 1.63; 95%CI, 1.06–2.50; $p = 0.026$).

Conclusions: The annual incidence of recurrent HSP was low. However, children who had underlying allergic rhinitis, presented with renal involvement, and received steroid treatment for > 10 days should be notified regarding the possibility of recurrence.

Keywords: Henoch-Scholein Purpura, Recurrent, Incidence, Steroid

Background

Henoch-Schönlein purpura (HSP) is the most common systemic vasculitis in children [1]. The incidence of HSP in children is approximately 6–22 per 100,000 person-years [1–4], which is higher than that in adult (3.4–14.3 per 100,000 person years) [5]. Most HSP symptoms, such as temporarily palpable purpura, gastrointestinal (GI) pain, and joint pain, are self-limited; however, intestinal obstruction, central nervous system involvement, and severe nephritis can also occur [1, 6–10]. The prognosis of HSP is generally good, but recurrence is common among children (recurrence rate, 2.7%–66.2%) [1, 11–16]. Various predictors for recurrence, including greater joint and gastrointestinal involvement at diagnosis, history of infection, elevated erythrocyte sedimentation rate, steroid treatment, and renal manifestations, have been identified but they are inconsistent [1, 12, 13].

Glucocorticoids used for HSP treatment do not prevent renal disease; therefore their use is controversial [17]. However, early treatment with glucocorticoids in HSP children may reduce the intensity or mean resolution time of joint or abdominal pain [18, 19]. Additionally, glucocorticoids should be tapered slowly to prevent the relapse of

* Correspondence: shuiwu624@gmail.com
[5]Department of Medicine, Mackay Medical College, No.45, Minsheng Rd., Tamsui Dist., New Taipei City 25160, Taiwan
[6]Audiology and Speech Language Pathology, Mackay Medical College, No.45, Minsheng Rd., Tamsui Dist., New Taipei City 25160, Taiwan
Full list of author information is available at the end of the article

symptoms. Although previous literature has mainly focused on the risk factors for renal involvement and long-term complications in patients with HSP, no standard protocol or long-term follow-up studies are available to clarify the impact of steroid on the clinical course or subsequent recurrence of HSP.

Furthermore, the few studies that focused on the average time to second episode of recurrence revealed discrepant results (range, 1–13.5 months) [12, 13]. Little is known regarding the third episode of recurrent HSP, and the long-term disease-free rate. However, these data are important in the decision making for adequate follow-up time. To clarify these aspects, data from a nationwide, population-based claims database, the Taiwan National Health Insurance Research Database (NHIRD), were used to investigate the mean duration between first and second HSP episodes, risk factors for recurrence, and the real-world use of steroids in patients with HSP.

Methods

Database

On March 1, 1995, the National Health Insurance (NHI) was established in Taiwan, achieving a coverage rate exceeding 99% among Taiwanese citizens. Each year, the Bureau of NHI provides data containing encrypted personal identifications, diagnoses, and healthcare utilizations to compose the Taiwan NHIRD [20]. In the NHIRD, diseases are coded according to the International Classifications of Disease, Ninth Revision, Clinical Modification (ICD-9-CM). A subset of the NHIRD, the Longitudinal Health Insurance Database (LHID), was used in our analysis. The LHID contains 3 million randomly selected enrollees from the NHIRD [21]. Distributions of age, gender, or healthcare costs between the LHID and the general population in Taiwan are not significantly different [22]. This study was reviewed and approved by the institutional Review Board of Mackay Memorial Hospital, Taipei, Taiwan (IRB approval number: 17MMHIS022e). The institutional review board exempted consent requirement.

Study sample

From the LHID and based on the criteria of the American College of Rheumatology [23], patients aged < 18 years with a first diagnosis of HSP (ICD-9-CM code 287.0) between January 1, 1997, and December 31, 2012, were identified from ambulatory, emergency, and inpatients claims data. Dates of the first HSP were defined as index dates. Patients diagnosed with HSP before December 31, 1996 were excluded. Among these subjects, those who received a second HSP diagnosis 3 months apart from the first HSP diagnosis were defined as having recurrent HSP (study subjects), which means a 3-months diagnosis-free interval between the first and second HSP diagnoses was required in order to define a recurrent HSP. The definition of our 3-months diagnosis-free interval t was based on findings from several epidemiological studies on HSP [12, 14, 24], in which they suggested that HSP commonly recurs within 2 to 3 months after the primary episode. Furthermore, glucocorticoids were suggested to be tapered over a 4 to 8 weeks time frame, to minimize the chance of precipitating a disease flare by overly aggressive medication tapering. Under such considerations, we found and excluded 10 patients with persistent HSP diagnosis and persistent steroid prescription in every follow-up outpatient visit during and after 3 months time because they may be seen as receiving continued treatment, instead of having relapse or recurrence. All patients included as recurrent HSP had records of HSP diagnosis-free interval for at least 3 months after the index date. Figure 1 shows the flow diagram of participant selection. Status and durations for steroid use (solu-medrol, solu-cortef, kidsolone, and prednisolone) were compared. All the generic names of steroid included in our analysis were attached in the supplement Additional file 1: Table S1. Corticosteroid exposure was characterized by the day of initial prescription and the duration of treatment. Children were divided into the following categories based on the time of initiating corticosteroids: (1) first dose prescribed within < 14 days of initial diagnosis,(2) first dose prescribed after day 14 of initial diagnosis, and (3) no receipt of steroids during the disease course. Fourteen days was chosen as the cutoff point for corticosteroid initiation to include patients with atypically late presentations or those with later worsened clinical course. The duration of corticosteroid use was defined as consecutive days of corticosteroids administration [25]. Currently, the recommended steroid treatment duration is 1–2 weeks for HSP [18]. However, there was no precise definition about the length of steroid therapy. So, we chose the median number of days in steroid use among our study subjects as the cutoff point to group patients with steroid use. For the sake of brevity, patients were categorized into those that used steroids for < 10 days (the shorter-term steroid use group); and ≥ 10 days (the longer-term steroid use group), respectively. HSP with renal involvement was defined as receiving a diagnosis of hematuria, proteinuria, nephritis, or nephrotic syndrome (ICD-9-CM codes 599.7, 791.0, and, 580–585) within 1 year after the first HSP diagnosis. Renal biopsy was defined by the ICD-9-CM codes 55.23 (Closed (percutaneous) (needle) biopsy of kidney) and 55.24 (Open biopsy of kidney)). Other clinical manifestations for HSP were defined as having the following diagnoses: joint pain (ICD-9-CM code 719.4×) or GI symptoms (ICD-9-CM codes 789, 787.0, 787.91, 558.9, and 578.9). Our covariates included demographic data (e.g., age, gender, and income levels) and diagnoses of asthma (ICD-9-CM code 493 and 494), allergic rhinitis (ICD-9-CM code 477.x), and atopic dermatitis (ICD-9-CM codes 691.8), which appeared

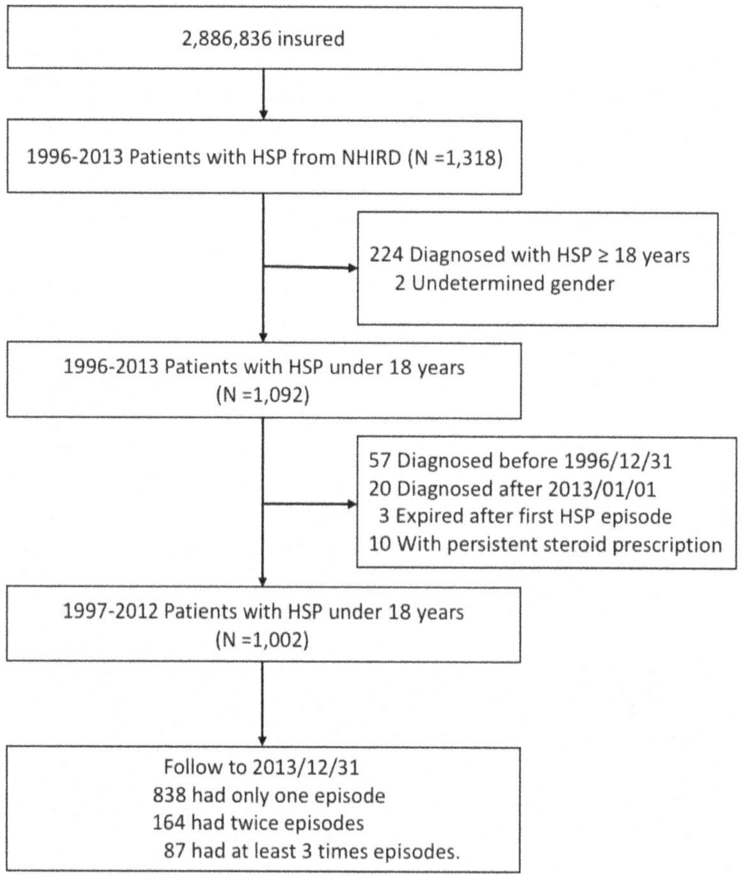

Fig. 1 Flow chart of study patients

before the diagnosis of the first HSP. All subjects were followed until December 31, 2013.

Statistical analysis

Data analysis was conducted using SPSS 18.0 software for descriptive and contingency tables (SPSS, Inc., Chicago, Illinois). Pearson's chi-squared tests were used for comparisons of categorical variables. The Kruskal-Wallis test was used to investigate average differences in age at HSP diagnosis and/or recurrence. Kaplan-Meier survival analysis and Cox proportional hazard models were used to estimate hazard ratios and adjust for other covariates. The event was the date of HSP recurrence. Censoring points were the end of follow-up or the date of withdrawal from the registry. $P < 0.05$ was considered statistically significant. This study was approved by the institutional review board of Mackay Memorial Hospital (IRB no: 17MMHIS022e).

Result

Recurrent rate and incidence

We identified 1002 patients aged < 18 years with a first diagnosis of HSP (index episode; Table 1; 50.8% females). Nearly 59.5% had HSP before 6 years of age, nearly one-fifth had recurrent events (secondary HSP), and nearly 10% ≥3 episodes of HSP. Recurrent HSP patients were predominantly male and younger aged (second recurrent HSP episode before 6 years of age). Furthermore, the third HSP episode occurred in higher proportions of individuals aged 7–12 years.

The incidence of the first HSP episode was 9.61per 100,000 person-years (male incidence, 4.82; female incidence,

Table 1 Henoch-Schönlein Purpura and recurrent events ($N = 1002$)

	One HSP episode ($n = 838$) n (%)	Two HSP episodes ($n = 164$) n (%)	Three HSP episodes ($n = 87$) n (%)
Gender			
Female	426 (50.8)	73 (44.5)	41 (47.1)
Male	412 (49.2)	91 (55.5)	46 (52.9)
Age, y			
0–6	499 (59.5)	82 (50.0)	37 (42.6)
7–12	268 (32.0)	71 (43.3)	43 (49.4)
13–18	71 (8.5)	11(6.7)	7 (8.0)

Abbreviations: *HSP* Henoch-Schönlein Purpura

4.79). The highest incidence (5.45 per 100,000 person-years) of first HSP was among the youngest age group (0–6 years).

The incidence of patients with secondary (recurrent) HSP was 7.05 per 100 person-years (male incidence, 8.29; female incidence, 4.96). The highest incidence (11.03 per 100 person-years) of recurrent HSP was among the youngest age group (0–6 years), and the lowest (2.87 per 100 person-years) was among the oldest age group (13–18 years).

Average time of steroid usage

Among the 1002 HSP patients, 342 (40.8%) used steroids during the first HSP episode. The average period of steroid use during the first HSP episode was 6.90 days. Among the 77 patients with a second HSP episode, 43 (55.8%) received steroid therapy. The average period of steroid use during the second HSP episode was 10. 09 days. Finally, among the 27 patients with a third HSP episode, 20 (74.1%) used steroids. The average period of steroid use during the third episode was 16.30 days. The percentage and duration of steroid use in each episode was listed in Additional file 2: Table S2.

Mean duration between first and second HSP episodes

The mean duration between first and second HSP episodes was 9.21 months (Fig. 2a); 47.0% patients with second HSP did not have a third HSP episode. The average time between the second and third HSP episodes was 6. 77 months (Fig. 2b).

Influence of age, clinical course, and steroid on the incidence of secondary HSP

Table 2 lists the hazard ratios for recurrent HSP obtained from univariate Cox proportional analysis. Compared with patients aged < 6 years, patients aged 7–12 years were more likely to have a second HSP episode. Recurrent HSP episodes were more likely to occur in those with underlying allergic rhinitis and renal involvement during the first HSP episode. Compared with patients who did not use steroids, patients who underwent steroid therapy for 14 days after the HSP diagnosis (late initiation) were more likely to have HSP recurrence. Furthermore, patients who used steroids for > 10 days had a higher likelihood of experiencing a second HSP episode. Joint pain and gastrointestinal symptoms during the first HSP course were not associated with a second HSP episode. Income levels and other comorbidities had no significant impact on the incidence of secondary HSP.

After adjusting for age, gender, and medical comorbidities, increased associations of renal involvement, underlying allergic rhinitis, and longer steroid therapy with the recurrence of HSP were still noted (Table 3). At the end of the 16-year cohort, patients without allergic rhinitis had less recurrent episodes than those with underlying allergic rhinitis (89.4% and 81.9% were free of recurrence, respectively; $P = 0.026$; Fig. 3a). A second HSP episode occurred in 93.3% patients without renal involvement and 72.0% patients with renal involvement(Fig. 3b). Patients with only the first HSP episode were further stratified into five subgroups according to the

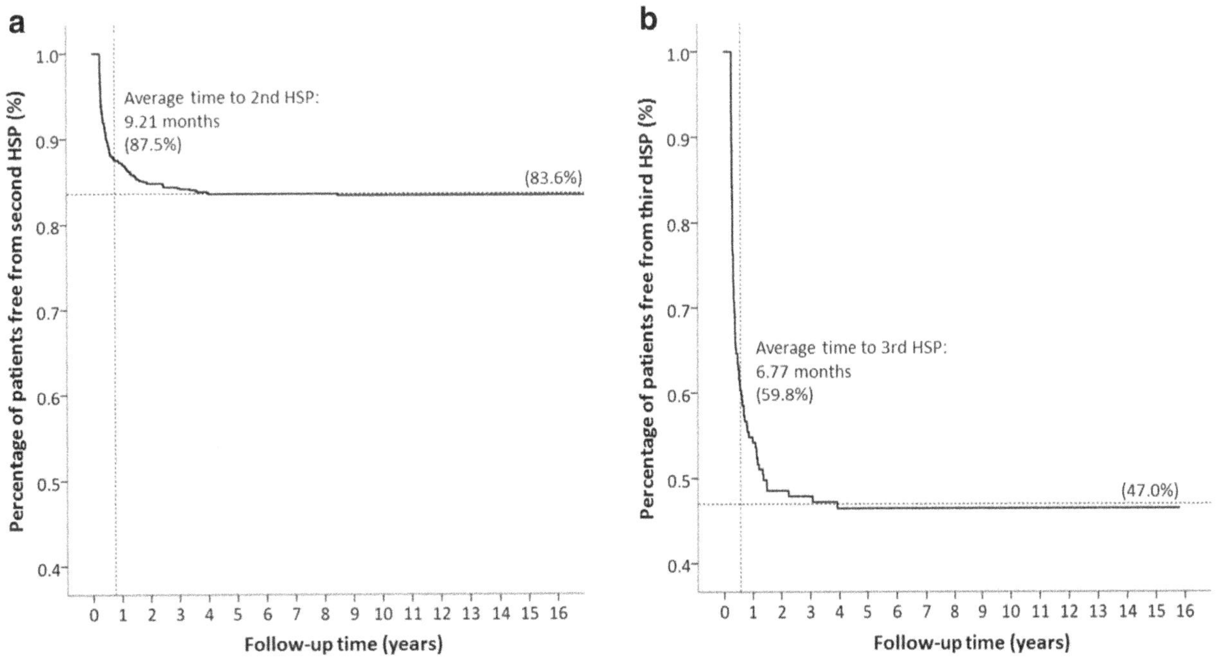

Fig. 2 Kaplan-Meier analysis. **a**, at the end of the 16-year cohort, 83.6% of patients remained free of a second HSP episode. The mean time between the first and the second HSP episodes was 9.21 months. **b**, among patients with second HSP, 47.0% of patients remained free of the third HSP episode. The average time from the second to the third HSP episode was 6.77 months

Table 2 Henoch-Schönlein Purpura events. (N = 1002)

	Only one Episode (n = 838), n (%)	Recurrent Episode (n = 164), n (%)	Crude HR (95% CI)[b]	p value[ʃ]
Sex				
Male	412 (49.2)	91 (55.5)	1.27(0.93–1.73)	0.131
Female	426 (50.8)	73 (44.5)	1.00	
Age, y				
Mean ± SD	6.85 ± 3.70	7.22 ± 3.37	1.03 (0.99–1.07)	0.224
0–6	499 (59.5)	82 (50.0)	1.00	
7–12	268 (32.0)	71 (43.3)	1.55 (1.13–2.13)	0.007
13–18	71 (8.5)	11 (6.7)	0.95 (0.51–1.79)	0.880
Economics Status				
Normal	771 (92.0)	154 (93.9)	1.00	
Low income	67 (8.0)	10 (6.1)	0.77 (0.40–1.45)	0.411
Comorbidities				
Asthma	356 (42.5)	68 (41.5)	0.97 (0.71–1.33)	0.866
Allergic rhinitis	627 (74.8)	139 (84.8)	1.80 (1.18–2.77)	0.006
Atopic dermatitis	221 (26.4)	47 (28.7)	1.13 (0.80–1.58)	0.484
Clinical course				
GI symptoms	799 (95.3)	161 (98.2)	2.50 (0.80–7.82)	0.116
Renal symptoms	57 (6.8)	36 (22.0)	3.15 (2.17–4.56)	< 0.001
Joint Pain	111 (13.2)	30 (18.3)	1.39 (0.94–2.07)	0.102
Initiation of Steroid[(1st)]				
No steroid use	496 (59.2)	67 (40.9)	1.00	
Early (< 14 days)	19 (2.3)	4 (2.4)	1.50 (0.55–4.12)	0.430
Late (≥ 14 days)	323 (38.5)	93 (56.7)	1.97 (1.44–2.70)	< 0.001
Duration of Steroid				
No steroid use	496 (59.2)	67 (40.9)	1.00	
SG (< 10 days)	284 (33.9)	48 (29.3)	1.20 (0.83–1.74)	0.329
LG(≥ 10 days)	58 (6.9)	49 (29.9)	4.98 (3.45–7.21)	< 0.001

Abbreviations: *HSP* Henoch-Schönlein Purpura, *SD* standard deviation, *SG* short-term group, LG long-term group, *HR* Hazard ratio
[ʃ]Cox proportional Regression Analysis
[b]Hazard ratio of 1.00 indicates reference group

initiation and duration of steroid therapy (Fig. 4). Percentages of patients without second HSP were 88.1% for the non-steroid group, 94.7% for the subgroup with steroid initiation within 14 days of diagnosis and steroid duration < 10 days, 85.0% for the subgroup with steroid initiation at ≥14 days after diagnosis and steroid duration < 10 days, 55.3% for the subgroup with steroid initiation at ≥14 days after diagnosis and steroid duration ≥10 days, and 25.0% for the subgroup with steroid initiation within 14 days of diagnosis and steroid duration ≥10 days (Fig. 4). Longer-term steroid use was associated with recurrent HSP regardless of early (< 14 days) or late (≥14 days) steroid initiation ($P < 0.001$, log-rank test).

Discussion

To our knowledge, this is the first population-based cohort study investigating the incidence and risk factors of recurrent HSP. Our results revealed that renal involvement, underlying allergic rhinitis, and steroid treatment for > 10 days were risk factors for HSP recurrence in children, regardless of age, sex, and income levels.

The recurrence rate (16.3%) in our study was within the range described by a previous study (2.7%–66.2%) [1, 12–16]. Reasons for discrepancies between our results and previous research may be partly related to different definitions of recurrence and patient selection. In this study, we defined our recurrent events as being re-diagnosed 3 months apart from the first HSP, which was also used by previous research, including one epidemiological HSP study in Taiwan [12, 14, 24]. Patients with a second diagnosis of HSP from both outpatient and in-patient departments were included in our study, whereas in previous studies, recurrence rates may have been underestimated if the definition of recurrent HSP was limited to patients readmitted for treatment [12, 16],

Table 3 Risk analysis of a second (Recurrent) Henoch-Schönlein Purpura episode

	Adjusted HR (95%CI)[b]	*p* value
Demographic factors		
Age, y	1.01 (0.96–1.05)	0.791
Comorbidities		
Allergic rhinitis	1.63 (1.06–2.50)	0.026
Clinical course		
Renal symptoms	2.41 (1.64–3.54)	< 0.001
Steroid initiation and duration[(1st)]		
No use record	1.00	
Initiation < 14 days and Duration ≤ 10 days	0.40 (0.06–2.90)	0.366
Initiation < 14 days and Duration > 10 days	8.13 (2.51–26.36)	< 0.001
Initiation ≥ 14 days and Duration ≤ 10 days	1.21 (0.83–1.76)	0.321
Initiation ≥ 14 days and Duration > 10 days	4.06 (2.76–5.96)	< 0.001

[b]Hazard ratio of 1.00 indicates reference group

because hospitalization is not always necessary for HSP patients unless complications (such as dehydration, severe abdominal pain, gastrointestinal bleeding, joint pain with ambulatory limitations, and renal insufficiency) occur. Conversely, recurrence may have been overestimated in studies that defined their recurrent episode as after at least 2–4 weeks of asymptomatic periods, because relapses of symptoms may occur after 4–6 weeks of spontaneous resolution [26]. Additionally, studies that defined recurrent episodes as asymptomatic for at least 2–4 weeks had the highest recurrent rate (33%–66%) [1, 7, 13, 15]. However, in children with HSP, relapses of symptoms occurred over 4–6 weeks before spontaneous resolution even in the absence of a complicated disease course [27].Thus, remission of symptoms for 2–4 weeks may not be adequate for HSP patients to affirm recovery. Furthermore, steroid therapy use may be another explanation for different recurrence rates between studies. In our study, the proportion of steroid use in first HSP was 40.8%. There might be an association between more steroid use and lower rates of recurrence. Lee et al. described a low recurrence rate of 5.2%, and the majority

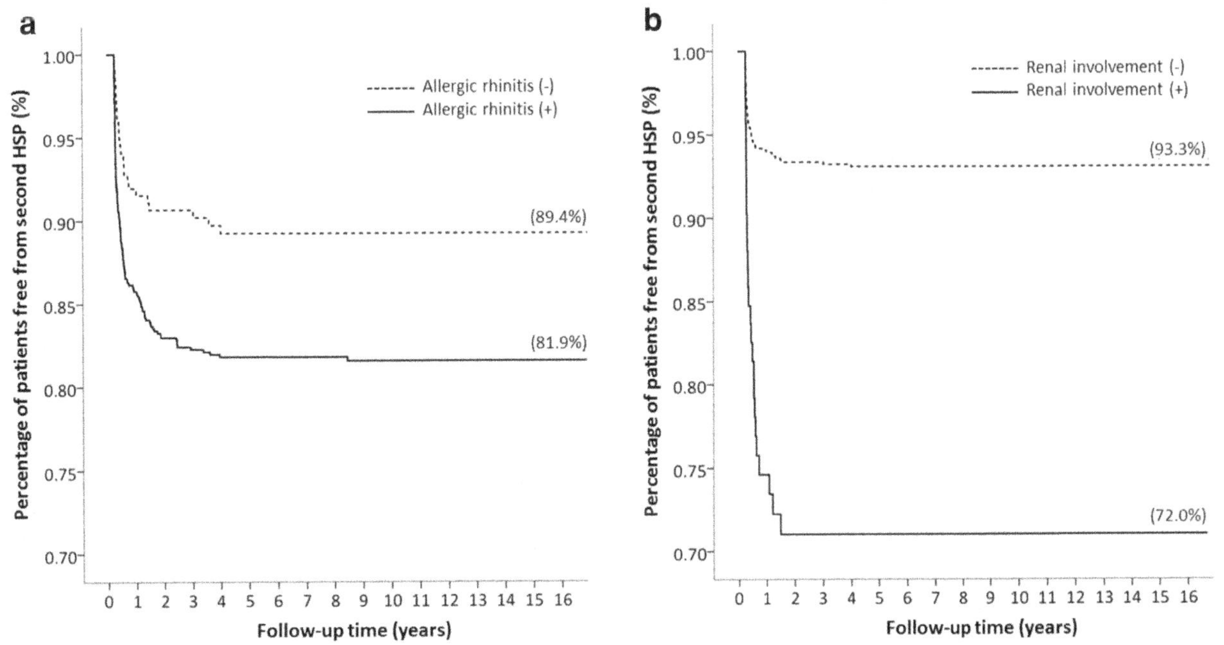

Fig. 3 Allergic rhinitis and renal involvement-specific Kaplan-Meier analysis. **a**, at the end of the 16-year cohort, the percentage of patients free of a second HSP episode was 89.4% in children without allergic rhinitis and 81.9% in those with allergic rhinitis. **b**, the percentage was 93.3% and 72.0% for patients without and with renal involvement, respectively

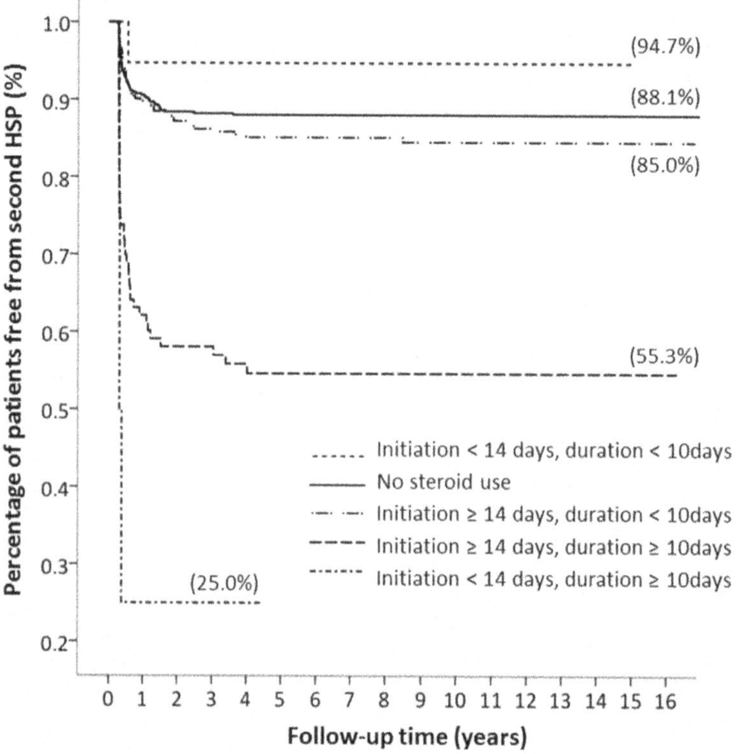

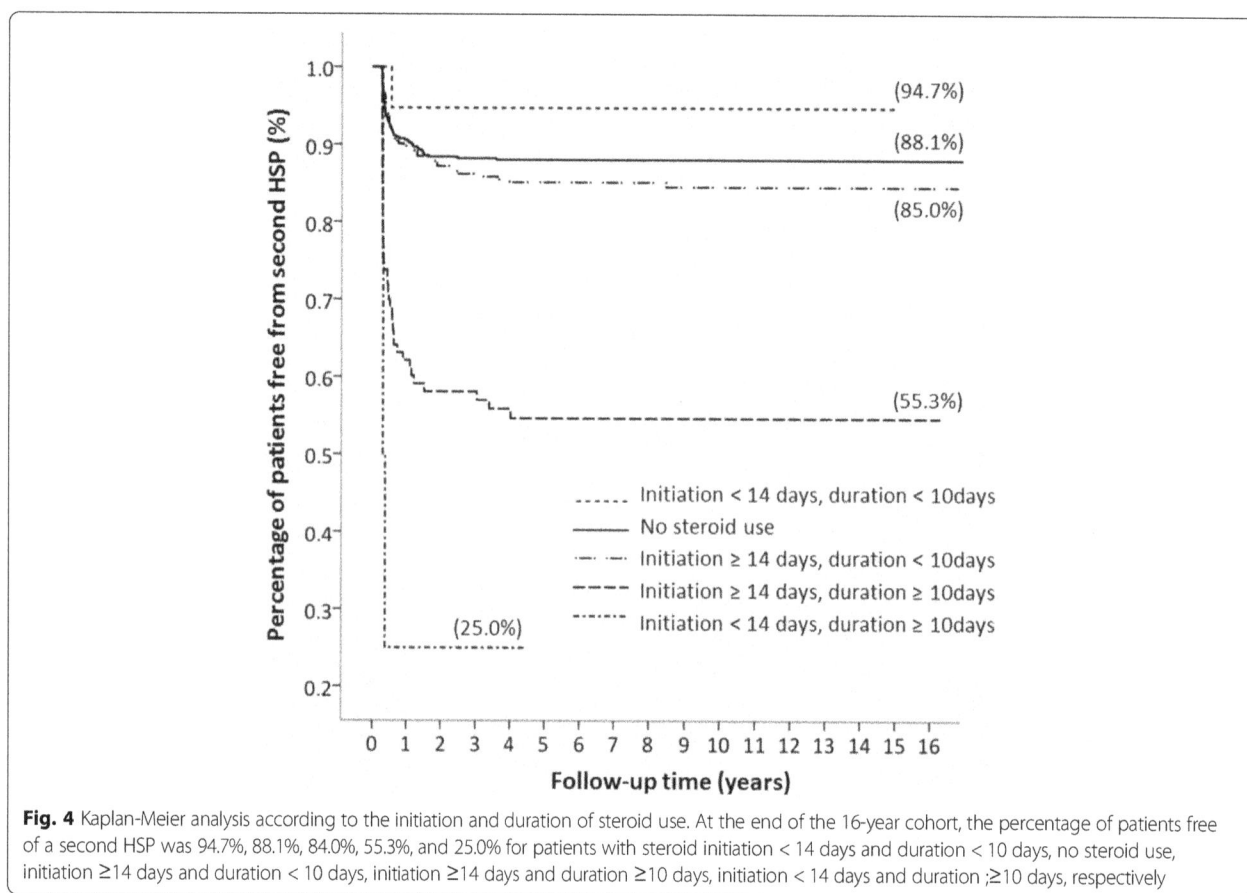

Fig. 4 Kaplan-Meier analysis according to the initiation and duration of steroid use. At the end of the 16-year cohort, the percentage of patients free of a second HSP was 94.7%, 88.1%, 84.0%, 55.3%, and 25.0% for patients with steroid initiation < 14 days and duration < 10 days, no steroid use, initiation ≥14 days and duration < 10 days, initiation ≥14 days and duration ≥10 days, initiation < 14 days and duration ;≥10 days, respectively

of patients (88.7%) from their study were treated with steroids [28]. Fretzayas et al. applied the strictest policy of using corticosteroids only in 18% of patients with a severe clinical course and reported the highest recurrence rate (66%) to date [15]. The choice of using steroids may be confounded by the disease severity. However, there was no significant difference in the initial clinical severity between the steroid-treated and non-steroid treated groups in Lee's report. Nevertheless, such observation requires further validation in different populations.

Our finding that allergic rhinitis was an independent risk factor for HSP was in line with studies reporting an increased risk of HSP in atopic children [29, 30]. However, no study has addressed the correlation between recurrent HSP and allergic diseases. For instance, elevated serum Th2-related cytokine levels (such as interleukin [IL]-4 and IL-5, and IgE) were reported in children with HSP [31–34]. Most HSP occurred after bacterial or viral infections, insect bites, or even food allergies, suggesting that allergic reactions predispose to HSP initiation [26, 35]. HSP is characterized by elevated serum IgA levels and vascular deposition of IgA immune complex, causing vascular necrosis mediated by IgE-sensitized mast cells [33]. For those with allergic rhinitis, the release of Th2-related cytokines results in chronic mucosal inflammation [36]. HSP patients with underlying allergic rhinitis may be more susceptible to chronic inflammatory status leading to a more intense immune response to causative antigens, thereby predisposing the recurrence of HSP. Moreover, the nasal mucosa (other than the bronchiole epithelium) is the first line of defense against pathogens [37]. The inability of the ailing mucosa to remove pathogens could forecast an infectious disease, which is a critical predisposing causative factor for HSP. This may partly explain why allergic rhinitis other than asthma or atopic dermatitis was a risk factor for recurrent HSP in this study. Further studies are needed to clarify the pathogenesis of this association.

Regarding the clinical manifestations of HSP, renal involvement remains a major concern because it may lead to permanent renal function impairment. In conformity with Jauhola et al. and Alfredo et al., who both reported higher recurrences in patients with nephritis but not in those with joint symptoms and GI manifestations [14, 38], our result revealed a higher risk of recurrence in patients with renal involvement (HR, 2.41). Additionally, the average time to recurrent episode in our patients with HSP nephritis was also shorter. Nevertheless, HSP nephritis affected 6.8% of patients in the current study, which is lower than the 10%–50% reported in previous literature [39] Moreover, our result that HSP nephritis occurred in 22% of patients with a recurrent episode was also lower than the 58.3% reported by Alfredo et al. [14]. Although the pathogenic mechanisms of HSP nephritis remain unclear, studies have described that galactose-deficient IgA1, recognized by antiglycan antibodies, might lead to the formation of circulating immune complexes and their mesangial deposition, resulting in renal injury among HSP patients [7].

Our study showed a significantly increased association between steroid use for > 10 days regardless of early initiation and the risk of recurrence. Steroids might have some treatment effects on HSP through their anti-inflammatory ability. Although early steroid therapy can ameliorate acute abdominal symptoms and mitigate short-term morbidity [18, 40–43], previous literature revealed conflicting results on the association between corticosteroid treatment and recurrence. Pamela et al. reported a non-significant protective effect of corticosteroids on recurrence rate [19]. However, Trapani et al. and Calvo-Rio et al. observed an opposite finding that emphasized an increased association between early corticosteroid use and the risk of relapse [1, 13]. In Trapani's case series of 150 patients, steroids were prescribed only in patients with a severe presentation, including 16 patients with severe abdominal and 3 patients with severe nephropathy. Their results of increased association might be explained by the fact that patients prescribed with corticosteroids had a more severe disease manifestation [1, 44], which is a risk factor for recurrence [44]. Currently, steroid therapy is suggested only in patients with nephritis and severe GI symptoms (dosage, 1–2 mg/kg/day). One might argue that our results of elevated recurrence rates in those with steroid use for > 10 days were associated with their disease severity. However, this may only partly explain our result because not all recurrences were associated with more severe clinical courses, such as renal involvement. Shin et al. also pointed out that there is a distinct group of multiple recurrent non-renal HSP [45]. Our findings indicate that the risk of recurrence might be associated with a longer duration of steroid use in certain patients. Thus, we hypothesized the mechanism that the longer use of steroid might indicate an "over-prescribing" of steroid, which might interfere with the clinical course, including the chance of recurrence. To date, there is no optimal recommendation for the duration of treatment. Expert opinions have suggested that steroids should be tapered slowly by < 25% per week to prevent relapse, thus, the overall duration of steroid treatment may easily exceeds 10 days and generally requires 4 weeks. Since the optimal duration and timing of steroid administration remains unanswered, further prospective randomized trials are needed to elucidate this possible underlying mechanism between longer-term steroid use and HSP recurrences.

The duration of follow-up in children with HSP for the early identification of possible recurrence is an important issue. In our study, the average duration between the first and second HSP episodes was 9.2 months (range, 4 months to 1 year in previous literature) [1, 8, 46]. Prais et al. described a longer duration of 13. 5 months between episodes [12]. The reason for the longer period in Prais's study may be because they only considered recurrences that required hospitalization in their analysis. We were the first study to report a 6.4-month average duration between the second and the third recurrences. Although there were only 6% of children with > 3 recurrences during our follow-up period, nearly half of the patients with second HSP had a third HSP event. Thus, for the early detection of recurrence, it may be worth considering following up patients with the first HSP episode for at least 9.2 months and those with a second HSP episode for another 6.4 months.

Strengths and limitations

A strength of the current study is the use of a nationwide, population-based dataset large enough to provide sufficient statistical power for detecting the association of interest. The distinctive feature of the data source strengthens the validity of the estimated disease incidences [47]. However, there were still several limitations in this study. First, although we have adjusted for covariates such as age, sex, income levels, and comorbidities, we were unable to control for information not recorded in the NHIRD, such as serum IgE and specific IgE levels, eosinophil counts, levels of albumin, triglyceride, urine protein, urine creatinine, infection pathogens, or genetic factors. Second, this population- based study mostly assessed the Han Chinese ethnic group, and the findings may not be generalized to other populations. Third, a proper definition of 'recurrence' was supposed to be defined as the occurrences of new symptoms after an initial remission, requiring the resumption of immunosuppressive therapy or an increased dose. Unfortunately, details of symptoms were not recorded in the NHIRD database. Besides, not every patient with HSP needs hospitalization or was prescribed with medications. As a consequence, we were unable to use symptoms or steroid prescription to define the disease episode or disease free intervals. However, the definition of our recurrent events as at least 3-months apart from the first HSP diagnosis was in accordance to previous research, and also considered the duration of tapering steroid. Although patients that never remitted from their first episode and not treated in the NHI system between the two diagnoses 3- months apart might be included as recurrent subject, such chances were small because over 99% of the citizens utilizes health care through the NHI program.

Conclusion

Ours was the first study to describe the incidence of recurrent HSP, and added evidence of increased associations of recurrent HSP and allergic rhinitis, renal involvement, and steroid treatment for > 10 days. These results can be considered observations from real-world conditions. Patients with the aforementioned clinical features were suggested to receive longer periods of follow-up than previously suggested for the early identification and management of recurrent HSP. In those with a second HSP episode, perhaps 6 more months of monitoring is also suggested for the early recognition of a third HSP recurrence. Further study is needed to clarify the underlying pathogenic mechanisms of these associations.

Abbreviations

CI: Confidence interval; GI: Gastrointestinal; HR: Hazard ratio; HSP: Henoch-Schönlein purpura; IgA: Immunoglobulin A; IgE: Immunoglobulin E; IL: Interleukin; LG: Long-term group; LHID: Longitudinal Health Insurance Database; NHI: National Health Insurance; NHIRD: Taiwan National Health Insurance Research Database; SD: Standard deviation; SG: Short-term group; Th1: T helper cell 1; Th2: T helper cell 2

Acknowledgements

The authors would like to thank Enago (http://www.enago.tw) for language editing and proofreading this manuscript. Thanks to the MacKay Memorial Hospital librarian Pei-Fang Shen for examining the references.

Authors' contributions

All authors have read and approved the final manuscript. WTL, SIW LCF and SHC conceived and designed the research; YWL and PLT analyzed the data; WTL wrote the paper. YHK, SDS and SIW performed the validation of the results.

Competing interests

All authors declare no conflict of interests.

Author details

[1]Division of Allergy, Immunology, Rheumatology Disease, Department of Pediatrics, Mackay Memorial Hospital, Hsinchu, Taiwan. [2]Division of Colorectal Surgery, Department of Surgery, Mackey Memorial Hospital, Taipei, Taiwan. [3]Department of Pediatrics, Mackay Memorial Hospital, Hsinchu, Taiwan. [4]Department of Medical Research, Mackay Memorial Hospital, Taipei, Taiwan. [5]Department of Medicine, Mackay Medical College, No.45, Minsheng Rd., Tamsui Dist., New Taipei City 25160, Taiwan. [6]Audiology and Speech Language Pathology, Mackay Medical College, No.45, Minsheng Rd., Tamsui Dist., New Taipei City 25160, Taiwan. [7]Department of Psychiatry, Mackay Memorial Hospital, No.45, Minsheng Rd., Tamsui Dist., New Taipei City 25160, Taiwan.

References

1. Trapani S, Micheli A, Grisolia F, Resti M, Chiappini E, Falcini F, De Martino M. Henoch Schonlein purpura in childhood: epidemiological and clinical analysis of 150 cases over a 5-year period and review of literature. Semin Arthritis Rheum. 2005;35(3):143–53.
2. Gardner-Medwin JM, Dolezalova P, Cummins C, Southwood TR. Incidence of Henoch-Schonlein purpura, Kawasaki disease, and rare vasculitides in children of different ethnic origins. Lancet. 2002;360(9341):1197–202.
3. Calvino MC, Llorca J, Garcia-Porrua C, Fernandez-Iglesias JL, Rodriguez-Ledo P, Gonzalez-Gay MA. Henoch-Schonlein purpura in children from northwestern Spain: a 20-year epidemiologic and clinical study. Medicine (Baltimore). 2001;80(5):279–90.
4. Watson L, Richardson AR, Holt RC, Jones CA, Beresford MW. Henoch schonlein purpura–a 5-year review and proposed pathway. PLoS One. 2012; 7(1):e29512.
5. Meiller MJL, Cavallasca JA, del Rosario Maliandi M, Nasswetter GG. Henoch-SchöNlein Purpura in Adults. Clinics (Sao Paulo, Brazil). 2008;63(2):273–6.
6. Garzoni L, Vanoni F, Rizzi M, Simonetti GD, Goeggel Simonetti B, Ramelli GP, Bianchetti MG. Nervous system dysfunction in Henoch-Schonlein syndrome: systematic review of the literature. Rheumatology (Oxford). 2009;48(12): 1524–9.
7. Lau KK, Suzuki H, Novak J, Wyatt RJ. Pathogenesis of Henoch-Schonlein purpura nephritis. Pediatr Nephrol. 2010;25(1):19–26.
8. Saulsbury FT. Henoch-Schonlein purpura in children. Report of 100 patients and review of the literature. Medicine (Baltimore). 1999;78(6):395–409.
9. Saulsbury FT. Clinical update: Henoch-Schonlein purpura. Lancet. 2007; 369(9566):976–8.
10. Tizard EJ. Henoch-Schonlein purpura. Arch Dis Child. 1999;80(4):380–3.
11. Blanco R, Martinez-Taboada VM, Rodriguez-Valverde V, Garcia-Fuentes M, Gonzalez-Gay MA. Henoch-Schonlein purpura in adulthood and childhood: two different expressions of the same syndrome. Arthritis Rheum. 1997; 40(5):859–64.
12. Prais D, Amir J, Nussinovitch M. Recurrent Henoch-Schonlein purpura in children. J Clin Rheumatol. 2007;13(1):25–8.
13. Calvo-Rio V, Hernandez JL, Ortiz-Sanjuan F, Loricera J, Palmou-Fontana N, Gonzalez-Vela MC, Gonzalez-Lamuno D, Gonzalez-Lopez MA, Armesto S, Blanco R, et al. Relapses in patients with Henoch-Schonlein purpura: analysis of 417 patients from a single center. Medicine (Baltimore). 2016;95(28): e4217.
14. Alfredo CS, Nunes NA, Len CA, Barbosa CM, Terreri MT, Hilario MO. Henoch-Schonlein purpura: recurrence and chronicity. J Pediatr. 2007;83(2):177–80.
15. Fretzayas A, Sionti I, Moustaki M, Papadimitriou A, Nicolaidou P. Henoch-Schonlein purpura: a long-term prospective study in Greek children. J Clin Rheumatol. 2008;14(6):324–31.
16. Anil M, Aksu N, Kara OD, Bal A, Anil AB, Yavascan O, Un B. Henoch-Schonlein purpura in children from western Turkey: a retrospective analysis of 430 cases. Turk J Pediatr. 2009;51(5):429–36.
17. Hahn D, Hodson EM, Willis NS, Craig JC. Interventions for preventing and treating kidney disease in Henoch-Schonlein Purpura (HSP). Cochrane Database Syst Rev. 2015;8 CD005128
18. Ronkainen J, Koskimies O, Ala-Houhala M, Antikainen M, Merenmies J, Rajantie J, Ormala T, Turtinen J, Nuutinen M. Early prednisone therapy in Henoch-Schonlein purpura: a randomized, double-blind, placebo-controlled trial. J Pediatr. 2006;149(2):241–7.
19. Weiss PF, Feinstein JA, Luan X, Burnham JM, Feudtner C. Effects of corticosteroid on Henoch-Schonlein purpura: a systematic review. Pediatrics. 2007;120(5):1079–87.
20. National Health Insurance Research Database T: Introduction to the National Health Insurance Research Database (NHIRD), Taiwan. 2006, http://www.nhri.org.tw/nhird/en/index.htm.
21. National Health Insurance Research Database TLHIDL: Taipei. 2008, http://w3.nhri.org.tw/nhird//en/Data_Subsets.html - S3.
22. National Health Insurance Research Database TRPotLHIDL: Taipei. 2009, http://w3.nhri.org.tw/nhird//date_cohort.htm.
23. Mills JA, Michel BA, Bloch DA, Calabrese LH, Hunder GG, Arend WP, Edworthy SM, Fauci AS, Leavitt RY, Lie JT, et al. The American College of Rheumatology 1990 criteria for the classification of Henoch-Schonlein purpura. Arthritis Rheum. 1990;33(8):1114–21.
24. Teng MC, Wang LC, Yu HH, Lee JH, Yang YH, Chiang BL. Kawasaki disease and Henoch-Schonlein purpura - 10 years' experience of childhood vasculitis at a university hospital in Taiwan. Journal of microbiology, immunology, and infection = Wei mian yu gan ran za zhi. 2012;45(1):22–30.

25. Weiss PF, Klink AJ, Localio R, Hall M, Hexem K, Burnham JM, Keren R, Feudtner C. Corticosteroids may improve clinical outcomes during hospitalization for Henoch-Schonlein purpura. Pediatrics. 2010;126(4):674–81.
26. Ackroyd JF. Allergic purpura, including purpura due to foods, drugs and infections. Am J Med. 1953;14(5):605–32.
27. Narayan H: Compendium for the antenatal care of high-risk pregnancies ISBN: 9780199673643 p47, published 30 July 2015.
28. Lee YH, Kim YB, Koo JW, Chung JY. Henoch-Schonlein Purpura in children hospitalized at a tertiary hospital during 2004-2015 in Korea: epidemiology and clinical management. Pediatr Gastroenterol Hepatol Nutr. 2016;19(3): 175–85.
29. Chen AC, Lin CL, Shen TC, Li TC, Sung FC, Wei CC. Association between allergic diseases and risks of HSP and HSP nephritis: a population-based study. Pediatr Res. 2016;79(4):559–64.
30. Wei CC, Lin CL, Shen TC, Li TC, Chen AC. Atopic dermatitis and Association of Risk for Henoch-Schonlein Purpura (IgA Vasculitis) and renal involvement among children: results from a population-based cohort study in Taiwan. Medicine (Baltimore). 2016;95(3):e2586.
31. Namgoong MK, Lim BK, Kim JS. Eosinophil cationic protein in Henoch-Schonlein purpura and in IgA nephropathy. Pediatr Nephrol. 1997;11(6):703–6.
32. Davin JC, Pierard G, Dechenne C, Grossman D, Nagy J, Quacoe M, Malaise M, Hall M, Jansen F, Chantraine JM, et al. Possible pathogenic role of IgE in Henoch-Schonlein purpura. Pediatr Nephrol. 1994;8(2):169–71.
33. Tsuji Y, Abe Y, Hisano M, Sakai T. Urinary leukotriene E4 in Henoch-Schonlein purpura. Clin Exp Allergy. 2004;34(8):1259–61.
34. Yano N, Endoh M, Miyazaki M, Yamauchi F, Nomoto Y, Sakai H. Altered production of IgE and IgA induced by IL-4 in peripheral blood mononuclear cells from patients with IgA nephropathy. Clin Exp Immunol. 1992;88(2): 295–300.
35. Burke DM, Jellinek HL. Nearly fatal case of Schoenlein-Henoch syndrome following insect bite. AMA Am J Dis Child. 1954;88(6):772–4.
36. Bradding P, Feather IH, Wilson S, Bardin PG, Heusser CH, Holgate ST, Howarth PH. Immunolocalization of cytokines in the nasal mucosa of normal and perennial rhinitic subjects. The mast cell as a source of IL-4, IL-5, and IL-6 in human allergic mucosal inflammation. J Immunol. 1993;151(7):3853–65.
37. Fokkens WJ, Scheeren RA. Upper airway defence mechanisms. Paediatr Respir Rev. 2000;1(4):336–41.
38. Jauhola O, Ronkainen J, Koskimies O, Ala-Houhala M, Arikoski P, Holtta T, Jahnukainen T, Rajantie J, Ormala T, Nuutinen M. Clinical course of extrarenal symptoms in Henoch-Schonlein purpura: a 6-month prospective study. Arch Dis Child. 2010;95(11):871–6.
39. Szer IS. Henoch-Schonlein purpura. Curr Opin Rheumatol. 1994;6(1):25–31.
40. Dudley J, Smith G, Llewelyn-Edwards A, Bayliss K, Pike K, Tizard J. Randomised, double-blind, placebo-controlled trial to determine whether steroids reduce the incidence and severity of nephropathy in Henoch-Schonlein Purpura (HSP). Arch Dis Child. 2013;98(10):756–63.
41. Davin JC, Coppo R. Pitfalls in recommending evidence-based guidelines for a protean disease like Henoch-Schonlein purpura nephritis. Pediatr Nephrol. 2013;28(10):1897–903.
42. Leung SP. Use of intravenous hydrocortisone in Henoch-Schonlein purpura. J Paediatr Child Health. 2001;37(3):309–10.
43. Szer IS. Gastrointestinal and renal involvement in vasculitis: management strategies in Henoch-Schonlein purpura. Cleve Clin J Med. 1999;66(5):312–7.
44. Shin JI, Park JM, Shin YH, Hwang DH, Kim JH, Lee JS. Predictive factors for nephritis, relapse, and significant proteinuria in childhood Henoch-Schonlein purpura. Scand J Rheumatol. 2006;35(1):56–60.
45. Shin JI, Kim JH, Lee JS. Comment on recurrent Henoch-Schonlein purpura in children. J Clin Rheumatol. 2007;13(4):244. author reply 244
46. Haroon M. Should children with Henoch-Schonlein purpura and abdominal pain be treated with steroids? Arch Dis Child. 2005;90(11):1196–8.
47. Lin HC, Chao PZ, Lee HC. Sudden sensorineural hearing loss increases the risk of stroke: a 5-year follow-up study. Stroke. 2008;39(10):2744–8.

18

Juvenile idiopathic arthritis managed in the new millennium: one year outcomes of an inception cohort of Australian children

Georgina Tiller[1*], Joanne Buckle[1,2], Roger Allen[1], Jane Munro[1,2], Peter Gowdie[1], Angela Cox[1] and Jonathan Akikusa[1,2]

Abstract

Background: The advent of new treatments for Juvenile Idiopathic Arthritis (JIA) has prompted interest in systematically studying the outcomes of patients treated in the 'modern era'. Such data provide both benchmarks for assessing local outcomes and important information for use in counselling families of newly diagnosed patients. While data are available for cohorts in Europe and North America, no such data exist for Australian patients.

The aim was to examine the demographics, treatment and outcomes at 12 months of an inception cohort of newly diagnosed patients with JIA at a single tertiary referral paediatric rheumatology centre in Australia.

Methods: Retrospective review of prospectively collected data from patients newly diagnosed with JIA between 2010 and 2014 at the Royal Children's Hospital in Melbourne.

Results: One hundred thirty four patients were included (62% female). Oligoarthritis was the single largest category of JIA (36%) and rheumatoid factor positive polyarthritis the least common (2%). Undifferentiated JIA accounted for 13% of patients and was the third largest category. Across the cohort 94% received NSAIDs, 53% oral steroids, 62% methotrexate and 15% a biologic DMARD. Intra-articular steroids were used in 62%, most commonly in the oligoarticular subtype (94%). 95% of patients achieved a joint count of zero at a median of 4.1 months, however flares occurred in 42%. At 12 months 65% had no active joint disease, though more than half remained on medication.

Conclusion: Australian children with JIA managed in the modern era have similar characteristics and achieve short term outcomes comparable to cohorts in Europe and North America, with high rates of joint remission in the first 12 months of follow-up but with a significant relapse rate and requirement for ongoing medication.

Keywords: Juvenile idiopathic arthritis, Cohort, Outcomes

Introduction

Juvenile idiopathic arthritis (JIA) is a heterogeneous group of conditions, characterized by the onset of persistent arthritis before the 16th birthday for which no cause can be identified [1]. It is the most common inflammatory rheumatic disease in childhood [2]. Recent reports of large prospective cohorts of patients with JIA from North America and Europe have led to an improved understanding of the early disease course, contemporary management and short-term outcomes of this condition [3–6]. In addition, these and other studies have contributed to the understanding that early disease course and response to treatment may predict outcome more accurately than disease category, making studies focused on the early disease period in the era of contemporary treatments increasingly important [7, 8].

In Australia, the estimated overall prevalence of JIA is 1–4 per 1000 children although national statistics and publications are limited [9, 10]. Despite its importance and relative frequency, there are no studies describing the outcome of children with JIA in Australia managed with current treatments. The aim of this study was to describe the clinical features, management, course and

* Correspondence: georgina.tiller@rch.org.au
[1]Department of Rheumatology, The Royal Children's Hospital, 50 Flemington Rd, Parkville, Melbourne, VIC 3052, Australia
Full list of author information is available at the end of the article

outcomes during the first 12 months of follow up, for an inception cohort of Australian children with JIA.

Patients and methods

We conducted a retrospective review of data from an inception cohort of children with JIA diagnosed between October 2010 and October 2014 at The Royal Children's Hospital (RCH), Melbourne, Australia. All children newly diagnosed with JIA during the relevant period and whose subsequent follow-up had been at the RCH were eligible for inclusion. All data had been prospectively documented in the Rheumatology Department database, a comprehensive clinical tool coded in Microsoft Access™ in which patient demographic details, diagnoses, clinic visits, medications, elective admissions for procedures and communications are recorded. At our institution, patients with a new diagnosis of JIA are followed routinely at least every three months for the first 12–18 months of their arthritis course. For the purposes of this study, patients followed less frequently than this over the relevant period were considered to have incomplete follow-up and were excluded. Acute hospital admissions between scheduled appointments were not included in this analysis.

For ease of analysis, data from the Rheumatology database were exported into an Excel ™ workbook. Exported data fields included patient demographics, assigned JIA category, medications, procedures, clinic visit dates and active joint count at each visit. The JIA category assigned by the treating rheumatologist was confirmed by the primary investigator (GT) using the International League of Associations for Rheumatology (ILAR) classification criteria. For the systemic category, where the ILAR classification was not met due to absence of active arthritis, the diagnosis was made by the treating paediatric rheumatologist. For the purposes of analysis, the two oligoarthritis categories (i.e. persistent and extended) were combined due to a small number of patients in the extended category.

The first visit was defined as the date of diagnosis of JIA. The 12-month visit was the date closest to 12 months from the date of first visit within a 2-month window. The time to zero joint count was calculated as the interval between the first visit and the date on which the treating rheumatologist recorded an active joint count of 0, which for the purposes of this study was considered to represent inactive arthritis. The date of first arthritis flare was the visit date at which a joint count was recorded as > 0 following the first visit at which the joint count had been 0. Uveitis at diagnosis was defined as uveitis detected prior to, or within one month of the diagnosis of JIA. The date of a first episode of uveitis was the visit at which uveitis was first documented by an ophthalmologist. Uveitis was recorded if present at any time during the 12 months of follow up and at the 12-month visit. For patients who did not reach examined outcomes in the first year of follow-up, additional data were collected up to the time at which the relevant outcome occurred or 36 months, whichever came first.

Medications were grouped as non-steroidal anti-inflammatories (NSAIDS), conventional disease modifying agents (cDMARDS) (ie. methotrexate, sulfasalazine, leflunomide), biologic disease modifying agents (bDMARDS) (ie. adalimumab, etanercept, infliximab, tocilizumab, anakinra), oral, intravenous (IV) and ophthalmic steroids. Medications were recorded as ever used in the 12 month follow up period, and in use at the 12 month visit. For cDMARDS and bDMARDS the time from first visit to commencement was calculated in months. Intra-articular steroid (IAS) injections were recorded as the number of visits for joint injections in the 12-month period of follow up. The time to first joint injection was calculated in months. Analysis was performed using descriptive statistics. Survival curves were used to examine medication exposure across the cohort.

The Royal Children's Hospital (RCH) Human Research Ethics Committee approved the study.

Results

One hundred sixty one patients were identified, of whom, 27 were excluded because of incomplete follow-up. Demographic and disease details of the 161 patients are given in Table 1. Of the 17 undifferentiated patients: 7 were males > 6 years, HLAB27 positive with a family history of psoriasis; 8 were oligo or poly arthritis with a family history of psoriasis with no other features; 2 were oligoarthritis with B27 and rheumatoid factor (RF) positivity. There were no statistically significant differences in age at diagnosis, gender and proportion of patients when comparing included and excluded patients.

Disease course

Details of the disease course of the cohort over the study period are provided in Table 2. In the 12 months following diagnosis, 127 (95%) of patients achieved an active joint count of zero on at least one occasion. The median time to achieve this outcome within the first 12 months was 3.1 months (Range 0.4–13.1 months) (Table 2). For the 7 (5%) who did not reach a joint count of zero, the median time to a joint count of zero was 18.5 months (range 15.2–32.0 months). Of this group, 4 (57%) were in the polyarticular RF negative JIA category. One patient, in the undifferentiated category, a 14 year old female with ANA and RF positive oligoarthritis, treated with two joint injections and methotrexate in the first 12 months, did not attain a zero-joint count during the 36 months of available follow up data.

Fifty six subjects (42%) had at least one arthritis flare from a joint count of zero. The median number of flares was 1 and the median time to flare was 3.6 months

Table 1 Demographics of the excluded patients and cohort presented in decreasing order of frequency of JIA category

	Number of excluded patients n (%)	Mean age excluded patients at diagnosis (years)	Female excluded patients n (%)	Number of included patients n (%)	Median age included patients at diagnosis (years)	Female included patients n (%)	Pre-diagnosis symptom period average months (range)	Median joint count baseline (range)	ANA positive n/n done (%)
Oligoarticular	12 (44)	7.5	7 (58)	48 (36)	3.4	34 (71)	3.9 (0.3–24.0)	2 (1–4)	36/47 (77)
Polyarticular RF-	1(4)	9.9	0 (0)	34 (25)	9.0	26 (76)	5.3 (0.5–24.0)	8 (1–42)	21/33 (64)
Undifferentiated	8 (30)	8.4	4 (50)	17 (13)	12.3	7 (41)	7.4 (0.5–24.0)	5 (1–43)	8/16 (50)
Enthesitis related arthritis	2(7)	10.8	0 (0)	13 (10)	13.9	1 (8)	11.2 (0.5–48.0)	2 (1–18)	0/7 (0)
Systemic	1(4)	3.2	0 (0)	10 (7)	8.4	7 (70)	1.4 (0.3–4.0)	5 (0–22)	3/8 (38)
Psoriatic arthritis	3(11)	11	1 (33)	9 (7)	9.3	5 (56)	9.9 (1.5–24.0)	5 (1–36)	2/7 (29)
Polyarticular RF +	0(0)	n/a	n/a	3 (2)	15.6	3 (100)	7.5 (3.8–12.1)	10 (7–44)	2/3 (67)
Overall	27	9.2	12 (44)	134	8.3	83 (62)	5.7 (0.3–48.0)	2 (0–44)	72/121 (60)

Table 2 Metrics of arthritis and uveitis activity of the cohort by JIA category for outcomes attained in the first twelve months

	Reached zero joint count in first year n (% of subtype)	Median time to zero joint count in the first twelve months (range)	Median joint count at 12 months (range)	Flared ever during first 12 months n (%)	Mdn time to flare from zero joint count (months)	Uveitis during first 12 months n (%)	Active uveitis at 12 months n (%)
Oligoarticular	48 (100)	2.8 (1.0–12.6)	0 (0–4)	15 (31)	3.2	8 (17)	5 (10)
Polyarticular RF -	30 (88)	5.3 (1.1–12.8)	0 (0–14)	16 (47)	3.5	0 (0)	0 (0)
Undifferentiated	16 (94)	3.9 (0.6–13.1)	0 (0–7)	11 (65)	3.9	0 (0)	0 (0)
Enthesitis related arthritis	11 (85)	6.6 (1.4–12.0)	1 (0–15)	5 (38)	5.5	0 (0)	0 (0)
Systemic	10 (100)	1.7 (0.4–8.1)	0 (0–8)	5 (50)	1.2	0 (0)	0 (0)
Psoriatic arthritis	9 (100)	7.6 (1.2–12.2)	0 (0–24)	4 (44)	3.1	1 (11)	1 (11)
Polyarticular RF +	3 (100)	5.9 (3.7–7.0)	0 (0–0)	0 (0)	n/a	0 (0)	0 (0)
Overall	127 (95)	3.1 (0.4–13.1)	0 (0–24)	56 (42)	3.6	9 (7)	6 (4)

(range 1.2–5.5 months). Of those patients that flared within the first 12 months, 30 (54%) were on a disease modifying medication at the time of the flare, most commonly methotrexate, 26 (50%).The JIA category with the highest proportion of arthritis flares was the undifferentiated group with 65% of patients flaring over the first 12 months. Where patients had first arthritis flares after the first 12 months of follow up, the median time to flare from zero joint count was 13.5 months and from first visit was 20.5 months. All the RF positive polyarthritis patients had arthritis flares, although none within the first 12 months of follow up. In this group, the median time to arthritis flare from a joint count of zero was 17.0 months (range 11.0–25.5 months). Of the 45 (34%) patients who never had an arthritis flare, 53% were in the oligoarthritis category. The proportion of oligoarthritis patients who had no arthritis flares in the first 12 months was 69%.

Uveitis occurred in 2 (1%) patients at diagnosis, 9 (7%) patients in the first 12 months of follow up. 89% of these patients were in the oligoarticular category. 100% of the patients with uveitis were ANA positive.

Medications

Table 3 details the exposure of the cohort to medications over the study period. Non-steroidal anti-inflammatory drugs were almost universally used (94%). Seventy-one patients (53%) were treated with oral corticosteroids at least once and 10 (7%) were treated with intravenous steroids. The median initial dose of oral steroids was 1 mg/kg/day (range 0.2–2) and the median duration of oral steroids, including the completed taper was 4 months (range 0.25–12 months). Eighty-three (62%) were treated with methotrexate, by far the most common cDMARD. Two patients were treated with sulfasalazine in the first 12 months, both of whom had also been treated with methotrexate. Across the whole cohort the median time to commencement of methotrexate was 0.9 months (Table 3). It was shortest in the RF positive polyarthritis category (median 0 months) and longest in patients with enthesitis related arthritis (ERA) (median 3.1 months) (Table 3, Fig. 1). Twenty patients (15%) were commenced on a bDMARD at a median of 5.5 months (Table 3). The patients with the highest rate of bDMARD commencement were in the polyarticular RF positive (33%), ERA (31%) and systemic (sJIA) (30%) categories. All patients with uveitis were treated with ophthalmic steroids during the first 12 months of follow up. Five (56%) were additionally commenced on methotrexate, either for arthritis or uveitis or both. None required addition of a bDMARD within that timeframe.

Sixty two percent of patients underwent at least one joint injection in the first year of follow up; the median time to first joint injection was 0.9 months (Range 0–11 months). Fifty four percent of patients undergoing intra-articular steroid therapy were in the oligoarticular category, 94% of whom had at least one joint injection in the year following diagnosis (Fig. 2). Ten patients (7%) required their first joint injection after the first 12 months of follow up. The median time to joint injection for this group was 21 months. Seven of these 10 patients were in the RF negative polyarthritis JIA category.

Outcome at twelve months

Seventy three percent of the cohort were on at least one medication at 12 months, with the two most common being methotrexate (79%) and NSAIDS (62%). Twenty-three (17%) were on oral corticosteroids. The JIA categories with the highest oral steroid use at 12 months were ERA (31%), sJIA(30%), and undifferentiated (29%). All but one patient (with systemic disease) commenced on a bDMARD remained on a bDMARD at 12 months.

Figure 3 outlines arthritis activity status according to medication use for each JIA category at the 12 month visit. Eighty-eight (66%) of patients had inactive arthritis. Thirty-six (41%) of these patients were of the oligoarticular subtype, of whom 75% had inactive arthritis at this time point. Of the 88 patients with inactive arthritis, 61% were on medications and 39% were off medication. All the RF factor positive polyarticular patients had inactive arthritis on medication at 12 months. Four patients (7%) with inactive arthritis at 12 months had active uveitis.

Of the 46 patients with active arthritis at 12 months, 96% were on medication. The two patients not on medication were awaiting intra-articular therapy. The categories with the highest proportion of patients with active arthritis at 12 months were, polyarticular RF negative (47%) and ERA (46%).

Six patients (4%) had active uveitis at 12 months: 2 had concurrent active arthritis on medication and 4 had inactive arthritis on medications.

Discussion

This study is the first report of early outcomes for Australian children newly diagnosed with JIA managed in the modern era of arthritis therapy. It demonstrates that Australian children with JIA have similar demographic features, disease course and medication exposure to those reported in large cohorts from Europe and North America [2–5] .

The sex distribution, proportion of patients within each JIA category and prevalence of ANA positivity concur with previously published cohorts [2, 4, 5]. Consistent with previous cohorts, the shortest and longest times from symptom onset to diagnosis were in the sJIA and ERA categories respectively [3, 11]. This likely reflects

Table 3 Medication exposure during first 12 months and at 12 months by JIA category

	Any	NSAIDS		Oral steroids		IV steroids	Methotrexate			bDMARD			Ocular steroids		Steroid joint injections	
	Ever n (%)	Ever n (%)	At 12 m n (%)	Ever n (%)	At 12 m n (%)	Number given IV steroids n(%)	Ever n (%)	Med. time to (m)	At 12 m n (%)	Ever n (%)	Med. time to (m)	At 12 m n (%)	Ever n (%)	At 12 m n (%)	Ever n (%)	Med joint injections per patient[a] (range)
Oligoarticular	43(90)	43 (90)	13 (27)	7 (15)	4 (8)	0 (0)	9 (19)	2.1	9 (19)	1 (2)	12.2	1 (2)	8(17)	4(8)	45 (94)	1 (0–3)
Polyarticular RF -	34 (100)	33 (97)	17 (50)	21 (62)	5 (15)	2 (6)	32 (94)	0.8	32 (94)	6 (18)	5.4	6 (18)	0 (0)	0 (0)	16 (47)	0 (0–4)
Undifferentiated	17 (100)	17 (100)	12 (71)	13 (76)	5 (29)	1 (6)	13 (76)	0	12 (71)	3 (18)	5.5	3 (18)	0 (0)	0 (0)	10 (59)	1 (0–2)
Enthesitis related arthritis	13 (100)	13 (100)	7 (54)	10 (76)	4 (31)	0 (0)	12 (92)	3.1	8 (62)	4 (31)	5.8	4 (31)	0 (0)	0 (0)	5 (38)	0 (0–3)
Systemic	10 (100)	9 (90)	5 (50)	10 (100)	3 (30)	6 (60)	7 (70)	0.5	6 (60)	3 (30)	2.4	2 (20)	0 (0)	0 (0)	2 (20)	0 (0–1)
Psoriatic arthritis	9 (100)	8 (89)	5 (56)	7 (78)	2 (22)	0 (0)	7 (78)	1.1	7 (78)	2 (22)	6.0	2 (22)	1 (11)	1 (11)	5 (56)	1 (0–1)
Polyarticular RF +	3 (100)	3 (100)	1 (33)	3 (100)	0 (0)	1 (33)	3 (100)	0	3 (100)	1 (33)	4.7	1 (33)	0 (0)	0 (0)	0 (0)	0 (0–0)
Overall	129 (96)	126 (94)	60 (45)	71 (53)	23 (17)	10 (7)	83 (62)	0.9	77 (57)	20 (15)	5.5	19 (14)	9 (7)	5 (4)	83 (62)	0 (0–4)

Key: *Med.* median; *NSAIDS* non-steroidal anti-inflammatory drugs; *bDMARD* biologic disease modifying anti-rheumatic drug
[a]Median number of elective admissions for joint injections per patient

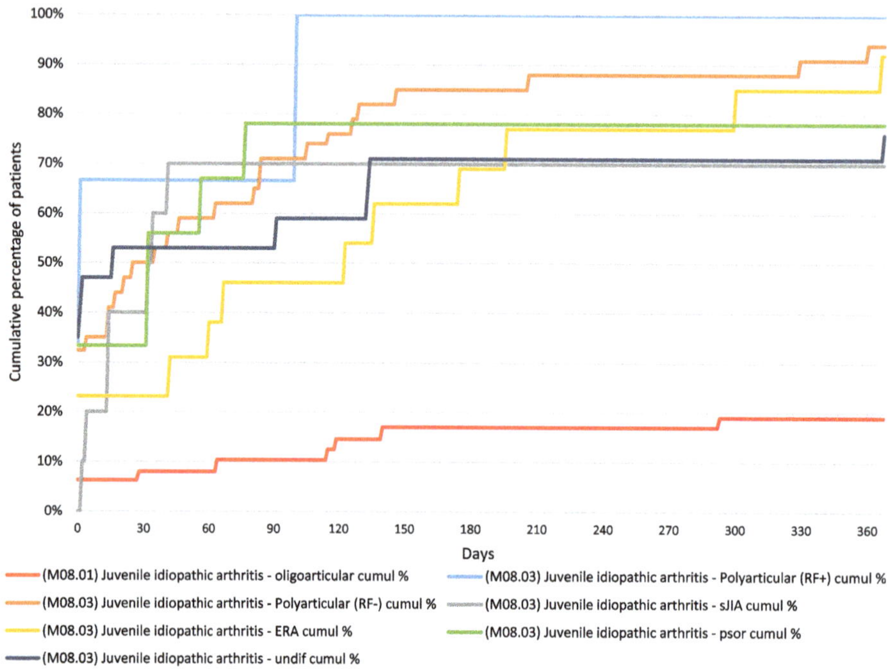

Fig. 1 Time to methotrexate commencement by JIA category

the common presentation of sJIA as an acute febrile illness, in contrast to the less dramatic symptoms of ERA, typically in adolescent boys, which may be incorrectly interpreted as non-inflammatory musculoskeletal pain or even ignored by the patients themselves. As expected, the systemic category was the only JIA category in which some patients had a zero joint count at diagnosis. It is well recognized that systemic features may precede joint disease in sJIA [12].

Most patients (95%) in our cohort achieved a joint count of zero in the first 12 months of follow up. This outcome was achieved relatively early, at a median time from

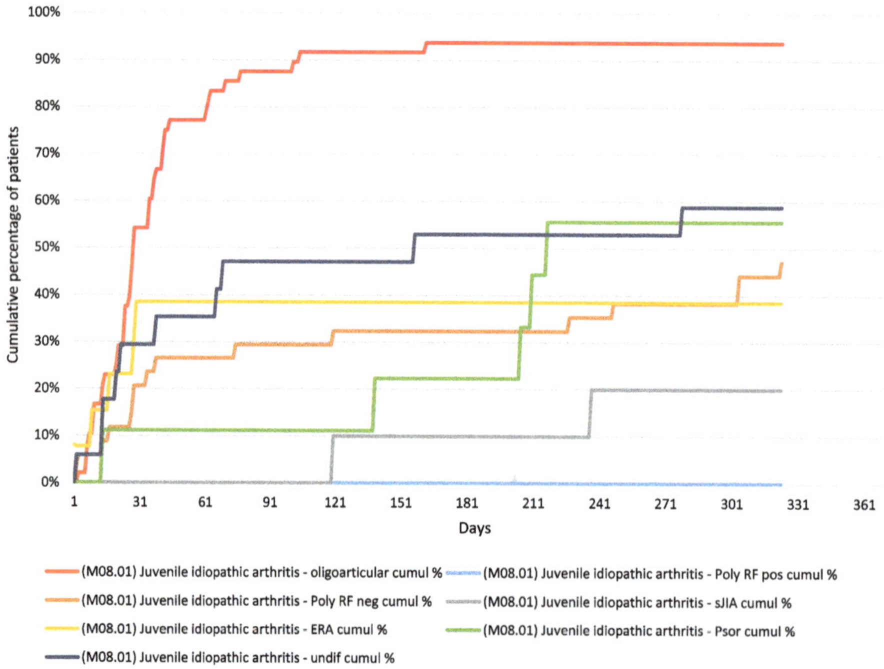

Fig. 2 Time to first intra-articular corticosteroid injection by JIA category

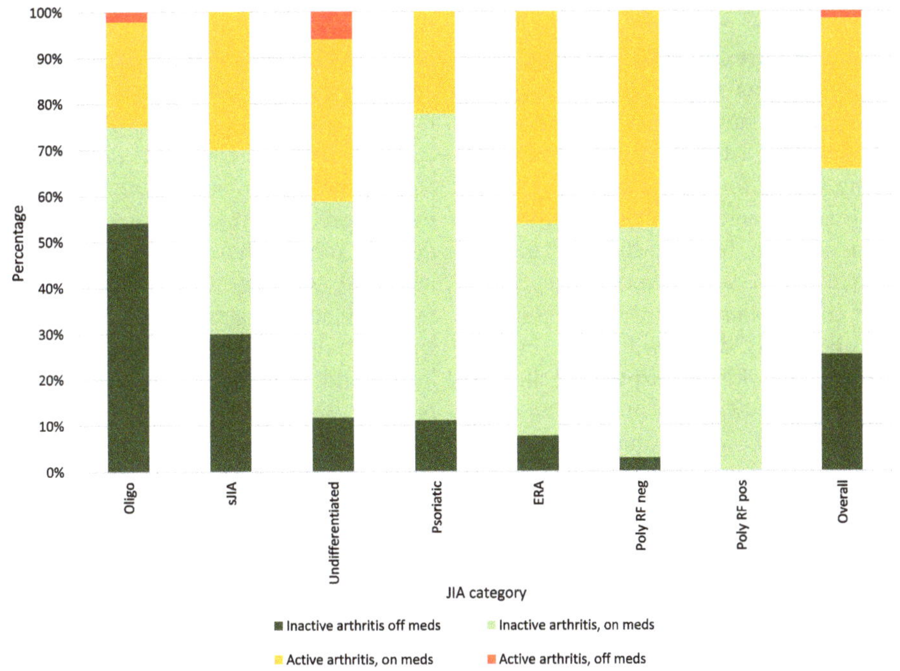

Fig. 3 Arthritis activity status by medication use at 1 year according to JIA category

diagnosis of 4.1 months. These figures are broadly comparable to those in the ReACCh-Out cohort in which ~ 91% of children achieved a zero joint count at a median of 7 months [5]. The slightly greater median time to zero joint count in that cohort may in part relate to the longer period over which this outcome was potentially captured [5]. The time to zero joint count was shortest in the sJIA and oligoarthritis categories (1.7 and 2.8 months, respectively). Early attainment of an active joint count of zero in ssJIA relative to the other categories was also found in the ReACCh-Out cohort [5]. In our patients, this likely reflects the early use of corticosteroids to control systemic disease in patients whose joint disease would not otherwise warrant their use (median joint count at baseline 0, range 0–8). The early response in the oligoarthritis group likely relates to the early use of intra-articular therapy with ~ 90% being injected within three months of diagnosis. This proportion is higher than reported in other cohorts in which rates of intra-articular corticosteroid use were just ~ 50–78% in the first year of follow-up [4, 5]. The higher rate of use of intra-articular steroid use in our patients may relate to ease of access - with 3 scheduled sedation lists and 1 general anaesthetic list per month at our centre - and physician preference. Our results would argue in favour of the early use of this therapy for this group of patients.

A surprising finding in our cohort is that approximately half of all patients received oral corticosteroids in the first year of follow up. This exposure is greater than reported in other cohorts, where oral corticosteroid use in the first year has ranged between 20 and 33% [4, 5, 13]. In our study oral steroids use was captured when an initial dosage was commenced and the date of the completed taper was then recorded. This gives an indication of exposure but makes accurate inferences regarding the cumulative exposure difficult. As expected, steroids were used most commonly in the sJIA and ERA categories and intravenous steroid use was most common in systemic disease. Oral steroids were used in significantly symptomatic patients as a 'bridging' measure while awaiting onset of action of DMARDS, or for joint injections. There were clear variations in practice relating to their use between clinicians, with rates of exposure per clinician patient group ranging between 25 and 50% (data not shown). Interestingly, despite the relatively high 'ever used' oral steroid exposure found in our cohort, the proportion of patients on oral steroids at 12 months (17%) was similar to the 14% reported in the German JIA cohort [4] and would be consistent with their short-term rather than long-term use.

The use of cDMARDS in our cohort was common; 63% of patients were commenced on a cDMARD in their first year of follow-up including 84% percent of non-oligoarticular and 25% of oligoarticular patients. The overall rate of cDMARDs use was broadly similar to those reported in the German (64.7% on methotrexate) and Canadian (47.6% on first DMARD) cohorts at the same time point [4, 5]. Our reported cDMARD use was higher than reported in the Childhood Arthritis and Rheumatology Research Alliance registry (CARRA), although the 30% cDMARD use in this study was in patients with less than 6 months of disease duration [13]. As in other cohorts, methotrexate was the cDMARD most commonly used and was started at a median of 0.7 months in non-oligoarticular disease and 2.1 months in oligoarticular disease, the latter consistent with its introduction following failure to achieve remission post early intra-articular steroid therapy. Fifteen percent of patients were commenced on biologic therapy; this is substantially more than the ~ 5% at 12 months reported in the ReACCH-Out cohort, and lower than the 38% of any biologic use in the newly diagnosed group in the CARRA cohort, but in line with the experience in the German cohort (22%) [4, 5, 13]. The median time to commencement of a bDMARD was 5.5 months, consistent with adherence to the requirements for accessing government-funded bDMARDS in Australia, which requires demonstration of failure to respond to a minimum of 3 months' methotrexate therapy [14]. 30% of the systemic arthritis group were commenced on a biologic agent, fewer than would be expected in the era of consensus treatment plans for systemic arthritis [13, 15]. This is likely multifactorial, reflecting a changing practice pattern as new guidelines and data emerge on the first line use of biologics in sJIA, and restrictions of access to biologic treatments for sJIA in Australia particularly at the start of data collection for this study [16]. Taken together these data are consistent with early aggressive treatment of JIA in the modern era, an approach based on predominantly adult data suggesting that early disease control improves long term outcomes in arthritis [17–19]. While the majority of our cohort achieved a zero joint count in the first year of follow-up, a significant minority (42%) subsequently flared. Despite this, across the cohort 65% of patients had inactive joint disease at 12 months although more than half remained on medication. Inactive joint disease off medication was uncommon (25%) except in patients with oligoarthritis (50%) and sJIA (30%), which were the two JIA categories most likely to experience a period of inactive disease in the German cohort [4]. These data suggest modern therapies in JIA are effective in controlling active joint disease in the majority of patients but that the underlying tendency to relapse - and therefore need for ongoing treatment - remains high.

The findings of this study should be interpreted taking into consideration several limitations. Compared to the cohorts in Germany and Canada our sample size is relatively small and from a single centre. Patient related outcomes, such as pain and quality of life, were not included as these data were not available. Similarly, disease remission as per the widely used 'Wallace criteria' [20] was not used as an outcome, because components of these criteria (such as acute phase reactants and physician global assessment of disease activity) are not routinely collected in every patient at every visit at our centre. Instead we chose to focus on active joint count which is documented at every visit and which, pragmatically, at most centres is the primary variable that drives contemporaneous treatment decisions in the majority of patients [21, 22]. Using the Juvenile Arthritis Disease Activity Score (JADAS) as an outcome measure, as has been done in other cohorts, may have strengthened our findings, and, we suspect, would have led to lower reported rates of inactive disease in our cohort [6, 22].

Our study also has a number of strengths. It provides 'real world' outcome data from consecutively diagnosed patients with JIA managed in a general rheumatology clinic at the largest paediatric rheumatology centre in Australia. Data were prospectively collected in a dedicated database used to record patient encounters in the clinic and, for each patient, joint counts were conducted by the same clinicians over time, negating the risk of inter-observer variability. The paediatric rheumatology department includes five rheumatologists, majority trained in North America, with experience ranging from 5 to 30 years, along with one supervised fellow. Finally, the primary outcome examined - zero joint count- is a concept that is easy to convey when discussing likely outcomes at the start of treatment, making our outcome data directly relevant to patients and their families.

Conclusions

We have shown that Australian children with JIA managed in the modern era have similar characteristics and achieve short term outcomes comparable to cohorts in North America and Europe. Whether their longer-term outcomes are similar is unknown. While the majority of patients achieve a zero joint count at least once within the first year of follow-up, relapses are common such that one third have active arthritis and three quarters require ongoing medication at 12 months. Ongoing research is required to further understand determinants of disease course and optimum management strategies.

Abbreviations

ANA: Anti-nuclear antibody; DMARD: Disease-modifying anti-rheumatic drug; ERA: Enthesitis related arthritis; IAS: Intra-articular steroid; ILAR: International League of Associations for Rheumatology; JIA: Juvenile idiopathic arthritis; NSAID: Non-steroidal anti-inflammatory drug; RCH: The Royal Children's Hospital; RF: Rheumatoid factor; sJIA: Systemic juvenile idiopathic arthritis

Acknowledgements

None.

Funding

No funding source.

Authors' contributions

All authors were involved in clinical care and the recording of data via the rheumatology database. All authors were invited to participate in peer review of the manuscript. All authors read and approved the final manuscript.

Competing interests

None to declare.

Author details

[1]Department of Rheumatology, The Royal Children's Hospital, 50 Flemington Rd, Parkville, Melbourne, VIC 3052, Australia. [2]Murdoch Childrens Research Institute, Melbourne, Australia.

References

1. Ravelli A. Juvenile idiopathic arthritis. Lancet (North American ed.). 2007; 369(9563):767.
2. Petty RE. Epidemiology of juvenile rheumatoid arthritis World. Pediatr Child Care. 1987;3:205–10.
3. Oen K, et al. Early outcomes and improvement of patients with juvenile idiopathic arthritis enrolled in a Canadian multicenter inception cohort. Arthritis care & research. 2010;62(4):527–36.
4. Sengler C, et al. The majority of newly diagnosed patients with juvenile idiopathic arthritis reach an inactive disease state within the first year of specialised care: data from a German inception cohort. RMD Open. 2015; 1(1):e000074.
5. Guzman J, et al. The outcomes of juvenile idiopathic arthritis in children managed with contemporary treatments: results from the ReACCh-out cohort. Ann Rheum Dis. 2015;74(10):1854–60.
6. Nordal E, et al. Ongoing disease activity and changing categories in a long-term nordic cohort study of juvenile idiopathic arthritis. Arthritis & Rheumatism. 2011;63(9):2809–18.
7. Bartoli M, et al. The magnitude of early response to methotrexate therapy predicts long-term outcome of patients with juvenile idiopathic arthritis. Ann Rheum Dis. 2008;67(3):370–4.
8. Wallace CA, et al. Trial of early aggressive therapy in polyarticular juvenile idiopathic arthritis. Arthritis & Rheumatism. 2012;64(6):2012–21.
9. The Australian Institute of Health and Welfare. Juvenile arthritis in Australia. Arthritis series no. 7. Cat. no. PHE 101. 2008 [cited 2016 Aug 31]; Available from: http://www.aihw.gov.au/publication-detail/?id=6442468170.
10. Manners P, Bower C. Worldwide prevalence of juvenile arthritis—why does it vary so much? J Rheumatol. 2002;29(7):1520–30.
11. Bowyer SL, et al. Health status of patients with juvenile rheumatoid arthritis at 1 and 5 years after diagnosis. J Rheumatol. 2003;30(2):394–400.
12. Behrens EM, et al. Evaluation of the presentation of systemic onset juvenile rheumatoid arthritis: data from the Pennsylvania systemic onset juvenile arthritis registry (PASOJAR). J Rheumatol. 2008;35(2):343–8.
13. Ringold S K.Y, Schanberg LE, Natter MD, Xie F, Ilowite N, Jones J, Mieszkalski K, Beukelman T, Patterns of Medication Use in Children with Juvenile Idiopathic Arthritis: Results from the Childhood Arthritis & Rheumatology Research Alliance Registry [abstract]. 2016: Arthritis Rheumatol.
14. DHHS A.G. Juvenile idiopathic arthritis: Initial PBS authority application. 2017 [cited 2017 13/11/12017]; Available from: https://www.humanservices.gov.au/organisations/health-professionals/forms/pb060.
15. Kimura Y, et al. Pilot study comparing the Childhood Arthritis & Rheumatology Research Alliance (CARRA) systemic juvenile idiopathic arthritis consensus treatment plans. Pediatr Rheumatol. 2017;15(1):23.
16. Nigrovic PA, et al. Anakinra as first-line disease-modifying therapy in systemic juvenile idiopathic arthritis: report of forty-six patients from an international multicenter series. Arthritis & rheumatism. 2011;63(2):545–55.
17. Anink J, et al. Two-year outcome of juvenile idiopathic arthritis in current daily practice: what can we tell our patients? Clinical & Experimental Rheumatology. 2012;30(6):972–8.
18. Tynjala P, et al. Aggressive combination drug therapy in very early polyarticular juvenile idiopathic arthritis (ACUTE-JIA): a multicentre randomised open-label clinical trial. Ann Rheum Dis. 2011;70(9):1605–12.
19. Boers M. Understanding the window of opportunity concept in early rheumatoid arthritis. Arthritis & Rheumatology. 2003;48(7):1771–4.
20. Wallace CA, Ruperto N, Giannini E. Preliminary criteria for clinical remission for select categories of juvenile idiopathic arthritis. J Rheumatol. 2004;31(11):2290–4.
21. Van Mater HA, et al. Psychometric characteristics of outcome measures in juvenile idiopathic arthritis: a systematic review. Arthritis care & research. 2012;64(4):554–62.
22. Consolaro A, et al. Development and validation of a composite disease activity score for juvenile idiopathic arthritis. Arthritis & Rheumatism. 2009; 61(5):658–66.

19

What do young people with rheumatic conditions in the UK think about research involvement? A qualitative study

Suzanne Parsons[1,2,3], Wendy Thomson[2,3,4,5], Katharine Cresswell[1,2,3], Bella Starling[2,6], Janet E. McDonagh[5,7,8*]
and on behalf of the Barbara Ansell National Network for Adolescent Rheumatology (BANNAR)

Abstract

Background: Involving people of all ages in health research is now widely advocated. To date, no studies have explored whether and how young people with chronic rheumatic conditions want to be involved in influencing health research. This study aimed to explore amongst young people with rheumatic conditions, 1) their experiences of research participation and involvement 2) their beliefs about research involvement and 3) beliefs about how young people's involvement should be organized in the future.

Methods: Focus groups discussions with young people aged 11–24 years with rheumatic conditions across the UK. Data was analysed using a qualitative Framework approach.

Results: Thirteen focus groups were held involving 63 participants (45 F: 18 M, mean age 16, range 10 to 24 years) across the UK. All believed that young people had a right to be involved in influencing research and to be consulted by researchers. However, experience of research involvement varied greatly. For many, the current project was the first time they had been involved. Amongst those with experience of research involvement, awareness of what they had been involved in and why was often low. Those who had previously participated in research appeared more positive and confident about influencing research in the future. However, all felt that there were limited opportunities for them to be both research participants and to get involved in research as public contributors.

Conclusions: These findings suggest that there is an on-going need to both increase awareness of research involvement and participation of young people in rheumatology as well as amongst young people themselves.

Keywords: Qualitative, Young people, Adolescent rheumatology, Rheumatic conditions, Patient involvement

Background

Involving people at all stages of health research (including young people) is now widely recommended [1]. In the UK, many grant and all ethics application processes now ensure that patient and public involvement (PPI) in research is embedded within them [2]. PPI is also advocated by professional bodies in general and specifically for young people. [3, 4].

* Correspondence: Janet.mcdonagh@manchester.ac.uk
[5]School of Biological Sciences, Faculty of Biology, Medicine and Health, The University of Manchester, Manchester, UK
[7]Arthritis Research UK Centre for Epidemiology, Centre for Musculoskeletal Research, Division of Musculoskeletal and Dermatological Sciences, Manchester, UK
Full list of author information is available at the end of the article

Within this study we defined involvement as "where members of the public are actively involved in research projects and in research organisations" [5] and participation as, "where patients and the public act as research participants".

Involving patients and the public in research helps ensure that research is designed around their needs and what is important to them [6]. However, it can be challenging to involve a diverse range of people [7]. This is particularly true with young people [8]. In view of the major sociocultural influences on adolescent health [9], representative sampling (in terms of socio-demographics- gender, ethnicity, culture and urban vs rural regional variations) is vital in studies of adolescents in general and when not feasible, the limitations of non-representative samples should be stated. In view of the wide variation of normal puberty, chronological age is a poor indicator of developmental status. Therefore, attention to the stages of adolescent development is required in any research involving young people. Ensuring such diversity may also result in part from a lack of confidence and/or inexperience amongst researchers regarding PPI [10], particularly with respect to young people in these particular developmental stages as although clinical research focusing on young people is rapidly evolving, it is still developing compared to research with adult populations [11].

The Barbara Ansell National Network for Adolescent Rheumatology (BANNAR) is a network of rheumatology professionals aiming to ensure that young people in the UK have the best chance to benefit from developments in the field of adolescent and young adult rheumatology [12]. A key priority for BANNAR is to involve young people in developing the network's research priorities.

This study aimed to explore (i) experiences of research participation and involvement (ii) beliefs about research involvement amongst young people with rheumatic conditions and (iii) beliefs about how young people's involvement should be organized in the future.

Data regarding their research priorities has been published elsewhere [13].

Methods

This was a qualitative study of young people with rheumatic conditions. Sixteen focus groups were planned (8 with 11–15 year olds and 8 with 16–24 year olds) in all four nations of the UK to capture the potential impact of differences in health service organisation on young people's experiences. The age ranges were chosen to reflect adolescent developmental stages i.e. early and mid-adolescence (11–15 years) and late adolescence and young adulthood (16–24 years).. Sixteen focus groups were conducted in all four nations of the UK to capture the potential impact of differences in health service organisation on young people's experiences. The methods for this project have already been reported in detail elsewhere [13, 14].

Recruitment

Rheumatology team members gave study information sheets to a broad range of eligible young people (in terms of age, gender, ethnicity, condition, research experience and socio-economic status). Inclusion criteria were English speaking 11–24 year olds, under the care of a rheumatologist with any chronic rheumatic condition.

Young people were also recruited via a UK based charity, Arthritis Care to ensure that young people who were not under the care of rheumatologists associated with BANNAR were involved [15]. As the aim of the project was to obtain the views from young people with any chronic rheumatic condition ie not specific to any particular disease, the only demographic details collected on individual participants were gender and age.

Focus groups were moderated by SP (a social scientist) and/or JMcD (a Paediatric Rheumatologist) who had no direct involvement in the clinical care of participants.

Focus group topic guide

The topic guide is described in detail elsewhere [14]. Focus groups lasted for up to 90 min and explored:

1. Experiences of research participation and involvement
2. Beliefs about the research process and young people's involvement in it
3. Beliefs about how young people's involvement should be organised in the future

Data management

Focus group recordings were transcribed verbatim, and pseudonyms were created for names, organisations and places.

The data was analysed thematically, using the Framework approach to qualitative data analysis [16]. Framework allowed both apriori and emergent themes to be included within the analysis. The study topic guide was used as a starting point for the thematic framework, and then SP, KC and JM read through the transcripts and identified recurrent themes to further develop the framework. This framework was then applied to the data and further refined where necessary.

Results

Thirteen focus groups were held across the UK (England 8; Scotland 2; Northern Ireland 2; Wales 1). The original aim had been to conduct 16 focus groups but data saturation was achieved after 11. We determined that no new ideas were generated via reviewing recordings and transcripts and early analyses of the data. We however conducted a further 2 focus groups to ensure that young people from all four nations of the UK had the opportunity to participate although no new ideas were identified in this groups.

Six groups were held with 11–15 year olds ($n = 30$) and seven with 16–24 year olds ($n = 33$). Participants' ages ranged from 11 to 24 years (mean = 16), 20 of whom were male and 43 female. Characteristics of participants are detailed in Table 1.

The themes which were identified are detailed in Table 2.

Table 1 Characteristics of participants [13]

	UK	England	Scotland	Northern Ireland	Wales
		Age group			
11–15 year olds	30	20	5	5	0
16–24 year olds	33	19	2	9	3
		Gender			
Male	20	15	2	3	0
Female	43	24	5	11	3

Young people's experiences of research participation
Young people's experience and understanding of research varied greatly. For example, some knew that they had been a research participant but could not recall the details of the research (Table 3a). This was due, in part, to the challenges of recalling childhood experiences when older (Table 3b) Some explained that their younger selves had been happy to leave the responsibility for understanding the details of the research to their parents. (Table 3c).

Some participants however had clear memories of the research with a number expressing concern about the lack of feedback they had received on findings (Table 3d, e and f). Others spoke about the importance of clearly understanding what they were contributing to the research (Table 3g).

For some young people, altruism was a key reason for their participation, as they believed that taking part was the 'right thing to do' and that it would be impossible for young people in their position in the future to be helped if they did not participate (Table 3h, i, j and k).

Table 2 Key themes identified with Framework analysis

- Young people's experiences of research participation
  - Experience of research participation as children
  - Feedback on research participation
  - Altruism as a motivator for research participation
- Beliefs about and experiences of young people being involved in research
  - Motivations for involvement
  - Role of experience of condition in involvement
  - Experience of involvement
- Challenges to, and facilitators of, young people's involvement
  - Being taken seriously by and listened to by researchers
  - Access to research and researchers
  - Clear roles and importance of co-production
  - Flexibility in involvement approaches
- Practical considerations when involving young people in research
  - Timing of involvement
  - Convenience of activity
  - Role of incentives
  - Patient-led versus researcher-led involvement

Finally, a considerable number of participants reported being interested in research participation but could not recall ever being asked to take part in clinical research until the reported study.

Beliefs about and experiences of, young people being involved in research
Young people believed that they offered a valuable, different perspective on the research process compared to adults (including researchers) (Table 4a and c). They felt that contributing the lived experience of their condition to the research process was valuable and essential, as many had significant experience of their illness and its treatment since disease onset in early childhood (Table 4c, d, e and f).

Experience of research involvement varied from considerable to no experience (Table 4g, h, i, j and k). Several reported prior involvement in advisory groups although they varied in their perceptions of the value of their contribution to such groups (Table 4h, I, j and k). As with research participation, altruism was a key driver for young people to become involved in shaping research (Table 4b).

Challenges to and facilitators of, young people's involvement All participants were able to discuss their beliefs on the best approaches to involving young people in research (Table 5a-f) even if they had no prior experience. They stressed the importance of co-production of research with researchers and believed that involvement should be driven and organised by public contributors when possible (Table 5d). Participants advocated using both online and face to face approaches to involvement in addition to gaining a greater understanding of young people's networks to facilitate their involvement (Table 5a, b and c). The use of social media was believed to be a key approach to facilitate the involvement of a wide range of young people in research (Table 5a).

Despite feeling that young people had a right to be involved, participants expressed uncertainty over the mechanisms by which young people could be involved in research and how this can best be supported (Table 4e). All believed that accessing information about research and research findings was challenging to both research participation and involvement (Table 5e).

Practical considerations when involving young people in research Timing of involvement opportunities was a key issue, with young people discussing the importance of their personal commitments being considered when involvement requests were made (Table 6a, b and c). They also discussed the importance of researchers not asking recently diagnosed young people to be involved

Table 3 Experience of Research Participation

	Examples of quotes
3a. Experience of research in childhood - Degree of understanding regarding the purpose of research when a child	F: I am 18 and I think I did one about a year and a half ago, and there was someone in the Children's Hospital that kept asking for my saliva yeah. It did become a running joke between me and my dad that she just wants my germs! So yeah, I think I have (England over 16)
3b. Experience of research in childhood - Challenges of recalling research participation in childhood	F: Yes I have when I was younger, I can't quite remember all the details, I think it was research in how metal joints affect the blood and that and when they test blood, they try and see whether or not they can judge how far…how worn out the joint is (Wales 16 and over)
3c. Experience of research in childhood - Parents taking control of research consent process when younger	F - The X study was okay because I was young enough that my mum came and kind of took control. (Northern Ireland 16 and over)
3d. Lack of feedback on research participation	F - The University one was slightly different. It was quite daunting, I had a one-to-one interview. Mine lasted just over three hours. But I could see the benefits of why I actually should do it, but I still haven't actually received anything back from it. Sometimes you need to see what's come off your participation. (Northern Ireland 16 and over)
3e. Lack of feedback on research participation	F: it is like taking a test and never getting your grade (Northern Ireland under 16)
3f. Lack of feedback on research participation	F – But I think it would be useful if people who have it know like what's been found so they kind of like have got an idea of where it is all going (England under 16)
3g. Importance of feeling that your contribution to research is meaningful	M- I think it's a trade-off between convenience and impact, if it's going to really be helpful or if it's really going to have a big impact. I feel that if I am just going to be a data point then it really doesn't impress me that it is important. It was conveyed to me that it was a really important factor in their research, I think I'd put a lot more effort into it (England over 16)
3h. Reasons for research participation - Altruism	Facilitator – Why did you decide to take part? M- Well I've got it may as well help other people who have it. (England over 16)
3i. Reasons for research participation – Altruism	F- I kind of decided, because it took me probably three or four years to get diagnosed, I was thinking whether if it was easier for someone else to just be diagnosed straight away, So that's kind of why I helped a bit. (England under 16)
3j. Reasons for research participation – Altruism	M- Not being rude but I think you are stupid if you don't take part in research. If you're upset about something and you want to get better, surely you would take part in something that might make you better in the long run and help others (England under 16)
3k. Reasons for research participation – Altruism – wanting to make things better	F: Exactly the reason I agreed to take part in this is so that young people won't be in the same situation I was when I was diagnosed. (Wales over 16)

F Female *M* Male (country, age group)

as they felt that at this time, young people would have too much to do to become familiar with their condition before they could consider research involvement (Table 6c). A further suggestion was for researchers to combine involvement with other activities young people are already doing (Table 6d).

Young people discussed how offering compensation could influence the types of people who became involved. Some felt that offering compensation could lead to people becoming involved who did not feel strongly about the research, and others that it would facilitate a wider range of people considering involvement (Table 6e).

Young people also had views regarding how involvement should be organised with some specifically advocating facilitation but that this ideally should be "patient-led" (Table 6f and g).

Discussion

To the best of our knowledge, this is the first study, to explore the experiences and beliefs of young people with rheumatic conditions about research involvement. Although young people felt that they had a right to be involved in research, experience of research involvement varied. This may reflect geographical variation in the research culture, i.e. the extent to which research participation and involvement of people in research were viewed as priorities and key elements of usual care by clinicians, researchers and their host institutions.

Young people also expressed a wish to increase their research awareness. This may have arisen in part due to difficulties in remembering whether they had taken part in research especially if what was involved was similar to usual care e.g. completing the Childhood Assessment Questionnaire [17].

If young people believe that they have a low awareness of research in general, then it is also likely to be difficult to increase their involvement as a public contributor. In this study some young people reported never being approached about research participation nor research involvement. This concurs with the findings of a previous

Table 4 Beliefs about and experiences of young people being involved in research

Theme	Example quotes
4a. Motivations for involvement – young people's views and experience are different than adults	F- I would do it because adults and people our age they think differently and they don't always consider the things that we consider and because we're the ones getting involved I think it's good that we have a say. (England under 16)
4b. Motivations for involvement - altruism	M- If someone came to me I'd instantly say, yeah, I'll take part in it. I don't care if it's a bit boring because it's for the benefit of others. So there needs to be like a Facebook page or something, you know like an online poll and stuff like that (England over 16)
4c.Experience as a young person – Providing a different perspective to researchers	M- I disagree because they should give ideas on how the research is done, because it's your opinion and if you're going through something you should have a say on what the researchers are actually focusing on, because it's happening to you. It would be useless if they were focusing on something that isn't important to you. (England under 16)
4d. Experience of condition- Importance and value of young people's experiences of their condition	F: Researchers think they are the best but sometimes they are not, young people have the problems in their body and they know more things about their condition than researchers do. (Northern Ireland under 16)
4e. Experience of condition - Importance and value of young people's experiences of their condition	M: I think also it is quite important that we have experience. We have experience in the service, we have experience with the doctors and we have kind of had all or quite a substantial part of our life in the service so we know what it is like and we have had good experiences and bad experiences. (England 16 and over)
4f. Experience of condition - Importance and value of young people's experiences of their condition to research	M: it is like a better thing as well, as you have the doctors who know about the thing, they know about condition and how to treat it but they don't know what it is like to cope with something like that. (Scotland 16 and over)
4g. Experiences of involvement - Involved but unclear what in	F – He's called M, he's 17 and he's been involved M – I think I have F – You've come on advisory groups for disease specific JIA and I'm sure there's questionnaires and stuff. You've done involvement and the research side (England over 16)
4h. Experiences of involvement – involved but in a limited way	Facilitator - the other question was whether you've ever given your thoughts on how research is done M- Yeah, once or twice, but that's only speaking to a researcher at the hospital, that just comes and talks to me (England under 16)
4i. Experiences of involvement – uncertain about whether played a useful role in advisory groups –	Two or three of you have said that you have taken part in advisory groups- have you had the chance to really have a say? F- I had a big rant one time, I don't know, it was like one of those next door. I went so off topic and just ranted about the NHS really. F- it's addressing things like mental health aspects, which might be more personal than information from blood samples (England over 16)
4j. Experiences of involvement – uncertainty on how or whether to input	M- I never talk during the advisory group thing … I just had nothing to say basically, They were saying things that I was thinking of saying but didn't end up saying because they got there first. (England over 16)
4k. Experiences of involvement - challenges to participating in advisory groups	F- The last one I think was one of the better ones, because as I said there was less people there, but also because it was kind of like, sometimes in the bigger groups you can hear someone say something that you disagree with, but it's a bit awkward because you don't know them well enough to disagree with them, because you just don't want to get into an argument. But that one, because we were basically all the same age and had the exact same thing, it was better. (England over 16)

F Female *M* Male (country, age group)

UK audit of paediatric and adolescent rheumatology services which reported that at least 60% of centres did not involve young people in research other than as research participants [14].

An interesting finding was that some young people who had actually been involved in shaping research did not always perceive this as involvement. One explanation for this may be the lack of feedback they received following their involvement, or it may reflect lack of clarity of their role during the participation and involvement processes.

A key strength of this study was the inclusion of 63 young people from a broad range of ages and from all four UK nations, thereby reflecting a range of service provision and research opportunities. The variation in the experiences of research involvement and participation was an important finding, validating our approach and highlighting the need to conduct a national study. However, recruitment for this study was poor in some areas particularly if there was not a PPI or transition coordinator who could help with recruitment. In the development phase of this research, a survey of the 25 main

Table 5 Challenges and facilitators to young people's involvement

5a. Flexible approaches to involvement – role of social media and online approaches	F-. So I mean you've Facebook, you've twitter, which I'm pretty sure at least everyone in this room has at least one. Even the younger group. There would be some way of getting in contact with them in that manner. And it's a free way of getting in contact with them; it can be monitored as well. And its instant results. And it means that you are not going to have the idea that you can't go along as you can't meet this person's schedule, not a problem, use that. (Northern Ireland over 16)
5b. Flexible approaches to involvement – role of social media and online approaches	F: Maybe consulting more groups like us, we can maybe video conference if you wanted to give it a group discussion about something and the same for all different regions. (Wales over 16)
5c. Continued importance of face to face involvement	M- Yeah I like face to face, because it's good to learn about other people, (England under 16)
5d. Clear roles and importance of co-production of research	M- I think both people should contribute and agree with what's going on... it shouldn't be just the doctors decision, it should be the patients' as well. (England over 16)
5e. Access to research and researchers	M: I think there is I don't know what the word is a barrier maybe between, you know, young people and researchers. And how you contact each other and even if we did sort of have to, how would we kind of work together? And put that into research. (Scotland over 16)
5f. Being taken seriously by researchers and feeling listened to	F- I think they have to take people who are actually suffering with it seriously, and how they are feeling it like, and they have to have some consideration for what they are doing. And to think whether it will actually benefit them in some way what they are actually researching into. (England over 16)

F Female *M* Male (country, age group)

paediatric rheumatology units identified that just five units had a team member with PPI included in their job description [14]. Furthermore, in order to limit recruitment bias, we adopted a maximum variety purposive sampling approach to sampling for this study. This aimed to encompass the range of AYA development by having focus groups for the first 2 stages (early and mid) and the latter 2 stages (late adolescence and young adulthood). We also involved centres in all 4 devolved nations of the UK in order to capture the range of services for this age group, in both urban and rural settings. There has been a significant growth in specialist services

Table 6 Practical considerations when involving young people in research

Theme	Example quotes
6a.Timing of involvement	M- I would probably say week days, because obviously people have like college or school or work or whatever. So like today (Saturday) there was no problem for me to come here (England over 16)
6b.Timing of involvement	F: Probably during holidays and all that, I have quite heavy workload with college and I have exams coming up and stuff so probably holiday kind of times. (Scotland over 16)
6c.Timing of involvement activity	F- I think as soon as you've been diagnosed, I think is probably the worst time, because I don't think you know the disease yourself. So I think if like in the future people are getting diagnosed, I think they should wait a while until they're familiar with their own disease before they start research. (England under 16)
6d.Convenience - Combining involvement with other things young people are doing	M- The most important thing about why you get involved with research is convenience, so try and maybe do what they did, because if I was to be asked to do this separately once every couple of months, I would probably think that this is going to be hassle. So rather than setting up a separate group, try and maybe go along to some other groups, like that lupus group or other support groups (England over 16)
6e.Incentives for involvement	M- People are going to be more receptive if they think there is a reward at the end. Because you could put out notices saying we need people to come and help and you'll only get those people who are actively involved or who actively seek out these type of opportunities. But if you set some sort of incentive, you may get people who think it's not the normal thing they do but they're willing to help out. (Northern Ireland over 16)
6f.Patient led or researcher led involvement	M: I think that it would be better if someone was there for ad/medical stuff as and when needed, but we were allowed to just get on with the thing. Like you might need someone to give stimulus and ask a couple of questions. But generally I think it should be like it is today, with just us talking, just the patients. (England 16 and over)
6g. Patient led or researcher led involvement	F: So it is interesting the continuity and management of it and stuff, so you set that up so it is a patient led thing and that is different to having a researcher-led thing, as researchers can't do a lot of obviously, it is time consuming… (England 16 and over)

F Female *M* Male (country, age group)

for this age group in recent years in the UK although significant delays in referral persist for certain conditions eg juvenile idiopathic arthritis [18]. To further maximise the diversity within our recruitment we recruited via charities in an attempt to recruit young people not being treated at centres with specific paediatric, adolescent and/or young adult rheumatology services. These young people potentially had less access to research opportunities.

However despite efforts to recruit a maximum variety sample, due to the relative small sample sizes required within qualitative research there will still be some limitations in terms of the diversity of the sample. For example, research-naïve young people or those with very mild disease and/or who are happy with their current care may not have perceived a study focused on beliefs about research involvement as being relevant to them. However we did successfully recruit such young people in this study. Another group less likely to engage in research are those young people who have become disengaged from their rheumatology care. Understanding their perspectives would be particularly valuable. Reasons for non-response are important in any research but particularly pertinent to adolescent health as some studies have shown that those who fail to respond have poorer outcomes compared to adult non-responders [19].

An important impact of this study is that, incorporating the clear advice regarding involvement in the current study, we have since established a national young person's advisory group to inform BANNAR research.

The group is called Your Rheum (https://yourrheum.org/) [20] and is currently holding face to face meetings several times a year and involving young people online in research.

Finally, whilst acknowledging the exploratory nature of the current study, one could argue that many of these findings are also true for adult populations. However, implementing change in the adolescent and young adult group in relation to involvement, just as in clinical care, requires developmentally appropriate approaches which change over time as young people grow and develop [11].

Young people identified a lack of opportunity or a perception of poor access to research and research involvement as a primary barrier to research involvement. This suggests that efforts are needed to increase researchers' awareness and understanding of PPI and its' likely impact. Increased awareness may increase researchers' confidence in involving young people in their work and lead to a wider range of research involvement opportunities becoming available. As part of this current project, models of good research involvement practice in this area beyond rheumatology were collated to serve as a future resource for researchers [21]. Since the Clinical Studies Group in Paediatric Rheumatology was established [22], research involvement outside of large teaching hospitals has significantly improved but further work is still required, if we consider the views of participants in the current study of their poor access to involvement opportunities. Investment into appropriate staffing for such initiatives is supported by the finding that recruitment to this particular study was better in those centres with a team member with PPI as part of their job description.

The findings from this exploratory study also suggest that further work is needed to increase young people's awareness of rheumatology research within the UK. The national paediatric rheumatology clinical studies group, which supports a portfolio of clinical studies across the UK states:

"All children and young people in the UK with a rheumatological condition may be given the opportunity to be enrolled in a clinical trial or well conducted clinical study from point of diagnosis onwards" [22].

The current study has revealed that it will be important to ensure both that the aims and purposes of young people's involvement in research are made clear to them as well as receiving feedback on both their involvement as well as their research participation. It will also be important to explore the language used to explain research participation and involvement to young people to gain some insights into why the nature of involvement is sometimes misconstrued.

In this current study, few young people had experience of being involved in influencing research, with those treated in large teaching hospitals being more likely to report having experience. Despite this finding, all young people strongly believed that they should be involved in research, particularly as they had lived experience of their condition and could provide a perspective which would otherwise not be available. Acknowledgement of the lived experience of young people with rheumatic disease is therefore as imperative for researchers as has also been reported for clinicians [23].

Understanding and evaluating the impact of patient and public involvement in general, and for young people is becoming an increasingly important issue. Evaluation frameworks for involvement have been developed for adults but it is still unclear whether they can be used effectively with young people [24]. The involvement of young people in research has been reported to have a positive impact on recruitment and retention [25]. However, Holland et al. cautions practitioners "against assuming that participatory research per se necessarily produces "better" research data, equalises power relations or enhances ethical integrity" [26]. Therefore, research is needed to explore how young people perceive their roles as active research partners in the context of chronic health conditions when involvement could potentially be an additional burden [27].

Conclusions

This exploratory study highlights the importance of further enhancing the culture of research in the adolescent and young adult age group, to increase young people's awareness of opportunities for both research participation and research involvement. In the UK, BANNAR and the YOURR project have made initial steps in doing so in rheumatology.

What is known about this subject?

Involving people of all ages in health research is now widely advocated. To date, no studies have explored whether and how young people with rheumatic conditions want to be involved in influencing health research.

What this study adds?

- This study highlights the need to increase the culture of research in some clinical specialities (including Rheumatology) to improve young people's access to research participation and involvement opportunities
- Providing support and training to researchers to increase their confidence in involving young people in their work is also likely to increase the number of research involvement opportunities available.
- Being flexible in the range of approaches used to involve young people in research may increase the likelihood that a more diverse group of young people will become involved.

Abbreviations

BANNAR: Barbara Ansell National Network for Adolescent Rheumatology.; BSPAR: British Society for Paediatric and Adolescent Rheumatology; CHAQ: Childhood Health Assessment Questionnaire; NHS: National Health Service; PPI: Patient and Public Involvement; YOURR: Young People's Opinions Underpinning Rheumatology Research

Acknowledgements

This article presents independent research funded by Arthritis Research UK BANNAR. The views expressed in this article are those of the authors and not necessarily those of the NHS, the National Institute for Health Research or Arthritis Research UK. We would like to thank all of the young people who took part in this study and the clinicians including members of the Barbara Ansell National Network for Adolescent Rheumatology, PPI coordinators and other individuals who facilitated their involvement. Arthritis Care for their support in the recruitment phase of the project.

Funding

We thank the Arthritis Research UK for their support: Arthritis Research UK grant number 20164; Centre for Epidemiology 20380 and Centre for Genetics and Genomics 20385.

Authors' contributions

JMcD wrote the successful application for funding. SP and JMcD co led on the writing of this manuscript and all authors read and approved the final version. JMcD and WT are the co-principal investigators with overall responsibility for the project. SP and JMcD moderated the focus groups. SP is the research associate who led the data analysis. JMcD, SP, WT, BS and KC were involved in data interpretation. KC is also the facilitator for the young people's involvement group Your Rheum. All authors read and approved the final manuscript.

Competing interests

"The authors declare that they have no competing interests".

Author details

[1]Public Programmes Team, Manchester University NHS Foundation Trust, Manchester, UK. [2]NIHR Manchester Biomedical Research Centre, Manchester University NHS Foundation Trust, Manchester, UK. [3]Manchester Academic Health Science Centre, Manchester, UK. [4]Arthritis Research UK Centre for Genetics and Genomics, Centre for Musculoskeletal Research, Division of Musculoskeletal and Dermatological Sciences, Manchester, UK. [5]School of Biological Sciences, Faculty of Biology, Medicine and Health, The University of Manchester, Manchester, UK. [6]Research and Innovation Division, Manchester University NHS Foundation Trust, Manchester, UK. [7]Arthritis Research UK Centre for Epidemiology, Centre for Musculoskeletal Research, Division of Musculoskeletal and Dermatological Sciences, Manchester, UK. [8]Centre for MSK Research, University of Manchester, Stopford Building 2nd floor, Oxford Rd, Manchester M13 9PT, UK.

References

1. Bate J, Ranasinghe N, Ling R, Preston J, Nightingale R, Denegri S. Public and patient involvement in paediatric research. Arch Dis Child Educ Pract Ed. 2016;101(3):158–61.
2. Elliott J. Health Research Authority strategy for Patient Involvement 2013; NHS Health Research Authority. (https://www.hra.nhs.uk/planning-and-improving-research/best-practice/involving-public/ (Accessed 12 Jan 2018) Accessed 27 May 2017).
3. Generation R website. http://generationr.org.uk/ (Accessed 12 Jan 2018).
4. Hunter L, Sparrow E, Modi N, Greenough A. Advancing child health research in the UK: the Royal College of Paediatrics and Child Health Infants' Children's and young People's research charter. Arch Dis Child. 2017 Apr; 102(4):299–300.
5. NIHR INVOLVE Jargon buster. http://www.invo.org.uk/resource-centre/jargon-buster/page/2/?letter=I (Accessed 12 Jan 2018).
6. Dudley L, Gamble C, Preston J, Buck D, EPIC Patient Advisory Group., Hanley B, Williamson P, Young B. What difference does patient and public involvement make and what are its pathways to impact? Qualitative study of patients and researchers from a cohort of randomised clinical trials. PLoS One. 2015;10(6):e0128817.
7. Boote J, Wong R, Booth A. 'Talking the talk or walking the walk?' A bibliometric review of the literature on public involvement in health research published between 1995 and 2009. Health Expect. 2015;18(1):44–57.
8. McDonagh JE, Dovey-Pearce G. Research methods in adolescents in. In: Thomet C, Moons P, Schwerzmann M, editors. "Adolescents with congenital heart disease". Switzerland: Springer International Publishing Switzerland; 2016. p. 207–21.
9. Viner RM, Ozer EM, Denny S, Marmot M, Resnick M, Fatsui A, Currie C. Adolescence and the social determinants of health. Lancet. 2012;379(9826):1641–52.
10. Dudley L, Gamble C, Allam A, Bell P, Buck D, Goodare H, Hanley B, Preston J, Walker A, Williamson P, Young B. A little more conversation please? Qualitative study of researchers' and patients' interview accounts of training for patient and public involvement in clinical trials. Trials. 2015;16(1):190.
11. Sammons HM, Wright K, Young B, Farsides B. Research with children and young people: not on them. Arch Dis Child. 2016 Dec;101(12):1086–9.
12. Barbara Ansell National Network for Adolescent Rheumatology website (BANNAR). http://bannar.org.uk/ (Accessed 12 Jan 2018).
13. Parsons S, Thomson W, Cresswell K, Starling B, JE MD. Barbara Ansell National Network for adolescent rheumatology. What do young people with rheumatic disease believe to be important to research about their condition? A UK-wide study. 2017;15(1):53.

14. Parsons S, Dack K, Starling B, Thomson W, McDonagh JE. Study protocol: determining what young people with rheumatic disease consider important to research (the young People's opinions underpinning rheumatology research-YOURR project). Research Involvement and Engagement. 2016;2(1):1.
15. Arthritis Care website. 2018. https://www.arthritiscare.org.uk/ (Accessed 28 Apr 2018).
16. Ritchie J, Lewis J. Qualitative research practice- a guide for social science students and researchers. London: Sage; 2003.
17. Nugent J, Ruperto N, Grainger J, Machado C, Sawhney S, Baildam E, Davidson J, Foster H, Hall A, Hollingworth P, Sills J, Venning H, Walsh JE, Landgraf JM, Roland M, Woo P, Murray KJ. Paediatric rheumatology international trials organisation. The British version of the childhood health assessment questionnaire (CHAQ) and the child health questionnaire (CHQ). Clin Exp Rheum. 2001;19(23):S163–7.
18. McErlane F, Foster HE, Carrasco R, Baildam EM, Chieng SE, Davidson JE, Ioannou Y, Wedderburn LR, Thomson W, Hyrich KL. Trends in paediatric rheumatology referral times and disease activity indices over a ten-year period among children and young people with juvenile idiopathic arthritis: results from the childhood arthritis prospective study. Rheumatology (Oxford). 2016;55(7):1225–34.
19. Mattila VM, Parkkari J, Rimpela A. Adolescent survey non-response and later risk of death. A prospective cohort study of 78609 persons with 11 year follow-up. BMC Public Health. 2007;7:87.
20. Your Rheum website - https://yourrheum.org/ (Accessed 28 Apr 2018).
21. Dack K, Williams H, Parsons S, Thomson W, McDonagh JE On behalf of the Barbara Ansell National Network for adolescent rheumatology. Summary of good practice when involving young people in health-related research. 2016 (available on www.bannar.org.uk, Accessed 12 Jan 2018).
22. Thornton J, Beresford MW, Clayton P. Improving the evidence base for treatment of juvenile idiopathic arthritis: the challenge and opportunity facing the MCRN/ARC Paediatric rheumatology clinical studies group. Rheumatology. 2008;47:563–6.
23. Hart RI, McDonagh JE, Thompson B, Foster HE, Kay L, Myers A, Rapley T. Being as normal as possible: how young people ages 16-25 years evaluate the risks and benefits of treatment for inflammatory arthritis. Arthritis Care Res (Hoboken). 2016 Sep;68(9):1288–94.
24. Public Involvement Impact Assessment Framework (Piiaff) http://piiaf.org.uk/ (Accessed 12 Jan 2018).
25. Shrewsbury VA, O'Connor J, Steinbeck KS, Stevenson K, Lee A, Hill AJ, Kohn MR, Shah S, Torvaldsen S, Baur LA. A randomised controlled trial of a community-based healthy lifestyle program for overweight and obese adolescents: the Loozit® study protocol. BMC Public Health. 2009 Apr 29;9(1):119.
26. Holland S, Renold E, Ross NJ, Hillman A. Power, agency and participatory agendas: a critical exploration of young people's engagement in participative qualitative research. Childhood. 2010;17:360–75.
27. Van Staa A, Jedeloo S, Latour JM, Trappenburg MJ. Exciting but exhausting: experiences with participatory research with chronically ill adolescents. Health Expect. 2010;13(1):95–107.

20

Frequency of CD19^{+}CD24^{hi}CD38^{hi} regulatory B cells is decreased in peripheral blood and synovial fluid of patients with juvenile idiopathic arthritis: a preliminary study

Qianzi Zhao and Lawrence K. Jung*

Abstract

Background: To understand the relationship between regulatory B cells (Bregs) and juvenile idiopathic arthritis (JIA), we analyzed the percentages of Bregs and their function in peripheral blood (PB) and synovial fluid (SF) of JIA patients.

Methods: Twenty-one JIA patients and 11 children with growing pain but without known rheumatic diseases as controls were included. The B cell phenotype and intracellular production of IL-10 of Bregs were assessed by flow cytometry. Mononuclear cells from PB and SF were stimulated to produce IL-10 in vitro for the identification of IL-10-producing regulatory B cells.

Results: The percentage of CD24^{hi}CD38^{hi} Bregs in the PB of JIA patients was significantly decreased compared to that in controls, and it was even lower in the SF of JIA patients compared to that in the PB. CD24^{hi}CD38^{hi} Bregs frequency was significantly lower in the PB of RF-positive patients than in RF-negative patients. Frequency of IL-10-producing regulatory B cells (B10 cells) was significantly lower in active JIA patients than that in inactive patients.

Conclusions: The inability of the host to produce enough regulatory B cells in PB and especially in SF of JIA patients may contribute to the disease, especially the local inflammation.

Keywords: B lymphocytes, Cytokines, Inflammation, Juvenile idiopathic arthritis, Synovial fluid

Background

Juvenile idiopathic arthritis (JIA) is the most common chronic rheumatic disease in children [1]. JIA is not one disease. Rather, International League of Associations for Rheumatology (ILAR) has classified it into 7 subtypes by the number of joints and the type of extra-articular involvement [2]. Children with JIA are at risk for joint damage, resulting in poor functional outcomes and decreased quality of life [3]. The pathogenesis of JIA is not known yet. Recent studies have suggested that B cells may have a role in these disorders. For example, B cell-related genes were up-regulated in JIA patients [4], and memory B cells were increased in oligoarticular and polyarticular JIA patients [5].

B cells are thought to play pathogenic role in the immune responses, due to their ability (a) to produce autoantibodies and (b) to act as antigen-presenting cells. However, evidences have accumulated showing that B cells can also down-regulate the immune response in both mouse and human [6–15]. Genetically B cell-deficient mice suffered more severe disease of experimental autoimmune encephalomyelitis [7]. When in vitro-activated B cells were transferred into mice in the collagen-induced arthritis mice model, they reduced the incidence and severity of disease [8, 13]. The term "regulatory B cells", shorted as Bregs, was used to define the B-cell subset with regulatory properties [9].

* Correspondence: Ljung@childrensnational.org
Division of Rheumatology, Children's National Medical Center, 111 Michigan Ave, NW, Washington, DC 20010, USA

There are several possible mechanisms by which B cells can regulate the immune responses [16–18]. Among these mechanisms, the ability to produce regulatory cytokine interleukin-10 (IL-10) is crucial in their regulatory function [8, 10, 12, 14, 16, 19–22]. Regulatory B cells that can produce IL-10 are termed as B10 cells. IL-10 is an anti-inflammatory cytokine that could regulate immune response by restoring Th1/Th2 balance and directly inhibit inflammatory cascade [23–25]. However, the ability of Bregs to suppress immune responses was not totally IL-10-dependent [10]. So B10 cells are a subgroup of regulatory B cells.

There is no unique surface marker to identify Bregs. $CD19^{+}CD24^{hi}CD38^{hi}$ [10, 14, 26, 27] and $CD19^{+}CD5^{+}CD1d^{hi}$ [28–31] have been used in different studies. It was reported that the majority of the $CD19^{+}CD5^{+}CD1d^{hi}$ B cells were contained within the $CD24^{hi}CD38^{hi}$ B cell subset [14]. Therefore, we utilized $CD19^{+}CD24^{hi}CD38^{hi}$ as a surface marker for Bregs in this study.

Deficiency of Bregs may lead to autoimmune diseases. Indeed, decreased Breg cells number or function have been identified in rheumatoid arthritis (RA) [32, 33], systemic lupus erythematosus (SLE) [10, 30], anti-neutrophil cytoplasmic antibodies (ANCA)-associated vasculitis [26, 34]. Transferred regulatory B cells could reduce disease activity in mouse arthritis model [8, 13]. Therefore, it is reasonable to hypothesize that Bregs may play a role in the pathogenesis of JIA. In this study, we test this hypothesis by analyzing the percentages of Bregs and their ability to produce IL-10 in peripheral bloods and synovial fluids of JIA patients.

Methods

Patients and controls

A total of 32 patients from the Division of Rheumatology of Children's National Medical Center were recruited in this study, including 21 JIA patients (13 poly-JIA, 5 oligo-JIA, 2 systemic, 1 psoriatic) and 11 children with growing pain but no known rheumatic diseases as controls. JIA patients were diagnosed according to the ILAR criteria [2]. Growing pain was diagnosed after known diseases were excluded with negative immunologic test findings. Peripheral blood (PB) samples were collected from the JIA patients and controls. One patient was followed longitudinally and PB samples were collected at both active and inactive phase. Synovial fluid (SF) samples were collected from 4 JIA patients who required intra-articular steroid injection as a part of treatment protocol. Of these subjects, both PB and SF samples were collected from 1 patient on the same day. Disease activity was assessed and inactive disease was defined according to Wallace's criteria [35]. Patients who didn't meet the definition for inactive disease were defined as having active disease. Demographic and clinical data of the patients were collected. The study was conducted in compliance with the Helsinki Declaration and ethical approval was obtained from the Institution Review Board of Children's National Medical Center (Pro00005055). All patients were enrolled after obtaining informed consent from parents and assent from patients older than 7 years old.

Human cell isolation and generation of B10 cells

Peripheral blood mononuclear cells (PBMCs) and synovial fluid mononuclear cells (SFMC) were isolated from heparin-treated PB and SF by Ficoll-Paque Plus (GE Healthcare, Uppsala, Sweden) gradient centrifugation. PBMCs and SFMCs were cultured in RPMI 1640 containing L-glutamine (Life Technologies, Paisley, UK) supplemented with 100 U/μg/ml penicillin/streptomycin (Life Technologies, Paisley, UK), and 10% fetal bovine serum in 48-well flat-bottom plates for 48 h at 37 °C in 5% CO_2. According to previous study [12], combination of CpG and CD40L stimulation could generate the most of B10 cells in human. Therefore, the cultured cells were stimulated with 10 μg/ml CpG ODN2006 (Invivogen, San Diego, USA) and 1 μg/ml CD40L (R&D Systems, Minneapolis, USA), or with phosphate-buffered saline (PBS) as control. For the last 6 h, 50 ng/ml phorbol myristate acetate (PMA) and 1 μg/ml ionomycin (Sigma-Aldrich, USA) were added to the stimulated cells; Brefeldin A (BFA, eBioscience, San Diego, USA), Golgi transport blocker, was added to all wells.

Surface markers and intracellular IL-10 detection

The following anti-human monoclonal antibodies (mAbs) were used for surface markers and intracellular IL-10 detection: fluorescein isothiocyanate (FITC)-conjugated anti-CD19; phycoerythrin (PE)-conjugated anti-CD24 (BD Biosciences, San Diego, USA); PE-Cyanine7-congugated anti-CD38; allophycocyanin (APC)-conjugated anti-IL-10 (Biolegend, San Diego, USA); and isotype-matched and fluorochrome-matched control antibodies. Cells were stained with combinations of CD19-FITC, CD24-PE and CD38-PE-Cy7 mAbs for surface phenotype. For intracellular IL-10 detection, cultured cells were washed, fixed, permeabilized, and stained with IL-10-APC mAb. APC-conjugated isotype control was used for gate setting for cytokine expression. Stained cells were analyzed on an eight-color FACSCanto II flow cytometer (BD Biosciences) using FACSDiva software (BD Biosciences).

Statistical analysis

Statistical analyses were performed using GraphPad Prism Version 6 (GraphPad Software, La Jolla, CA, USA). Chi-square tests were performed for discrete variables. Student *t* test was used for parametric test when comparing two groups with equal variances. Welch's *t* test was used for parametric test when comparing two groups with unequal variances. Mann-Whitney *U*-test was used for non-parametric test when comparing two groups. Spearman's correlation was performed to determine correlation. A p value of < 0.05 was considered statistically significant.

Results

Clinical characteristics of study subjects

The demographic and clinical features of 21 JIA patients and 11 controls are summarized in Table 1. There was no significant difference between the 2 groups with the exception that none of the control subjects were positive for rheumatoid factor. Table 2 shows the demographic and clinical features of 4 JIA patients from whom SF samples were collected.

CD24hiCD38hi B cell levels were reduced in PB of JIA patients and even lower in SF

Peripheral blood and synovial fluid mononuclear cells from subjects were phenotypically analyzed by flow cytometry for their expression of CD19, CD24, and CD38 surface markers. B cells were defined as $CD19^+$ lymphocytes. Within $CD19^+$ B cells gate, $CD24^{hi}CD38^{hi}$ cells were defined as $CD24^{hi}CD38^{hi}$ Bregs. The gate strategy for $CD19^+CD24^{hi}CD38^{hi}$ cells was illustrated by a representative staining of cells in a healthy control subject (Fig. 1a). The percentages of $CD24^{hi}CD38^{hi}$ Bregs subset were calculated as the ratios of gated targeted cells to total $CD19^+$ B cells. The results were expressed as mean values ± standard deviation (SD).

Table 1 Demographic and clinical features of JIA patients and controls

Characteristics	JIA patients	Controls
Number	21[a]	11
Gender, Female:Male (n:n)	12:9	6:5
Age (years)	10.9 ± 1.1	12.4 ± 1.1
Duration of disease (years)	3.7 ± 0.7	NA
Treatment when sampled; n	NSAID, MTX, anti-TNF;4 NSAID, Anti-TNF; 3 MTX, anti-TNF;1 Anti-TNF;4 NSAID; 7 None; 2[b]	None; 5 NSAID alone;6
RF Pos:Neg (n)	4:14[c]	0:11
PB White blood cell count ($\times 10^9$/L)	7.62 ± 0.66	6.19 ± 0.54
PB Lymphocyte count ($\times 10^9$/L)	3.06 ± 0.31	2.24 ± 0.12

[a]One patient was sampled at both active and inactive phase
[b]Patients were sampled when diagnosis was made and before treatment was given
[c]RF was not tested in 3 patients
JIA juvenile idiopathic arthritis, *MTX* methotrexate, *NA* not applicable, *Neg* negative, *NSAID* non-steroidal anti-inflammation drug, *Pos* positive, *RF* rheumatoid factor, *TNF* tumor necrosis factor, *PB* peripheral blood

As shown in Fig. 1b, we observed a significant decrease in the levels of $CD24^{hi}CD38^{hi}$ Bregs in the PB of JIA patients compared to those in controls (16.11 ± 1.09% vs. 23.83 ± 1.73%, $p < 0.001$). An even more significant decrease was seen in the SF of JIA patients compared to those in the PB (3.23 ± 1.92% vs. 16.11 ± 1.09%, $p < 0.0001$). The data of PB and SF samples from the same patient supported this result. The percentage of $CD24^{hi}CD38^{hi}$ Bregs in the SF was lower than that in the PB of the same patient collected on the same day (1.41% vs. 13.00%) (Fig. 1c). Of note, there was no significant difference of B cells percentages in PB between JIA patients and controls (15.22 ± 1.28% vs. 16.35 ± 1.22, $p = 0.5788$). However, B cells population in SF was significantly decreased compared with PB (1.47 ± 0.27% vs. 15.22 ± 1.28%, $p = 0.0001$). Probably due to this decrease, $CD24^{hi}CD38^{hi}$ Bregs subset was almost absent in SF mononuclear cells (SFMCs). In peripheral blood mononuclear cells (PBMCs) of JIA patients, the percentage of $CD24^{hi}CD38^{hi}$ Bregs was 2.41 ± 0.27%, while this percentage was 0.04 ± 0.02% in SFMCs, which was highly significant ($p = 0.0004$).

We next examined the frequencies of $CD24^{hi}CD38^{hi}$ Bregs in poly-JIA and non-poly-JIA patients. As in total JIA patients, the frequencies of $CD24^{hi}CD38^{hi}$ Bregs in poly-JIA and non-poly-JIA patients were significantly decreased compared with controls ($p < 0.01$ and $p < 0.05$, respectively) (Fig. 1b). No significant difference of frequency of $CD24^{hi}CD38^{hi}$ Bregs was observed between poly and non-poly JIA patients ($p = 0.6177$).

Next, we examined whether $CD24^{hi}CD38^{hi}$ Bregs level correlated with disease activity or treatment. Treatments for all patients are shown in Table 1. As shown in Fig. 2a, there was no significant difference in the $CD24^{hi}CD38^{hi}$ Bregs levels between active JIA and inactive JIA patients ($p = 0.6238$). In addition, no difference of $CD24^{hi}CD38^{hi}$ Bregs level was observed between patients with and without methotrexate(MTX) or TNF antagonist treatment ($p = 0.1358$, $p = 0.1469$, respectively) (Table 3).

$CD24^{hi}CD38^{hi}$ Breg cells levels were associated with RF in PB of JIA patients

We further examined the possible correlations between the frequencies of $CD24^{hi}CD38^{hi}$ Bregs and laboratory parameters. As shown in Fig. 2b, a significantly lower frequency of $CD24^{hi}CD38^{hi}$ Bregs was found in the PB of RF-positive patients than in RF-negative patients (10.81 ± 1.80% vs. 17.11 ± 1.14%, $p < 0.05$). However, no significant correlation was found between the frequencies of $CD24^{hi}CD38^{hi}$ Bregs and ESR (Spearman's $r = -0.5108$, $p = 0.0519$) (Fig. 2c).

Table 2 Demographic and clinical features of JIA patients from whom synovial fluid samples were collected

No.	Subtype	Gender	Age (years)	Duration of disease (years)	RF	Treatment when sampled
1	Oligoarticular	M	1.2	0.1	Neg	None[a]
2	Oligoarticular[b]	M	8	2.1	Neg	NSAID
3	Polyarticular	F	8	4	Neg	NSAID
4	Psoriatic	M	15	1	Neg	NSAID, MTX, anti-TNF

[a]This patient was sampled when diagnosis was made and before treatment was given
[b]Peripheral blood sample was collected from the patient the same day synovial fluid sample was collected
F female, *JIA* juvenile idiopathic arthritis, *M* male, *MTX* methotrexate, *NA* not applicable, *Neg* negative, *NSAID* non-steroidal anti-inflammation drug, *RF* rheumatoid factor, *TNF* tumor necrosis factor

IL-10-producing regulatory B cells (B10 cells) percentages in JIA patients was increased in the poly-JIA patients although had no difference in JIA patients as a group

As a subgroup of Bregs, B10 cells level was also examined in PB and SF of JIA patients and PB of controls. By ex vivo stimulation of CpG + CD40L for 48 h and PMA + ionomycin for the last 6 h, intracellular production of IL-10 by $CD19^+$ B cells was observed, while few B cells produced IL-10 when cultured with PBS only (Fig. 3a). A representative experiment showing intercellular IL-10 staining of B cells in a JIA patient is shown in Fig. 3a.

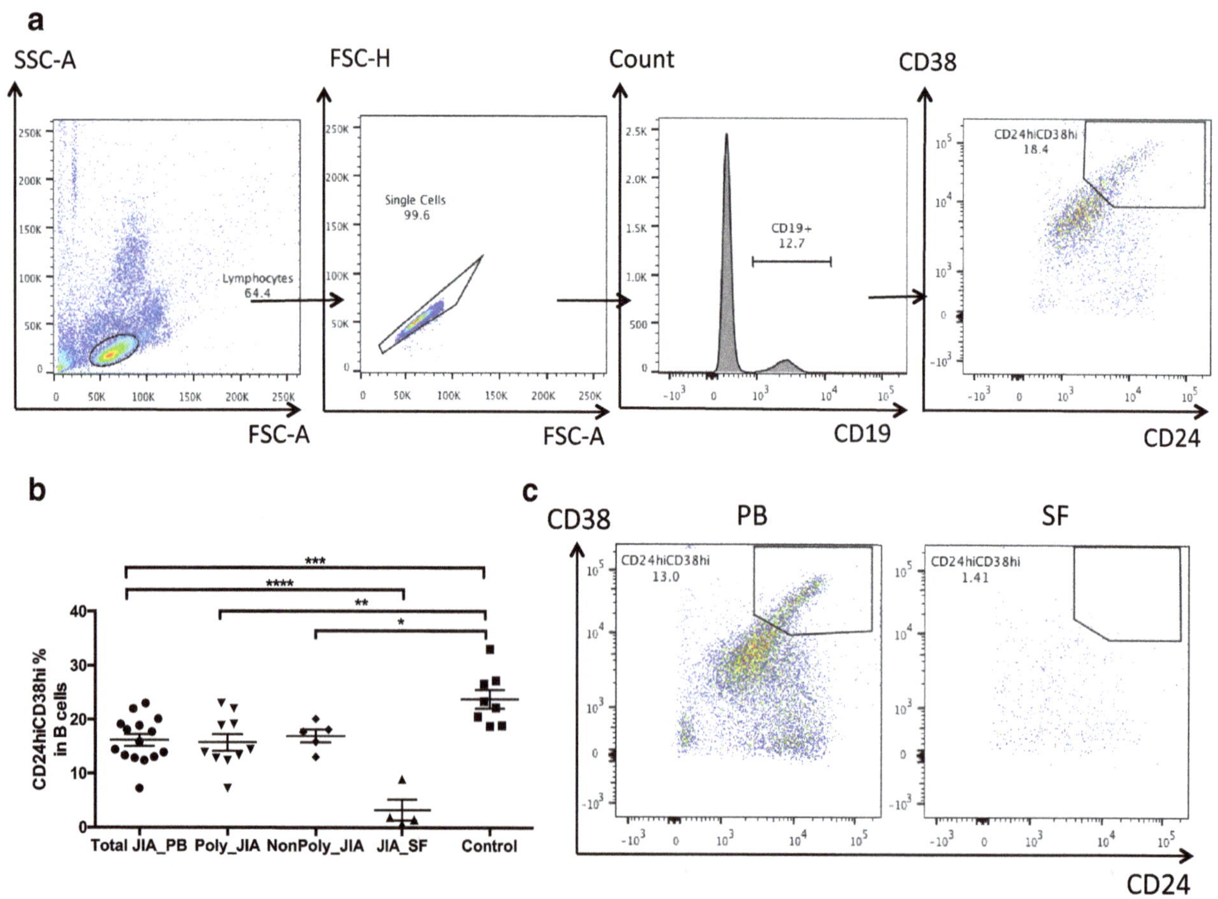

Fig. 1 Frequencies of $CD24^{hi}CD38^{hi}$ Bregs in juvenile idiopathic arthritis (JIA) patients and controls. **a** The gate strategy for $CD19^+CD24^{hi}CD38^{hi}$ cells in the peripheral blood (PB) of one control. B cells were defined as $CD19^+$ lymphocytes. Within $CD19^+$ B cells gate, $CD24^{hi}CD38^{hi}$ cells were defined as $CD24^{hi}CD38^{hi}$ Bregs. **b** $CD24^{hi}CD38^{hi}$ Bregs frequencies in total B cells were compared in PB of total, poly and non-poly JIA patients, synovial fluid (SF) of JIA patients, and PB of controls. The frequency of $CD24^{hi}CD38^{hi}$ Bregs in the PB of total JIA patients was significantly decreased compared to those in controls ($p = 0.0007$), and it was even much lower in the SF of JIA patients compared to that in the PB ($p < 0.0001$). **c** The percentage of $CD24^{hi}CD38^{hi}$ Bregs in the SF of one patient was lower than that in the PB of the same patient collected on the same day. *$p < 0.05$, **$p < 0.01$, ***$p < 0.001$, ****$p < 0.0001$

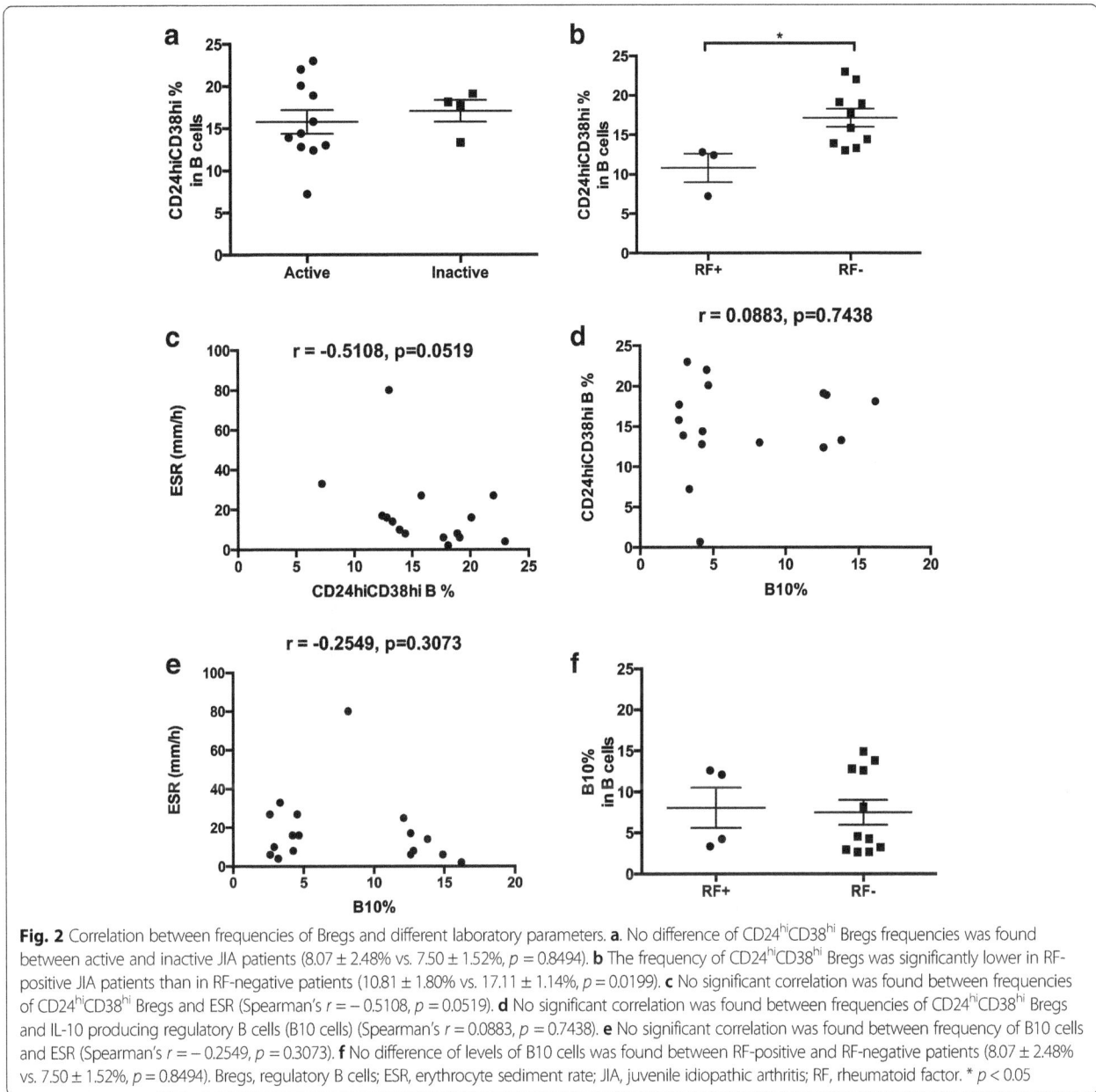

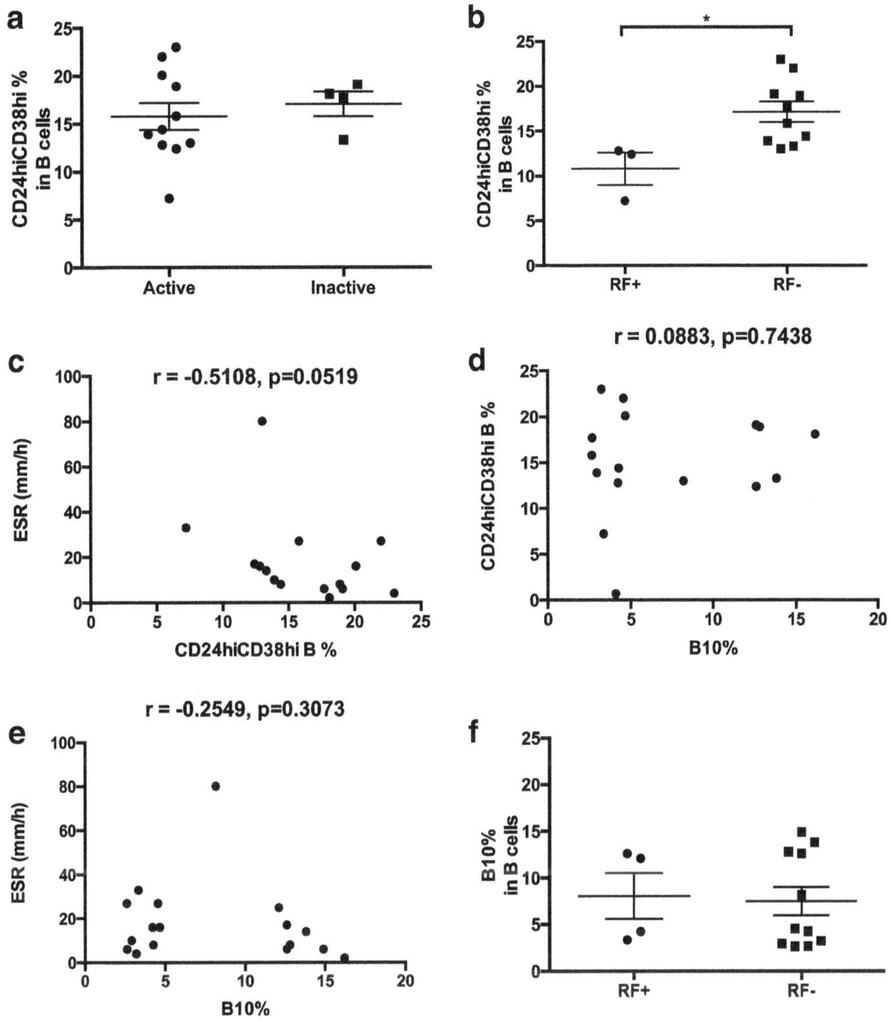

Fig. 2 Correlation between frequencies of Bregs and different laboratory parameters. **a**. No difference of $CD24^{hi}CD38^{hi}$ Bregs frequencies was found between active and inactive JIA patients (8.07 ± 2.48% vs. 7.50 ± 1.52%, $p = 0.8494$). **b** The frequency of $CD24^{hi}CD38^{hi}$ Bregs was significantly lower in RF-positive JIA patients than in RF-negative patients (10.81 ± 1.80% vs. 17.11 ± 1.14%, $p = 0.0199$). **c** No significant correlation was found between frequencies of $CD24^{hi}CD38^{hi}$ Bregs and ESR (Spearman's $r = -0.5108$, $p = 0.0519$). **d** No significant correlation was found between frequencies of $CD24^{hi}CD38^{hi}$ Bregs and IL-10 producing regulatory B cells (B10 cells) (Spearman's $r = 0.0883$, $p = 0.7438$). **e** No significant correlation was found between frequency of B10 cells and ESR (Spearman's $r = -0.2549$, $p = 0.3073$). **f** No difference of levels of B10 cells was found between RF-positive and RF-negative patients (8.07 ± 2.48% vs. 7.50 ± 1.52%, $p = 0.8494$). Bregs, regulatory B cells; ESR, erythrocyte sediment rate; JIA, juvenile idiopathic arthritis; RF, rheumatoid factor. * $p < 0.05$

Unlike the remarkable reduction of $CD24^{hi}CD38^{hi}$ Bregs levels in JIA patients, there was no significant difference of B10 cells levels between the PB of JIA patients and controls (7.43 ± 0.99% vs. 4.56 ± 0.71%, $p = 0.0527$) (Fig. 3b). In SF of JIA patients the B10 cells level was not significantly different from that in PB (4.32 ± 1.14% vs. 7.43 ± 0.99%, $p = 0.2419$) either. However, when we examined B10 cells frequency in the poly-JIA subgroup, we noticed a significant increase compared with controls ($p = 0.0249$) (Fig. 3b).

Table 3 Regulatory B cells percentages in different treatment subgroups

	No DMARD	DMARD	p value	No anti-TNF	Anti-TNF	p value
B cells (%)	14.96 ± 0.87 ($n = 14$)	16.19 ± 4.48 ($n = 6$)	0.7006	13.41 ± 1.07 ($n = 8$)	16.61 ± 2.20 ($n = 12$)	0.2757
$CD24^{hi}CD38^{hi}$ Bregs (% in B cells)	17.11 ± 1.12 ($n = 11$)	13.38 ± 2.43 ($n = 4$)	0.1358	18.08 ± 1.42 ($n = 6$)	14.80 ± 1.45 ($n = 9$)	0.1469
B10 cells (% in B cells)	7.25 ± 1.14 ($n = 14$)	7.73 ± 2.30 ($n = 5$)	0.8408	6.16 ± 1.48 ($n = 7$)	8.09 ± 1.34 ($n = 12$)	0.3683

Bregs regulatory B cells, *B10 cells* IL-10 producing regulatory B cells, *DMARD* disease-modifying antirheumatic drug, *JIA* juvenile idiopathic arthritis, *PB* peripheral blood, *SF* synovial fluid, *TNF* tumor necrosis factor

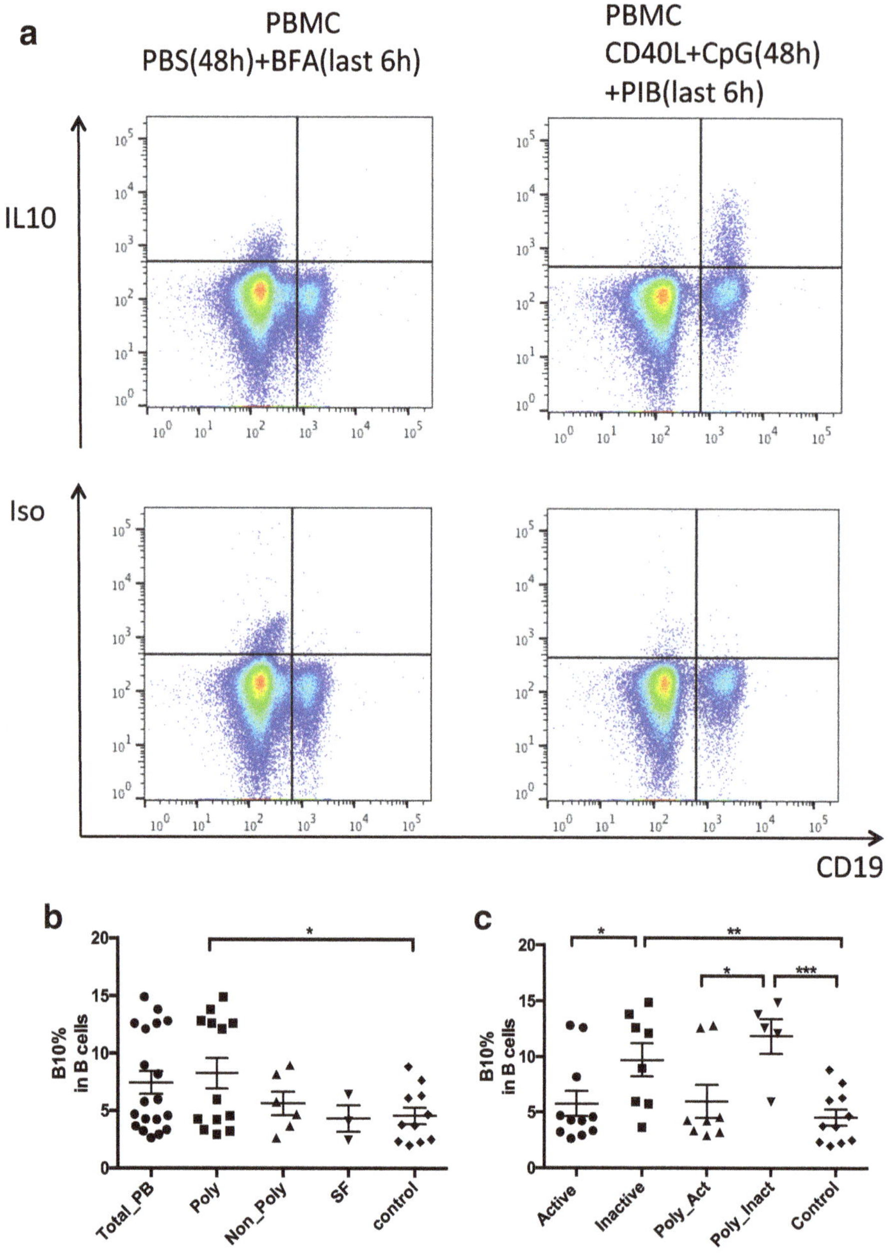

Fig. 3 Frequencies of IL-10 producing regulatory B (B10) cells in juvenile idiopathic arthritis (JIA) patients and controls. **a** Representative intracellular IL-10 staining in B cells in peripheral blood (PB) of one JIA patient with/without stimulation of CpG + CD40L for 48 h and phorbol 12-myristate 13-acetate+ionomycin+brefeldin A (PIB) for the last 6 h (right). Few B cells produced IL-10 when cultured with PBS only (left). Isotype controls were used to set up the negative population (lower). **b** Comparison of B10 cells frequencies in PB of different groups of JIA patients, synovial fluid (SF) of JIA patients, and PB of controls (left). **c** Comparison of B10 cells frequencies in active and inactive patients. BFA, brefeldin A; CD40L, CD40 ligand; Iso, isotype; PBMC, peripheral blood mononuclear cells; PBS, phosphate-buffered saline; PIB, phorbol 12-myristate 13-acetate +ionomycin+brefeldin A; poly-JIA, polyarticular juvenile idiopathic arthritis. *$p < 0.05$, **$p < 0.01$,***$p < 0.001$

B10 cells frequency in JIA patients was associated with disease activity

We then examined whether the frequencies of B10 cells correlate with disease activity. Significantly lower frequency of B10 cells was found in active JIA patients compared with that in inactive patients ($5.77 \pm 1.13\%$ vs. $9.72 \pm 1.49\%$, $p < 0.05$), while no significant difference was found between active patients and controls ($5.77 \pm 1.13\%$ vs. $4.56 \pm 0.71\%$, $P = 0.3762$) (Fig. 3c). One patient was followed longitudinally and the same trend was noted: the percentage of B10 cells increased from 2.93% when active and increased to 5.96% when inactive, supporting the association between B10 level and JIA disease activity.

Same trend was also found in poly-JIA patient. As shown in Fig. 3c, when we subdivided poly-JIA patients into active and inactive subgroups, we observed a significantly lower frequency of B10 cells in the active poly-JIA subgroup compared with inactive poly-JIA subgroup (6.00 ± 1.48 vs. 11.87 ± 1.56, $p = 0.0239$), while no significant difference was found between B10 cells frequencies in the active poly-JIA subgroup and controls ($p = 0.3531$).

When we compared the frequencies of B10 cells with different treatment groups, no significant difference was observed between groups with and without MTX or TNF antagonist ($p = 0.8408$, $p = 0.3683$, respectively) (Table 3).

There is no notable correlation between Bregs levels and B10 cells levels

Since B10 cells are a specific subgroup of Bregs, we examined whether there was a correlation between the level of $CD24^{hi}CD38^{hi}$ Bregs and the level of B10 cells in JIA patients. As shown in Fig. 2d, no notable correlation was observed ($p = 0.7438$). Also, there was no correlation between the level of B10 cells and ESR level ($p = 0.3073$) (Fig. 2e). No difference of levels of B10 cells was found between RF-positive and RF-negative patients ($8.07 \pm 2.48\%$ vs. $7.50 \pm 1.52\%$, $p = 0.8494$) (Fig. 2f).

Discussion

In this study, we found that $CD24^{hi}CD38^{hi}$ Bregs percentage was remarkably lower in the peripheral blood of JIA patients compared with control, and it was even much lower in the SF of JIA patients. This decrease was seen in both the poly-JIA and nonPoly-JIA groups. Also, reduced PB $CD24^{hi}CD38^{hi}$ Bregs levels were associated with patients with positive RF. In contrast, B10 cells, a special subgroup of regulatory B cells that could produce IL-10, were not reduced in PB and SF of JIA patients compared with controls, but it was associated with disease activity. The B10 cells level was significantly lower in active JIA patients than in inactive patients; this finding is also true in the poly-JIA subgroup.

Peripheral blood $CD24^{hi}CD38^{hi}$ Bregs deficiencies have been described in several autoimmune diseases, including RA [32, 33], SLE [10, 30] and ANCA-associated vasculitis [26, 34]. In this study, we have not only showed a decreased level of $CD24^{hi}CD38^{hi}$ Bregs in the PB of JIA patients, but also the deficiency of these cells in the synovial fluid of JIA patients. In SFMCs, $CD24^{hi}CD38^{hi}$ Bregs subset was almost absent and was as low as 1.6% of that in the PBMCs.

Taken together, those findings suggest that $CD24^{hi}CD38^{hi}$ Bregs may be critical in controlling inflammation in JIA and the inability of the host to produce enough of them in PB and especially in SF may contribute to the disease. Moreover, even if the patients had inactive disease, the $CD24^{hi}CD38^{hi}$ Bregs level was still significantly lower than control, and there was no significant difference between active and inactive patients, suggesting that the reduced $CD24^{hi}CD38^{hi}$ Bregs was inherent in the JIA patients.

In addition, we noticed that in the RF-positive patients, the $CD24^{hi}CD38^{hi}$ Bregs level was lower than that in RF-negative patients.This suggests that Bregs may play a role in regulating the production of autoantibody such as RF. This concept is supported by a murine model of transplantation tolerance, wherein the production of alloantibodies was significantly reduced by adoptive transfer of Bregs [36].

It is interesting that despite the decrease of $CD24^{hi}CD38^{hi}$ Bregs, B10 cells levels were not decreased in PB and SF of JIA patients compared with controls, and there was no notable correlation between $CD24^{hi}CD38^{hi}$ Bregs levels and B10 cells levels in JIA patients. This result might suggest that although $CD24^{hi}CD38^{hi}$ Bregs were numerically deficient in JIA patients, their inherent ability to produce IL-10 was not compromised. This lack of correlation between phenotypically defined Breg cell subset and B10 cells has already been reported in adults [33, 34, 37]. The reason might be that B10 cells are not restricted to the $CD24^{hi}CD38^{hi}$ B cell subset, and other B cells subsets might contain more of them [33].

Interestingly, we observed an association of disease activity with B10 cells in JIA patients, although we didn't observe a difference between the levels of B10 cells in PB of total JIA patients and controls. The B10 cells frequency was significantly lower in all active patients than in inactive patients. This was also true in poly-JIA subgroup of patients. The increase in the B10 cells in inactive patients may be indicative of a successful pathophysiological response to the inflammation. Kalampokis et al. [38] have recently reported the number of B10 cells in JIA patients and in health children. Similar to our result, they didn't find a significant difference of B10 levels between JIA group and controls. However, they didn't observe a significant difference of total IL-10-producing B cells levels between active and inactive patients. This discrepancy may be due to different definition for "inactive disease". In our study, we used the more strict criteria to define inactive disease as an active joint count of 0, absence of uveitis and a PGA < 10 mm with normal ESR [35], while Kalampokis et al.. used only one criterion of PGA < 10 mm. Our result suggests that the status of disease activity is a very important consideration when one studies the B10 cells in JIA.

Our study showed that patients with active JIA had less B10 cells frequency compared with patients with inactive disease. This is consistent with the results in patients with RA [14, 33]. We didn't find a correlation between $CD24^{hi}CD38^{hi}$ Bregs or B10 cells levels and MTX or TNF treatment in JIA patients. This is consistent with the result of Kalampokis et al... This result suggests that MTX or TNF treatment might not help to correct the altered immunological balance in JIA patients. Glaesener et al showed that the $CD24^{hi}CD38^{hi}$ transitional B cells was significantly decreased in patients receiving MTX compared with untreated patients [39]. In our study, we didn't see a significant difference of $CD24^{hi}CD38^{hi}$ B cells percentages between patients with and without MTX treatment. The difference in our conclusion may be rooted in the fact that their study-subject composition was different from ours. In Glaesener et al's study, the dominant group of patients was oligo-JIA patients (68%). In our study, poly-JIA patients were the dominant group (62%). Our poly-JIA patients required both MTX and anti-TNF treatment while none receiving only MTX; whereas in their study, the group receiving just MTX were predominantly oligo-JIA subjects (71%). Due to our small sample size, we could not perform detailed analysis of effect of MTX alone.

Conclusions

- Regulatory B cells a relatively new area of research compared with regulatory T cells. In recent years, emerging data support their importance in diverse normal and pathologic processes.
- Our study showed for the first time that $CD24^{hi}CD38^{hi}$ Bregs percentage was remarkably lower in the peripheral blood of JIA patients compared with healthy control, and it was even lower in the synovial fluid of JIA patients.
- Also, the regulatory B10 cells level was inversely correlated with disease activity.
- Our study suggests that the inability of the host to produce enough regulatory B cells in PB and especially in SF of JIA patients may contribute to the local inflammation.
- These findings provide new insights in the pathogenesis of autoimmune diseases and may suggest a novel approach to control the disease processes.
- One caveat about our finding is that the numbers of SF samples and subgroup subjects were small in this preliminary study. Further studies with a larger sample size and more longitudinal follow up will be needed to confirm the findings reported here.

Abbreviations

ANCA: Anti-neutrophil cytoplasmic antibodies; ANOVA: One-way analysis of variance; APC: Allophycocyanin; B10 cells: IL-10-producing regulatory B cells; BFA: Brefeldin A; Bregs: Regulatory B cells; ESR: Erythrocyte sediment rate; FITC: Fluorescein isothiocyanate; IL-10: Interleukin-10; ILAR: International League of Associations for Rheumatology; JIA: Juvenile idiopathic arthritis; mAbs: Monoclonal antibodies; MTX: Methotrexate; PBMCs: Peripheral blood mononuclear cells; PBS: Phosphate-buffered saline; PE: Phycoerythrin; PGA: Physician Global Assessment; PMA: Phorbol myristate acetate; Poly-JIA: Polyarticular juvenile idiopathic arthritis; RA: Rheumatoid arthritis; RF: Rheumatoid factor; SF: Synovial fluid; SLE: Systemic lupus erythematosus; TNF-α: Tumor Necrosis Factor-α

Acknowledgements

The authors appreciate the help of Drs. T. Ronis and H. Srinivasalu in recruiting subjects and patients to this study. We want to express our gratitude to Dr. Yang Liu for his support and advice. Finally, we want to thank the patients and their parents/guardians for their willingness to participate in this study.

Funding

This work was supported by a Pilot research grant from the Center for Cancer and Immunology at Children's Research Institute.

Authors' contributions

QZ collected samples and data, performed cell culture and flow cytometry examination, performed statistical analysis, analyzed and interpreted the data, and wrote the manuscript. LJ the corresponding author, did conception and designed the study, recruited subjects, analyzed and interpreted the data, and revised the manuscript. Both authors read and approved the final manuscript.

Competing interests

The authors declare that they have no competing interests.

References

1. Peterson LS, Mason T, Nelson AM, O'Fallon WM, Gabriel SE. Juvenile rheumatoid arthritis in Rochester, Minnesota 1960-1993. Is the epidemiology changing? Arthritis Rheum. 1996;39:1385–90.
2. Petty RE, Southwood TR, Manners P, Baum J, Glass DN, Goldenberg J, et al. International league of associations for rheumatology classification of juvenile idiopathic arthritis: second revision, Edmonton, 2001. J Rheumatol. 2004;31:390–2.
3. Ringold S, Seidel KD, Koepsell TD, Wallace CA. Inactive disease in polyarticular juvenile idiopathic arthritis: current patterns and associations. Rheumatology (Oxford). 2009;48:972–7.
4. Barnes MG, Grom AA, Thompson SD, Griffin TA, Luyrink LK, Colbert RA, et al. Biologic similarities based on age at onset in oligoarticular and polyarticular subtypes of juvenile idiopathic arthritis. Arthritis Rheum. 2010;62:3249–58.
5. Marasco E, Aquilani A, Cascioli S, Moneta GM, Caiello I, Farroni C, et al. Switched memory B cells are increased in Oligoarticular and Polyarticular juvenile idiopathic arthritis and their change over time is related to response to tumor necrosis factor inhibitors. Arthritis Rheumatol. 2018;70:606–15.
6. Katz SI, Parker D, Turk JL. B-cell suppression of delayed hypersensitivity reactions. Nature. 1974;251:550–1.
7. Wolf SD, Dittel BN, Hardardottir F, Janeway CA Jr. Experimental autoimmune encephalomyelitis induction in genetically B cell-deficient mice. J Exp Med. 1996;184:2271–8.
8. Mauri C, Gray D, Mushtaq N, Londei M. Prevention of arthritis by interleukin 10-producing B cells. J Exp Med. 2003;197:489–501.
9. Mizoguchi A, Bhan AK. A case for regulatory B cells. J Immunol. 2006;176: 705–10.
10. Blair PA, Norena LY, Flores-Borja F, Rawlings DJ, Isenberg DA, Ehrenstein MR, et al. CD19(+)CD24(hi)CD38(hi) B cells exhibit regulatory capacity in healthy individuals but are functionally impaired in systemic lupus erythematosus patients. Immunity. 2010;32:129–40.
11. DiLillo DJ, Matsushita T, Tedder TF. B10 cells and regulatory B cells balance immune responses during inflammation, autoimmunity. and cancer Ann N Y Acad Sci. 2010;1183:38–57.
12. Iwata Y, Matsushita T, Horikawa M, Dilillo DJ, Yanaba K, Venturi GM, et al. Characterization of a rare IL-10-competent B-cell subset in humans that parallels mouse regulatory B10 cells. Blood. 2011;117:530–41.
13. Yang M, Deng J, Liu Y, Ko KH, Wang X, Jiao Z, et al. IL-10-producing regulatory B10 cells ameliorate collagen-induced arthritis via suppressing Th17 cell generation. Am J Pathol. 2012;180:2375–85.
14. Flores-Borja F, Bosma A, Ng D, Reddy V, Ehrenstein MR, Isenberg DA, et al. CD19+CD24hiCD38hi B cells maintain regulatory T cells while limiting TH1 and TH17 differentiation. Sci Transl Med. 2013;5:173ra23.
15. Menon M, Blair PA, Isenberg DA, Mauri C. A Regulatory feedback between

Plasmacytoid dendritic cells and regulatory B cells is aberrant in systemic lupus erythematosus. Immunity. 2016;44:683–97.
16. Mizoguchi E, Mizoguchi A, Preffer FI, Bhan AK. Regulatory role of mature B cells in a murine model of inflammatory bowel disease. Int Immunol. 2000;12:597–605.
17. Knoechel B, Lohr J, Kahn E, Abbas AK. The link between lymphocyte deficiency and autoimmunity: roles of endogenous T and B lymphocytes in tolerance. J Immunol. 2005;175:21–6.
18. Wei B, Velazquez P, Turovskaya O, Spricher K, Aranda R, Kronenberg M, et al. Mesenteric B cells centrally inhibit CD4+ T cell colitis through interaction with regulatory T cell subsets. Proc Natl Acad Sci U S A. 2005;102:2010–5.
19. Brummel R, Lenert P. Activation of marginal zone B cells from lupus mice with type a(D) CpG-oligodeoxynucleotides. J Immunol. 2005;174:2429–34.
20. Lenert P, Brummel R, Field EH, Ashman RF. TLR-9 activation of marginal zone B cells in lupus mice regulates immunity through increased IL-10 production. J Clin Immunol. 2005;25:29–40.
21. Fillatreau S, Sweenie CH, McGeachy MJ, Gray D. Anderton SM. B cells regulate autoimmunity by provision of IL-10. Nat Immunol. 2002;3:944–50.
22. Bouaziz JD, Calbo S, Maho-Vaillant M, Saussine A, Bagot M, Bensussan A, et al. IL-10 produced by activated human B cells regulates CD4(+) T-cell activation in vitro. Eur J Immunol. 2010;40:2686–91.
23. Fiorentino DF, Zlotnik A, Mosmann TR, Howard M, O'Garra A. IL-10 inhibits cytokine production by activated macrophages. J Immunol. 1991;147:3815–22.
24. O'Farrell AM, Liu Y, Moore KW, Mui AL. IL-10 inhibits macrophage activation and proliferation by distinct signaling mechanisms: evidence for Stat3-dependent and -independent pathways. EMBO J. 1998;17:1006–18.
25. Grunig G, Corry DB, Leach MW, Seymour BW, Kurup VP, Rennick DM. Interleukin-10 is a natural suppressor of cytokine production and inflammation in a murine model of allergic bronchopulmonary aspergillosis. J Exp Med. 1997;185:1089–99.
26. Aybar LT, McGregor JG, Hogan SL, Hu Y, Mendoza CE, Brant EJ, et al. Reduced CD5(+) CD24(hi) CD38(hi) and interleukin-10(+) regulatory B cells in active anti-neutrophil cytoplasmic autoantibody-associated vasculitis permit increased circulating autoantibodies. Clin Exp Immunol. 2015;180:178–88.
27. Simon Q, Pers JO, Cornec D, Le Pottier L, Mageed RA, Hillion S. In-depth characterization of CD24(high)CD38(high) transitional human B cells reveals different regulatory profiles. J Allergy Clin Immunol. 2016;137:1577–84. e10
28. Yanaba K, Bouaziz JD, Haas KM, Poe JC, Fujimoto M. Tedder TF. A regulatory B cell subset with a unique CD1dhiCD5+ phenotype controls T cell-dependent inflammatory responses. Immunity. 2008;28:639–50.
29. Matsushita T, Yanaba K, Bouaziz JD, Fujimoto M, Tedder TF. Regulatory B cells inhibit EAE initiation in mice while other B cells promote disease progression. J Clin Invest. 2008;118:3420–30.
30. Wang L, Zhao P, Ma L, Shan Y, Jiang Z, Wang J, et al. Increased interleukin 21 and follicular helper T-like cells and reduced interleukin 10+ B cells in patients with new-onset systemic lupus erythematosus. J Rheumatol. 2014;41:1781–92.
31. Ma L, Liu B, Jiang Z, Jiang Y. Reduced numbers of regulatory B cells are negatively correlated with disease activity in patients with new-onset rheumatoid arthritis. Clin Rheumatol. 2014;33:187–95.
32. Cui D, Zhang L, Chen J, Zhu M, Hou L, Chen B, et al. Changes in regulatory B cells and their relationship with rheumatoid arthritis disease activity. Clin Exp Med. 2015;15:285–92.
33. Daien CI, Gailhac S, Mura T, Audo R, Combe B, Hahne M, et al. Regulatory B10 cells are decreased in patients with rheumatoid arthritis and are inversely correlated with disease activity. Arthritis Rheumatol. 2014;66:2037–46.
34. Todd SK, Pepper RJ, Draibe J, Tanna A, Pusey CD, Mauri C, et al. Regulatory B cells are numerically but not functionally deficient in anti-neutrophil cytoplasm antibody-associated vasculitis. Rheumatology (Oxford). 2014;53:1693–703.
35. Wallace CA, Ruperto N, Giannini E. Preliminary criteria for clinical remission for select categories of juvenile idiopathic arthritis. J Rheumatol. 2004;31:2290–4.
36. Moreau A, Blair PA, Chai JG, Ratnasothy K, Stolarczyk E, Alhabbab R, et al. Transitional-2 B cells acquire regulatory function during tolerance induction and contribute to allograft survival. Eur J Immunol. 2015;45:843–53.
37. Lepse N, Abdulahad WH, Rutgers A, Kallenberg CG, Stegeman CA, Heeringa P. Altered B cell balance, but unaffected B cell capacity to limit monocyte activation in anti-neutrophil cytoplasmic antibody-associated vasculitis in remission. Rheumatology (Oxford). 2014;53:1683–92.
38. Kalampokis I, Venturi GM, Poe JC, Dvergsten JA, Sleasman JW, Tedder TF. The regulatory B cell compartment expands transiently during childhood and is contracted in children with autoimmunity. Arthritis Rheumatol. 2017;69:225–38.
39. Glaesener S, Quach TD, Onken N, Weller-Heinemann F, Dressler F, Huppertz HI, et al. Distinct effects of methotrexate and etanercept on the B cell compartment in patients with juvenile idiopathic arthritis. Arthritis Rheumatol. 2014;66:2590–600.

Inpatient burden of juvenile dermatomyositis among children in the United States

Michael C. Kwa[1], Jonathan I. Silverberg[2] and Kaveh Ardalan[3*]

Abstract

Background: Juvenile dermatomyositis (JDM) is a rare autoimmune disease that causes significant morbidity and quality of life impairment. Little is known about the inpatient burden of JDM in the US. Our goal was to determine the prevalence and risk factors for hospitalization with juvenile dermatomyositis and assess inpatient burden of JDM.

Methods: Data on 14,401,668 pediatric hospitalizations from the 2002–2012 Nationwide Inpatient Sample (NIS) was analyzed. ICD-9-CM coding was used to identify hospitalizations with a diagnosis of JDM.

Results: There were 909 and 495 weighted admissions with a primary or secondary diagnosis of JDM, respectively. In multivariable logistic regression models with stepwise selection, female sex (logistic regression; adjusted odds ratio [95% confidence interval]) (2.22 [2.05–2.42]), non-winter season (fall: 1.18[1.06–1.33]; spring (1.13 [1.01–1.27]; summer (1.53 [1.37–1.71]), non-Medicaid administered government insurance coverage (2.59 [2.26–2.97]), and multiple chronic conditions (2–5: 1.41[1.30–1.54]; 6+: 1.24[1.00–1.52]) were all associated with higher rates of hospitalization for JDM. The weighted total length of stay (LOS) and inflation-adjusted cost of care for patients with a primary inpatient diagnosis of JDM was 19,159 days and $49,339,995 with geometric means [95% CI] of 2.50 [2.27–2.76] days and $7350 [$6228–$8674], respectively. Costs of hospitalization in primary JDM and length of stay and cost in secondary JDM were significantly higher compared to those without JDM. Notably, race/ethnicity was associated with increased LOS (log-linear regression; adjusted beta [95% confidence interval]) (Hispanic: 0.28 [0.14–0.41]; other non-white: 0.59 [0.31–0.86]) and cost of care (Hispanic: 0.30 [0.05–0.55]).

Conclusion: JDM contributes to both increased length of hospitalization and inpatient cost of care. Non-Medicaid government insurance was associated with higher rates of hospitalization for JDM while Hispanic and other non-white racial/ethnic groups demonstrated increased LOS and cost of care.

Keywords: Juvenile dermatomyositis, Epidemiology, Cost of care

Background

Juvenile dermatomyositis (JDM) is a rare autoimmune disease characterized by proximal muscle weakness concurrent with specific cutaneous manifestations. [1] In the United States, JDM has an estimated incidence of 2–4 per million children per year. [2] While improved management of the disease has led to reduced mortality in recent years, up to 40% JDM patients continue to have active disease despite treatment. [3, 4] Ongoing disease activity, cumulative damage, and aggressive immunosuppressive treatments remain a concern for long term outcomes and quality of life. [4] Previous studies have compared cost of specific JDM treatment regimens [5], evaluated the inpatient burden of adult dermatomyositis [6], and examined economic burden of other childhood inflammatory conditions such as JIA [7]. However, little is known about the inpatient burden of JDM in the United States. As a result, use of a

* Correspondence: kaveh.ardalan@northwestern.edu
[3]Division of Rheumatology, Departments of Pediatrics and Medical Social Sciences, Ann & Robert H. Lurie Children's Hospital of Chicago/Northwestern University Feinberg School of Medicine, 225 E Chicago Ave Box 50, Chicago, IL 60611, USA
Full list of author information is available at the end of the article

comprehensive, national inpatient database could help to elucidate the economic burden posed by JDM.

Previous studies found racial/ethnic and socioeconomic differences in hospitalization rates and outcomes for stroke [8], cardiovascular disease [9], asthma [10], acute respiratory illness [11], pemphigus [12], and adult dermatomyositis [6]. We hypothesized that JDM is also associated with similar racial/ethnic and socioeconomic differences, possibly related to lack of insurance coverage and reduced access to specialty care, such as rheumatology and dermatology. In the present study, we analyzed the prevalence and predictors of hospitalization, cost of care and length of stay in US patients with JDM.

Methods

Data source

The 2002–2012 Nationwide Inpatient Sample (NIS) provided by the Healthcare Cost and Utilization Project (HCUP) from the Agency for Healthcare Research and Quality (AHRQ) was analyzed. Each year of NIS contains an approximately 20% stratified representative sample of all inpatient hospitalizations in the United States. Sample weights were created by NIS that factored the sampling design of hospitals in the US. These sample weights are needed to provide representative estimates of hospital discharges across the whole country. All data were de-identified and no attempts were made to identify any of the individuals in the database. All parties with access to the HCUP were compliant to HCUP's formal data use agreement. This study was deemed exempt by the institutional review board at Northwestern University.

Identification of JDM

The databases were searched for a primary and/or secondary diagnosis of JDM using the International Classification of Diseases, Ninth Revision, Clinical Modification (*ICD-9-CM)* code 710.3. The primary diagnosis was defined in NIS as the condition chiefly responsible for admission to the hospital for care. A previous study validated the use of the discharge diagnosis code 710.3 in the inpatient setting for the study of dermatomyositis. [13] Patients with *ICD-9-CM* diagnostic codes of 701.0/ 710.1 (scleroderma), 710.0 (systemic lupus erythematosus), 710.4 (polymyositis), 710.8 (mixed connective tissue disease), and 710.9 (undifferentiated connective tissue disease) were excluded to minimize misclassification. The control group included all hospitalizations without any diagnosis of JDM, yielding a representative cohort of US pediatric hospitalizations.

Data processing and statistics

All data analyses and statistical processes were performed using SAS version 9.4 (SAS Institute, Cary, NC). Analyses of survey responses were performed using SURVEY procedures. Weighted prevalence (95% confidence intervals [CI]) of hospitalization either with a primary or secondary *ICD-9-CM* code of JDM were determined. The hospital cost for inpatient care was calculated based on the total charge of the hospitalization and the cost-to-charge ratio estimated by HCUP. All costs were adjusted for inflation to the year 2014 according to the Consumer Price Index from the United States Bureau of Labor Statistics. [14] Summary statistics were generated for length of stay (LOS), inflation-adjusted cost-of-care, including sum, mean and 95% confidence interval (CI) for hospitalizations with a primary, secondary or no diagnosis of JDM.

Three different regression models were constructed. [1] Survey logistic regression models were used to determine the predictors of hospitalization for JDM. The dependent variable was hospitalization with a primary diagnosis of JDM vs. no JDM. Linear regression models with log-transformed [2] cost of care or [3] length of stay (LOS) as the dependent variables were used to determine the predictors of cost of hospitalization and length of stay LOS. Cost of care and LOS were log-transformed because they were not normally distributed. The independent variable was a primary diagnosis of JDM vs. no JDM. Other independent variables included age (0–5, 6–11, 11–17), season of admission (fall, winter, spring, summer), sex (male, female), race/ethnicity (White, Black, Hispanic, Other[Asian, Native American, and other racial/ethnic groups]), health insurance coverage (Medicaid, private, self-pay, no charge/charity, non-Medicaid government administered insurance programs [e.g. KidCare, Children's Health Insurance Program (CHIP), other federal/state/local government]) number of comorbid chronic conditions (0–1, 2–5, ≥6), hospital location (metropolitan [≥1 urban cluster of population ≥ 50,000] >1million, fringe/metro < 1 million, micropolitan [≥1 urban cluster of population 10,000-49,999], not metropolitan or micropolitan), hospital region (Northeast, Midwest, South and West), and an indicator for calendar year (2002–2003, 2004–2005, 2006–2007, 2008–2009, 2010–2011, 2012). Chronic conditions were defined by HCUP as lasting ≥12 months and meeting one or both of the following: (a) places limitations on self-care, independent living, and social interactions (b) results in the need for ongoing intervention with medical products, services, and special equipment. [15] Chronic condition count was calculated and provided by HCUP. Crude odds ratios (OR), beta-coefficients and 95% CI were estimated. Multivariate regression models were constructed using stepwise selection (alpha = 0.1) from the abovementioned covariates. Adjusted OR, beta coefficients and 95% CI were estimated. All statistical models included discharge trend weights, sample strata that account for hospital's census region or division, ownership/control, location/teaching and bedsize that were provided by NIS and clustering by individual hospital. Complete case-analysis was performed. A two-sided *P*-value < 0.05 was considered statistically significant.

Results

Juvenile dermatomyositis patient and hospital characteristics

Overall, there were 14,401,668 pediatric discharges captured in the NIS between the years 2002–2012. 4,879,511 pediatric discharges remained after exclusion of live births and other connective tissue diseases. There were 909 and 495 admissions with a primary or secondary diagnosis of JDM (weighted frequencies of 4317 and 2321, respectively). The weighted prevalences of primary and secondary hospitalization for JDM ranged from 144.0–228.8 and 71.9–133.8 per million patients per year (Fig. 1). Hospitalization rates for patients with a primary or secondary diagnosis of JDM did not significantly increase after 2003 compared with years 2002–2003 (generalized linear models, $P < 0.05$; Fig. 1).

Pediatric patients with a primary or secondary diagnosis of JDM were significantly older than those without such a diagnosis (mean [standard deviation] age, 8.77 [0.25] and 10.23 [0.30] vs. 6.19[0.05] years). Hospitalizations with a primary diagnosis of JDM were associated with older patient age compared to hospitalizations without a primary diagnosis of JDM (survey logistic regression; OR [95% CI]) (6–11: 5.79 [4.23–7.93]; 11–17: 2.57 [1.87–3.51]) (Table 1). Patients who were admitted for a primary diagnosis of JDM were more likely to be female (2.17 [1.74–2.71]), receive financial coverage from non-Medicaid government administered insurance programs (2.59 [2.26–2.97]) compared to private insurance, and have multiple chronic conditions (2–5: 1.89 [1.45–2.45]), but were less likely to have Medicaid (0.66 [0.54–0.81]) compared to private insurance. Primary admissions for JDM were less likely to occur in hospitals in nonmetropolitan areas (fringe area or metropolitan area with < 1 million people: 0.65 [0.43–0.99]; micropolitan: 0.30 [0.15–0.57]; not metropolitan or micropolitan: 0.24 [0.13–0.45]) and more likely to occur during the summer (1.44 [1.15–1.80]).

In multivariate logistic regression models with stepwise selection, non-white race, Medicaid insurance, self-pay, non-metropolitan area, and Midwest and South regions were all associated with lower rates of admission for JDM patients compared to those without a primary diagnosis of JDM, whereas older age, female sex, non-Medicaid government administered insurance coverage, multiple chronic conditions, non-winter seasons and West region were all associated with higher rates of admission for JDM compared to those without a primary diagnosis of JDM (Table 1).

Reasons for secondary admission

The top 3 primary admission diagnoses for patients with a secondary diagnosis of JDM were: cellulitis of leg (rank, prevalence [95% CI]) (#1, 4.38% [3.46–5.30]), cellulitis of arm (#2, 4.22% [3.31–5.12]), and pneumonia (#3, 3.66% [2.81–4.51]). Meanwhile, the top 3 primary admission diagnoses for inpatients without a diagnosis of JDM were: pneumonia (#1, 5.24% [5.23–5.25]), acute bronchiolitis due to RSV (#2, 3.34% [3.33–3.35], and asthma with exacerbation (#3, 3.04% [3.03–3.05]) (Table 2).

The frequency of diagnosis codes for the most common symptoms in JDM as documented in other studies [16, 17] was also analyzed (Table 3). Compared to non-JDM patients, ten of the most common symptoms (rash, muscle weakness, muscle pain, fever, dysphagia,

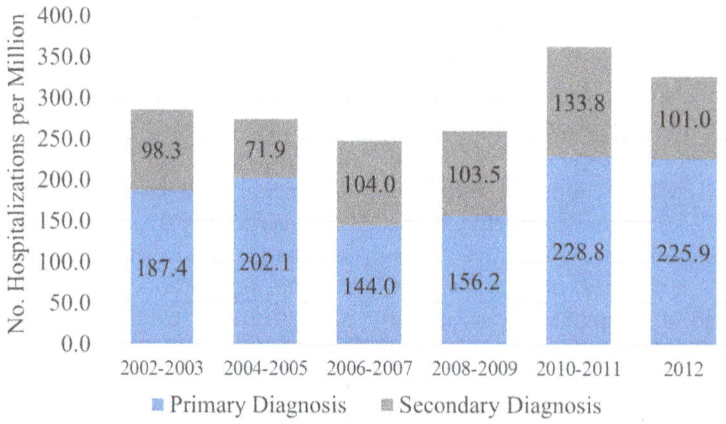

Fig. 1 Annual prevalence of hospitalizations for patients with primary/secondary diagnoses of juvenile dermatomyositis (JDM). Survey weighted logistic regression was performed to compare the prevalence of hospitalization for JDM over time. Hospitalization rates for patients with a primary or secondary diagnosis of JDM did not significantly increase after 2003 compared with years 2002–2003 (generalized linear models, $P < 0.05$)

Table 1 Associations of hospitalization for JDM in US children

Variable	Primary diagnosis of JDM							
	No		Yes					
	Freq	Row Percent [95% CI]	Freq	Percent [95% CI]	Crude OR [95% CI]	*P*	Adjusted OR [95% CI]	*P*
Age								
0–5	12,470,783	55.00 [54.35–55.64]	1077	25.18 [19.85–30.52]	Reference	–	Reference	–
6–11	3,371,272	14.87 [14.65–15.09]	1686	39.42 [33.59–45.25]	5.79 [4.23–7.93]	<.0001	4.62 [4.18–5.10]	<.0001
11–17	6,832,983	30.13 [29.47–30.80]	1514	35.39 [29.87–40.91]	2.565 [1.872–3.514]	<.0001	1.86 [1.67–2.06]	<.0001
Season								
Fall	5,305,485	25.01 [24.89–25.14]	958	25.29 [21.95–28.64]	1.21 [0.97–1.52]	0.0980	1.18 [1.06–1.33]	0.004
Winter	6,135,926	28.93 [28.69–29.17]	916	24.18 [20.81–27.54]	Reference	–	Reference	–
Spring	5,007,154	23.61 [23.51–23.71]	892	23.53 [20.49–26.57]	1.19 [0.97–1.46]	0.0931	1.13 [1.01–1.27]	0.0349
Summer	4,761,755	22.45 [22.29–22.61]	1023	27.00 [23.73–30.27]	1.44 [1.15–1.80]	0.0015	1.53 [1.37–1.71]	<.0001
Gender								
Female	10,343,988	54.16 [54.03–54.30]	2753	64.74 [59.70–69.70]	2.170 [1.739–2.708]	<.0001	2.22 [2.05–2.42]	<.0001
Male	12,222,939	45.84 [45.70–45.97]	1499	35.26 [30.21–40.30]	Reference	–	Reference	–
Race								
White	9,127,707	51.60 [49.63–53.57]	1712	51.83 [43.21–60.45]	Reference	–	Reference	–
Black	2,970,647	16.79 [15.48–18.11]	529	16.02 [11.32–20.71]	0.949 [0.650–1.388]	0.7889	0.83 [0.73–0.94]	0.0026
Hispanic	3,975,465	24.47 [20.45–24.50]	811	24.56 [17.39–31.72]	1.088 [0.731–1.619]	0.6781	1.01 [0.91–1.13]	0.8044
Other	1,615,416	9.13 [8.24–10.03]	251	7.60 [3.71–11.48]	0.828 [0.462–1.485]	0.5271	0.60 [0.51–0.71]	<.0001
Insurance								
Medicaid	10,669,493	46.42 [45.17–47.66]	1530	35.47 [30.99–39.95]	0.658 [0.538–0.805]	<.0001	0.71 [0.65–0.78]	<.0001
Private insurance	10,435,364	45.40 [44.06–46.74]	2273	52.71 [47.02–58.40]	Reference	–	Reference	–
Self-pay	855,164	3.72 [3.28–4.16]	105	2.44 [0.21–4.66]	0.564 [0.226–1.408]	0.2197	0.57 [0.43–0.76]	<.0001
No charge	43,330	0.19 [0.12–0.26]	9	0.20 [0.00–0.48]	0.903 [0.226–3.606]	0.8850	1.91 [0.97–3.76]	0.0595
Non-Medicaid government program	888,190	3.86 [3.53–4.20]	396	9.18 [5.08–13.29]	2.047 [1.253–3.344]	0.0043	2.59 [2.26–2.97]	<.0001
Number of Chronic Conditions								
0–1	16,472,397	71.53 [70.36–72.70]	2479	57.42 [50.81–64.03]	Reference	–	Reference	–
2 to 5	5,928,336	25.74 [24.77–26.72]	1682	38.96 [33.40–44.52]	1.885 [1.451–2.449]	<.0001	1.41 [1.30–1.54]	<.0001
6+	627,835	2.73 [2.48–2.97]	156	3.62 [1.47–5.76]	1.653 [0.844–3.236]	0.1426	1.24 [1.00–1.52]	0.046
Hospital Location								
Metropolitan >1million	7,153,680	37.36 [33.68–41.04]	19,300	51.32 [40.24–62.41]	Reference	–	Reference	–
Fringe/Metro < 1 million	9,216,267	48.13 [44.80–51.47]	1624	43.19 [32.59–53.79]	0.653 [0.431–0.989]	0.0443	0.70 [0.64–0.77]	<.0001

Table 1 Associations of hospitalization for JDM in US children *(Continued)*

Variable	Primary diagnosis of JDM							
	No		Yes					
	Freq	Row Percent [95% CI]	Freq	Percent [95% CI]	Crude OR [95% CI]	*P*	Adjusted OR [95% CI]	*P*
Micropolitan	1,736,350	9.07 [8.20–9.94]	139	3.69 [1.48–5.91]	0.296 [0.154–0.572]	0.0003	0.27 [0.21–0.35]	<.0001
Not metropolitan or micropolitan	1,041,038	5.44 [4.92–5.95]	67	1.79 [0.73–2.86]	0.240 [0.127–0.454]	<.0001	0.25 [0.18–0.34]	<.0001
Region								
Northeast	4,281,720	18.59 [15.96–21.23]	814	18.87 [7.69–30.04]	Reference	–	Reference	–
Midwest	4,853,593	21.08 [17.99–24.16]	883	20.45 [10.90–29.99]	0.956 [0.463–1.976]	0.9035	0.82 [0.71–0.94]	0.0047
South	8,992,204	39.05 [35.41–42.69]	1450	33.59 [21.57–45.61]	0.848 [0.421–1.708]	0.6441	0.83 [0.74–0.94]	0.0020
West	4,901,051	21.28 [18.32–24.25]	1170	27.10 [15.36–38.84]	1.255 [0.599–2.632]	0.5470	1.23 [1.11–1.36]	<.0001

Missing data was encountered in 74,174 (1.7%) for age, 400,342(10.5%) for season, 96,625 (2.3%) for sex, 1,120,507 (26.2%) for race, 8898, (0.2%) for insurance, 0 (0.0%) for number of chronic conditions, 830,247 (19.7%) for hospital location, and 0 (0.0%) for region

There was no significant differences of missing values for season ($p = 0.37$), race/ethnicity ($p = 0.76$), or hospital location ($p = 0.14$) between hospitalizations with a primary, secondary, or no diagnosis of JDM. 95% *CI* 95% confidence interval; *OR* odds ratio

Table 2 Top five primary diagnoses of patients admitted with secondary or no diagnosis of JDM

Rank	ICD-9-CM Code	Primary diagnosis	Weighted Frequency	Prevalence [95% CI]
Secondary diagnosis of JDM				
1	6826	Cellulitis of Leg	101.62064	4.38%[3.46–5.30]
2	6823	Cellulitis of Arm	97.86453	4.22%[3.31–5.12]
3	486	Pneumonia	84.98956	3.66%[2.81–4.51]
4	V5789	Rehabilitation procedure NEC	84.56049	3.64%[2.77–4.51]
5	88	Other arthropod-borne disease	52.25267	2.25%[1.58–2.93]
No diagnosis of dermatomyositis				
1	486	Pneumonia	1,206,317	5.24%[5.23–5.25]
2	46,611	Acute Bronchiolitis Due to RSV	768,637	3.34%[3.33–3.35]
3	49,392	Asthma, unspecified, with exacerbation	700,180	3.04%[3.03–3.05]
4	46,619	Acute Bronchiolitis Due to Other Infectious Organism	561,443	2.44%[2.43–2.45]
5	5409	Acute appendicitis w/o mention of peritonitis	550,923	2.39%[2.39–2.40]

ICD-9-CM International Classification of Diseases, Ninth Revision, Clinical Modification; 95% CI 95% confidence interval; RSV respiratory syncytial virus; NEC Not Elsewhere Classifiable

Table 3 Primary or Secondary Diagnoses of Most Common Symptoms in Patients with Secondary and No diagnosis of JDM from 2002 to 2012

Rank	*ICD-9-CM* Code[a]	Diagnosis	Weighted Frequency	Row Prevalence [95% CI]
710.3 as Secondary Diagnosis				
1	782.1	Rash	44	1.87 [0.65–3.10]
2	728.87	Muscle Weakness	40	1.72 [0.39–3.05]
3	729.1	Muscle Pain	30	1.30 [0.33–2.28]
4	780.6	Fever	96	4.14 [2.26–6.01]
5	787.20	Dysphagia	45	1.94 [0.43–3.46]
6	784.42	Dysphonia	0	–
7	789.00	Abdominal Pain	23	0.97 [0.11–1.83]
8	CCS 204	Arthritis NOS	80	3.44 [1.86–5.02]
9	709.3	Calcinosis	27	1.14 [0.06–2.23]
10	578.1	Melena	8	0.36 [0.00–0.86]
11	783.0	Anorexia	10	0.43 [0.00–1.04]
No Diagnosis of 710.3				
1	782.1	Rash	166,932	0.73 [0.68–0.77]
2	728.87	Muscle Weakness	8152	0.04 [0.03–0.04]
3	729.1	Muscle Pain	31,879	0.14 [0.13–0.15]
4	780.6	Fever	621,463	2.70 [2.53–2.87]
5	787.20	Dysphagia	64,240	0.28 [0.23–0.32]
6	784.42	Dysphonia	1836	0.01 [0.00–0.01]
7	789.00	Abdominal Pain	159,317	0.69 [0.65–0.73]
8	CCS 204	Arthritis NOS	136,958	0.59 [0.56–0.63]
9	709.3	Calcinosis	1025	0.0044 [0.0036–0.0053]
10	578.1	Melena	59,509	0.26 [0.24–0.28]
11	783.0	Anorexia	67,501	0.29 [0.25–0.33]

[a]Excluded repeat diagnosis of JDM

ICD9-CM International Classification of Diseases, Ninth Revision, Clinical Modification; 95% CI 95% confidence interval; NOS Not Otherwise Specified abdominal pain, arthritis, calcinosis, melena, and anorexia) were more frequent in JDM patients. However, the prevalence of *ICD-9-CM* codes for these symptoms within the dataset was lower than documented prevalence of these symptoms within other published studies [16, 17].

Length of stay

Patients with JDM spent a weighted total of 19,159 days and 18,218 days in the hospital for their JDM or other reasons, respectively. LOS in the hospital was 39% longer for hospitalizations with a secondary diagnosis (geometric mean [95% CI]: 3.75 [3.27–4.30] days) ($p <$ 0.0001) compared with hospitalizations without a diagnosis of JDM while hospitalizations were not prolonged for a primary diagnosis (2.50 [2.27–2.76]) when compared with hospitalizations without a diagnosis of JDM (2.70 [2.66–2.75]). This pattern of prolonged LOS for hospitalizations with a secondary diagnosis of JDM was consistent across all years (Fig. 2).

In multivariate weighted linear regression models of log-transformed LOS, increased LOS in patients with a primary diagnosis of JDM was associated with race/ethnicity (beta coefficient [95% CI]) (Hispanic: 0.28 [0.14–0.41]; Other: 0.59 [0.31–0.86]), type of insurance (Medicaid: 0.16 [0.01–0.31]), multiple chronic conditions (2–5: 0.41 [0.29–0.52]; 6+: 0.94 [0.63–1.26]), micropolitan location (0.59 [0.27–0.90]), and South region (0.34 [0.12–0.56]) (Table 4). Note that since LOS was log transformed, coefficients from regression models of log-transformed LOS are not the same scale as raw LOS.

Cost of care

The weighted total inflation-adjusted cost-of-care for patients with a primary and secondary inpatient diagnosis of JDM was $49,339,995 and $49,784,853 respectively. The actual total cost is likely higher as 106 patients had a missing value for charge and cost. The inflation-adjusted cost of care for hospitalization was 64% higher for hospitalizations with a primary diagnosis (geometric mean [95% CI]: $7350 [$6228–$8674] and 64% higher for a secondary diagnosis ($7352 [$6331–$8537]) of JDM than those with no diagnosis of JDM (4479 [$4295–$4671] ($p < 0.0001$ for both). This pattern of higher costs for hospitalizations for JDM was consistent for every year within the cohort.

In multivariate linear regression models of log-transformed cost of care, increased cost-of-care in patients with a primary diagnosis of JDM was associated with race/ethnicity (beta coefficient [95% CI] Hispanic: 0.30 [0.05–0.55]) and multiple chronic conditions (2–5: 0.36 [0.17–0.55]; 6+: 1.01 [0.39–1.63]).

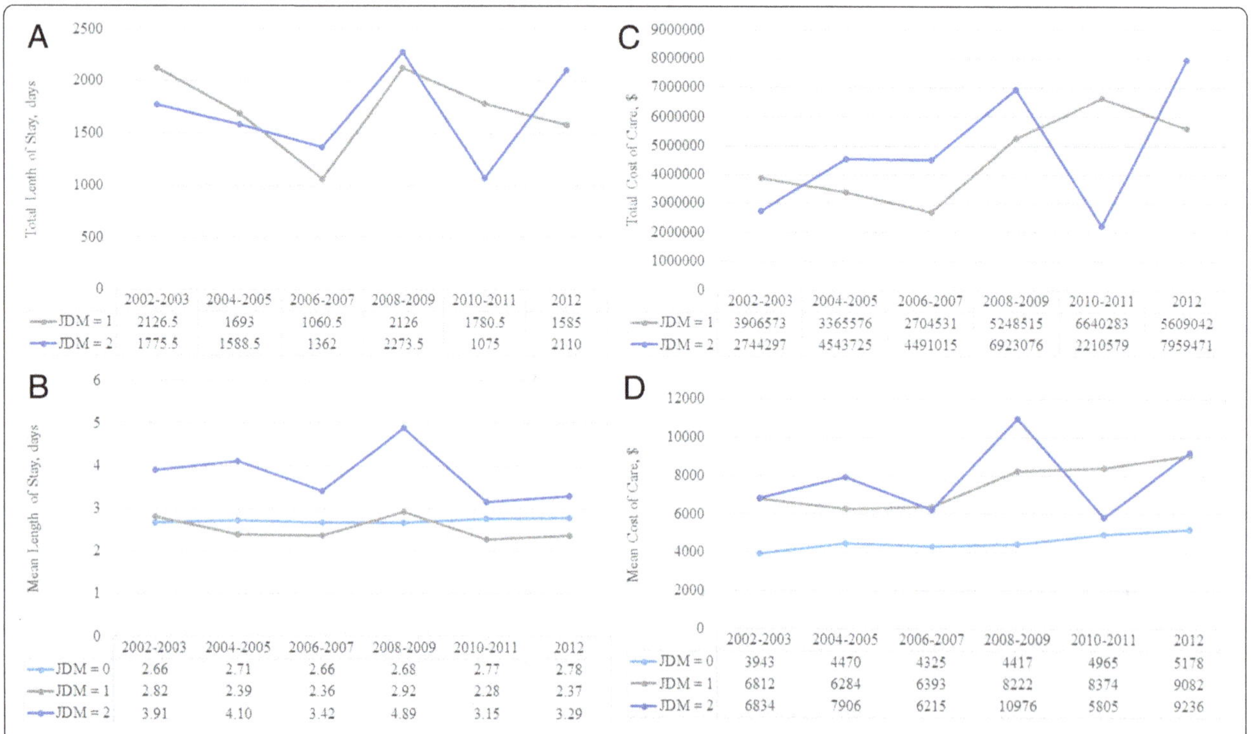

Fig. 2 Length of stay and costs of hospitalization with primary/secondary diagnoses for juvenile dermatomyositis (JDM). (**a**) Total and (**b**) geometric mean length of hospital stay and (**c**) total and (**d**) geometric mean inflation-adjusted cost of inpatient care are presented for 2002–2003, 2004–2005, 2006–2007, 2008–2009, 2010–2011 and 2012. *jdm* 0: no JDM. *jdm* 1: primary dx of JDM. *jdm* 2: secondary dx of JDM

Table 4 Predictors of Length of Stay and Cost of Care for Hospitalizations with a Primary Diagnosis of JDM-

	Length of Stay			Cost of Care		
	LSM	Adj Beta [95% CI][a]	*p*-value	LSM	Adj Beta [95% CI]*	*p*-value
Age						
0–5	1.72	0 [ref]	–	9.47	0 [ref]	–
6–10	1.51	−0.22[− 0.34--0.09]	0.001	9.43	− 0.03[− 0.24–0.17]	0.7459
11–17	1.69	− 0.04[− 0.19–0.12]	0.6417	9.64	0.18[− 0.07–0.42]	0.1536
Season						
Fall	1.62	−0.05[− 0.16–0.06]	0.3442	9.57	0.00[− 0.24–0.23]	0.9674
Winter	1.67	0 [ref]	–	9.57	0 [ref]	–
Spring	1.6	−0.07[− 0.15–0.01]	0.0853	9.45	− 0.13[− 0.35–0.09]	0.2514
Summer	1.66	− 0.01[− 0.11–0.08]	0.7552	9.46	− 0.11[− 0.33–0.10]	0.3131
Gender						
Female	1.64	0.01[− 0.09–0.11]	0.8992	9.54	0.05[− 0.13–0.23]	0.5914
Male	1.63	0 [ref]	–	9.49	0 [ref]	–
Race						
White	1.38	0 [ref]	–	9.32	0 [ref]	–
Black	1.55	0.17[− 0.12–0.46]	0.2395	9.44	0.12[− 0.21–0.45]	0.4806
Hispanic	1.66	0.28 [0.14–0.41]	<.0001	9.62	0.30 [0.05–0.55]	0.0168
Other	1.96	0.59 [0.31–0.86]	<.0001	9.68	0.36[−0.07–0.79]	0.0993
Insurance						
Medicaid	1.62	0.16 [0.01–0.31]	0.0386	9.32	0.02[−0.21–0.25]	0.8646
Private insurance	1.46	0 [ref]	–	9.3	0 [ref]	–
Self-pay	1.7	0.24[−0.07–0.55]	0.1316	9.52	0.22[−0.67–1.10]	0.6276
No charge	2.11	0.65[−0.06–1.37]	0.0739	10.48	1.18[−0.56–2.93]	0.1833
Non-Medicaid government program	1.3	−0.16[− 0.29--0.04]	0.0085	8.95	−0.34[− 0.63--0.06]	0.0196
Number of Chronic Conditions						
0–1	1.19	0 [ref]	–	9.06	0 [ref]	–
2 to 5	1.59	0.41 [0.29–0.52]	<.0001	9.42	0.36 [0.17–0.55]	0.0002
6+	2.13	0.94 [0.63–1.26]	<.0001	10.07	1.01 [0.39–1.63]	0.0014
Hospital Location						
Metropolitan >1million	1.46	0 [ref]	–	9.52	0 [ref]	–
Fringe/Metro < 1 million	1.41	−0.04[−0.14–0.05]	0.3704	9.35	−0.17[− 0.36–0.02]	0.0835
Micropolitan	2.04	0.59 [0.27–0.90]	0.0003	9.87	0.35[−0.20–0.91]	0.2128
Not metropolitan or micropolitan	1.64	0.19[−0.69–1.07]	0.6753	9.31	−0.20[− 0.98–0.58]	0.6082
Region						
Northeast	1.62	0 [ref]	–	9.35	0 [ref]	–
Midwest	1.51	−0.10[−0.29–0.09]	0.285	9.63	0.28[−0.04–0.59]	0.0875
South	1.95	0.34 [0.12–0.56]	0.0024	9.63	0.28 [0.00–0.56]	0.0529
West	1.47	−0.15[−0.35–0.05]	0.1342	9.44	0.09[−0.17–0.35]	0.5113
Year						
2002–2003	1.79	0 [ref]	–	9.55	0 [ref]	–
2004–2005	1.64	−0.15[−0.31–0.02]	0.0785	9.44	−0.11[− 0.44–0.23]	0.5253
2006–2007	1.53	−0.26[− 0.47--0.05]	0.0146	9.34	− 0.21[− 0.57–0.15]	0.2445
2008–2009	1.73	−0.06[− 0.24–0.11]	0.4759	9.61	0.06[− 0.29–0.40]	0.7548
2010–2011	1.51	− 0.18[− 0.49–0.14]	0.2666	9.39	−0.16[− 0.52–0.20]	0.3796
2012	1.61	−0.28[− 0.43--0.13]	0.0003	9.75	0.20[− 0.14–0.54]	0.2469

Missing data was encountered in 74,174 (1.7%) for age, 400,342(10.5%) for season, 96,625 (2.3%) for sex, 1,120,507 (26.2%) for race, 8898, (0.2%) for insurance, 0 (0.0%) for number of chronic conditions, 830,247 (19.7%) for hospital location, 0 (0.0%) for region, and 0 (0.0%) for year

There were no significant differences of missing values for season ($p = 0.37$), race/ethnicity ($p = 0.76$), or hospital location ($p = 0.14$) between hospitalizations with a primary, secondary, or no diagnosis of JDM. LSM least squares mean; 95% *CI* 95% confidence interval

[a]Coefficients from regression models of log-transformed LOS or cost of care should be interpreted with caution as the transformed variables are not the same scale as the raw variables

Discussion

The present study finds that JDM incurs a significant inpatient burden, with primary diagnoses having a higher cost of care (approximately $3000 more per hospitalization) and secondary diagnoses having longer hospitalizations and cost of care (also approximately $3000 more per hospitalization) compared to no diagnosis of JDM. The higher cost of care is likely related to additional workup required for diagnosis, disease comorbidity and treatment regimen required for the disease. Previous studies have suggested that infection may play a role in both the development [18] and recurrence [19, 20] of JDM episodes. In our study, we found increased rates of infection i.e. cellulitis among JDM patients. Multiple mechanisms may make individuals with JDM more prone to infection with pathogens such as staphylococcus. Skin breakdown, seen in JDM patients with calcinosis and cutaneous ulceration, may serve as a nidus for infection. In addition, underlying immune dysregulation such as granulocyte chemotactic defects may contribute to infection risk. [21] The long-term use of immunosuppressants (e.g. corticosteroids, methotrexate) likely also contributes to infection risk. A novel finding that 'other arthropod-borne diseases' represented the 5th most common primary diagnosis among patients with a secondary diagnosis of JDM (Table 2) deserves further study to determine the strength of this association, whether the code refers specifically to arthropod-borne diseases per se versus chief complaints (e.g. cutaneous eruptions, other infections) for which arthropod-borne diseases are on the differential diagnosis, or an outlier due to readmission of a few inpatients with JDM who happened to have had arthropod-borne diseases. JDM patients within our study were also shown to have higher rates of comorbid chronic conditions. Emerging literature supports the finding that JDM patients are often medically complex. For example, we recently found in a separate study that inpatients with JDM had increased odds of multiple cardiovascular and cerebrovascular comorbidities. [22] It is likely that sequelae of JDM itself, adverse effects of treatment (e.g. infections, side effects of steroids), and concomitant autoimmunity contribute to higher chronic condition counts in JDM, with further study needed to better clarify the exact comorbidities in this population. In addition, while current treatment regimens favoring rapid and aggressive management, such as those involving high-dose intravenous pulse methylprednisone therapy, improve outcomes and prognosis of the disease [23], they may also contribute to inpatient costs. Unfortunately, we did not have access to specific diagnostic tests and medications used during hospitalizations, as these were not recorded within the NIS. As a result, future studies are needed to determine specific contributors to inpatient costs. Notably, annual prevalence for both primary and secondary diagnoses have not increased over time as opposed to trends seen in adult dermatomyositis. [6] Future studies are needed to assess whether disease pathophysiology or management may explain the differences in these trends.

There were significant age, sex, seasonal, financial, and regional differences in hospitalization for JDM. In particular, higher rates of hospitalization were found in JDM patients who were older, female, received non-Medicaid government administered insurance coverage (e.g. KidCare, CHIP, other federal/state/local government programs), hospitalized in metropolitan areas, and hospitalized in non-winter seasons when compared to the control group. Hospitalization rates were highest for the 6–11 year old age group, which corresponds to the average age of onset (approximately 7 years) found in other studies. [18, 24] Higher rates of hospitalization in females are likely related to females having higher overall disease prevalence. [2, 18] Hospitalizations for JDM were more likely to occur in non-winter seasons, which stand in stark contrast to the higher frequency of winter admissions seen in control patients. This finding reinforces that ultraviolet light and other environmental exposures may play a role in disease pathogenesis and exacerbation, which corroborates the view that JDM can be a photosensitive condition [25–27] and that JDM patients should be advised to routinely use sunscreen. [28]

Financial coverage and regional differences in hospitalizations may point to differences in access to care for different patient populations. Notably, patients were more likely to be hospitalized if they were covered under government programs, excluding Medicaid. These alternative programs often represent efforts at the state/local level to provide assistance for children of lower income families. As a result, increased risk of hospitalization for patients with these alternative forms of coverage may represent the decreased access to care that lower income families face. Paradoxically, hospitalizations rates were lower among JDM patients with Medicaid coverage. As a result, further research is needed to evaluate how differences in group characteristics and social determinants of health between those covered under different government programs may contribute to differences in outcomes as seen in this study. Additionally, the majority of hospitalizations occurred in metropolitan locations. This speaks to multiple potential issues, including access to outpatient care in urban settings and lack of pediatric rheumatologists in more rural settings requiring treatment at large referral centers in urban areas, both of which may be attributable to a limited supply of pediatric rheumatologists [29] and pediatric subspecialists in general. [30] This is further reinforced by the fact that hospitalizations for JDM in micropolitan locations resulted in an 80% longer LOS compared to metropolitan locations. Further research is needed to evaluate how distribution and access to the pediatric rheumatology workforce affects patient outcomes.

Interestingly, race/ethnicity did not play a major role in increased hospitalizations, contrasting trends seen across other diseases, including adult dermatomyositis [6], pemphigus [12], and psoriasis [31] where racial/ethnic differences did affect rates of hospitalization. However, race was an important contributor to inpatient burden in terms of both length of stay and cost, with Hispanic patients having an estimated 32% longer hospitalization and 35% higher cost of care and other non-white racial groups (excluding Black and Hispanic patients) having 80% longer hospitalizations. These differences in length of stay and costs of care may point to differences in disease manifestations or severity among different races/ethnicities. Indeed, previous studies have found differences in human leukocyte antigen (HLA) frequencies among different ethnic groups, with the HLA-DQA1*0501 allele having a high frequency in Hispanic JDM patients. [32] In addition, studies have suggested that differences between patient HLA subtype and autoantibody associations may help predict disease subtype and severity. [33] Alternatively, access to care may be contributing to racial/ethnic differences. However, one study, which found that minority race and lower family income were associated with worse outcomes—as measured by Childhood Health Assessment Questionnaire, patient global scores, and health-related quality of life scores—did not find associations between race and proxy measures of access to care e.g. time to diagnosis, disease duration, and treatment. [34] In our own study, we did not find that Black patients experienced a difference in hospitalization, length of stay, or cost of care, although we did find that these outcomes differed among other minority groups. Further research examining the relationship of race/ethnicity to outcomes in JDM are warranted.

Strengths of this study include an analysis of a nationally representative sample of all payer data over a period of 11 years with over 14 million pediatric records. JDM patients were identified using the previously validated *ICD-9-CM* codes for dermatomyositis in the inpatient setting. [13] Limitations of this study include the inability to distinguish between different degrees of disease severity or specific clinical features. This limited our ability to examine how differences between individual hospitals and patient characteristics might contribute to LOS and cost of care. Due to the structure of the NIS dataset, it was not possible to determine how many of the hospitalizations were due to readmissions or transfers between hospitals. In addition, cost analysis did not include costs of physician services, out-of-pocket expenses or outpatient costs. Thus the total economic burden of JDM is likely much higher. In addition, while common symptoms for JDM were higher among the JDM cohort, little additional insight could be gleaned due to lack of symptom coding within the database, as prevalence of these codes was much lower than documented prevalence of these symptoms. [16, 17] There was a large frequency of missing data for season, race/ethnicity, and hospital location in NIS. However, there were no significant differences of missing values between hospitalizations with a primary, secondary or no diagnosis of dermatomyositis. Finally, geographic variation was considered by four Health Resources and Services Administration regions. Controlling for region did not attenuate the observed seasonal, racial/ethnic, or hospital location differences. However, future studies using more granular distinctions of geographic location would be useful to further validate these seasonal, racial, and hospital location differences.

Conclusions

The findings of this study indicate that the inpatient burden of JDM is extensive. Cost was higher for patients with primary JDM while both length of stay and cost were higher for secondary dermatomyositis versus those without. Older age, female sex, non-winter season, non-Medicaid administered government insurance coverage, and metropolitan area were associated with higher rates of hospitalization for JDM while race/ethnicity was more influential in resulting in increased LOS and cost of care, particularly in Hispanic populations. Future research is needed to identify how factors such as access to care may relate to the financial, regional, and racial differences found within this study.

Abbreviations

AHRQ: Agency for Healthcare Research and Quality; CI: Confidence Intervals; HCUP: Healthcare Cost and Utilization Project; HLA: Human Leukocyte Antigen; ICD-9-CM: International Classification of Diseases, Ninth Revision, Clinical Modification; JDM: Juvenile dermatomyositis; LOS: Length of Stay; NEC: Not Elsewhere Classifiable; NIS: Nationwide Inpatient Sample; NOS: Not Otherwise Specified; OR: Odds Ratio; RSV: Respiratory Syncytial Virus

Acknowledgments

Not applicable.

Funding

This publication was made possible with support from the Agency for Healthcare Research and Quality (AHRQ), grant number K12HS023011, and the Dermatology Foundation.

Author's contributions

Study concept and design: JIS, KA. Acquisition of Data: JIS and MK. Analysis and interpretation of data: JIS, MK, KA. Drafting of the manuscript: JIS and MK. Critical revision of the manuscript for important intellectual content: KA. Statistical analysis: JIS and MK. Obtained funding: JIS. All authors read and approved the final manuscript.

Competing interests
Dr. Ardalan has had travel costs for participation in a biomarker workshop reimbursed on one occasion by ReveraGen BioPharma in an amount less than $600. The authors declare that they have no other competing interests to declare.

Author details
[1]Department of Dermatology, Northwestern University Feinberg School of Medicine, Chicago, IL 60611, USA. [2]Departments of Dermatology, Preventive Medicine and Medical Social Sciences, Northwestern University Feinberg School of Medicine, Chicago, IL 60611, USA. [3]Division of Rheumatology, Departments of Pediatrics and Medical Social Sciences, Ann & Robert H. Lurie Children's Hospital of Chicago/Northwestern University Feinberg School of Medicine, 225 E Chicago Ave Box 50, Chicago, IL 60611, USA.

References

1. Brown V, Pilkington C, Feldman B, Davidson J. An international consensus survey of the diagnostic criteria for juvenile dermatomyositis (JDM). Rheumatology. 2006;45(8):990–3.
2. Mendez EP, Lipton R, Ramsey-Goldman R, Roettcher P, Bowyer S, Dyer A, et al. US incidence of juvenile dermatomyositis, 1995–1998: results from the National Institute of Arthritis and Musculoskeletal and Skin Diseases registry. Arthritis Care Res (Hoboken). 2003;49(3):300–5.
3. Huber AM, Lang B, LeBlanc C, Birdi N, Bolaria RK, Malleson P, et al. Medium- and long-term functional outcomes in a multicenter cohort of children with juvenile dermatomyositis. Arthritis Rheum. 2000;43(3):541–9.
4. Ravelli A, Trail L, Ferrari C, Ruperto N, Pistorio A, Pilkington C, et al. Long-term outcome and prognostic factors of juvenile dermatomyositis: a multinational, multicenter study of 490 patients. Arthritis Care Res (Hoboken). 2010;62(1):63–72.
5. Klein-Gitelman MS, Waters T, Pachman LM. The economic impact of intermittent high-dose intravenous versus oral corticosteroid treatment of juvenile dermatomyositis. Arthritis Care Res (Hoboken). 2000;13(6):360–8.
6. Kwa MC, Ardalan K, Laumann AE, Silverberg JI. Predictors of hospitalization. Arthritis Care Res (Hoboken): Length of Stay and Costs of Care Among Adults with Dermatomyositis in the United States; 2017.
7. Gidman W, Meacock R, Symmons D. The humanistic and economic burden of juvenile idiopathic arthritis in the era of biologic medication. Curr Rheumatol Rep. 2015;17(5):31.
8. Boan AD, Feng WW, Ovbiagele B, Bachman DL, Ellis C, Adams RJ, et al. Persistent racial disparity in stroke hospitalization and economic impact in young adults in the buckle of stroke belt. Stroke. 2014;45(7):1932–8.
9. Mochari-Greenberger H, Mosca L. Racial/ethnic differences in medication uptake and clinical outcomes among hospitalized cardiovascular patients with hypertension and diabetes. Am J Hypertens. 2014;28(1):106–12.
10. Curtis LM, Wolf MS, Weiss KB, Grammer LC. The impact of health literacy and socioeconomic status on asthma disparities. J Asthma. 2012;49(2):178–83.
11. Iwane MK, Chaves SS, Szilagyi PG, Edwards KM, Hall CB, Staat MA, et al. Disparities between black and white children in hospitalizations associated with acute respiratory illness and laboratory-confirmed influenza and respiratory syncytial virus in 3 US counties—2002–2009. Am J Epidemiol. 2013;177(7):656–65.
12. Hsu D, Brieva J, Silverberg JI. Costs of care for hospitalization for pemphigus in the United States. JAMA Dermatol. 2016;152(6):645–54.
13. Kwa MC, Ardalan K, Laumann AE, Nardone B, West DP, Silverberg JI. Validation of international classification of disease codes for the epidemiological study of dermatomyositis. Arthritis Care Res (Hoboken). 2016.
14. Statistics USDoLBoL. CPI detailed report June 2015.
15. Chronic Condition Indicator (CCI) for ICD-9-CM: Agency for Healthcare Research and Quality; 2016 [updated May 2016. Available from: https://www.hcup-us.ahrq.gov/toolssoftware/chronic/chronic.jsp#pubs.
16. Pachman LM, Hayford JR, Chung A, Daugherty CA, Pallansch MA, Fink CW, et al. Juvenile dermatomyositis at diagnosis: clinical characteristics of 79 children. J Rheumatol. 1998;25(6):1198–204.
17. Gowdie PJ, Allen RC, Kornberg AJ, Akikusa JD. Clinical features and disease course of patients with juvenile dermatomyositis. Int J Rheum Dis. 2013;16(5):561–7.
18. Pachman LM, Lipton R, Ramsey-Goldman R, Shamiyeh E, Abbott K, Mendez EP, et al. History of infection before the onset of juvenile dermatomyositis: results from the National Institute of Arthritis and Musculoskeletal and Skin Diseases research registry. Arthritis Care Res (Hoboken). 2005;53(2):166–72.
19. Massa M, Costouros N, Mazzoli F, De Benedetti F, La Cava A, Le T, et al. Self epitopes shared between human skeletal myosin and Streptococcus pyogenes M5 protein are targets of immune responses in active juvenile dermatomyositis. Arthritis Rheum. 2002;46(11):3015–25.
20. Martini A, Ravelli A, Albani S, Viola S, Scotta MS, Magrini U, et al. Recurrent juvenile dermatomyositis and cutaneous necrotizing arteritis with molecular mimicry between streptococcal type 5 M protein and human skeletal myosin. J Pediatr. 1992;121(5):739–42.
21. Moore EC, Cohen F, Douglas SD, Gutta V. Staphylococcal infections in childhood dermatomyositis--association with the development of calcinosis, raised IgE concentrations and granulocyte chemotactic defect. Ann Rheum Dis. 1992;51(3):378.
22. Silverberg JI, Kwa L, Kwa MC, Laumann AE, Ardalan K. Cardiovascular and cerebrovascular comorbidities of juvenile dermatomyositis in US children: an analysis of the National Inpatient Sample. Rheumatology. 2018;57(4):694–702.
23. Fisler RE, Liang MG, Fuhlbrigge RC, Yalcindag A, Sundel RP. Aggressive management of juvenile dermatomyositis results in improved outcome and decreased incidence of calcinosis. J Am Acad Dermatol. 2002;47(4):505–11.
24. McCann L, Juggins A, Maillard S, Wedderburn L, Davidson J, Murray K, et al. The juvenile dermatomyositis National Registry and repository (UK and Ireland)—clinical characteristics of children recruited within the first 5 yr. Rheumatology. 2006;45(10):1255–60.
25. Sun C, Lee J-H, Yang Y-H, Yu H-H, Wang L-C, Lin Y-T, et al. Juvenile dermatomyositis: a 20-year retrospective analysis of treatment and clinical outcomes. Pediatr Neonatol. 2015;56(1):31–9.
26. Rider LG, Wu L, Mamyrova G, Targoff IN, Miller FW. Environmental factors preceding illness onset differ in phenotypes of the juvenile idiopathic inflammatory myopathies. Rheumatology. 2010;49(12):2381–90.
27. Shah M, Targoff IN, Rice MM, Miller FW, Rider LG. Brief report: ultraviolet radiation exposure is associated with clinical and autoantibody phenotypes in juvenile myositis. Arthritis Rheum. 2013;65(7):1934–41.
28. Enders FB, Bader-Meunier B, Baildam E, Constantin T, Dolezalova P, Feldman BM, et al. Consensus-based recommendations for the management of juvenile dermatomyositis. Ann Rheum Dis. 2017;76(2):329–40.
29. Henrickson M. Policy challenges for the pediatric rheumatology workforce: Part I. Education and economics. Pediatr Rheumatol Online J. 2011;9(1):23.
30. Jewett EA, Anderson MR, Gilchrist GS. The pediatric subspecialty workforce: public policy and forces for change. Pediatrics. 2005;116(5):1192–202.
31. Hsu DY, Gordon K, Silverberg JI. The inpatient burden of psoriasis in the United States. J Am Acad Dermatol. 2016.
32. Reed AM, Stirling JD. Association of the HLA-DQA1* 0501 allele in multiple racial groups with juvenile dermatomyositis. Hum Immunol. 1995;44(3):131–5.
33. Wedderburn L, McHugh NJ, Chinoy H, Cooper R, Salway F, Ollier W, et al. HLA class II haplotype and autoantibody associations in children with juvenile dermatomyositis and juvenile dermatomyositis–scleroderma overlap. Rheumatology. 2007;46(12):1786–91.
34. Phillippi K, Hoeltzel M, Robinson AB, Kim S. Investigators RRACLR. Race, Income, and Disease Outcomes in Juvenile Dermatomyositis. J Pediatr. 2017;184:38–44. e1.

22

Clinical study of children with cryofibrinogenemia: a retrospective study from a single center

Hsiao-Feng Chou[1], Yu-Hung Wu[2], Che-Sheng Ho[3] and Yu-Hsuan Kao[4*]

Abstract

Background: This study aimed to evaluate the demographic, clinical features, laboratory data, pathology and other survey in pediatric patients with cryofibrinogenemia.

Methods: A 12-year retrospective chart review identified eight pediatric patients at Mackay Memorial Hospital, Taipei, Taiwan.

Results: The female-to-male ratio was 3:1. The mean age at symptom onset and of diagnosis was 10.3 ± 4.6 years and 12.3 ± 4 years, respectively. One child (12.5%) had primary cryofibrinogenemia. The common symptoms were purpura, arthralgia, and muscle weakness (100%). On laboratory examination, cryofibrinogen was positive in all patients. All patients had increased anti-thrombin III while 87.5% and 62.5% had abnormal protein S and protein C, respectively. All eight also complained of neurologic symptoms. One had vertebral artery narrowing, two showed increased T2-weighted signal intensity on the thalamus or white matter, and one had acute hemorrhagic encephalomyelitis on brain magnetic resonance imaging.

Conclusions: This study reports on the presentations of cryofibrinogenemia, which is rare in children. Most cases are associated with autoimmune disease and have severe and complex presentations. Central nervous system involvement is common.

Keywords: Cryofibrinogenemia, Children, Central nervous system

Background

Cryofibrinogenemia is a rare hematologic disorder wherein plasma forms a cryoprecipitate that consists of fibrinogen, fibrin, fibronectin, factor VII, and smaller amounts of various plasma proteins. Cryofibrinogen precipitates at a low temperature (4 °C) and re-dissolves on warming to (37 °C) [1]. Its exact pathogenesis has not been elucidated. A first hypothesis is that there is a defect in the fibrinolytic process, with high plasma levels of α1 antitrypsin and α2-macroglobulin (protease inhibitors), and delayed lysis of euglobulin. But since elevated plasma α1-antitrypsin and α2-macroglobulin levels are not found in other studies, a second hypothesis favors an increased thrombin-binding capacity and clot formation. Both hypotheses lead to thrombotic occlusions of medium and small vessels, leading to amplified hyper-viscosity, reflex vasospasms, and vascular stasis [2].

The most common symptoms of cryofibrinogenemia are due to cutaneous ischemia and include purpura, livedo reticularis, blisters, tissue necrosis, and ulceration. Systemic symptoms have been reported to be glomerulonephritis and thrombophlebitis [3]. Cases involving children have rare been reported. This is a retrospective review on pediatric patients diagnosed with cryofibrinogenemia in a tertiary medical center in Taiwan.

* Correspondence: evakao65@gmail.com
[4]Section of Immunology, Rheumatology and Allergy, Department of Pediatrics, Mackay Memorial Hospital, No. 92, Sec. 2, Zhong-shan N. Rd, Taipei City 10449, Taiwan
Full list of author information is available at the end of the article

Methods

After a review of the diagnostic criteria and clinical features, a medical chart review of eight patients younger than 18 years with a diagnosis of cryofibrinogenemia at the pediatric department of Mackay Memorial Hospital, Taipei, Taiwan, between May 2010 and July 2015. The diagnostic criteria originally proposed by essential and supportive evidence. Essential evidence included: 1) appropriate clinical presentation of sudden onset of skin changes and constitutional symptoms, with or without thrombosis, bleeding, or exposure to cold; 2) presence of cryofibrinogen in plasma; and 3) absence of cryoglobulins. Essential cryofibrinogenemia meant no secondary causes of cryofibrinogens and no evidence of other vaso-occlusive diseases.

Supportive evidence was non-specific and not compulsory. However, when present along with essential evidence, supportive evidence improved diagnostic accuracy. Supportive evidence included: 1) angiogram with abrupt occlusion of small to medium sized arteries; 2) typical skin biopsy findings of cryofibrinogen plugging vessels, leukocytoclastic vasculitis, or dermal necrosis; and 3) elevated serum levels of α1-antitrypsin and α2-macroglobulin [3].

Data were collected and charted in terms of sex, age at onset, initial complaints, presenting features, laboratory values, electrophysiologic examinations, imaging studies (i.e., angiography and magnetic resonance imaging [MRI]), and skin biopsy.

The clinical symptoms evaluated were defined as follows: 1) skin manifestations, including purpura, Raynaud phenomenon, skin necrosis or ulceration, livedo reticularis, urticaria, gangrene, sensitivity to cold, and ecchymosis; 2) neurologic involvement (e.g. muscle weakness, numbness, headache, vertigo, dizziness, seizures, dysuria, and dysphonia); 3) arthralgia, fever, and myalgia; and 4) other systemic symptoms like dyspnea, chest pain, abdominal pain, hematochezia, menorrhea, bone pain, or insomnia.

The laboratory examinations included platelet count, Prothrombin time (PT), activated partial thromboplastin time (aPTT), von Willebrand factor (vWF), serum immunoglobulin A (IgA), cryofibrinogen, cryoglobulin, α1 anti-trypsin, and other immunological examinations. Hepatitis C virus (HCV) antigen, anti-HCV, hepatitis B virus (HBV) surface antigen (HBsAg), and anti-HBV antibodies were measured. Proteinuria, hematuria, and serum creatinine were also recorded.

Systemic involvements were evaluated by several examinations. Skin biopsy was performed for establish the diagnosis. Arthritis indicated joint swelling with two or more of erythema, local heat, tenderness, or limited range of motion. In the peripheral and central nervous system (CNS), neuritis indicated peripheral neuropathy on nerve conduction velocity (NCV), while patients presented with numbness, weakness, or pain. Brain and spine MRI, electromyogram (EMG), somato-sensory evoked potential (SSEP), brainstem auditory evoked potential (BAEP), and visual evoked potential (VEP) were performed according CNS symptoms and signs.

In the respiratory system, pulmonary embolism and acute respiratory distress syndrome (ARDS) were recorded. Renal involvement was indicated by proteinuria, hematuria, or elevated serum creatinine.

Arterial thrombosis was confirmed clinically and by angiogram of the lower limbs, superior mesentery artery, and celiac artery. The associated autoimmune diseases were diagnosed based on the following criteria: systemic lupus erythematosus (SLE) was defined accorded to the 1997 revised criteria of the American College of Rheumatology [4]; juvenile idiopathic arthritis (JIA) was defined by the International League of Associations for Rheumatology criteria [5]; juvenile dermatomyositis (JDM) was according to the criteria of Bohan and Peter in 1975 [6]; Behcet's disease was diagnosed according to the International Study Group for Behcet's disease in 1990 [7] and cutaneous mastocytosis was according to the criteria of a consensus proposal of Valent et al. in 2001 [8].

Results

The female-to-male ratio was 3:1. The mean age at symptom onset was 10.3 ± 4.6 months (range, 2.5–18. 5 years). The mean age at diagnosis was 12.3 ± 4 months (range, 4–18.6 years). Based on the symptoms identified, the most common initial symptoms were arthralgia and myalgia. The most common symptoms were purpura, muscle weakness, and arthralgia (Table 1). The skin manifestations were shown in Fig. 1.

On laboratory examination, cryofibrinogen was positive and cryoglobulin was negative in seven children (87.5%). Three patients with α1 anti-trypsin checked had negative results (Table 3). In addition, anti-thrombin III was increased in all patients. The other frequent laboratory abnormality was abnormal protein S (87.5%), increased protein C (5/8, 62.5%), decreased C3 (4/8; 50%), and abnormal C4 (4/ 8; 50%). Other immunologic results had relatively lower proportion of abnormal values. None of the eight children had hepatitis B or C virus infection (Table 2).

Four patients received skin biopsy and one revealed micro-thrombi on small arterioles (Fig. 2). Angiograms were performed on four patients and all revealed abnormal findings that included vessel narrowing or decreased arterial flow rate on the lower extremities, renal arteries, or celiac trunks (Table 3, Fig. 3).

All eight patients had neurologic symptoms, the most common of which was muscle weakness (Table 1). On electro-physiologic examinations, NCV revealed neuropathic change on three of seven (42.9%) patients, compatible with multi-neuritis. The VEP showed prolonged P100 in two patients who complained of blurred vision or diplopia. The EEG showed spikes or cortical dysfunction on three of four patients (75%) who presented with chronic headache or consciousness disturbance. Three patients who received SSEP examinations had normal findings (Table 2).

Table 1 Clinical symptoms and demographic features children

Case	1		2 (primary)		3		4		5		6		7		8		Total	
Sex	M		F		F		F		M		F		F		F		Female/male ratio 3:1	
Age of onset (yrs)	9.4		13.6		11.4		9.6		2.5		12.4		18.5		14.6		Mean (SD) age at on set (yrs) 10.3 ± 4.6	
Age at diagnosis (yrs)	9.6		13.8		11.6		10.6		4		13.6		18.6		17.1		Mean (SD) at diagnosis (yrs) 12.3 ± 4	
Expired on (yrs)	10.4		Loss to follow up		12.1		10.8		(−)		(−)		19		17.6			
Clinical symptoms																	All patients	
Initial/Total																	Initial, n	Total, n
Myalgia	(+)	(+)	(+)	(+)	(+)	(+)	(+)	(+)	(−)	(−)	(−)	(+)	(−)	(+)	(+)	(+)	5	7
Fever	(−)	(+)	(−)	(+)	(−)	(+)	(−)	(−)	(−)	(−)	(−)	(−)	(−)	(+)	(−)	(−)	0	4
Arthralgia	(+)	(+)	(+)	(+)	(+)	(+)	(+)	(+)	(+)	(+)	(+)	(+)	(−)	(+)	(+)	(+)	7	8
Skin manifestations																		
Purpura	(−)	(+)	(+)	(+)	(−)	(+)	(+)	(+)	(−)	(+)	(−)	(+)	(+)	(+)	(−)	(+)	3	8
Raynaud phenomenon	(−)	(+)	(−)	(−)	(−)	(−)	(−)	(−)	(−)	(−)	(−)	(−)	(−)	(−)	(−)	(−)	0	1
Skin necrosis or ulceration	(−)	(+)	(−)	(−)	(−)	(+)	(−)	(−)	(+)	(+)	(−)	(−)	(−)	(+)	(−)	(+)	1	5
Livedo reticularis	(−)	(+)	(−)	(−)	(+)	(+)	(−)	(−)	(−)	(−)	(−)	(−)	(−)	(+)	(−)	(−)	1	3
Urticaria	(−)	(−)	(+)	(+)	(−)	(−)	(−)	(−)	(−)	(−)	(−)	(−)	(−)	(+)	(+)	(+)	2	3
Gangrene	(−)	(+)	(−)	(−)	(−)	(+)	(−)	(−)	(−)	(−)	(−)	(−)	(−)	(+)	(−)	(+)	0	4
Sensitivity to cold	(−)	(−)	(+)	(+)	(−)	(−)	(−)	(+)	(−)	(−)	(−)	(+)	(−)	(+)	(−)	(+)	1	5
Ecchymosis	(−)	(+)	(−)	(−)	(−)	(+)	(−)	(+)	(−)	(+)	(−)	(+)	(+)	(+)	(−)	(+)	1	7
Neurological involvement																		
Muscle weakness	(+)	(+)	(−)	(+)	(+)	(+)	(+)	(+)	(−)	(+)	(−)	(+)	(−)	(+)	(−)	(+)	3	8
Numbness	(−)	(+)	(−)	(−)	(−)	(+)	(−)	(+)	(−)	(−)	(−)	(+)	(−)	(+)	(−)	(+)	0	6
Headache	(−)	(+)	(−)	(+)	(+)	(+)	(−)	(+)	(−)	(−)	(+)	(+)	(+)	(+)	(+)	(+)	4	7
Vertigo	(−)	(−)	(−)	(+)	(−)	(+)	(−)	(−)	(−)	(−)	(−)	(+)	(−)	(+)	(+)	(+)	1	5
Dizziness	(−)	(+)	(−)	(+)	(+)	(+)	(−)	(+)	(−)	(−)	(+)	(+)	(+)	(+)	(+)	(+)	4	7
Seizure	(−)	(−)	(−)	(−)	(−)	(+)	(−)	(−)	(−)	(−)	(−)	(−)	(−)	(+)	(−)	(+)	0	3
Blurred vision	(−)	(−)	(−)	(−)	(−)	(−)	(−)	(−)	(−)	(−)	(−)	(+)	(+)	(+)	(−)	(+)	1	3
Urinary retention	(−)	(−)	(−)	(−)	(−)	(−)	(−)	(−)	(−)	(−)	(−)	(−)	(−)	(−)	(−)	(+)	0	1
Others																		
Dyspnea	(+)	(+)	(−)	(−)	(+)	(+)	(−)	(+)	(−)	(+)	(−)	(+)	(−)	(+)	(−)	(+)	2	7
Chest pain	(+)	(+)	(−)	(−)	(+)	(+)	(−)	(+)	(−)	(+)	(−)	(+)	(−)	(+)	(−)	(+)	2	7
Abdominal pain	(+)	(+)	(−)	(+)	(+)	(+)	(−)	(−)	(−)	(+)	(+)	(+)	(−)	(+)	(−)	(+)	3	7
Hematochezia	(−)	(−)	(−)	(−)	(−)	(−)	(−)	(−)	(−)	(+)	(−)	(+)	(−)	(−)	(−)	(+)	0	3
Menorrhea	(−)	(−)	(−)	(−)	(−)	(−)	(−)	(−)	(−)	(−)	(−)	(−)	(−)	(−)	(−)	(+)	0	1
Bone pain	(−)	(−)	(−)	(−)	(−)	(−)	(−)	(−)	(−)	(−)	(−)	(−)	(−)	(−)	(+)	(+)	1	1
Insomnia	(−)	(+)	(−)	(+)	(−)	(−)	(−)	(−)	(−)	(−)	(−)	(+)	(−)	(+)	(−)	(+)	0	5

On imaging studies, four of seven (57.1%) patients who underwent brain MRI had abnormal findings (Fig. 4). One patient revealed vertebral artery narrowing. Two others had increased T2-weighted signal intensity on the thalamus or white matter. Another revealed multiple hyper-intense with central hypo-intense lesions on T2-paired images on the thalamus and white matter, indicating hemorrhage in the demyelinating lesions. Diffusion-weighted imaging revealed restriction (increasing signal) in this area (Fig. 4).

Other frequent involvements were the gastrointestinal (GI) and respiratory systems. Although seven of the eight patients had complained of recurrent abdominal pain, several kinds of GI examinations (e.g. plain abdominal X-ray, abdominal sonogram, and upper or lower GI series) were

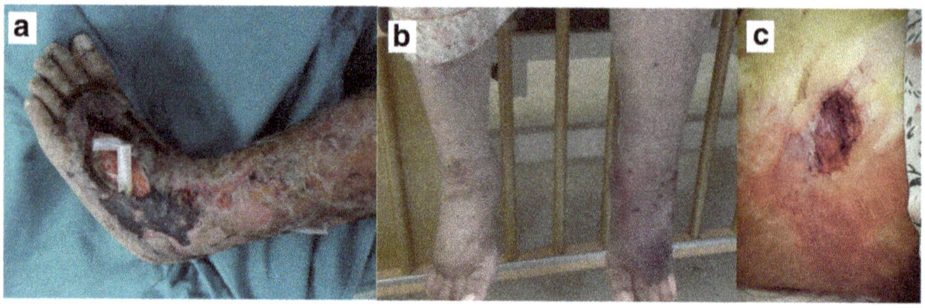

Fig. 1 a) Extensive purpura and gangrene on the left foot (Case 7). **b**) Ecchymosis and swelling on the left foot (Case 3). **c**) Ulcer on the buttocks (Case 3)

usually normal. One patient underwent abdominal MRI, which revealed inflammatory change in the middle jejunal loop, probably related to vasculitis.

In the respiratory system, seven patients complained of dyspnea or chest pain. One presented with pulmonary emboli on lung perfusion scan. Four patients suffered from acute respiratory distress syndrome and expired in the end stage. Three (37.5%) had renal involvement, with proteinuria, hematuria, or renal insufficiency.

As regards associated disease, One patient (12.5%) was primary cryofibrinogenemia (Cases 2) and six had co-morbid JIA, SLE, Behcet's disease, JDM, and cutaneous

Table 2 Immunological laboratory examinations

Case	1	2	3	4	5	6	7	8	No. Positive/No. All checked	(%)
Cryofibrinogen	(+)	(+)	(+)	(+)	(+)	(+)	(+)	(+)	8/8	(100)
Cryoglobulin	(+)	(–)	(–)	(–)	(–)	(–)	(–)	(–)	0/8	(0)
α1-antitrypsin	ND	ND	(–)	ND	ND	(–)	ND	(–)	0/3	(0)
PT/aPTT(initial)	(–)	(–)	(–)	(–)	(–)	(–)	(–)	(–)	0/8	(0)
Bleeding time	(–)	ND	ND	ND	ND	ND	ND	ND	0/1	(0)
IgA	(–)	(–)	(–)	(–)	(–)	(–)	ND	(–)	0/7	(0)
Platelet count	(–)	(–)	(–)	(–)	(–)	(–)	(–)	(–)	0/7	(0)
vWF	ND	(–)	I	(–)	(–)	I	(–)	(–)	2/7	(28.5)
C3	(–)	D	(–)	(–)	D	(–)	D	D	4/8	(50)
C4	(–)	(–)	(–)	D	(–)	D	I	D	4/8	(50)
Protein C	I	(–)	(–)	I	I	(–)	I	I	5/8	(62.5)
Protein S	I	(–)	D	D	D	D	D	I	7/8	(87.5)
Anti-thrombin III	I	I	I	I	I	I	I	I	8/8	(100)
Lupus anticoagulant	(–)	ND	(+)	(–)	(+)	(–)	(–)	(–)	2/7	(28.5)
RA factor	(–)	(–)	(+)	(–)	(–)	(+)	(–)	(+)	3/8	(37.5)
Antinuclear Factor	(–)	(–)	(–)	(–)	(–)	(–)	(–)	(+)	1/8	(12.5)
Anti-cardiolipin IgG	(–)	(–)	(–)	(–)	(+)	(–)	(–)	(–)	1/8	(12.5)
Anti-cardiolipin IgM	(–)	(–)	(–)	(–)	(+)	(–)	(–)	(–)	1/8	(12.5)
anti-ENA (all)	(–)	(–)	(–)	(–)	(+)	(–)	(–)	(–)	1/8	(12.5)
Anti CCP	ND	ND	ND	(–)	(–)	(–)	(–)	(–)	0/5	(0)
ANCA-C	(–)	(–)	ND	ND	(–)	(–)	(–)	(–)	0/6	(0)
ANCA-P	(–)	(–)	ND	ND	(–)	(–)	(–)	(–)	0/6	(0)
Anti-β2 GP1 IgG	(–)	(–)	(–)	(–)	(–)	(–)	(–)	(–)	0/8	(0)
Anti-β2 GP1 IgM	(–)	(–)	(–)	(–)	(–)	(–)	(–)	(–)	0/8	(0)
Anti-ds DNA	(–)	(–)	(–)	(–)	(–)	(–)	(–)	(–)	0/8	(0)
Anti-SSA	(–)	(–)	(–)	(–)	(–)	(–)	(–)	(–)	0/8	(0)
Anti-SSB	(–)	(–)	(–)	(–)	(–)	(–)	(–)	(–)	0/8	(0)

CCP cyclic citrullinated peptide, *ANCA-C* cytoplasmic anti-neutrophil cytoplasmic antibody, *ANCA-P* peri-nuclear anti-neutrophil cytoplasmic antibody, *Anti-β2 GP1* Anti-β2-glycoprotein I, *ENA* extractable nucleic antigen, *SSA* Sjögren's-syndrome-related antigen-A, *Anti-SSB* Sjögren's-syndrome-related antigen-B

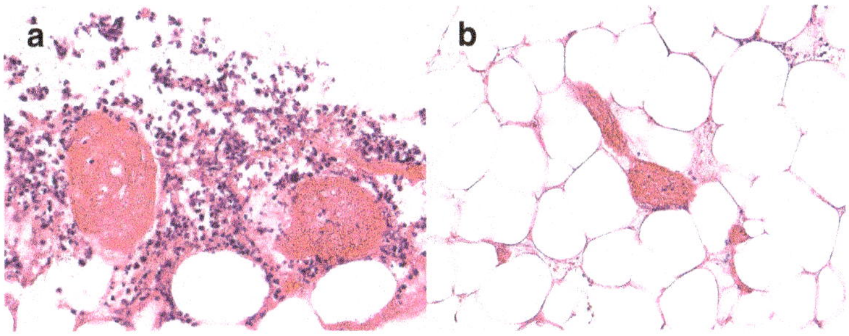

Fig. 2 Skin histopathology showed micro-thrombi and deposition within the lumen of blood vessel (**a**, **b**) (Case 7) (400X, H&E stain)

mastocystosis (Table 3). Three of these six had mixed autoimmune disease. There were five (62.5%) mortalities (Table 1).

Discussion

Cryofibrinogenemia is very rare in children. In review of literature, only Geest et al. reported primary cryofibrinogenemia in a family with 2 children. They presented with only mild skin manifestations as purpura and bullae [9]. Compared to common clinical manifestations, purpura and arthralgia are more prevalent than in previous review articles (purpura 0–78%; arthralgia 6.25–58%). Nevertheless, muscle weakness has not been previously mentioned [2]. This kind of disease is difficult to diagnose in children because initial complaints are variable and non-specific. We approached this disease from the perspective of purpura. The platelet count of all patients was normal. According to the follow-up non-thrombocytopenia purpura

Table 3 Systemic involvement and underline disease

Case No.	1	2	3	4	5	6	7	8	No. Abnormal/Total	%
Skin biopsy	(+)	(−)	ND	ND	(+)	ND	ND	(−)	2/4	50
Renal involvement									3/8	37.5
Proteinuria	(−)	(−)	(−)	(−)	(+)	(+)	(−)	(−)	2/8	25
Hematuria	(−)	(−)	(−)	(+)	(+)	(+)	(−)	(−)	3/8	37.5
Renal insufficiency	(−)	(−)	(−)	(−)	(−)	(−)	(−)	(+)	1/8	12.5
Arthritis	(+)	(+)	(+)	(+)	(+)	(+)	(+)	(+)	8/8	100
Thrombotic events	(−)	(−)	(+)	(+)	(−)	(+)	(+)	(+)	5/8	62.5
Angiogram	ND	ND	(+)	(+)	ND	(+)	ND	(+)	4/4	100
Respiratory involvement										
Pulmonary embolism	(+)	ND	(−)	ND	(−)	ND	(−)	ND	1/4	25
ARDS	(+)	(−)	(+)	(+)	(−)	(−)	(+)	(−)	4/8	50
Neurological involvement										
Multineuritis	(+)	(−)	(+)	ND	(−)	(−)	(−)	(+)	3/7	42.9
Brain MRI	(−)	(−)	(+)	(+)	ND	(−)	(+)	(+)	4/7	57.1
Spine MRI	ND	ND	(−)	ND	ND	ND	ND	(−)	0/2	0
SSEP	ND	(−)	(−)	ND	ND	(−)	ND	ND	0/3	0
EMG	ND	(−)	ND	ND	ND	ND	(+)	ND	1/2	50
EEG	ND	(+)	(−)	ND	ND	ND	(+)	(+)	3/4	75
BAEP	ND	(−)	ND	ND	ND	(−)	(−)	(+)	1/4	25
VEP	ND	ND	ND	ND	ND	ND	(+)	(+)	2/2	100
Associated disease										
Autoimmune disease	CG	(−)	JIA	JIA	JIA, JDM, SLE	JIA	B, SLE, JIA	CM, JIA, B	6/8	75
HCV/HBV infection	(−)	(−)	(−)	(−)	(−)	(−)	(−)	(−)	0	0

(+) = abnormal; (−) = normal; ND = not done

ARDS acute respiratory distress syndrome, *NCV* nerve conduction velocity, *EMG* electromyogram, *SSEP* somatosensory evoked potential, *BAEP* brainstem auditory evoked potential, *VEP* visual evoked potential, *HCV* hepatitis C virus infection, *HBV* hepatitis B virus infection, *CG* cryoglobulinemia, *JIA* juvenile idiopathic arthritis, *JDM* juvenile dermatomyositis, *SLE* systemic lupus erythematosus, *B* Behcet's disease, *CM* Cutaneous mastocytosis

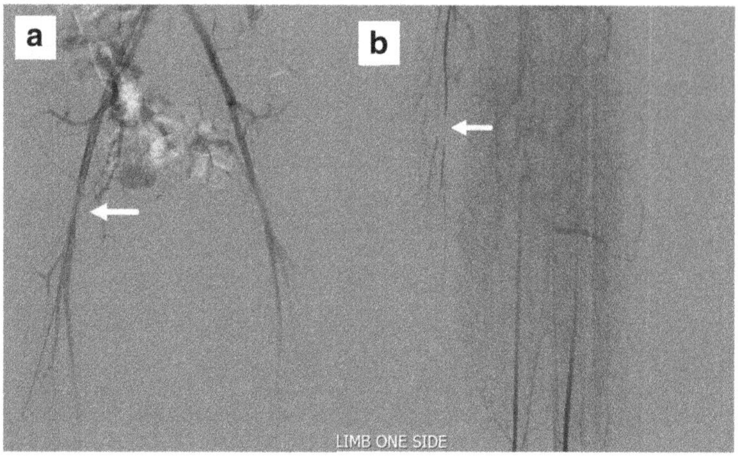

Fig. 3 Angiogram demonstrated narrowing on the right femoral artery (black arrow) (Case 7; **a**) and incomplete obstruction of medium-sized arteries on the knee (white arrow) (Case 4; **b**)

survey, all patients exhibited normal PT/aPTT. Thus, we considered vWF disease, platelet dysfunction, and vascular disease to have caused purpura. Although PLT dysfunction and vWF diseases are typically congenital, those cases diagnosed in the patients were acquired. Therefore, the purpura caused by vascular diseases was examined. Although Henoch–Schonlein purpura (HSP) is the most common disease causing vascular purpura in children, we confirmed diagnoses of cryofibrinogenemia after an extensive survey [10]. Other children complained of long-term and recurring pain at multiple sites on the body, with symptoms such as arthralgia, myalgia, bone pain, numbness, abdominal pain, and headache; however, these have even been regarded as psychiatric problems.

In laboratory studies, an immunologic role for cryofibrinogenemia is suggested by the possible presence of immunoglobulins in the precipitate and of complement deposits in vessel walls. There are excess circulating immunoglobulins or immune complexes produced during pathologic conditions (e.g. infection, cancer, inflammatory, and collagen diseases) [2]. Although most cases (87.5%) in this study is secondary cryofibrinogenemia,

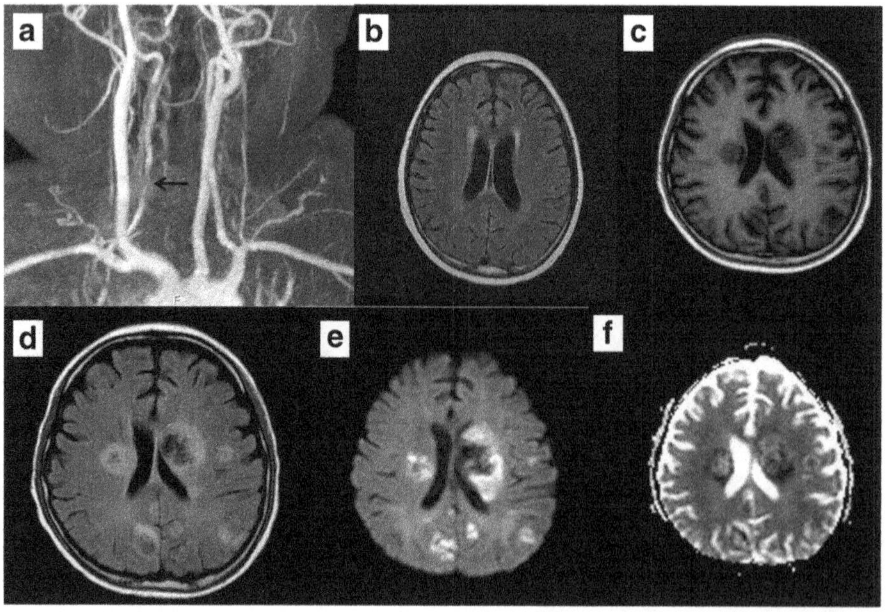

Fig. 4 Brain magnetic resonance imaging (MRI). **a**) MR angiogram showed right vertebral artery narrowing (arrow) (Case 3). **b**) Axial T2-weighted flair MRI imaging demonstrated hyper-intense lesion on the peri-ventricular white matter (TR/TE: 9002/135.4 ms) (Case 3). **c–f**) Acute hemorrhagic encephaomyelitis (Case 8). Axial T2-weighted flair showed multiple hyper-intense with central hypo-intense lesions on the thalamus and white matter (T1-weighted flair: TR/TE: 2000/20 ms; T2-weighted flair: TR/TE: 8000/125 ms; ADC and DWI: TR/TE: 6000/72.89 ms)

the abnormal rate of autoimmune antibody is relatively low. In our study, autoantibodies are usually negative in the initial stage and became positive after treatment. Thus, we speculated that autoantibodies are fixed in the vessel walls and released into circulation after treatment; however, this requires further study.

What mechanisms cause the increased protein C and anti-thrombin III levels in cryofibrinogenemia? This issue has not been discussed in previous studies. We speculated that it may reflect compensation for a temporary hypercoagulatory state of the body. Furthermore, there is no case of cryofibrinogenemia with HBV or HCV infection in our study. This may be due to the HBV vaccination prophylaxis and low possibility of viral exposure in children in Taiwan.

In terms of neurologic involvement, the proportion of multi-neuritis in this study is 42.9%, slightly higher than in previous reports (4.1–22%) [2]. The patients here have higher proportions of CNS involvement, which is rare in previous studies. Only one previous study mentions central nerve system involvement in cryofibrinogenemia. Dunsker et al. reported primary cryofibrinogenemia in a patient who presented with pseudo-tumor cerebri. He suffered from headache, blurred vision, and papillary edema. Venograms revealed cerebral venous thrombosis [11].

In this study, patients with CNS involvement presented as large artery narrowing, parenchymal involvement, and hemorrhage in demyelinating lesions on the white matter and basal ganglion. The last is compatible with acute hemorrhagic encephalomyelitis (AHEM), considered a hyper-acute sub-form of acute disseminated encephalomyelitis. It is frequently a fulminant inflammatory hemorrhagic demylination of the CNS white matter. Death from brain edema is common within one week of the onset of encephalopathy. The pathogenesis is known as acute vasculitis with subsequent vessel occlusion [12]. The patient here (Case 8) with AHEM presented with consciousness disturbance and repeated seizures. Herpes simplex virus infection is identified by laboratory examinations. Thus, these three kinds of brain MRI findings are all compatible with vasculopathy.

In respiratory system involvement, seven of eight (87.5%) patients have complained of dyspnea and chest pain. But chest x-rays often reveal no abnormality. Pulmonary embolism can occur (Case 1), but ARDS is the most frequent complication causing mortality. On the other hand, abdominal pain is also a frequent complaint but determining the underlying problem is difficult. Abdominal vasculitis is proven by angiography or MRI. The rate of renal involvement in this study is also slightly higher than in previous reports (4–22%) [2].

Conclusions

In conclusion, this study reports on the presentations of cryofibrinogenemia, which is rare in children. Most pediatric cases are associated with autoimmune diseases and have more severe and complex presentations. Although rarely reported previously, CNS involvement is common in our study. When children complain of persistent unexplained pain on multiple sites with purpura or ecchymosis, cryofibrinogenemia should be considered and further investigated.

Abbreviations

aPTT: activated thromboplastin time; ARDS: acute respiratory distress syndrome; BAEP: brainstem auditory evoked potential; CNS: central nervous system; EMG: electromyogram; GI: gastrointestinal; HBsAg: Hepatitis B virus surface antigen; HBV: hepatitis B virus; HCV: hepatitis C virus; IgA: immunoglobulin A; JDM: juvenile dermatomyositis; JIA: juvenile idiopathic arthritis; MRI: magnetic resonance imaging; NCV: nerve conduction velocity; PT: prothrombin Time; SLE: systemic lupus erythematosus; SSEP: somato-sensory evoked potential; VEP: visual evoked potential; vWF: von Willebrand factor

Acknowledgements

The authors cordially thank Dr. Gene Alzona Nisperos and Dr. Malcolm Higgins for writing assistance.

Funding

The authors disclose there is no funding source involvement in this article.

Authors' contributions

HFC analyzed and interpreted the patient data and was the major contributor in writing the manuscript. YHW performed the histological examination of the skin, which was important to make disease diagnosis. CSH contributed to the neurological care of patients. YHK, who was the attending physician, managed all patients mentioned in this article and revised it critically for important content. All authors read and approved the final manuscript.

Competing interests

The authors declare that they have no competing interests.

Author details

[1]Song Zhan Clinics, No.88, Songlong Rd, Taipei City 110, Taiwan. [2]Department of Dermatology, Mackay Memorial Hospital, No. 92, Sec. 2, Zhong-shan N. Rd, Taipei City 10449, Taiwan. [3]Section of Neurology, Department of Pediatrics, Mackay Memorial Hospital, No. 92, Sec. 2, Zhong-shan N. Rd, Taipei City 10449, Taiwan. [4]Section of Immunology, Rheumatology and Allergy, Department of Pediatrics, Mackay Memorial Hospital, No. 92, Sec. 2, Zhong-shan N. Rd, Taipei City 10449, Taiwan.

References

1. Saadoun D, Elalamy I, Ghillani-Dalbin P, Sene D, Delluc A, Cacoub P. Cryofibrinogenemia: new insights into clinical and pathogenic features. Am J Med. 2009;122:1128–35.
2. Michaud M, Pourrat J. Cryofibrinogenemia. J Clin Rheumatol. 2013;19:142–8.

3. Amdo TD, Welker JA. An approach to the diagnosis and treatment of cryofibrinogenemia. Am J Med. 2004;116:332–7.
4. Hochberg MC. Updating the American college of rheumatology revised criteria for the classification of systemic lupus erythematosus. Arthritis Rheum. 1997;40:1725.
5. Petty RE, Southwood TR, Baum J, Bhettay E, Glass DN, Manners P, et al. Revision of the proposed classification criteria for juvenile idiopathic arthritis: Durban, 1997. J Rheumatol. 1998;25:1991–4.
6. Bohan A, Peter JB. Polymyositis and dermatomyositis (first of two parts). N Engl J Med. 1975;292:344–7.
7. International Study Group for Behçet's Disease. Criteria for diagnosis of Behçet's disease. Lancet. 1990;335:1078–80.
8. Valent P, Horny HP, Escribano L, Longley BJ, Li CY, Schwartz LB, et al. Diagnostic criteria and classification of mastocytosis: a consensus proposal. Leuk Res. 2001;25:603–25.
9. van Geest AJ, van Dooren-Greebe RJ, Andriessen MP, Blomjous CE, Go IH. Familial primary cryofibrinogenemia. J Eur Acad Dermatol Venereol. 1999;12: 47–50.
10. Leung AK, Chan KW. Evaluating the child with purpura. Am Fam Physician. 2001;64:419–28.
11. Dunsker SB, Torres-Reyes E, Peden JC Jr. Pseudo-tumor cerebri associated with idiopathic cryofibrinogenemia. Report of a case. Arch Neurol. 1970;23: 120–7.
12. Tenembaum S, Chitnis T, Ness J, Hahn JS. International pediatric MS study group. Acute disseminated encephalomyelitis. Neurology. 2007;68(16 Suppl 2):S23–36.

Health-related quality of life in children with inflammatory brain disease

Elina Liu[1,2], Marinka Twilt[1,3,4*], Pascal N. Tyrrell[5], Anastasia Dropol[1,3,4], Shehla Sheikh[6], Mark Gorman[7], Susan Kim[7,8], David A. Cabral[9], Rob Forsyth[10], Heather Van Mater[11], Suzanne Li[12], Adam M. Huber[13], Elizabeth Stringer[13], Eyal Muscal[14], Dawn Wahezi[15], Mary Toth[16], Pavla Dolezalova[17], Katerina Kobrova[17], Goran Ristic[18] and Susanne M. Benseler[1,3,4]

Abstract

Objective: To quantify the impact of inflammatory brain diseases in the pediatric population on health-related quality of life, including the subdomains of physical, emotional, school and social functioning.

Methods: This was a multicenter, observational cohort study of children (< 18 years of age) diagnosed with inflammatory brain disease (IBrainD). Patients were included if they had completed at least one Health Related Quality of Life Questionnaire (HRQoL). HRQoL was measured using the Pediatric Quality of Life Inventory Version 4.0 (PedsQL) Generic Core Scales, which provided a total score out of 100. Analyses of trends were performed using linear regression models adjusted for repeated measures over time.

Results: In this study, 145 patients were included of which 80 (55%) were females. Cognitive dysfunction was the most common presenting symptoms (63%), and small vessel childhood primary angiitis of the CNS was the most common diagnosis (33%). The mean child's self-reported PedsQL total score at diagnosis was 68.4, and the mean parent's proxy-reported PedsQL score was 63.4 at diagnosis. Child's self-reported PedsQL scores reflected poor HRQoL in 52.9% of patients at diagnosis. Seizures or cognitive dysfunction at presentation was associated with statistically significant deficits in HRQoL.

Conclusion: Pediatric IBrainD is associated with significantly diminished health-related quality of life. Future research should elucidate why these deficits occur and interventions should focus on improving HRQoL in the most affected subdomains, in particular for children presenting with seizures and cognitive dysfunction.

Keywords: Pediatrics, Inflammatory brain disease, CNS vasculitis, Health-related quality of life, Quality of life

Introduction

Childhood inflammatory brain diseases (IBrainDs) encompass a group of devastating conditions with high disease burden presenting with substantial neurological dysfunction in previously healthy children [1–4]. IBrainDs result from immune system activation against structures within the central nervous system (CNS), including both the brain and spinal cord, resulting in inflammation. Types of IBrainD affecting children include small vessel childhood primary angiitis of the CNS (SV-cPACNS), anti-N-methyl-D-aspartate (NMDA) receptor encephalitis, multiple sclerosis (MS), and Rasmussen's encephalitis. These conditions often present acutely with one or more neurological symptoms, including cognitive and behavioural dysfunction, seizure, hallucination and hemiparesis [1, 4–7]. Systematic use of immunosuppressive therapy has improved survival and reduced long-term neurological deficits in childhood IBrainD, though significant burden of illness still exists [5].

Health-related quality of life (HRQoL) is a concept which considers the multidimensional contributions of physical, emotional and social functioning when defining wellbeing [8]. In pediatric populations especially, HRQoL has become an important central outcome, requiring separate evaluation from traditional medical definitions of

* Correspondence: marinka.twilt@ahs.ca; marinkatwilt@gmail.com
[1]Rheumatology, Department of Pediatrics, Alberta Children's Hospital, 2888 Shaganappi Trail NW, Calgary, AB T3B 6A8, Canada
[3]Cumming School of Medicine, University of Calgary, Calgary, AB, Canada
Full list of author information is available at the end of the article

outcome such as mortality [8–10]. It is increasingly used in both drug trials, and the clinical setting, to guide treatment and rehabilitation decisions [8, 9]. The Pediatric Quality of Life Inventory Version 4.0 Generic Core Scales (PedsQL) is a validated questionnaire that assesses pediatric HRQoL under four subdomains of functioning: physical, emotional, social and school [9]. Thus, poor PedsQL scores can reflect outcomes such as depression, fatigue, poor school participation, and social strains, which are difficult to quantify using other outcome scales but are critical considerations for assessing the long-term burden of IBrainD.

HRQoL in children with IBrainD has not yet been systematically evaluated. Although there is a perceived high disease burden for children with IBrainD and their families, there is limited existing literature. The impact of IBrainD on HRQoL, the clinical phenotypes associated with poor HRQoL, the subdomains of functioning most affected in IBrainD, and the relationship between early and late measures of HRQoL are not currently known.

Therefore, the aims of the study were to [1] describe the characteristics of patients with IBrainD, including clinical phenotype and HRQoL, [2] compare both the burden of IBrainD on the different subdomains within HRQoL, and patient perspectives of HRQoL against parent/proxy perspectives in children with IBrainD and [3] identify trajectories and risk factors for impaired HRQoL.

Patients and methods

Patients

This BrainWorks study was a multicenter, observational cohort study of children diagnosed with IBrainD between August 2001 and August 2016. BrainWorks is an international multicenter collaborative study aimed at increasing recognition, promoting rapid diagnostic evaluation and optimizing treatment for pediatric IBrainD. For new patients enrolled in BrainWorks, measurement of outcomes occurred at pre-specified intervals, including diagnosis. Patients from the BrainWorks study were included if they met diagnostic criteria for an IBrainD as defined by the treating physician at 18 years of age or younger, and had completed at least one HRQoL Questionnaire.

Demographic and clinical features

Age at diagnosis, gender, and time to diagnosis were evaluated. Diagnosis was categorized into small vessel childhood primary angiitis of the CNS (SV-cPACNS), angiography -positive non-progressive childhood primary angiitis of the CNS (APNP-cPACNS), angiography-positive progressive childhood primary angiitis of the CNS (APP-cPACNS), antibody-mediated IBrainD, demyelinating IBrainD, granulomatous IBrainD, Moyamoya phenotype, Secondary CNS vasculitis, T-cell mediated IBrainD, and unclassified IBrainD. Anti-NMDA receptor encephalitis, Hashimoto's encephalopathy, anti-glutamic acid decarboxylase antibody encephalitis, mycoplasma-associated encephalitis and neuromyelitis optica were categorized under antibody-mediated IBrainD.

Disease activity, damage and neurological functioning

Neurological clinical features at time-of-diagnosis collected to the BrainWorks database included presence of seizures (focal, generalized, or status epilepticus), hemiparesis and cognitive dysfunction. Cognitive dysfunction included memory loss and behavioural abnormality.

Estimated disease activity and estimated damage were measured as separate continuous variables using the physician global assessment (PGA). Disease activity is determined based on the presence of symptoms and positive markers of disease activity, whereas estimated damage is an estimate of permanent structural damage and functional impairment. Both scores were reported by physicians on a visual analog scale out of 10 cm, where 0 cm represented no disease activity/estimated damage and 10 cm represented high disease activity/estimated damage.

Neurological functioning was characterized using the pediatric stroke outcome measure (PSOM), which assesses neurological and functional deficit across 5 subscales: right sensorimotor, left sensorimotor, language production, language comprehension and cognitive/behavioural deficit [11]. Overall neurological deficit in the PSOM is scaled out of 10, with each subscale measured out of 2. Higher values represent greater deficit. PSOM score at 12 months was assessed as a discrete variable, with any subscale score greater than 0.5 indicating the presence of neurological dysfunction.

Health-related quality of life (HRQoL)

HRQoL was captured using the PedsQL, a validated tool built of two 23-question surveys; one self-report for pediatric patient completion, and one proxy-report for completion by the patient's parent or caregiver [12]. Both PedsQL questionnaires were routinely completed at time-of-diagnosis and at each follow-up clinical visit, clinical situation permitting. Total PedsQL score was calculated for each report by taking the sum-total average of item scores across the four subdomains [9]. PedsQL scores were reported on a 0–100 scale, with higher scores representing superior HRQoL.

The four subdomains of PedsQL are physical (8 items), emotional (5 items), social (5 items) and school (5 items) functioning. A score can be reported for each subdomain by taking a sum-total average of the individual item scores within the subdomain. Alternatively, many sources often report only two subdomain scores: physical functioning and psychosocial functioning, where the psychosocial subdomain is a sum-total average of the item scores from the emotional, social and school functioning sections of the questionnaire. All subdomain PedsQL scores are also reported on a 0–100 scale, with higher scores representing superior HRQoL.

Poor HRQoL was defined as a child's self-reported PedsQL score of ≤70, or a parent-proxy reported PedsQL score ≤ 65. Various studies have established PedsQL cut-off scores to differentiate good quality of life from notable impairment in quality of life, with the most frequent cut-off scores reported to be in the range of 70–79 [9, 13–15]. The cut-off scores for this study were chosen based on a study by Kim et al., which concluded that a PedsQL cut-off score of 70 separated patients with low symptoms and high quality of life from those with moderate-to-severe symptoms, and a study by Varni et al., which used PedsQL child self-reported total scores of 69.1 and a PedsQL parent proxy-reported total scores of 65.4 as "meaningful cut-off point(s) for impaired HRQoL", at one standard deviation below the mean PedsQL score for healthy children [9, 14].

Outcomes

The primary outcome assessed was the pediatric HRQoL, defined by PedsQL total score. Secondary outcomes were the HRQoL subdomains of physical, emotional, social and school functioning.

Statistical analysis

Descriptive statistics for demographic and clinical variables are reported as means and standard deviation or medians with interquartile range for continuous variables and frequencies/proportions for categorical variables. Univariable linear regression models with a maximum likelihood algorithm for parameter estimation were used to test the association between PedsQL scale and summary scores with age at diagnosis, time to diagnosis, and estimated damage at diagnosis as well as the association between gender and the presence of hemiparesis, cognitive/behavioural dysfunction, or seizures at diagnosis and PedsQL scores at diagnosis. Regression models were adjusted for repeated measures with an autoregressive covariance structure in order to establish whether these relationships changed statistically significantly with time (log transformed). Parameter estimate and its standard error are reported, where parameter estimate represents the change ratio for each increase of 1 unit in the independent variable (unless otherwise indicated). Parameter estimates were used to estimate the difference between PedsQL scores of patients with different presentations at time of diagnosis to account for the longitudinal analysis and the variable PedsQL questionnaire completion. All statistical test results were considered significant at the $P < .05$ level. SAS 9.4 for Windows (SAS Institute Inc., Cary, NC, USA) was used for all analyses.

Results

Patients

A total of 145 patients from 13 international sites were included in the study; 80 (55%) female and 65 (45%) male; median age at diagnosis 10.3 years (range = 0.4–18.2 years); median time to diagnosis 1.2 months (range = 0–120 months); median follow-up of 24 months (range = 0–160 months) in the proxy-reports, and 28 months (range = 0–160 months) in the self-reports. The most common diagnoses were SV-cPACNS (48 children, 33%), antibody-mediated IBrainD (28 children, 18%), and APNP-cPACNS (22 children, 15%). One patient died. Patient demographic data are summarized in Table 1.

Clinical presentation

The most frequently reported symptoms at diagnosis were; cognitive/behavioural dysfunction 91 (63%) patients, seizures 65 (45%), stroke 64 patients (44%). The median disease activity score at diagnosis was high at 8.0 (range = 0–10), captured in 116 patients (80%). Neurologic function 1 year after diagnosis was measured in 106 patients; 43 (41%) poor outcome and 63 good outcome (59%). Clinical phenotypes and outcomes of the patient population are summarized in Table 2.

Health related quality of life

A total of 145 patients completed at least one PedsQL questionnaire; at time of diagnosis, 34 child self reports and 39 parent proxy reports were completed. At 1 year

Table 1 Patient demographics for 145 pediatric patients with inflammatory brain disease

Female. Number (%)	80 (55%)
Age at diagnosis, years. Median (range)	10.3 (0.4–18.2)
Diagnosis	
Small vessel cPACNS	48 (33%)
Angiography positive, non-progressive cPACNS	22 (15%)
Angiography positive, progressive cPACNS	8 (6%)
Antibody-mediated IBrainD	26 (18%)
Anti-NMDA receptor encephalitis	13 (9%)
Other antibody-mediated	13 (9%)
Secondary IBrainD	12 (8%)
Secondary CNS Vasculitis	10 (7%)
Demyelinating	4 (3%)
Granulomatosis IBrainD	2 (1%)
Moyamoya-like	1 (1%)
T-cell mediated IBrainD	2 (1%)
IBrainD NYD	10 (7%)
Time to diagnosis, months. Median (range)	1.2 (0–150)

Legend: *Acronyms*: *CNS* Central nervous system, *cPACNS* Childhood primary angiitis of the central nervous system, *IBrainD* Inflammatory brain disease, *NYD* Not yet determined

Table 2 Clinical phenotypes and outcomes for 145 pediatric patients with inflammatory brain disease

Clinical phenotypes at diagnosis	
Presenting symptoms	
Cognitive Dysfunction	91 (63%)
Seizures	65 (45%)
Hemiparesis	64 (44%)
Disease activity	
Number of patients with disease activity measurements	116 (80%)
Median (Range)	8.0 (0–10)
Estimated damage	
Number of patients with estimated damage measurements	98 (68%)
Median (Range)	1.0 (0–8)
Poor health-related quality of life	
Child's self-reported	53% (18/34)
Parent's proxy-reported	49% (19/39)
Outcomes	
Survival	144/145 (99%)
Neurologic function at 1 year	
Number of patients with neurologic function measurements	106 (73%)
Good	63/106 (59%)
Poor	43/106 (41%)
Poor health-related quality of life at 1 year	
Child's self-reported	34% (16/47)
Parent's proxy-reported	35% (17/48)

Legend: Disease activity and estimated damage were measured using the physician global assessment (PGA). The PGA is measured on a continuous scale from 0 to 10, with 0 representing no disease activity/damage, and 10 representing severe disease activity/damage. Neurologic function was measured using the pediatric stroke outcome measure (PSOM), with the presence of significant dysfunction in any of the 5 subdomains (right sensorimotor, left sensorimotor, language production, language comprehension and cognitive/behavioural deficit) indicating poor neurologic function

after diagnosis 47 child self reports and 48 parent proxy reports were completed. A total of 98 patients completed a PedsQL questionnaire at more than one time point. Reasons for inability to complete the PedsQL were language limitations, poor medical status, lack of request by contributing physicians, or death.

The mean PedsQL scores at diagnosis were below the threshold reflecting poor HRQoL for both the child's self-reported (mean 68.4 (range = 20.7–98.9)) and the parent proxy-reported (mean 63.4 (range = 13.0–98.9)). A total of 73 PedsQL questionnaires were completed at diagnosis: 34 child's self-report and 39 parent's proxy-report. Poor HRQoL at diagnosis was reported in 53% (18/34) of children, defined by PedsQL total scores less than or equal to 70, and 48% (19/39) of parents, defined by PedsQL scores of less than or equal to 65.

Mean PedsQL scores trended upward 1 year after diagnosis. A total of 95 PedsQL questionnaires were completed at 1 year after diagnosis; 47 child's self-reports and 48 parent's proxy-reports. The mean child's self-reported PedsQL score 1 year after diagnosis was 72.5 (range = 6.3–98.9), while the mean parent proxy-reported PedsQL score was 66.7 (range = 14.1–95.65). A total of 34% (16/47) of children and 35% (17/48) of parents reported poor HRQoL 1 year after diagnosis.

HRQoL at diagnosis and at 1 year after diagnosis are described in Table 2.

HRQoL subdomain functioning from parent and child perspectives at time-of-diagnosis

The mean child self-reported PedsQL subdomain score at diagnosis were; 67.9 (range = 9.4–100.0) physical functioning, 70.9 (range = 35.0–100.0) emotional functioning, 56.3 (range = 0.0–100.0 school functioning, and 78.7 (range = 0.0–100.0) social functioning. The mean parent proxy-reported PedsQL subdomain scores at diagnosis were; 61.4 (range = 0.0–100.0) physical functioning, 63.8 (range = 20.0–100.0) emotional functioning, 57.4 (range = 0.0–100.0) school functioning, and 74.0 (range = 0.0, 100.0) social functioning (see Fig. 1).

Predictors of impaired HRQoL

The impact of patient characteristics and presenting clinical features on trajectories of HRQoL is summarized in Table 3, with increased risk of impaired HRQoL reflected by more negative parameter estimates.

Children with seizures at diagnosis had an increased risk of poor HRQoL, with dramatic impairments in both physical and psychosocial functioning subdomains. Child's self-reported total PedsQL score at time-of-diagnosis was 15.6 points lower ($p < 0.01$) in children who had seizures at diagnosis, while the parent's proxy-reported total PedsQL score at diagnosis was 11.5 points lower ($p < 0.01$), when compared to patients without seizures. PedsQL physical subdomain score at time-of-diagnosis was lower by 13.4 points ($p < 0.01$) in the child self-report in patients with seizures at diagnosis, and 9.9 points lower at time-of-diagnosis in the parent proxy-report, though not statistically significant ($p = 0.10$). Compared to patients without seizures at diagnosis, the child self-reported psychosocial subdomain PedsQL score at time-of-diagnosis was lower by 16.2 points ($p < 0.01$) in patients with seizures at diagnosis, and the parent proxy-reported psychosocial subdomain PedsQL score at diagnosis was lower by 12.4 points ($p < 0.01$). All reported values are parameter estimates at time-of-diagnosis.

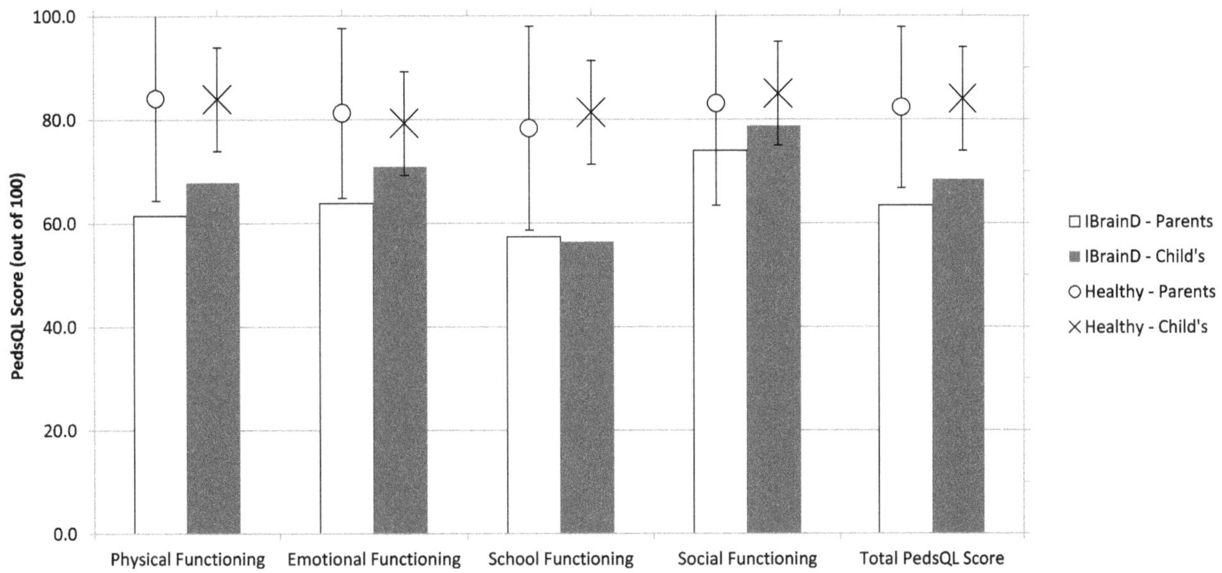

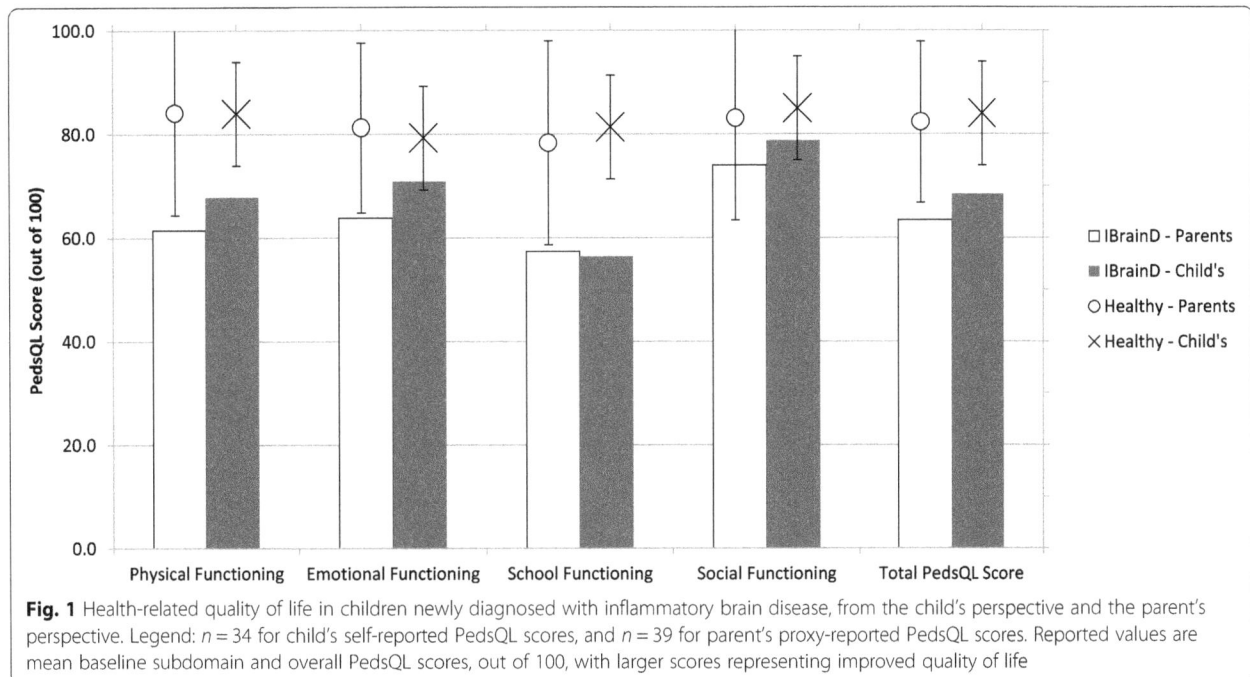

Fig. 1 Health-related quality of life in children newly diagnosed with inflammatory brain disease, from the child's perspective and the parent's perspective. Legend: $n = 34$ for child's self-reported PedsQL scores, and $n = 39$ for parent's proxy-reported PedsQL scores. Reported values are mean baseline subdomain and overall PedsQL scores, out of 100, with larger scores representing improved quality of life

Presenting with cognitive (and/or behavioural) dysfunction was a significant risk factor for impaired functioning across all subdomains. When compared to patients whithout cognitive dysfunction, the child self-reported total PedsQL in patients presenting with cognitive dysfunction was 15.0 points lower ($p < 0.01$) at time-of-diagnosis, the PedsQL physical subdomain score was 14.4 points lower ($p < 0.01$), and PedsQL psychosocial score was 15.3 points lower ($p < 0.01$). In the parent proxy-reports, cognitive dysfunction was associated with a decrease in the total PedsQL at time-of-diagnosis of 15.2 points ($p < 0.01$), and decrease in the psychosocial PedsQL at time-of-diagnosis of 17.7 points ($p < 0.01$). Cognitive dysfunction trended with a physical subdomain score at time-of-diagnosis 11.4 points lower than for those without cognitive dysfunction ($p = 0.07$). All reported values are parameter estimates at time-of-diagnosis, and are presented in Table 3.

Hemiparesis at diagnosis was not found to be a risk factor for impaired HRQoL.Male and female pediatric IBrainD patients did not have statistically different perceptions of physical or psychosocial functioning.

Trajectories of HRQoL

Overall HRQoL, physical functioning, and psychosocial functioning were found to improve with time for all pediatric IBrainD patients, reflected by improving PedsQL scores with increasing log-transformed time from diagnosis. The relative improvement in HRQoL varied according to presenting features.

From the child's perspective, improvement in HRQoL over time was seen in pediatric patients presenting with seizures or with cognitive/behavioural dysfunction relative to patients without these presenting features. This improvement was not observed from the parent's viewpoint. Regression models adjusted for repeated measures showed that the overall HRQoL impairment for pediatric IBrainD patients presenting with seizures decreased with time ($\beta = 2.7$, SE $= 1.4$, $p = 0.05$). From a separate model completed using the same methodology, patients with cognitive/behavioural dysfunction at diagnosis were found to self-report decreased overall HRQoL impairment ($\beta = 3.5$, SE $= 1.5$, $p = 0.02$), as well as decreased impairment in psychosocial functioning over time ($\beta = 3.6$, SE $= 3.9$, $p = 0.02$), when compared to patients without cognitive/behavioural dysfunction at diagnosis. Parent-perceived impairment in psychosocial functioning was found to decrease with log-transformed time for patients with cognitive dysfunction at diagnosis ($\beta = 8.0$, SE $= 3.9$, $p = 0.04$).

By contrast, according to children's self-reports, there was no improvement in physical functioning in patients presenting with either seizures or cognitive dysfunction compared to IBrainD patients who presented without these clinical features. Impairments in psychosocial functioning were not seen to decrease with time in patients presenting with seizures, relative to IBrainD patients without these clinical features. Parents did not perceive a decrease in impairment in overall HRQoL with increasing log-transformed time, for patients with seizures or cognitive dysfunction at diagnosis, compared to reports from parents of IBrainD patients without these clinical features. Parents also did not perceive decreased impairment in psychosocial functioning with increased log-transformed

Table 3 Impact of baseline patient characteristics and presenting clinical features on trajectories of health-related quality of life (HRQoL) over time

	Child self-reported HRQoL Parameter estimate β (SE[b])	*P* value	Parent proxy-reported HRQoL Parameter estimate β (SE[b])	*P* value
Predictors for impaired overall HRQoL trajectories over time				
Female Gender (vs. Male)	−7.6 (4.6)	0.10	−3.8 (4.4)	0.39
Seizures	−15.6 (4.6)[a]	< 0.01	−11.5 (4.4)	< 0.01
Cognitive Dysfunction	− 15.0 (4.8)[a]	< 0.01	−15.2 (4.6)	< 0.01
Hemiparesis	−2.9 (4.6)	0.53	−2.5 (4.4)	0.58
Predictors for impaired physical functioning trajectories over time				
Female Gender (vs. Male)	−8.9 (5.6)	0.12	−7.8 (5.9)	0.19
Seizures	−13.4 (5.7)	0.02	−9.9 (6.0)	0.10
Cognitive Dysfunction	−14.4 (5.9)	0.02	−11.4 (6.2)	0.07
Hemiparesis	−7.3 (5.7)	0.20	−1.7 (5.9)	0.77
Predictors for impaired psychosocial functioning trajectories over time				
Female Gender (vs. Male)	−7.1 (4.7)	0.13	−1.6 (4.3)	0.71
Seizures	−16.2 (4.7)	< 0.01	−12.4 (4.3)	< 0.01
Cognitive Dysfunction	−15.3 (4.9)[a]	< 0.01	−17.7 (4.4)[a]	< 0.01
Hemiparesis	−0.1 (4.7)	0.98	−0.1 (4.7)	0.44

Legend: Health-related quality of life (HRQoL) was measured using PedsQL 4.0 Generic Core Scales. Child-reported HRQoL was measured using the child self-reporting PedsQL questionnaire. PedsQL scores are between 0 and 100, with higher values representing better HRQoL. Negative changes in HRQoL associated with a clinical phenotype therefore represent risk factors for impaired HRQoL. 464 child self-reported PedsQL questionnaires were completed and used in this analysis. Each parameter estimate was derived from a separate, univariable linear regression model, adjusted for time, evaluating the impact of the predictor alongside time on HRQoL. Regression models were adjusted for repeated measures with an autoregressive covariance structure to establish whether these relationships changed statistically significantly with time

$n = 145$ patients

[a]asterisk indicates that the HRQoL impairment associated with the presence of the clinical variable at diagnosis is time-dependent, with the gap in HRQoL between patients with the clinical variable at diagnosis and patients who do not have the clinical variable at diagnosis decreasing with increasing time. This was only assessed in clinical parameters with statistically significant parameter estimates

[b]*SE* Standard error

time for patients with seizures at diagnosis compared to patients without seizures at diagnosis.

Continuous variables with associations with HRQoL

Improvement of HRQoL, reflected by improved PedsQL scores, was associated with older age at diagnosis, increased time between presentation and diagnosis, lower estimated damage at diagnosis, and higher estimated disease activity at diagnosis. Only the association between improvement of HRQoL and higher initial disease activity was statistically significant ($\beta = 8.0$, SE $=3.9$, $p = 0.04$). These trends were not found to significantly change with time.

Discussion

This is the first study to systematically evaluate the impact of pediatric IBrainD on both overall HRQoL and its various subdomains. HRQoL is a multi-dimensional measurement used to estimate burden of disease. In the context of pediatric IBrainD, HRQoL will be critical in ensuring effective dialogue with affected children and families, and shaping future rehabilitation efforts. In IBrainD, the various subdomains of HRQoL are significantly impacted, with the greatest burden of disease in children presenting with cognitive/behavioural dysfunction or seizures.

HRQoL in pediatric patients with IBrainD is significantly impaired, with mean PedsQL scores at diagnosis consistently dramatically lower than mean PedsQL scores in healthy children, as reported by Varni et al., reflecting significant burden of disease [9]. Based on greater than 5000 child self-reports, Varni et al. determined the mean total PedsQL score in healthy children to be 83.9 (SD = 12.5) [9]. This is almost 25% higher than the mean PedsQL score for children with IBrainD. School functioning was found to be the most affected PedsQL subdomain at baseline; Varni et al.'s healthy pediatric population had a mean PedsQL score almost 1.5 times greater than children newly diagnosed with IBrainD [9]. Social functioning was found to be the least affected of all the subdomains, with healthy children scoring 8% higher than pediatric IBrainD patients [9]. The mean physical and emotional subdomain PedsQL scores for healthy children as reported by Varni et al. were 24 and 12% higher, respectively, than those calculated for pediatric patients newly diagnosed with IBrainD [9]. This follows a similar trend to pediatric patients with MS; in a study by MacAllister, 46% of pediatric patients with MS self-reported physical impairment, 42% academic impairment, 28% emotional impairment, and only 14% social impairment at baseline [16]. A study by Russell et al. following adolescents with sports-related concussions found the greatest impairments at clinical presentation to be in the physical and cognitive subdomains [17]. School functioning for patients with IBrainD is especially affected at time of diagnosis, potentially due to extensive school absences owing to hospitalization. Consequently, attention should be given to determine if poor school functioning in children with IBrainD recovers with time or if additional cognitive rehabilitation services are required.

Children presenting with seizures or cognitive/behavioural dysfunction have an especially high risk of long-term impairment of HRQoL, with reduced mean PedsQL scores across all subdomains of HRQoL. These findings were consistent with findings in a study of children following acquired brain injury, where post-injury cognition/learning impairment was associated with worse overall HRQoL, particularly in the psychosocial domain, and post-injury behavioural impairment was moderately associated with reduced psychosocial functioning [18]. It may be postulated that seizures and cognitive/behavioural dysfunction fit within a phenotypic cluster associated with certain conditions previously identified to have poorer prognoses; for example, concentration difficulties, cognitive dysfunction, and mood/personality changes were found to be more common in the APP-cPACNS population, whereas hemiparesis was found to occur more frequently in the APNP-cPACNS cohort and seizures were common in SV-cPACNS [1, 19]. Alternatively, the prognosis of pediatric IBrainD patients with hemiparesis may be more favorable as a result of high availability and routine utilization of targeted physical rehabilitation efforts for children with physical impairment. In comparison, rehabilitation efforts and social services targeting children with seizures or pathological cognitive and/or behavioural dysfunction is typically limited or absent. Though mean HRQoL tended to increase for all patients, as consistent with the 'response shift' process [20], the impairments in functioning associated with seizures were found to persist through time, and the diminished quality of life associated with behavioural/cognitive dysfunction was found to recover only very slowly. More rigorous and targeted attention and intervention should be initiated at diagnosis for this group of patients.

There are a number of limitations to this study. One limitation concerns generalizability to children with IBrainD presenting with severe disability, as acutely hospitalized children with significant impairment were often unable to complete the PedsQL questionnaires. As a result, the true impact was likely underestimated in this study. Specifically, the self-reported pediatric HRQoL for children with cognitive dysfunction at diagnosis was likely significantly poorer than reported, as this population likely encountered significant barriers understanding and completing the PedsQL questionnaires. In addition, while the results are applicable to IBrainD as a whole, they may not be generalizable to all distinct disease subtypes, explaining the variability of patient presentations. For example, while some IBrainDs have abrupt and severe symptom onset, others progress more insidiously, often resulting in a prolonged time to diagnosis. Separation of these disease subtypes may be considered for future studies. Finally, the BrainWorks study was a largely unfunded, international, multi-center study, and accordingly, adherence to study guidelines was variable, resulting in missing and incomplete data. However, as this study is the first to evaluate HRQoL in pediatric IBrainD patients using validated study instruments, it is the only information to date pertaining to the impact of any of the pediatric IBrainDs on perceptions of functioning and disability. Analysis of this data provides valuable initial documentation of the burden of IBrainD.

Conclusion

This study is the first to evaluate the burden of pediatric IBrainD on the HRQoL. While differences of opinion exist regarding whether the greatest value from the PedsQL tool is ascertained through the objective components, such as observation of activity and interaction by parents via the parent-proxy report, or via the subjective component that allows the child to self-report their own experience of impairment, it is agreed upon that the PedsQL can provide valuable insight into the patient experience of illness [10]. IBrainD was found to result in significant HRQoL impairment, with the greatest disabilities in the school functioning and physical functioning subdomains at diagnosis. Children presenting with seizures and cognitive dysfunction were found to have a higher risk of impairment, both at diagnosis and in the future, mandating improvements in rehabilitation and social service strategies targeting these patients. While rehabilitation programs targeting physical deficits are currently robust, there is a clear unmet demand for rehabilitation for children with pathologic cognitive or behavioral dysfunction, targeting psychosocial recovery. Future work should strive to improve the prognosis for children with IBrainD, especially those presenting with risk factors for increased burden of disease. Identification of patients with increased risk of poor HRQoL should be followed by the provision of targeted rehabilitation, which aims to improve functioning in the subdomains predicted to have weak recovery.

Abbreviations

APNP-cPACNS: Angiography-positive non-progressive childhood primary angiitis of the CNS; APP-cPACNS: Angiography-positive progressive childhood primary angiitis of the CNS; cPACNS: Childhood primary angiitis of the CNS; HRQoL: Health-related quality of life; IBrainD: Inflammatory brain disease; MS: Multiple sclerosis; NMDA: N-methyl-D-aspartate; PedsQL: Pediatric Quality of Life Inventory Version 4.0; PedVas: Pediatric Vasculitis Initiative; PGA: Physician global assessment; PSOM: Pediatric stroke outcome measure; SD: Standard deviation; SV-cPACNS: Small vessel childhood primary angiitis of the CNS

Acknowledgements

This BrainWorks cohort study was conducted in the context of the Pediatric Vasculitis Initiative (PedVas) and the authors would like to thank and acknowledge the PedVas Investigator Network. We also thank Dr. Arno Ebner and Dr. Angela Robinson for their contribution of subjects to the BrainWorks Registry subsequently utilized in the analysis of this study.

Funding

CRA-Roche Research Studentship for Elina Liu. The BrainWorks registry was established in 2007 and received research support by the CIHR-funded study, the Pediatric Vasculitis Initiative (PedVas) (TR@-119188), from 2012 to 2018.

Financial disclosure

No financial relationships relevant to this article to disclose.

Authors contributions

All co-authors contributed patients, revised the manuscript and signed off on the final version of the Manuscript. EL, MT, AS, SB, PT were responsible for the concept of the study, the data collection, data analysis, data interpretation and manuscript draft. All authors read and approved the final manuscript.

Competing interests

The authors declare that they have no competing interests.

Author details

[1]Rheumatology, Department of Pediatrics, Alberta Children's Hospital, 2888 Shaganappi Trail NW, Calgary, AB T3B 6A8, Canada. [2]School of Medicine, Queen's University, Kingston, ON, Canada. [3]Cumming School of Medicine, University of Calgary, Calgary, AB, Canada. [4]Alberta Children's Hospital Research Institute, Calgary, AB, Canada. [5]Department of Medical Imaging and Department of Statistical Sciences, University of Toronto, Toronto, ON, Canada. [6]Department of Rheumatology, Hospital for Sick Children, Toronto, ON, Canada. [7]Boston's Children Hospital, Boston, MA, USA. [8]Benioff Children's Hospital, University of California, San Francisco, California, USA. [9]BC Children's Hospital, Vancouver, BC, Canada. [10]Institute of Neuroscience, Newcastle University, Newcastle upon Tyne, UK. [11]Duke Children's Hospital & Health Centre, Durham, North Carolina, USA. [12]Joseph M. Sanzari Children's Hospital, Hackensack, NJ, USA. [13]IWK Health Centre and Dalhousie University, Halifax, NS, Canada. [14]Texas Children's Hospital, Houston, TX, USA. [15]Children's Hospital at Montefiore, Bronx, New York, USA. [16]Akron Children's Hospital, Akron, OH, USA. [17]Charles University in Prague, Prague, Czech Republic. [18]Mother and Child Health Care Institute of Serbia, Belgrade, Serbia.

References

1. Twilt M, Benseler SM. Childhood inflammatory brain diseases: pathogenesis, diagnosis and therapy. Rheumatology (Oxford). 2014;53(8):1359–68.
2. Twilt M, Benseler SM. CNS vasculitis in children. Mult Scler Relat Disord. 2013;2(3):162–71.
3. Cellucci T, Benseler SM. Central nervous system vasculitis in children. Curr Opin Rheumatol. 2010;22(5):590–7.
4. Bigi S, Hladio M, Twilt M, Dalmau J, Benseler SM. The growing spectrum of antibody-associated inflammatory brain diseases in children. Neurol Neuroimmunol Neuroinflamm. 2015;2(92):1–9.
5. Twilt M, Benseler SM. The spectrum of CNS vasculitis in children and adults. Nat Rev Rheumatol. 2012;8:97–107.
6. Dalmau J, Gleichman AJ, Hughes EG, Rossi JE, Peng XY, Lai MZ, et al. Anti-NMDA-receptor encephalitis: case series and analysis of the effects of antibodies. Lancet Neurol. 2008;7(12):1091–8.
7. Cellucci T, Tyrrell PN, Twilt M, Sheikh S, Benseler SM. Distinct phenotype clusters in childhood inflammatory brain diseases: implications for diagnostic evaluation. Arthritis Rheumatol. 2014;66(3):750–6.
8. de Wit M, Hajos T. Health-related quality of life. In: Gellman MD, Turner JR, editors. Encyclopedia of behavioral medicine. New York, NY: Springer New York; 2013. p. 929–31.
9. Varni JW, Burwinkle TM, Seid M, Skarr D. The PedsQL 4.0 as a pediatric population health measure: feasibility, reliability, and validity. Ambul Pediatr. 2003;3(6):329–41.
10. Eiser C. Morse R. a review of measures of quality of life for children with chronic illness. Arch Dis Child. 2001;84:205–11.
11. Kitchen L, Westmacott R, Friefeld S, MacGregor D, Curtis R, Allen A, et al. The pediatric stroke outcome measure: a validation and reliability study. Stroke. 2012;43(6):1602–8.
12. Varni JW, Seid M, Smith Knight T, Burwinkle T, Brown J, Szer IS. The PedsQL in pediatric rheumatology: reliability, validity, and responsiveness of the pediatric quality of life inventory generic Core scales and rheumatology module. Arthritis Rheum. 2002;46(3):714–25.
13. Huang IC, Thompson LA, Chi YY, Knapp CA, Revicki DA, Seid M, et al. The linkage between pediatric quality of life and health conditions: establishing clinically meaningful cutoff scores for the PedsQL. Value Health. 2009;12(5):773–81.
14. Kim J, Chung H, Amtmann D, Salem R, Park R, Askew RL. Symptoms and quality of life indicators among children with chronic medical conditions. Disabil Health J. 2014;7(1):96–104.
15. Lundberg V, Lindh V, Eriksson C, Peterson S, Eurenius E. Health-related quality of life in girls and boys with juvenile idiopathic arthritis: self- and parental reports in a cross-sectional study. Pediatr Rheumatol. 2012;10(33):1–8.
16. MacAllister WS, Christodoulou C, Troxell R, Milazzo M, Block P, Preston TE, et al. Fatigue and quality of life in pediatric multiple sclerosis. Mult Scler. 2009; 15(12):1502–8.
17. Russell K, Selci E, Chu S, Fineblit S, Ritchie L, Ellis M. Longitudinal assessment of health-related quality of life following adolescent sports-related concussion. J Neurotrauma. 2017;34(13):2147–53.
18. Ilmer EC, Lambregts SA, Berger MA, de Kloet AJ, Hilberink SR, Roebroeck ME. Health-related quality of life in children and youth with acquired brain injury: two years after injury. Eur J Paediatr Neurol. 2016;20(1):131–9.
19. Benseler SM. Central nervous system Vasculitis in children. Curr Rheumatol Rep. 2006;8:442–9.
20. Sprangers MAG, Scwartz CE. Integrating response shift into health-related quality of life research: a theoretical model. Soc Sci Med. 1999;48:1507–15.

24

Long-term follow-up of autologous hematopoietic stem cell transplantation for refractory juvenile dermatomyositis: a case-series study

Jia Zhu, Gaixiu Su, Jianming Lai, Boya Dong, Min Kang, Shengnan Li, Zhixuan Zhou and Fengqi Wu*

Abstract

Objective: To follow up the refractory juvenile dermatomyositis (JDM) with autologous hematopoietic stem cell transplantation (AHSCT) in a long time and to investigate whether AHSCT is effective and safe to treat refractory JDM.

Methods: We collected the AHSCT and follow-up data of three patients with refractory JDM who received autologous peripheral blood CD34+ cell transplantation in our hospital between June 2004 and July 2015. Those data include: hight, weight, routine blood and urine tests, ESR, CK, ALT, AST, LDH, renal functional tests, lymphocyte subpopulations, HRCT and muscle MRI. The last follow-up was done in June 2017.

Results: All three patients had complete remission and could stop prednisone after 3–12 months. None of them relapsed at 144, 113 and 23 months follow-up. Twelve months after their AHSCT, all of their monitoring indexes have returned to normal and they have stopped all medications. Until the date of this article, none of them relapsed or need medicine.

Conclusion: Our study suggests that AHSCT is safe and effective in treating refractory JDM, and it can provides long term drug-free survival. However, more cases are needed for further confirmation.

Keywords: Follow-up, Autologous hematopoietic stem cell transplantation, Juvenile dermatomyositis

Introduction

Juvenile dermatomyositis (JDM) is a chronic autoimmune inflammatory disorder of unknown aetiology that mainly affects muscle and skin. The gold standard treatment for JDM is corticosteroids, along with immunomodulatory therapies, which are used to counteract disease activity, prevent mortality, and reduce long-term disability [1]. Although these medications have led to a significant improvement in prognosis, JDM management remains challenging due to the adverse effects associated with conventional therapies and the occurrence of refractory disease.

Autologous hematopoietic stem cell transplantation (AHSCT) as a treatment for autoimmune diseases (AD) was initiated in 1996, and more than 2000 patients with AD have been treated till 2016. The majority of AD being treated with AHSCT are multiple sclerosis (MS), juvenile idiopathic arthritis (JIA), systemic sclerosis (SSc), Crohn's disease and so on. There was an overall 85% 5-year survival and 43% progression-free survival. Around 30% of AD patients had complete remission [2]. The major advantage of AHSCT in treating AD is to eliminate the autoimmune T cell cells clones and alter the natural course of the disease [3].

Therefore, we believe that AHSCT could be a therapeutic option for refractory JDM. However, there are only a few case reports about JDM/DM patients who have recovered with successful AHSCT [4–6] and no articles about the long-term results. Herein, we report the treatment and follow-up of three patients with refractory JDM who received AHSCT in our department since 2004.

* Correspondence: fengqiwu112@2008.sina.com
Division of Rheumatology and Immunology, The Affiliated Children's Hospital, Capital Institute of Pediatrics, Beijing 100020, China

Methods

We retrospectively collected AHSCT and follow-up data of three patients with refractory JDM who received autologous peripheral blood CD34+ cell transplantation between June 2004 and July 2015, including height, weight (according to the criteria of standardised curve of growth of Chinese children by Hui et al. [7, 8], routine blood and urine tests, erythrocyte sedimentation rate (ESR), creatine kinase (CK), alanine transaminase (ALT), aspartate aminotransferase (AST), lactate dehydrogenase (LDH), renal functional tests, lymphocyte subpopulations, lung high resolution computed tomography (HRCT), muscle magnetic resonance imaging (MRI) and academic record in their class ranking. Those three patients were the only JDM patients who received AHSCT between June 2004 and June 2017 in our hospital. We searched our medical records with keywords "myositis" and "transplantation". In June 2017, we did the last follow-up for all of them.

We diagnosed those three patients (2 females, 1 male) with severe and refractory JDM based on the clinical and laboratory criteria proposed by Bohan and Peter [9, 10]. In 2012, the AD guidelines by European Group for Blood and Marrow Transplantation recommended that hematopoietic stem cell transplantation (HSCT) should be considered as a second line therapeutic option or beyond for AD patients with severe progression despite standard and/or approved therapy (level II) [11]. Therefore, all of our three patients met this criteria for HSCT treatment. Some of them failed conventional medication; some had progressive or frequent relapsing disease, which indicated poor prognosis; some had important organs involvement, resulting in a life-threatening condition; and some were intolerable to the toxic side effect of therapeutic drugs.

Mobilisation and collection of autologous CD34+ cells of peripheral blood

CTX (3–4 g/m^2) was admitted intravenously for 2 days. Recombinant human granulocyte colony-stimulating factor (G-CSF) 5 μg/(kg.d) was used for mobilisation when WBC decreased to the lowest level. On the fourth day after using G-CSF, we collected mononuclear cells of peripheral blood with a CS-300 blood cell separator,CD34+ cells with CliniMACS cell separator, and removed 3 to 4 logarithmic degree CD3+ cells.

Preparative regimen

For pretransplant conditioning, high dose CTX (50 mg/kg) was given for 4 days from day − 6 to day − 3. Rabbit antithymocyte globulin (ATG, Saida Company, France) 3.5 mg/(kg•d) was given for 3 days, from day − 4 to day − 2. In day − 2, melphalan 100 mg/(kg•d) was given once. After transplantation of frozen-thawed CD34+ cells on day 0, G-CSF was administered from day 2.

Treatment and follow-up after transplantation

Immunodepressants were stopped after transplantation, but low doses of glucocorticoids was given continuously and tapered gradually. Antibiotics, such as sulfamethoxine, ganciclovir and fluconazole, were used to prevent infection. IVIG was given monthly for 6 months. The patients were evaluated in the outpatient rheumatology department every 1–3 months for half year, then every 6–12 months till June 2017.

Results

The data of three cases

Patient 1 was a 4-year-old male. The onset of the disease was 20 months before the transplantation. He presented with symmetrical proximal muscle weakness, dyspnea, dysphagia and dysphonia. On physical examination, his muscle strength was as following: right lower extremity proximal 1–2/5, distal 3/5; left lower extremity proximal 3/5, distal 4/5; upper extremities proximal 3/5, distal 4/5. He had positive Gottron's sign and heliotrope rash. His laboratory results showed: CK 1200 U/L (0–195 U/L); negative antinuclear antibody (ANA). Electromyogram (EMG) showed myogenic damage. Muscle MRI showed diffuse muscle involvement of proximal legs. HRCT showed mild pulmonary interstitial disease. A left quadriceps biopsy showed extensive muscle atrophy, focal necrosis, small vessel wall degeneration and thickening, fibrous thrombosis, and fatty tissue hyperplasia. Initially we gave him intravenous immunoglobulin (IVIG) (2.0 g/kg per month for 3 months), cyclophosphamide (CTX) (1 g/m^2 body surface area monthly intravenously for 6 months), and high-dose methylprednisolone (MP) (20 mg/kg per day for 3 days) followed with prednisone 2 mg/kg daily. After 6 months of treatment, his rash, expiratory dyspnea, dysphagia and dysphonia improved, but muscle weakness remained. Therefore, we recommended AHSCT and he received the transplantation in June 2005.

Patient 2 was a 7-year-old girl. The onset of the disease was 31 months before AHSCT. Her symptoms included fever, muscle weakness, dysphonia, dyspnea and dysphagia. On physical examination, her muscle power was as following: right lower extremities proximal 2/5, distal 4/5; upper extremities proximal 3/5, distal 3/5. Gottron's sign is positive. Her laboratory results showed serum CK 500 U/L (0–195 U/L) and negative ANA. EMG showed myogenic damage. Muscle MRI showed diffuse muscle enhancement of proximal legs and limbs. HRCT showed severe pulmonary parenchyma and interstitial disease. A right quadriceps biopsy showed denatured, broken and dissolved muscle, along with focal chronic inflammatory cells and positive Masson staining. We intubated her and placed her on a ventilator, and simultaneously gave her IVIG (2.0 g/kg per month•3 months), CTX (1 g/m^2 body surface area intravenously monthly for 6 months), high-dose MP (20 mg/kg daily for 5 days) and followed by prednisone 2 mg/kg daily. Two weeks later, her dyspnea improved, and tracheal intubation was removed. One month later, her dysphagia and dysphonia improved. But the improvement of muscle weakness and rash was not obvious. So we gave her methotrexate (MTX) 15 mg/ m^2 body surface area and cyclosporine A (CsA). Nine months after the initial treatment, her muscle weakness and rash were not improved. Therefore, we recommended AHCST and she received the transplant in January 2008.

Patient 3 was a two and half years old female. The onset of JDM was 6 months before the transplant. She presented with muscle weakness and dysphagia. On physical examination, her muscle strength was as following: lower extremities proximal 2/5, distal 3/5; upper extremities proximal 2/5, distal 3/5. Gottron's sign was positive. Her laboratory tests showed high serum CK 2569 U/L (normal: 0–195 U/L) and negative antinuclear antibody. EMG showed myogenic damage. Muscle MRI showed diffuse muscle involvement of proximal legs. HRCT showed spot shadow in left lung, and focal interlobular septal thickening. Parents refused muscle biopsy. Initially, we gave her IVIG (2.0 g/kg per month•3 months), CTX (1 g/m^2 body surface area intravenously monthly for 5 months), high-dose MP (20 mg/kg daily • 5 days), followed by prednisone 2 mg/kg daily. After 5 months of treatment, her rash and dysphagia improved, but muscle weakness remained the same. Therefore, we recommended AHCST, and the girl received the transplant in July 2015.

Reconstitution of hematopoietic function

Three to eight days after the AHSCT, the leukocyte and lymphocyte levels of all 3 patients decreased to the lowest level (0.01×10^9/L). The platelets decreased to 5–10×10^9/L. Haemoglobin (HGB) decreased to 30–60 g/L. 10 to 14 days after AHSCT, the neutrophils increased to more than 1.0×10^9/L. 14 to 16 days after the AHSCT, the platelets came back to 20×10^9/L. Those results indicated that AHSCT for all three patients were succeeded.

Follow-up of patients' condition

Immunological reconstitution

The immunological function was obviously inhibited after the auto-PBHSCT (Fig. 1). The number of CD4 and CD8 cells remained low within 3 months after the transplantation. 6 months later, the number of CD4+ and CD8+ cells returned to normal.

Clinical manifestation

In the first 6 months after AHSCT, muscle weakness and rash improved slowly for all three patients. However, after 6 months, the improvement was much faster. About 12 months later, all of their monitoring indexes, including immunological function, CK, AST, height, weight and academic record in their class ranking, returned to normal without taking any medication. They remained stable without relapse till this article was written.

Patient 1 has been followed up for 144 months. He didn't show any sign of JDM relapsing, and his immunological function was normal. All of his medications were stopped after HSCT. At last follow-up, his height was 170 cm, and body weight was 50 kg. He went to school as an ordinary student and performed well in class (Fig. 2).

Patient 2 has been followed up for 113 months. During that time, she had no sign of JDM activation. Her immunological function was normal, and she did not take any medication anymore. Her height was 160 cm, and her weight was 42 kg. Her menarch was at 14, and period was regular, 5–7/30 days, with normal volume. She went to school as others and performed well in class (Fig. 3).

Patient 3 has been followed up for 23 months. She had no sign of JDM activation. Her immunological function was normal, and she did not take any medication anymore. Her height was 105 cm, and her weight was 15 kg. She went to kindergarten, and performed well (Fig. 4).

Transplantation-related complications

Patient 1 had fever and cough because of Epstein–Barr virus infection 7 days after the transplantation. He was cured with 3-week introvanous ganciclovir. Patient 2 had no complication after the transplantation. Patient 3 had CMV infection 32 days after the transplantation and recovered with 5-week introvanous ganciclovir. No other complications were found in our three patients. There were no deaths and no graft-versus-host disease in our cases.

Discussion

Our three patients presented with a typical cutaneous change of JDM with diffuse muscle involvement. Since they were not cured by conventional immunosuppressive, they all met the creation for refractory JDM. Till now, it is very difficult to treat refractory JDM. Many researchers have contributed to find out new treatment. In 2011, Pediatric Rheumatology International Trials Organisation (PRINTO) studied 145 patients with recent-onset JDM and 130 patients with one disease flare. It found out that cyclosporine and IVIG were preferred for treating relapse in Europe [12]. In 2012, the Childhood Arthritis and Rheumatology Research Alliance (CARRA) put forward three consensus protocols, including steroids, methotrexate and IVIG, in order to optimize the baseline standard therapy for patients with moderate to severe JDM [13]. However, those medications have unavoidable toxic side effects, such as weight gain, growth delay, gonadoinhibitory and so on. Therefore, we would like to find out a new way to cure refractory JDM, based

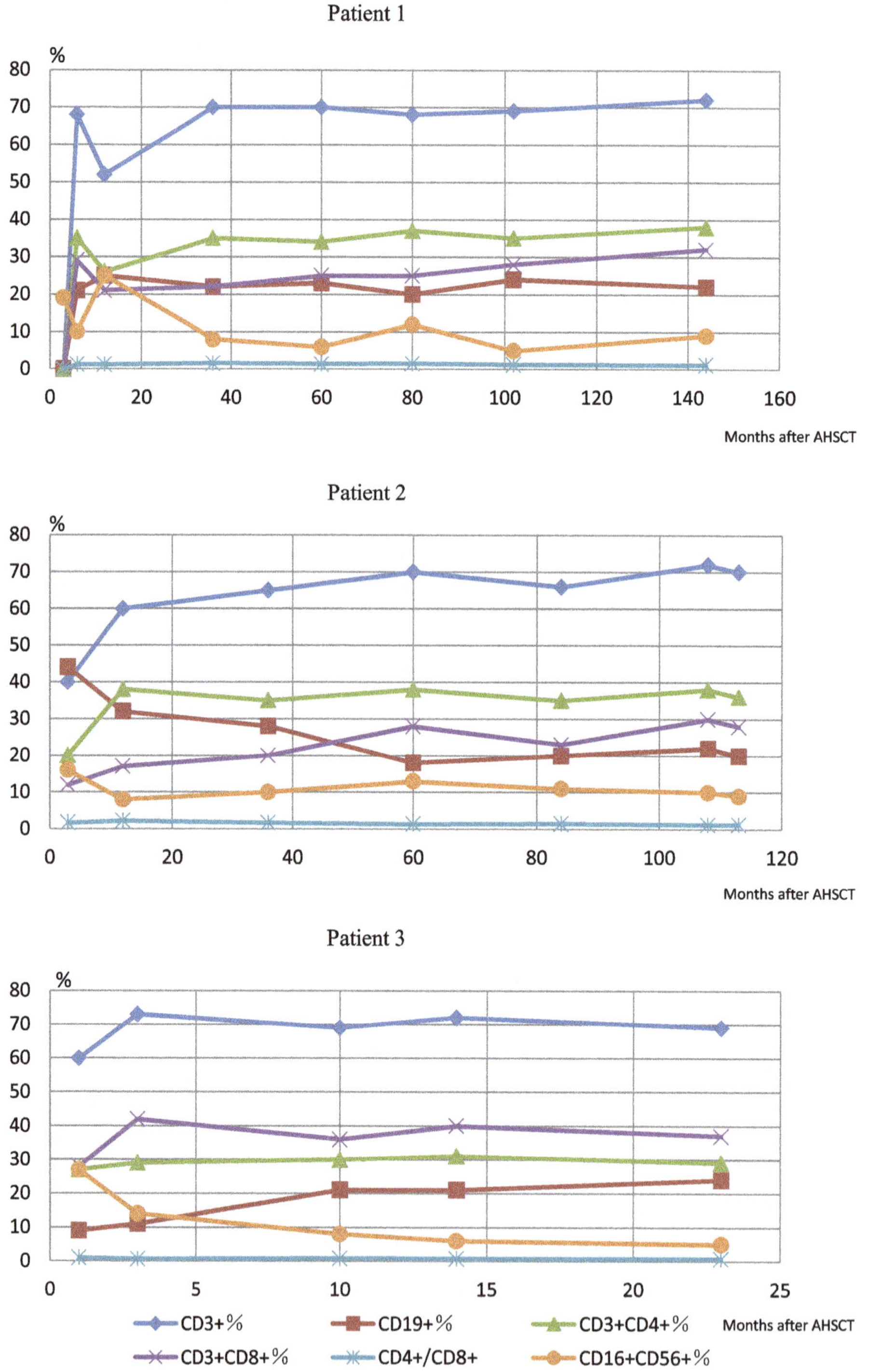

Fig. 1 The proportion of different cells in peripheral blood of three patients after AHSCT

on its possible pathogenesis. Although the aetiology of JDM remains unclear, current theories propose a combination of environmental triggers, immune dysfunction and specific tissue responses as possible causes [14]. Many literatures point out that JDM is a true inflammatory small vessel vasculitis, and cytokines, such as interferons and tumor necrosis factor α, play an important role in the pathogenesis [1, 15]. Besides, literatures showed AHSCT was safe for children [7, 16]. Therefore, we thought that autologous HSCT might be effective and safe for refractory JDM.

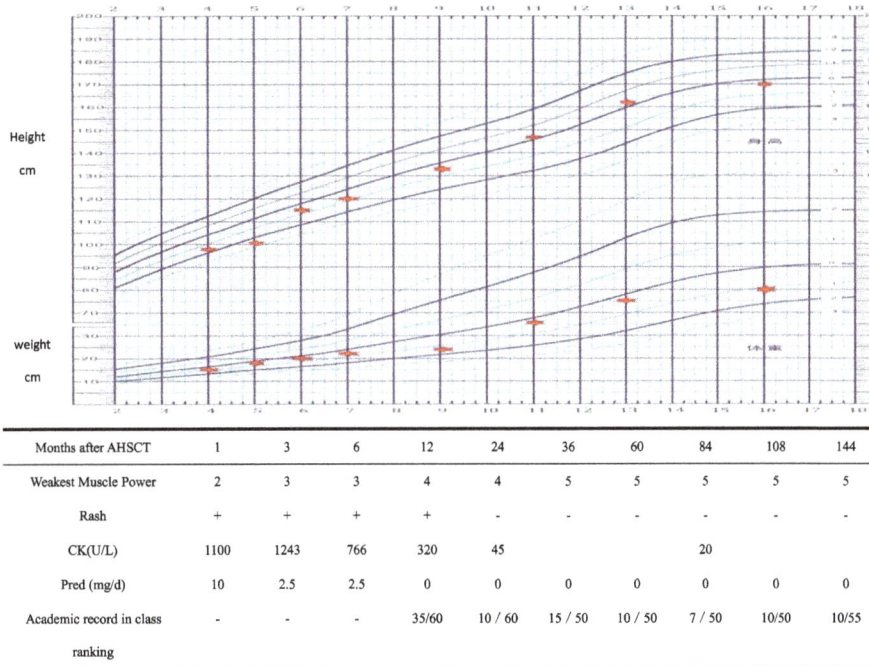

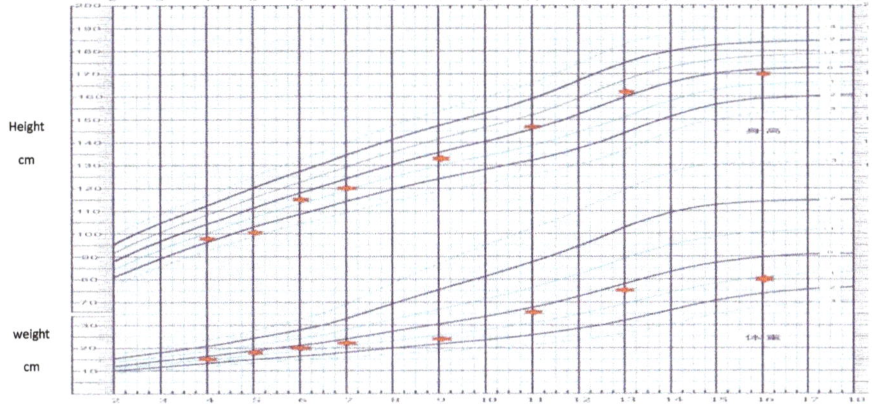

Months after AHSCT	1	3	6	12	24	36	60	84	108	144
Weakest Muscle Power	2	3	3	4	4	5	5	5	5	5
Rash	+	+	+	+	-	-	-	-	-	-
CK(U/L)	1100	1243	766	320	45			20		
Pred (mg/d)	10	2.5	2.5	0	0	0	0	0	0	0
Academic record in class ranking	-	-	-	35/60	10 / 60	15 / 50	10 / 50	7 / 50	10/50	10/55

Fig. 2 Patient 1's height, weight and other clinical characteristics after AHSCT

Autologous HSCT was first reported to treat DM/PM in 2000 [17]. Until now, only 11 cases were reported (Table 1), and 5 of them were children. All of these patients had tried a lot of conventional drugs before HSCT and some of them tried biotherapy (4 cases used rituximab, 2 cases used infliximab, 1 case used alemtuzumab) without any improvement. All of our three patients had tried conventional medicatons for 6 to 31 months before HSCT, but none of them used biologics. During 2005–2008, biologics was rarely used in

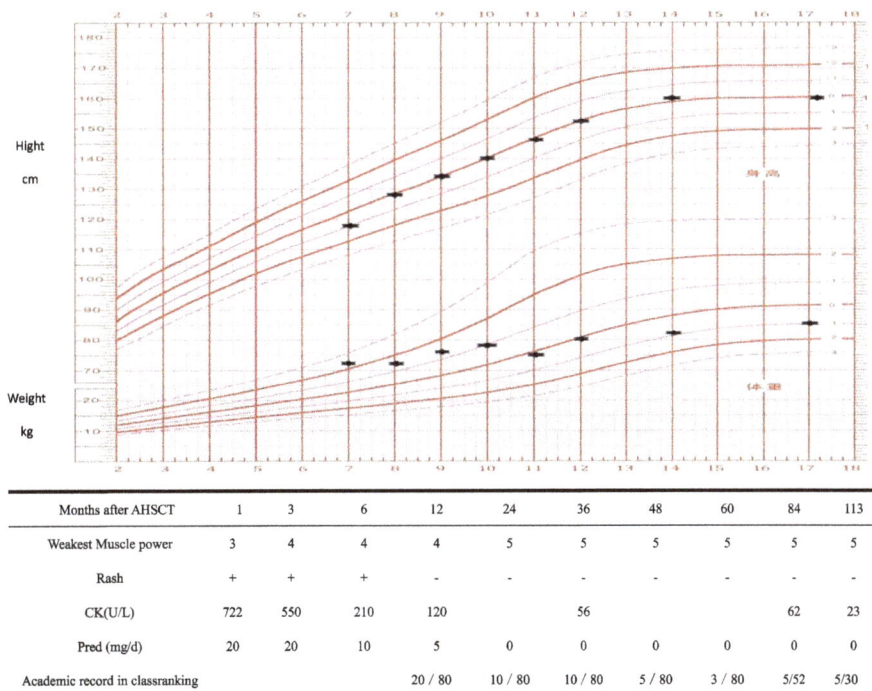

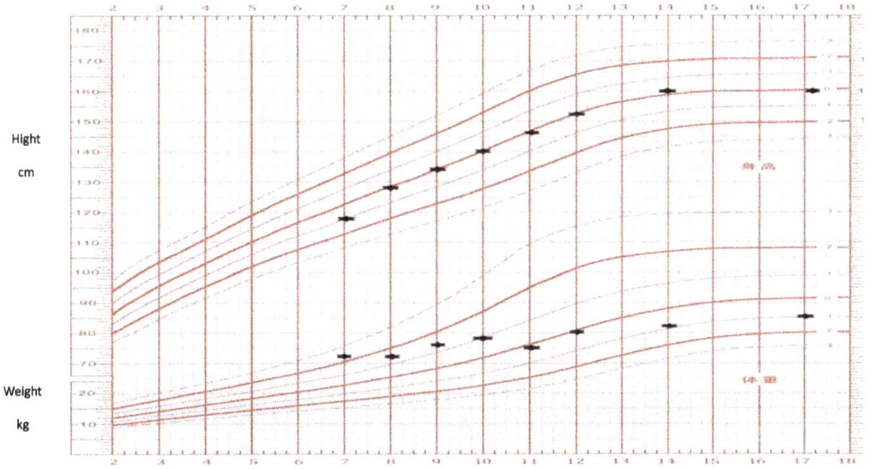

Months after AHSCT	1	3	6	12	24	36	48	60	84	113
Weakest Muscle power	3	4	4	4	5	5	5	5	5	5
Rash	+	+	+	-	-	-	-	-	-	-
CK(U/L)	722	550	210	120		56			62	23
Pred (mg/d)	20	20	10	5	0	0	0	0	0	0
Academic record in classranking				20 / 80	10 / 80	10 / 80	5 / 80	3 / 80	5/52	5/30

Fig. 3 Patient 2's height, weight and other clinical characteristics after AHSCT

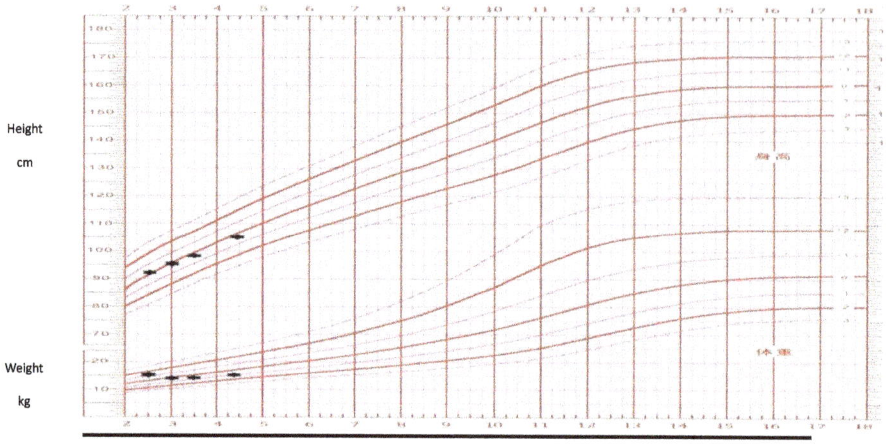

Months after AHSCT	1	3	6	12	23
Weakest Muscle power	3	4	4	4	5
Rash	+	+	-	-	-
CK(U/L)	2890	778	210	190	35
Pred (mg/d)	8	2	0	0	0

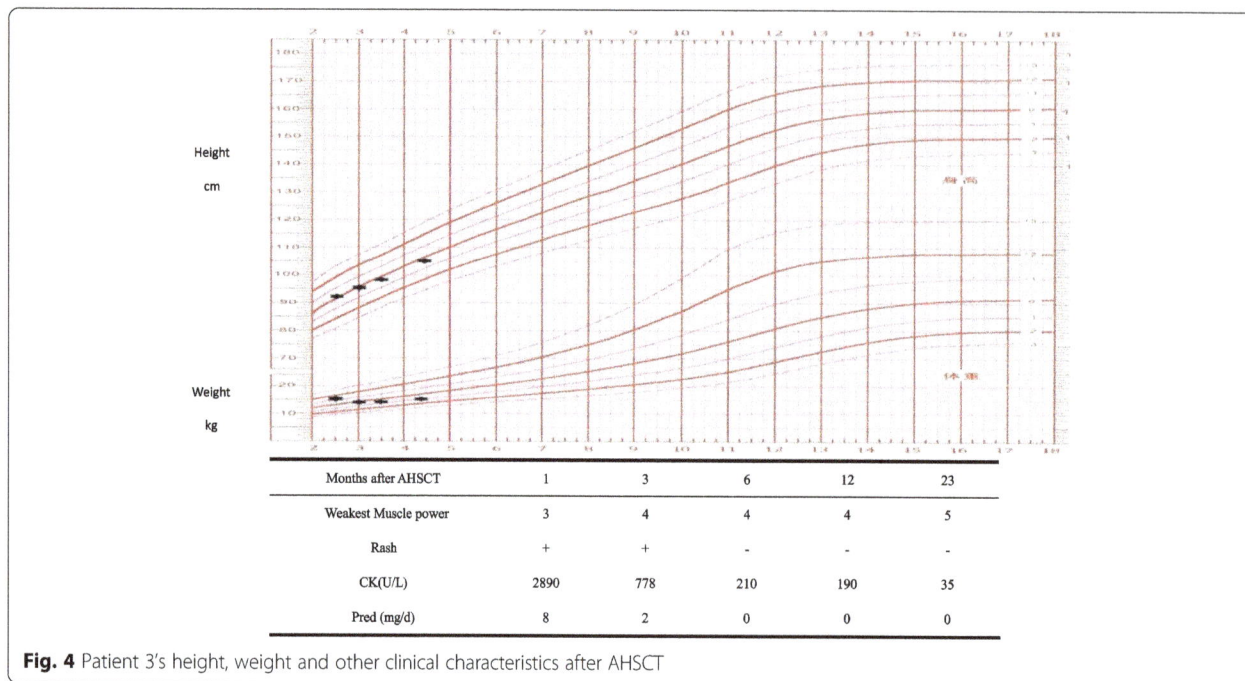

Fig. 4 Patient 3's height, weight and other clinical characteristics after AHSCT

China, and its efficacy in dermatomyositis is not confirmed [15].Therefore, our three patients did not try biologics. [4–6, 17–21]. After AHSCT, 13 cases had improved (13/14), and only one case (1/14) did not. There was no death. Therefore, we and articles verified together that AHSCT was an effective and safe way to treat refractory DM/PM patients.

Stem cells were mobilized by application of 2 g/m^2 cyclophosphamide and subsequent administration of granulocyte colonystimulating factor (G-CSF) in our cases, the same as in reported articles. Chakraverty chose DEX, vincristine and Adriamycin, because his patient had combined multiple myeloma [4]. The conditioning regimens were different among articles. However, CTX and

Table 1 The clinical characteristics of ten cases of DM/PM treated with AHSCT in articles

First Author/Year	diseases	*n*	Gender	age	Treatment before HSCT[a]	Mobilization	Conditioning	Improve	Follow-up (months)	complication
Baron, 2000 [17]	PM	1	Female	28	Pred, AZA, MTX, CTX	CTX + G-CSF	ATG, CTX	yes	12	severe ARDS; fevers and chills by ATG
Chakraverty,2001 [4]	DM	1	Male	46	DEX, vincristine, adriamycin	CTX + G-CSF	melphalan	yes	18	severe mucositis
Bingham, 2001 [21]	PM	1	Female	38	Pred, CTX, CsA, AZA, IVIG, plasmapheresis	CTX + G-CSF	–	yes	24	no
Oryoji, 2005 [5]	DM	1	Female	54	Pred, CsA, CTX	CTX + G-CSF	CTX	Yes	12	Cytomegalovirus antigenemia
Henes, 2009 [18]	PM	1	Male	32	Pred, AZA, MTX, CsA, MMF, IVIG, CTX, alemtuzumab, RTX, IFX	CTX + G-CSF	CTX, ATG	Yes	36	No
Holzer, 2010 [19]	JDM	2	Female	12	Pred, MTX, CsA, IVIG, RTX	CTX + G-CSF	ATG, CTX, fludarabine	yes	26	No
				8	Pred, MTX, CTX, RTX, tacrolimus	CTX + G-CSF	ATG, CTX, fludarabine	Yes	13	No
Storek, 2013 [6]	DM	1	Male	22	Pred, IVIG, AZA, MMF, CTX, CsA, IFX, RTX	CTX + G-CSF	CTX, ATG	no	3	No
Enders,2015 [20]	JDM	3	–	–	–	–	–	Yes	36–60	–

[a] *Pred* is prednisone, *CTX* is cyclophosphamide, *IVIG* is intravenous immunoglobulin, *MTX* is methotrexate, *CsA* is cyclosporine A, *RTX* is rituximab, *IFX* is infliximab, *MMF* is mycophenolate mofetida

ATG were included in almost all regiments. For our three cases, we used CTX, ATG and melphalan as the conditioning regimen, because my first patient (patient 1) received AHSCT in 2005. At that time, no successful case was reported about JDM treated by HSCT. Since our patient responded poorly to immunosuppressants, we gave him an intensive conditioning. All of our three patients were successfully transplanted and improved. After AHSCT, patient 1 and patient 3 developed virus infection, but no other complication or death. According to articles (Table 1), reported complications include three virus infection (3/11), one mycobacterium avium infection (1/11), one acute respiratory distress syndrome (1/11), one ATG allergy (1/11) and one mucositis (1/11). 5 out of 10 patients had no complication after transplantation. No death was reported (0/14). Therefore, we concluded that AHSCT would be a safe treatment for DM/PM.

Our follow-up time was the longest in the literatures. After AHSCT, our 3 patients only received oral prednisone for 3–12 months. Their muscle weakness and rash improved gradually. Twelve months later, all of their monitoring indexes returned to normal and they are not taking any medications. Until this article was written, they all stayed medication free and had no relapse. In 2010, the European Group for Blood and Marrow Transplantation released a long-term follow-up result, including SSc, lupus and JIA, but no exact data of DM/PM. It showed that the 5-year overall survival rate was more than 76%, the transplant related mortality was less than 11% [22]. In 2017, the European Society for Blood and Marrow Transplantation Autoimmune Diseases Working Party recommended that AHSCT should be considered after careful evaluation of patients' medical condition [23]. However, these articles did not clarify whether those patients had long-term immunosuppressive medications or glucocorticoids after transplantation. Our study could show AHSCT is able to cure refractory DM, and may provide long-term drug free survival.

Our study still had some limitations. Firstly, we did not do validated clinical scores, and we just focused on the weakest muscle, which makes it a little difficult to compare with other studies of treatments in this field. Secondly, the follow-up time of the three children was not identical. We will improve our work in future.

Conclusion

Treatment of refractory JDM is challenging. Long-term use of corticosteroids and immunosuppressive agents may cause severe adverse reactions and psychological problem in children. Although there were only a few articles about AHSCT in treating JDM, our study supports that this method could be an effective and safe to treat refractory JDM and provide long-term drug free survival. However, we will need more clinical data to confirm it in the future.

Abbreviation

AD: autoimmune diseases; AHSCT: autologous hematopoietic stem cell transplantation; ALT: alanine transaminase; ANA: antinuclear antibody; AST: aspartate aminotransferase; ATG: antithymocyte globulin; CARRA: Childhood Arthritis and Rheumatology Research Alliance; CK: creatine kinase; CsA: cyclosporine A; CTX: cyclophosphamide; EMG: Electromyogram; ESR: erythrocyte sedimentation rate; G-CSF: granulocyte colony-stimulating factor; HGB: Haemoglobin; HRCT: high resolution computed tomography; HSCT: hematopoietic stem cell transplantation; IVIG: intravenous immunoglobulin; JDM: juvenile dermatomyositis; JIA: juvenile idiopathic arthritis; LDH: lactate dehydrogenase; MP: methylprednisolone; MRI: magnetic resonance imaging; MS: multiple sclerosis; MTX: methotrexate; PRINTO: Pediatric Rheumatology International Trials Organisation; SSc: systemic sclerosis

Acknowledgements

Thank you very much for our colleagues from Department of Hematology in Capital Institute of Pediatrics. During the process of transplantation, you had done so much work.

Funding

The study was funded by The National Natural Science Fund of China (81701618/H1008); Beijing Municipal Administration of Hospital's Youth Programme(QML20171301); Beijing Talents Fund (2014000021469G225); Science Foundation of Capital Institute of Pediatrics(PY-2017-06).

Authors' contributions

All authors were involved in drafting the article or revising it critically for important intellectual content, and all authors approved the final version to be published. Dr. Zhu and Wu had full access to all of the data in the study and take responsibility for the integrity of the data and the accuracy of the data analysis.Study conception and design. J Z, G S, F W. Acquisition of data. J L, M K, S L, Z Z, J Z, F W. Analysis an interpretation of data. J Z, F W, B D. All authors read and approved the final manuscript

Competing interests

The authors declare that they have no competing interests.

References

1. Pagnini I, Vitale A, Selmi C, Cimaz R, Cantarini L. Idiopathic inflammatory myopathies: an update on classification and treatment with special focus on juvenile forms. Clin Rev Allergy Immunol. 2017;52(1):34–44.
2. Tyndall A, van Laar JM. Stem cell transplantation and mesenchymal cells to treat autoimmune diseases. Presse Med. 2016;45(6 Pt 2):e159–69.
3. Ramaswamy S, Jain S, Ravindran V. Hematopoietic stem cell transplantation for auto immune rheumatic diseases. World J Transplant. 2016;6(1):199–205.
4. Chakraverty R, Rabin N, Peggs K, Robinson S, Duncan JR, Yong K. Dermatomyositis and sarcoid-like reaction associated with multiple myeloma treated effectively by high-dose chemotherapy and autologous peripheral blood stem cell transplantation. Bone Marrow Transplant. 2001;27(11):1215–7.

5. Oryoji K, Himeji D, Nagafuji K, Horiuchi T, Tsukamoto H, Gondo H, et al. Successful treatment of rapidly progressive interstitial pneumonia with autologous peripheral blood stem cell transplantation in a patient with dermatomyositis. Clin Rheumatol. 2005;24(6):637–40.
6. Storek J, LeClercq SA, Aaron SL. Lack of sustained response of advanced dermatomyositis to autologous haematopoietic cell transplantation. Scand J Rheumatol. 2013;42(5):421–2.
7. Su G, Luan Z, Wu F, Wang X, Tang X, Wu N, et al. Long-term follow-up of autologous stem cell transplantation for severe paediatric systemic lupus erythematosus. Clin Rheumatol. 2013;32(12):1727–34.
8. Wulffraat NM, de Kleer IM, Prakken B. Refractory juvenile idiopathic arthritis: using autologous stem cell transplantation as a treatment strategy. Expert Rev Mol Med. 2006;8(26):1–11.
9. Bohan A, Peter JB. Polymyositis and dermatomyositis (second of two parts). N Engl J Med. 1975;292:403–7.
10. Bohan A, Peter JB. Polymyositis and dermatomyositis (first of two parts). N Engl J Med. 1975;292:344–7.
11. Snowden JA, Saccardi R, Allez M, Ardizzone S, Arnold R, Cervera R, et al. Haematopoietic SCT in severe autoimmune diseases: updated guidelines of the European group for blood and marrow transplantation. Bone Marrow Transplant. 2012;47(6):770–90.
12. Hasija R, Pistorio A, Ravelli A, Demirkaya E, Khubchandani R, Guseinova D, et al. Therapeutic approaches in the treatment of juvenile dermatomyositis in patients with recentonset disease and in those experiencing disease flare: an international multicenter PRINTO study. Arthritis Rheum. 2011; 63:3142–52.
13. Huber AM, Robinson AB, Reed AM, Abramson L, Bout-Tabaku S, Carrasco R, et al. Subcommittee of the Childhood Arthritis and Rheumatology Research Alliance Consensus treatments for moderate juvenile dermatomyositis: beyond the first two months. Results of the second childhood arthritis and rheumatology research Alliance consensus conference. Arthritis Care Res. 2012;64:546–53.
14. Wedderburn LR, Rider LG. Juvenile dermatomyositis: new developments in pathogenesis, assessment and treatment. Best Pract Res Clin Rheumatol. 2009;23:665–78.
15. Papadopoulou C, Wedderburn LR. Treatment of juvenile dermatomyositis: an update. Paediatr Drugs. 2017;19(5):423–34.
16. Milanetti F, Abinun M, Voltarelli JC, Burt RK. Autologous hematopoietic stem cell transplantation for childhood autoimmune disease. Pediatr Clin N Am. 2010;57(1):239–71.
17. Baron F, Ribbens C, Kaye O, Fillet G, Malaise M, Beguin Y. Effective treatment of Jo-1-associated polymyositis with T-cell-depleted autologous peripheral blood stem cell transplantation. Br J Haematol. 2000;110(2):339–42.
18. Henes JC, Heinzelmann F, Wacker A, Seelig HP, Klein R, Bornemann A, et al. Antisignal recognition particle-positive polymyositis successfully treated with myeloablative autologous stem cell transplantation. Ann Rheum Dis. 2009;68(3):447–8.
19. Holzer U, van Royen-Kerkhof A, van der Torre P, Kuemmerle-Deschner J, Well C, Handgretinger R, et al. Successful autologous stem cell transplantation in two patients with juvenile dermatomyositis. Scand J Rheumatol. 2010;39(1):88–92.
20. Enders FB, Delemarre EM, Kuemmerle-Deschner J, van der Torre P, Wulffraat NM, Prakken BP, et al. Autologous stem cell transplantation leads to a change in proinflammatory plasma cytokine profile of patients with juvenile dermatomyositis correlating with disease activity. Ann Rheum Dis. 2015;74(1):315–7.
21. Bingham S, Griffiths B, McGonagle D, Snowden JA, Morgan G, Emery P. Autologous stem cell transplantation for rapidly progressive Jo-1-positive polymyositis with long-term follow-up. Br J Haematol. 2001;113(3):840–1.
22. Farge D, Labopin M, Tyndall A, Fassas A, Mancardi GL, Van Laar J, et al. Autologous hematopoietic stem cell transplantation for autoimmune diseases: an observational study on 12 years' experience from the European Group for Blood and Marrow Transplantation Working Party on autoimmune diseases. Haematologica. 2010;95:284–92.
23. Farge D, Burt RK, Oliveira MC, Mousseaux E, Rovira M, Marjanovic Z, et al. Cardiopulmonary assessment of patients with systemic sclerosis for hematopoietic stem cell transplantation: recommendations from the European Society for Blood and Marrow Transplantation Autoimmune Diseases Working Party and collaborating partners. Bone Marrow Transplant. 2017;52(11):1495–503.

25

Dutch juvenile idiopathic arthritis patients, carers and clinicians create a research agenda together following the James Lind Alliance method: a study protocol

Casper G. Schoemaker[1,2,3,22*], Wineke Armbrust[4,5], Joost F. Swart[1,5,6], Sebastiaan J. Vastert[1,6], Jorg van Loosdregt[1,6], Anouk Verwoerd[1,6], Caroline Whiting[7], Katherine Cowan[7], Wendy Olsder[8], Els Versluis[2], Rens van Vliet[1,2], Marlous J. Fernhout[1,2], Sanne L. Bookelman[2], Jeannette Cappon[9,10], J. Merlijn van den Berg[11,5], Ellen Schatorjé[12,13,5], Petra C. E. Hissink Muller[14,15,5], Sylvia Kamphuis[15,5], Joke de Boer[16,6], Otto T. H. M. Lelieveld[17,10], Janjaap van der Net[18,10,6], Karin R. Jongsma[19], Annemiek van Rensen[20], Christine Dedding[21] and Nico M. Wulffraat[1,6]

Abstract

Background: Research on Juvenile Idiopathic Arthritis (JIA) should support patients, caregivers/parents (carers) and clinicians to make important decisions in the consulting room and eventually to improve the lives of patients with JIA. Thus far these end-users of JIA-research have rarely been involved in the prioritisation of future research.

Main body: Dutch organisations of patients, carers and clinicians will collaboratively develop a research agenda for JIA, following the James Lind Alliance (JLA) methodology. In a 'Priority Setting Partnership' (PSP), they will gradually establish a top 10 list of the most important unanswered research questions for JIA. In this process the input from clinicians, patients and their carers will be equally valued. Additionally, focus groups will be organised to involve young people with JIA. The involvement of all contributors will be monitored and evaluated. In this manner, the project will contribute to the growing body of literature on how to involve young people in agenda setting in a meaningful way.

Conclusion: A JIA research agenda established through the JLA method and thus co-created by patients, carers and clinicians will inform researchers and research funders about the most important research questions for JIA. This will lead to research that really matters.

Keywords: Juvenile Idiopathic Arthritis (JIA), Research agenda, James Lind Alliance, Patient involvement

Background

Research priority setting involving the end-users of knowledge is clearly needed in order to formulate research questions that can really make a difference [1–3]. In a recent review, Odgers et al. reported a substantial increase in the number of research priority setting initiatives in paediatric chronic disease since 2010, generating a broad range of priorities shared across multiple conditions [4]. Unfortunately, the methodology was generally inadequately described. This lack of clarity raises concerns over the legitimacy and relevance of identified priorities. Odgers et al. suggested that the available systematic methods of priority setting should be used more often [4].

Patient and parent/caregiver (carer) involvement in establishing research priorities is crucial in generating a research agenda that encompasses the full spectrum of issues that affects paediatric patients with chronic

* Correspondence: C.G.Schoemaker-3@umcutrecht.nl
[1]Pediatric Rheumatology and Immunology, Wilhelmina Children's Hospital, University Medical Center Utrecht, Utrecht, Netherlands
[2]Netherlands JIA Patient and Parent Organisation, member of ENCA, Amsterdam, The Netherlands
Full list of author information is available at the end of the article

disease [5–9]. Thus far, their involvement in research priority appears to be limited. Only approximately one-in-four studies reported some parental/caregiver involvement, and only 5% involved children directly [4]. Furthermore, qualitative research showed that the involvement of patients and carers seems to be challenging: real co-design does not happen by itself [3]. Therefore, precautionary measures need to be taken to empower patients and carers [7], and their involvement in the process should be monitored and evaluated [4, 10].

As noted above, understanding young people's research priorities is crucial to develop research that is in tune with their needs [4, 11, 12]. However, some researchers have reported challenges to collaborating with young people in health research [12–14]. More recently, there appears to be increasing efforts to involve children and adolescents in research priority setting [7, 11, 12, 15]. Parsons et al. organised 13 focus groups involving young people with rheumatic diseases, aged 11–24, to explore what they believed to be important research questions regarding their condition [12, 16]. They provided evidence that even younger adolescents (11–15 years) are equipped to discuss and prioritise scientific research even if they are relatively research naive [16].

In 2018 four Dutch organisations of patients, parents and clinicians will start to establish a research agenda for Juvenile Idiopathic Arthritis (JIA). The research agenda was initiated by the Netherlands JIA patient and parent organisation (Dutch Juvenile Arthritis Association: DJAA), a member organisation of the European Network for Children with Arthritis (ENCA). Three other Dutch organisations are involved: the Dutch network organisation for young arthritis patients (16–30 years old) Youth-R-Well.com, the Dutch Association for Pediatric Rheumatology (DAPR) and the Dutch Health Professionals in Pediatric Rheumatology (DHPPR). The project will be based at the Pediatric Rheumatology and Immunology department of the Wilhelmina Children's Hospital (WKZ) in Utrecht. DAPR, DJAA and WKZ funded the project. Amsterdam UMC will develop and lead the focus groups for young people with JIA, and enable them to have effective and fulfilling participation in the whole process. PGO-support, a Dutch networking organisation for patient organisations will issue an independent process evaluation of the PSP. The Department of Medical Ethics at the Julius Center of the UMC Utrecht will perform the research concerning the process evaluation.

In this paper, the project is outlined briefly. We discuss how we will address the aforementioned questions on the use of systematic methods and the feasibility of meaningful patient and caregiver participation in research agenda setting. Formulating a research agenda is not a goal in itself [2, 17]. Finally, we will describe how we aim to inspire researchers and research funders by the defined priorities when preparing for and guiding funding new research projects.

Main text

In a recent review on patient and public engagement in priority setting, Manafo et al. described four highly structured deliberative methods that are inclusive and objectively based, specific to the priorities of all stakeholders engaged in the process [5]. Two of these methods have successfully been applied in the Netherlands: The Dialogue Method and the James Lind Alliance (JLA) Priority Setting Partnerships [18, 19]. Both methods are clearly suited for this purpose [5, 20]. Eventually, we chose the JLA method as it proved to be very effective in implementing agendas in calls for research. United Kingdom's National Institute for Health Research (NIHR) and several funding charities, for example Marie Curie, the Multiple Sclerosis Society and Parkinson's UK, have adopted the research agendas as an important part of their research funding strategy [21].

The James Lind Alliance (JLA) is a non-profit initiative established in the United Kingdom (UK) in 2004 by Sir Iain Chalmers [22]. The JLA team is positioned at the NIHR Evaluation, Trials and Studies Coordinating Centre (NETSCC), based at the University of Southampton in the UK. The goal of the JLA is to bring together the end users of scientific knowledge – patients, carers and clinicians – to jointly formulate a research agenda for a disease or type of care. In a so-called 'Priority Setting Partnership' (PSP) they gradually establish a top-10 list of the most important unanswered questions for their health area of interest [23].

Until now about 70 different Top 10s have been published. More information on the content and the background of these Top 10s can be found on the JLA website [24]. In 2015, Chalmers and colleagues compared the prioritised unanswered questions of several PSPs to the research questions they found in registered clinical trials. They demonstrated that the JLA method identifies questions and themes that are not yet being addressed in current studies [2].

The JLA method consists of 5 steps: setting up the steering group, gathering uncertainties, data processing and verifying uncertainties, interim priority setting, and final priority setting (see Table 1). In a free internet-based Guidebook the JLA method has been described in more detail [23]. Following these five steps, it takes approximately twelve to eighteen months to formulate a research agenda [23].

A PSP is led by a steering group (10–15 people) that coordinates the PSP and organises the activities [23]. The Dutch JIA-PSP steering group will be led by a carer and a pediatric rheumatologist. The steering group will include representatives of patients (i.c. adult JIA-patients),

Table 1 The priority setting process in the James Lind Alliance methodology

Step in the process	Description
1. Setting up the steering group	A PSP is led by a steering group that coordinates the PSP and organises the activities. It will include representatives of patients, carers and clinicians.
2. Gathering uncertainties	An electronic survey questionnaire is distributed widely. Patients, carers and clinicians will be asked: "What questions would you like answered to improve the health and wellbeing of people with JIA?" For young people with JIA focus groups will be organised. Research recommendations stated in systematic reviews and clinical guidelines are searched for as well (i.c. the Dutch JIA-medication guideline and the European SHARE initiative).
3. Data processing and verifying uncertainties	Out-of-scope submissions are removed. The eligible submissions are categorised and rephrased as researchable questions. Duplicates and very similar submissions are combined. Questions that have already been answered in relevant good quality research will be removed.
4. Interim priority setting	The long list of in-scope verified uncertainties goes into an electronic interim priority setting survey. Patients, carers and clinicians are asked to choose (and possibly also rank) the 10 uncertainties from the list that are most important in their experience. Completed interim prioritisation results are grouped into patients, carers and clinicians, and separate scores kept to ensure fair weighting of the constituent groups. The top 25–30 questions are taken to the final workshop.
5. Final priority setting	In a final day-long workshop, 20–30 people (patients, carers and clinicians) discuss the questions and gradually agree on the final order of priority of the list, focusing especially on agreeing a 'Top 10'. The Top 10 will be published on the JLA website, and in a peer reviewed journal.

carers (i.c. parents) and clinicians (i.c. pediatric rheumatologists, ophthalmologists, physiotherapists and nurses,). The four previously mentioned organisations recruited their members for the steering group. Four groups – pediatric rheumatologists, other health professionals, patients and parents – will be equally represented in the steering group. The two PSP Leaders made a selection for the pediatric rheumatologists, and invited one of the centers to invite one of their nurse practitioners, in order to achieve a balanced representation of clinicians of all 6 academic centres including their affiliated rehabilitation centre within the steering group. These decisions were made in collaboration with the chairs of both organisations. Furthermore, all Dutch centers for pediatric rheumatology will be represented in this steering group. A MD PhD-student coordinates the JIA-PSP, reviews the data collected, identifies the existing research evidence, and formulates potential research questions with input from the steering group. The PSP will be supported and guided by a trained JLA Adviser [23].

According to Odgers et al., the JLA approach may not be very well suited to children with chronic disease [4]. It demands creative and developmentally appropriate strategies to empower children to reflect on their situation, and how research could benefit them and to articulate their priorities [25, 26]. Inspired by the work of Parsons et al. we will organise additional focus group meetings involving children and adolescents with JIA. This established qualitative method allows the participants to draw from other participant's knowledge and allows for a conversation among peers [25].

Specific themes and research questions formulated by these young patients will be added to our dataset of uncertainties from the survey. In the focus groups the young patients will discuss how they wish to be involved in the process and which arrangements need to be made in order for them to participate successfully. The results of the focus group will be discussed in the second meeting of the steering group. This may change the involvement of young patients in the process onwards.

Some precautionary measures to empower patients and carers are built into the JLA method. Patients and carers take part in the steering group. We will ensure that the chairing of the steering group is fair and neutral so as not to favour one group over another. The final priority setting workshop of the PSP is attended by patients and carers as well as clinicians and the opinions of all people at the workshop are valued equally [23]. The JLA supports an adapted Nominal Group Technique for PSPs choosing their priorities during the final workshop. One benefit of this technique is that it prevents the domination of discussion by a single person and encourages the participation of less assertive members. There is no hierarchy between the different participants; no one individual or group's views or experiences are more valid than another's. Nominal Group Technique is a well-established and well-documented approach to decision making. Despite these measures, engaging patients and carers in the complexities of health science based discussions of uncertainty is challenging [27]. To empower patients and carers in the steering group, most of them received a two-day training as a patient partner in research [28].

A process evaluation with a specific focus on the ethical aspects of the decision-making process is conducted parallel to the priority setting process [10, 27]. In the process evaluation, issued by PGOsupport and executed by a researcher from the Julius Center, attention will be paid to the inclusion of different stakeholders, their influence on the priority setting as well as facilitating and limiting factors for equal deliberation between the different stakeholders. For this, the researcher from the Julius Center will observe all key meetings during the project and perform additional interviews among the stakeholder groups. Important deliverables include evaluation of the suitability of the JLA method for patient organisations that aim to take a role as partner and/or driving force in scientific research; identification of critical success factors during the process in relation to patient representation; identification of specific requirements for appropriate involvement of children and adolescents. PGOsupport will disseminate the results of the evaluation via the relevant media in order to inform other patient organisations that consider a similar approach.

Formulating a research agenda for JIA is not a goal in itself. It is important that researchers and research funders are inspired by the defined priorities when preparing for and funding new research projects. Therefore all Dutch academic centers for pediatric rheumatology will be represented in the steering group. We will present our results at a 2019 meeting of a large Dutch/Canadian research project on personalised medicine, UCAN CAN-DU, funded by the Netherlands Organisation for Health Research and Development ZONMW, the Canadian Institutes of Health Research (CIHR) and Dutch Arthritis Foundation (ReumaNederland), to inspire further JIA-research. Funding agencies will be invited for our final workshop. Members and ambassadors of the Dutch JIA-PSP are involved in European organisations like ENCA, Paediatric Rheumatology European Society (PReS) and the European League Against Rheumatism (EULAR). Collectively, these measures will ensure the optimal implementation of the research agenda in different "layers" of research.

Conclusions

In 2018 four Dutch organisations for JIA-patients, parents, pediatric rheumatologists and health professionals will initiate a PSP for JIA, following the JLA methodology. This research agenda, will be established in 2019, and will improve the relevance of JIA-research in the Netherlands and beyond. This will not only benefit patients, parents and clinicians in the consulting room, but also the JIA-researchers themselves since their research will really matter to the people that need it most.

Abbreviations

CIHR: Canadian Institutes of Health Research; DAPR: Dutch Association for Pediatric Rheumatology; DHPPR: Dutch Health Professionals in Pediatric Rheumatology; DJAA: Dutch Juvenile Arthritis Association:; ENCA: European Network for Children with Arthritis; EULAR: European League Against Rheumatism; JIA: Juvenile Idiopathic Arthritis; JLA: James Lind Alliance; NETSCC: NIHR Evaluation, Trials and Studies Coordinating Centre; NIHR: National Institute for Health Research (NIHR); PGOsupport: Dutch networking organisation for patient organisations; PReS: Paediatric Rheumatology European Society; PSP: Priority Setting Partnership; UCAN CAN-DU: Canada – Netherlands Personalized Medicine Network in Childhood Arthritis and Rheumatic diseases; WKZ: Wilhelmina Children's Hospital; Youth-R-Well.com: Dutch network organisation for young arthritis patients (16–30 years old); ZONMW: Netherlands Organisation for Health Research and Development

Authors' contributions

CGS wrote the manuscript. All authors revised and approved the final manuscript.

Competing interests

The authors declare that they have no competing interests.

Author details

[1]Pediatric Rheumatology and Immunology, Wilhelmina Children's Hospital, University Medical Center Utrecht, Utrecht, Netherlands. [2]Netherlands JIA Patient and Parent Organisation, member of ENCA, Amsterdam, The Netherlands. [3]National Institute for Public Health and the Environment (RIVM), Bilthoven, The Netherlands. [4]University Medical Center Groningen (UMCG), Beatrix Childrens Hospital, Dept Pediatric Rheumatology and Immunology, University of Groningen, Groningen, The Netherlands. [5]Dutch Association for Pediatric Rheumatology, Amsterdam, The Netherlands. [6]Faculty of Medicine, Utrecht University, Utrecht, The Netherlands. [7]James Lind Alliance, National Institute for Health Research Evaluation, Trials and Studies Coordinating Centre (NETSCC), based at the University of Southampton, Southampton, UK. [8]Youth-R-Well.com, Young Patient Organisation, The Netherlands, member of EULAR PARE, Amsterdam, The Netherlands. [9]Reade, Centre for Rehabilitation and Rheumatology, Department Rehabilitation, Amsterdam, The Netherlands. [10]Dutch Health Professionals in Pediatric Rheumatology (DHPPR), Amsterdam, The Netherlands. [11]Paediatric rheumatology, Emma Children's Hospital, University Medical Centre Amsterdam, Amsterdam, The Netherlands. [12]Paediatric Rheumatology, Amalia Children's Hospital, Radboudumc, Nijmegen, The Netherlands. [13]Paediatric Rheumatology, St. Maartenskliniek, Nijmegen, The Netherlands. [14]Paediatric Rheumatology, Leiden University Medical Centre, Leiden, The Netherlands. [15]Paediatric Rheumatology, Sophia Children's Hospital, Erasmus University Medical Centre, Rotterdam, The Netherlands. [16]Department of Ophthalmology, University Medical Centre Utrecht, Utrecht, The Netherlands. [17]University Medical Center Groningen, Center for Rehabilitation, University of Groningen, Groningen, The Netherlands. [18]Child Development and Exercise Center, Division of Pediatrics. Wilhelmina Children's Hospital, University Medical Centre Utrecht, Utrecht, The Netherlands. [19]Julius Center for Health Sciences and Primary Care Utrecht, University Medical Center Utrecht, Utrecht, The Netherlands. [20]PGOsupport, Dutch Networking Organisation for Patient Organisations, Utrecht, The Netherlands. [21]Department of Medical Humanities, Amsterdam UMC, Amsterdam, The Netherlands. [22]Department of Paediatric Rheumatology, University Medical Centre Utrecht, Wilhelmina Children's Hospital, Room KC.03.063.0, P.O. box 85090, 3508 AB Utrecht, The Netherlands.

References

1. Macleod MR, et al. Biomedical research: increasing value, reducing waste. Lancet. 2014;383(9912):101–4.
2. Crowe S, et al. Patients', clinicians' and the research communities' priorities for treatment research: there is an important mismatch. Res Involv Engagem. 2015;1:2.
3. Abma TA, Broerse JE. Patient participation as dialogue: setting research agendas. Health Expect. 2010;13(2):160–73.
4. Odgers HL, et al. Research priority setting in childhood chronic disease: a systematic review. Arch Dis Child. 2018. https://doi.org/10.1136/archdischild-2017-314631.
5. Manafo E, et al. Patient and public engagement in priority setting: a systematic rapid review of the literature. PLoS One. 2018;13(3):e0193579.
6. Tong A, et al. Children's experiences of living with juvenile idiopathic arthritis: a thematic synthesis of qualitative studies. Arthritis Care Res (Hoboken). 2012;64(9):1392–404.
7. Bate J, et al. Public and patient involvement in paediatric research. Arch Dis Child Educ Pract Ed. 2016;101(3):158–61.
8. Gomez-Ramirez O, et al. A recurring rollercoaster ride: a qualitative study of the emotional experiences of parents of children with juvenile idiopathic arthritis. Pediatr Rheumatol Online J. 2016;14(1):13.
9. Eyckmans L, et al. What does it mean to grow up with juvenile idiopathic arthritis? A qualitative study on the perspectives of patients. Clin Rheumatol. 2011;30(4):459–65.
10. Bryant J, et al. Health research priority setting in selected high income countries: a narrative review of methods used and recommendations for future practice. Cost Eff Resour Alloc. 2014;12:23.
11. McDonagh JE, Bateman B. 'Nothing about us without us': considerations for research involving young people. Arch Dis Child Educ Pract Ed. 2012;97(2):55–60.
12. Parsons S, et al. Study protocol: determining what young people with rheumatic disease consider important to research (the young People's opinions underpinning rheumatology research - YOURR project). Res Involv Engagem. 2016;2:22.
13. Bird D, Culley L, Lakhanpaul M. Why collaborate with children in health research: an analysis of the risks and benefits of collaboration with children. Arch Dis Child Educ Pract Ed. 2013;98(2):42–8.
14. van Staa A, et al. Exciting but exhausting: experiences with participatory research with chronically ill adolescents. Health Expect. 2010;13(1):95–107.
15. Tunnicliffe DJ, et al. Healthcare and research priorities of adolescents and young adults with systemic lupus erythematosus: a mixed-methods study. J Rheumatol. 2017;44(4):444–51.
16. Parsons S, et al. What do young people with rheumatic disease believe to be important to research about their condition? A UK-wide study. Pediatr Rheumatol Online J. 2017;15(1):53.
17. Abma TA, et al. Patient involvement in research programming and implementation: a responsive evaluation of the dialogue model for research agenda setting. Health Expect. 2015;18(6):2449–64.
18. Broerse JE, et al. Involving burn survivors in agenda setting on burn research: an added value? Burns. 2010;36(2):217–31.
19. van Furth EF, van der Meer A, Cowan K. Top 10 research priorities for eating disorders. Lancet Psychiatry. 2016;3(8):706–7.
20. Schoemaker CG, Prakken ABJ, Furth EF. Patients and physicians creating a research agenda together: the method of the British James Lind Alliance. Ned Tijdschr Geneeskd. 2017;161(0):D1764.
21. JLA. Funded research. 2018; Available from: http://www.jla.nihr.ac.uk/making-a-difference/funded-research.htm. Accessed 1 Sept 2018.
22. Chalmers I. The James Lind initiative. J R Soc Med. 2003;96(12):575–6.
23. JLA. JLA Guidebook. 2018; Available from: www.jla.nihr.ac.uk/jla-guidebook. Accessed 1 Sept 2018.
24. JLA. Top 10s of priorities for research. 2018; Available from: http://www.jla.nihr.ac.uk/top-10-priorities. Accessed 1 Sept 2018.
25. Dedding CW, et al. Kinderen en jongeren actief in wetenschappelijk onderzoek. Ethiek, methoden en resultaten van onderzoek met en door jeugd. Houten: LannooCampus; 2013.
26. Schalkers I, Dedding CW, Bunders JF. '[I would like] a place to be alone, other than the toilet'—Children's perspectives on paediatric hospital care in the Netherlands. Health Expect. 2015;18(6):2066–78.
27. Madden M, Morley R. Exploring the challenge of health research priority setting in partnership: reflections on the methodology used by the James Lind Alliance pressure ulcer priority setting partnership. Res Involv Engagem. 2016;2:12.
28. de Wit MP, et al. European league against rheumatism recommendations for the inclusion of patient representatives in scientific projects. Ann Rheum Dis. 2011;70(5):722–6.

Methotrexate in juvenile idiopathic arthritis: advice and recommendations from the MARAJIA expert consensus meeting

Giovanna Ferrara[1†], Greta Mastrangelo[2†], Patrizia Barone[3], Francesco La Torre[4], Silvana Martino[5], Giovanni Pappagallo[6], Angelo Ravelli[7], Andrea Taddio[8], Francesco Zulian[9], Rolando Cimaz[2*] On behalf of the Rheumatology Italian Study Group

Abstract

Background: Conventional pharmacological therapies for the treatment of juvenile idiopathic arthritis (JIA) consist of non-biological, disease-modifying antirheumatic drugs, among which methotrexate (MTX) is the most commonly prescribed. However, there is a lack of consensus-based clinical and therapeutic recommendations for the use of MTX in the management of patients with JIA. Therefore, the **M**ethotrexate **A**dvice and **R**ecommend**A**tions on **J**uvenile **I**diopathic **A**rthritis (MARAJIA) Expert Meeting was convened to develop evidence-based recommendations for the use of MTX in the treatment of JIA.

Methods: The preliminary executive committee identified a total of 9 key clinical issues according to the population, intervention, comparator, outcome (PICO) approach, and performed an evidence-based, systematic, literature review. During the subsequent Expert Meeting, the relevant evidence was assessed and graded, and 10 recommendations were made.

Results: Recommendations relating to the efficacy, optimal dosing and route of administration and duration of treatment with MTX in JIA, and to the issue of folic acid supplementation to prevent MTX side effects, use of MTX in the treatment of chronic JIA-associated uveitis, combination treatment with biologic agents, and the use of vaccinations in patients with JIA were developed. The selected topics were considered to represent clinically important issues facing clinicians caring for patients with JIA. Evidence was insufficient to formulate recommendations for the use of biomarkers predictive of treatment response.

Conclusions: These consensus recommendations provide balanced and evidence-based recommendations designed to have broad value for physicians and healthcare clinicians involved in the clinical management of patients with JIA.

Keywords: Juvenile idiopathic arthritis, Methotrexate, Consensus

Background

Juvenile idiopathic arthritis (JIA) is one of the most common chronic conditions of childhood. JIA comprises a group of heterogeneous forms of arthritis characterized by persistent joint inflammation lasting longer than 6 weeks and beginning before the age of 16 years and has an unknown cause [1]. According to the classification criteria of the International League of Associations for Rheumatology (ILAR), the term JIA covers seven mutually exclusive categories with differences in their clinical presentation, disease course and treatment response, namely systemic arthritis, oligoarthritis, polyarthritis (rheumatoid factor negative), polyarthritis (rheumatoid factor positive), psoriatic arthritis, enthesitis-related arthritis, and undifferentiated arthritis [1]. Conventional pharmacological therapies consist of non-biological, disease-modifying antirheumatic drugs (DMARD), among which methotrexate (MTX) is the most commonly prescribed [2].

* Correspondence: rolando.cimaz@meyer.it
†Giovanna Ferrara and Greta Mastrangelo contributed equally to this work.
[2]Rheumatology Unit, Anna Meyer Children Hospital and University of Florence, University of Florence, Florence, Italy
Full list of author information is available at the end of the article

To date, despite the wide use of MTX, there is a lack of consensus-based clinical and therapeutic recommendations for the use of MTX in the management of patients with JIA. Only two papers, one recently-published article from the Spanish Society of Paediatric Rheumatology (Sociedad Española de Reumatología Pediátrica; SERPE) [3], and an older article by the Pediatric Immunology and Rheumatology Division of the Centre for Child Health, Heinrich-Heine-University, Düsseldorf, Germany [4] currently deal with this task.

Thus, the aim of our group was to develop evidence-based recommendations for the use of MTX in the treatment of juvenile idiopathic arthritis. To this end, the **M**ethotrexate **A**dvice and **R**ecommend**A**tions on **J**uvenile **I**diopathic **A**rthritis (MARAJIA) Expert Meeting was convened in Milan, Italy.

Methodology

Development of the research topics

Establishing recommendations requires the use of formal methods, such as the nominal group technique (NGT), which is based on discussions by an Expert Panel to gather opinions and define a degree of consensus for each statement.

A preliminary executive committee comprising Rolando Cimaz, Giovanna Ferrara and Greta Mastrangelo was responsible for identifying key clinical issues using the PICO (Population – Intervention – Comparator - Outcome) system [5], with the aim of: 1) defining research questions, and 2) developing criteria for selecting studies to be reviewed by the Expert Panel in the development of clinical and therapeutic recommendations for the management of MTX in patients with JIA. The PICO framework is designed to help researchers to achieve relevant and precise questions that can be answered in a systematic review structure, and allows improved specificity and conceptual clarity of the clinical question by splitting the questions into smaller manageable components which are more straightforward to identify in the literature search process.

The approach facilitates the identification of a precise definition of a group of participants (**Population**), clear reporting of the drug exposures (**Intervention**) and the control group interventions (**Comparator**) under consideration, and well-defined and clearly specified **Outcomes** of the intervention being assessed. Finally, the type of **Study design** to be included in the review should be reported.

The executive committee identified nine clinically important research topics relating to the use of MTX in JIA using a structured PICO process. The topics covered efficacy and safety, dosages, routes of administration, tapering, and discontinuation of MTX, folic acid supplementation, efficacy in JIA-associated uveitis, add-on therapy with biologic drugs, biomarkers, and vaccination. The selected topics were considered to represent clinically important issues facing clinicians caring for patients with JIA.

Strategy for the literature search

A systematic search using PubMed and the Cochrane Library for human studies published in English until the present was conducted on the 30th of November 2016. The keywords used in the search were "juvenile idiopathic arthritis" and "methotrexate" ("arthritis, juvenile"[MeSH Terms] OR ("arthritis"[All Fields] AND "juvenile"[All Fields]) OR "juvenile arthritis"[All Fields] OR ("juvenile"[All Fields] AND "idiopathic"[All Fields] AND "arthritis"[All Fields]) OR "juvenile idiopathic arthritis"[All Fields]) AND ("methotrexate"[MeSH Terms] OR "methotrexate"[All Fields]).

Study selection and data extraction

All papers found with the first search were initially selected as appropriate to the intended purpose on the basis of the title. Papers inconsistent with the main topic (for example for disease or drug) were excluded. A second revision and selection was made reading the abstracts of remaining papers. Then all studies identified were read in their full text.

Critical appraisal of identified studies

Each of the included studies was assessed for level of evidence using Oxford criteria for evidence-based levels of evidence [6]. The levels of evidence used in the analyses are summarized in Table 1. Evidence levels are indicative of quality regarding confidence and study design. In

Table 1 Levels of evidence [6]

Levels of evidence	
1	Systematic review of all relevant randomized clinical trials or *n*-of-1 trials
2	Randomized trial or observational study with dramatic effect
3	Non-randomized controlled cohort/follow-up study (observational)
4	Case series, case-control study, or historically controlled study
5	Mechanism-based reasoning (expert opinion, based on physiology, animal or laboratory studies)
Grades of recommendation	
A	Consistent level 1 studies
B	Consistent level 2 or 3 studies, or extrapolations from level 1 studies
C	Level 4 studies, or extrapolations from level 2 or 3 studies
D	Level 5 evidence or troubling, inconsistent or inconclusive studies of any level

defining the recommendations, the experts' assessment of the clinical conclusions of the studies was combined with the definition of the evidence levels.

Consensus process

Expert panel composition

The Expert Panel participating in the MARAJIA Expert Consensus Meeting held in Milan, Italy on the 12th of April, 2017 to identify recommendations for the use of MTX in the treatment of JIA consisted of Patrizia Barone, Rolando Cimaz, Francesco La Torre, Silvana Martino, Angelo Ravelli, Andrea Taddio, and Francesco Zulian, under the methodological guidance of Giovanni Pappagallo. Giovanna Ferrara and Greta Mastrangelo were involved in formulating the PICO research topics and drafting the recommendation statements.

All experts were pediatric rheumatologists, the majority from tertiary centers with longstanding expertise in pediatric rheumatic diseases.

Formulation of clinical recommendations

During the meeting, the Expert Panel considered the supporting research identified using the targeted literature search and formulated specific recommendation statements for each research topic. Ten clinical and therapeutic recommendations for the management of MTX were drafted and presented to the meeting with their supporting scientific evidence for discussion and voting by the Expert Panel towards reaching consensus.

The strength and relevance of the published evidence in support of a clinical intervention or treatment approach was evaluated, in addition taking into consideration the personal clinical experience of the panel participants. Each participant was required to express his or her expert opinion by rating the statement according to the following 7-point scale: 1) completely disagree; 2) somewhat disagree; 3) disagree a little; 4) neither agree nor disagree; 5) agree a little; 6) somewhat agree; 7) completely agree. A score of 6 or 7 was defined as "In favor", 3, 4 or 5 as "Uncertain", and 1 or 2 "Against".

Through this process, all research statements achieved acceptance, with a second round of voting not required for any statement. One hundred percent agreement (a unanimous score of 7 on the 7-point scale) was obtained on 5 statements (Statements 2, 3, 4, 7 and 8) and 83% agreement on Statements 1 and 6 (7 or 6) and Statement 5 (7 or 6 with a single score of 5 from one Advisor). The research questions are detailed in Table 2.

Research strategy and evidence selection

We obtained 843 references in our literature search. Among these, we selected 209 relevant references, of which 33 were clinical trials, 51 reviews, 1 Cochrane meta-analysis and 124 articles of other types.

A total of 472 references were excluded because they were judged not to be relevant, 139 because the studies were mainly about biologic drugs and there was an insufficient focus on MTX, and 23 because they were published in non-European languages. Six articles (2 clinical trials, 1 review, and 3 articles of other types) were subsequently included from an updated literature search (28 February 2017). A flow diagram of the study selection process is shown in Fig. 1.

Methotrexate in juvenile idiopathic arthritis: Recommendations for use

A summary of the recommendations for the use of MTX in JIA for each of the PICO research questions is presented in Table 2.

Research question 1: Efficacy and safety of methotrexate in juvenile idiopathic arthritis

Recommendation 1. *MTX is recommended as the first-line treatment in oligoarthritis that persists despite nonsteroidal anti-inflammatory drugs (NSAIDs) and intraarticular steroid (IAS) therapy, and in polyarticular disease (Evidence Grade 1A).*

MTX is also recommended in systemic arthritis with predominant joint inflammation, without active systemic features (Evidence Grade 4C).

Recommendation 2. *Clinical and laboratory monitoring of MTX toxicity is recommended every 4–8 weeks initially, and then every 12–16 weeks, unless risk factors are present (Evidence Grade 4C).*

PICO framework: P: children affected by JIA; I: administration of MTX; C: placebo or other therapies (salazopyrin, oral steroids, NSAIDs); O: efficacy and safety.

MTX is the most widely used DMARD in the treatment of JIA. A folic acid analog and an inhibitor of several different enzymes in the folate pathway, MTX exerts immunomodulatory and anti-inflammatory actions. Its efficacy was first demonstrated in a randomized controlled trial more than two decades ago [7]. MTX has been studied in further controlled clinical trials [8, 9] and has been established as the most common first-line DMARD treatment according to several national treatment guidelines [10–13]. In particular, considering the categories of JIA, NSAIDs and IAS therapy remain the first choice in oligoarthritis [1]. Furthermore, a recent multicenter, prospective, randomized, open-label trial [14] found that concomitant administration of MTX did not augment the effectiveness of intra-articular corticosteroid therapy.

MTX is recommended as first-line treatment in polyarthritis, and in systemic arthritis with predominant joint inflammation [2, 8, 11, 15]. However, initiation of sulfasalazine (SSZ) is recommended following IAS or an adequate

Table 2 Summary of recommendations for the use of methotrexate in juvenile idiopathic arthritis

PICO research questions and recommendations	Grade of evidence	Supporting references
Research question 1: Efficacy and safety of methotrexate in juvenile idiopathic arthritis		
1. MTX is recommended as the first-line treatment in oligoarthritis that persists despite nonsteroidal anti-inflammatory drugs (NSAIDs) and intraarticular steroid (IAS) therapy, and in polyarticular disease	1A	[2–4, 7–15, 20, 21, 23–25]
MTX is also recommended in systemic arthritis with predominant joint inflammation, without active systemic features	4C	[2–4, 7–15, 20–25]
2. Clinical and laboratory monitoring of MTX toxicity is recommended every 4-8 weeks initially, and then every 12-16 weeks, unless risk factors are present	4C	[1, 4, 12, 21, 26–38, 40–42]
Research question 2: Dosages of methotrexate in juvenile idiopathic arthritis		
3. A dose of 10-15 mg/m^2/week is recommended.	5D	[7, 9, 42]
Further increases in MTX dosage have not been associated with additional therapeutic benefit	1A	
Research question 3: Route of administration of methotrexate in juvenile idiopathic arthritis		
4. MTX may be given orally or subcutaneously once a week. If high doses (15 mg/m^2/week) are requested, the subcutaneous route is preferable due to increased bioavailability	4C	[9, 21, 43–49]
Research question 4: Tapering and discontinuation of methotrexate in juvenile idiopathic arthritis		
5. MTX could be discontinued after 6 months of stable remission	1A	[50–52]
Research question 5: Folic acid supplementation for the prevention of methotrexate toxicity in patients with juvenile idiopathic arthritis		
6. Folic or folinic acid supplementation is recommended to prevent MTX side effects.	1A	[53–57, 59–62]
The advised dose is approximately one third of the MTX dose, at least 24 hours after the weekly dose of MTX for folinic acid; for folic acid 1 mg/day skipping the day when MTX is administered	4C	
Research question 6: Efficacy of methotrexate in uveitis associated with juvenile idiopathic arthritis		
7. MTX is recommended for the treatment of JIA-related uveitis refractory to topical treatment	4C	[63–72, 74–79]
Research question 7: Add-on therapy with biologic drugs in juvenile idiopathic arthritis not responding to methotrexate		
8. The combination of MTX with a TNF-α inhibitor is recommended in patients who had an inadequate clinical response to MTX alone	3B	[11, 48, 80, 83–85, 88, 89]
Combination therapy is safe and may reduce the development of anti-drug antibodies	2B	[83, 88–90]
Research question 8: Molecular elements and genetic markers of response to methotrexate in juvenile idiopathic arthritis – Biomarkers		
9. No recommendation is made regarding the use of biomarkers in current clinical practice		[91–101]
Research question 9: Use of vaccination in patients with juvenile idiopathic arthritis treated with methotrexate		
10. Vaccination with non-live vaccines is not contraindicated during MTX treatment	2B	[101–119]
No recommendation can be formulated for live-attenuated vaccines, but the available data for measles, mumps, rubella (MMR) booster indicate that it is safe and adequately immunogenic		

Abbreviations: *IAS* intra-articular steroid, *JIA* juvenile idiopathic arthritis, *MMR* measles, mumps, rubella, *MTX* methotrexate, *NSAIDs* nonsteroidal anti-inflammatory drugs, *TNF-α* tumor necrosis factor-α

trial of NSAIDs for patients with the enthesitis-related arthritis category of JIA, with moderate activity [11]. Sulfasalazine has never been compared with MTX in treating JIA.

Currently, there are no published recommendations for the treatment of juvenile spondyloarthropathies. The ACR recommendations for the management of JIA suggest the use of sulfasalazine for patients with enthesitis-related arthritis. This recommendation is based on clinical experience and data from adult patients with ankylosing spondylitis. However, in the adult population it has been shown that sulfasalazine is ineffective in axial disease, while several observational studies have found that tumor necrosis factor (TNF)-α inhibitors are beneficial in juvenile spondyloarthropathies [16–19]. Furthermore, a recent randomized controlled trial demonstrated the efficacy of adalimumab in enthesitis-related arthritis [16, 18]. Available studies suggest that TNF-α inhibitors should be used when sulfasalazine is ineffective or earlier in moderate or highly active axial disease with established radiographic damage, such as erosions or joint-space narrowing.

MTX has been shown to be an effective drug in the indication, with 65–90% of patients successfully responding to treatment [9, 20–22]. MTX also significantly improved a wide range of health-related quality-of-life components, particularly in the physical domains [23].

Despite what has previously been reported in adult patients, MTX may also slow the radiologic progression of

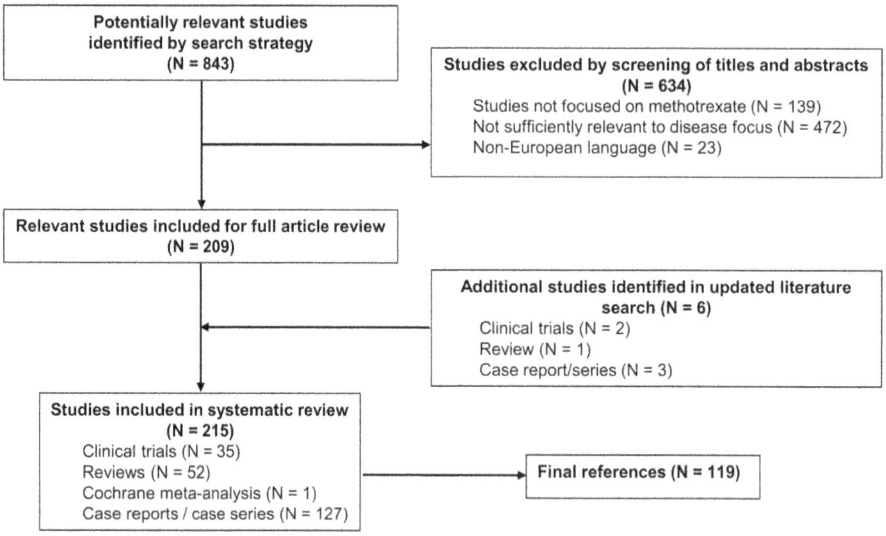

Fig. 1 Study selection process flow diagram

disease in JIA, acting as a disease-modifying drug, although the studies available involved few children [24, 25].

During 30 years of its use, MTX has shown a good safety profile, with few severe side effects reported [26]. Nevertheless, more than half of children were reported to have difficulties in taking it [27, 28]. The most common side effect of MTX include nausea or vomiting and abnormalities in liver function tests, the latest reported in 10–20% of patients [29, 30]. However, the transaminase levels usually normalize one or two weeks after stopping therapy. Others symptoms are mouth sores, rash, diarrhea and laboratory abnormalities such as leukopenia and hypogammaglobulinemia that may predispose to infections. Alopecia is seen in some patients, but hair grows back after stopping the medication. Since photosensitivity has been reported, limiting sun exposure and the use of sunscreen is advised. It is worth remembering that MTX is teratogenic, and it is necessary to use contraception while taking the drug and for 3–6 months after discontinuation [29].

MTX may cause cirrhosis and lung fibrosis, but these are extremely rare and have been reported only in adults with other comorbidities [31–33]. In the literature there are also few reports of lymphoma in children treated with MTX [34–36], but it has not been possible to determine whether these observations were merely coincidental, were causally linked to MTX, or were related to the underlying disease process. The issue of whether MTX treatment is an independent risk factor for various malignancies is controversial and remains unresolved. Long-term prospective cohort studies are needed to define the risk of hematological or other malignancies in MTX-treated patients.

Nodulosis is a rare MTX adverse event that has been described in JIA (accelerated nodulosis in two teenagers with rheumatoid factor [RF]-positive juvenile rheumatoid arthritis and one 3-year-old girl with systemic-onset disease). The nodules developed within six months after the initiation of MTX treatment and regressed after discontinuing therapy, or were successfully treated with hydroxychloroquine or colchicine [37–39].

Regarding laboratory monitoring in patients with JIA, there is only one guideline by Ortiz-Alvarez et al., derived from the American College of Rheumatology (ACR) guidelines for monitoring MTX toxicity in adults. They suggest a complete and differential blood count, liver function tests and albumin and serum creatinine levels every 4–8 week initially, and then every 12–16 week, unless risk factors are present [40]. Other authors also recommended hepatitis and varicella-zoster virus serology and tuberculin test before starting therapy [4]. MTX is contraindicated in children with reduced renal function.

Bulatović et al. [27] designed and validated the MTX Intolerance Severity Score (MISS) questionnaire to identify patients with MTX intolerance. The items investigated were: abdominal signs and symptoms (pain, nausea, vomiting) and behavioral symptoms (restless, crying, irritability, and refusal of MTX) before and after the administration of MTX. A cut-off score of 6 yielded the best sensitivity (88%) and specificity (80%). They found there was no difference in efficacy between the various routes of MTX administration. However, half of the 297 patients were MTX-intolerant. This was especially the case in patients who received parenteral MTX, who experienced more anticipatory behavioral symptoms prior to administration, compared to patients receiving oral MTX. However, the difference in the prevalence of gastrointestinal symptoms was not great.

Van Dijkhuizen et al. [41] also found more side effects among patients who received parenteral MTX. On the other hand, Klein et al. [21] found no difference in the prevalence of side effects between oral and parenteral MTX.

Overall, analysis of available studies and clinical experience of the participating experts show that MTX is usually well tolerated in patients with JIA.

Research question 2: Dosages of methotrexate in juvenile idiopathic arthritis

Recommendation 3. *A dose of 10–15 mg/m^2/week is recommended (Evidence Grade 5D). Further increases in MTX dosage have not been associated with additional therapeutic benefit (Evidence Grade 1A).*

PICO framework: P: children affected by JIA on treatment with MTX; I: low dosage of MTX (< 10 mg/m^2/week); C: high dosage of MTX (> 10 mg/m^2/week); O: efficacy and safety.

The therapeutic range of MTX for JIA is 8.5–15 mg/m^2/week. The first study by Giannini et al. showed that a dose of 5 mg/m^2/week was not superior to placebo, while 15 mg/m^2/week was superior to 10 mg/m^2/week [7].

Children seem to tolerate much higher doses than adults, and some series have described using 20 to 25 mg/m^2/week or 1.1 mg/kg/week in children with resistant disease with relative safety in the short-term [42]. However, a multinational, randomized controlled study confirmed this therapeutic range and showed no benefit of doses above 15 mg/m^2/week [9].

Research question 3: Route of administration of methotrexate in juvenile idiopathic arthritis

Recommendation 4. *MTX may be given orally or subcutaneously once a week. If high doses (15 mg/m^2/week) are requested, the subcutaneous route is preferable due to increased bioavailability (Evidence Grade 4C).*

PICO framework: P: children affected by JIA on treatment with MTX; I: subcutaneous administration of MTX; C: oral administration of MTX; O: efficacy, safety, and tolerability.

There is significant intraindividual and interindividual variability in the absorption and pharmacokinetics of MTX after oral administration [43, 44].

A pharmacokinetic study showed that factors such as age, body weight, creatinine clearance, gender, dose, and fasting state significantly influenced the absorption of MTX in adults with rheumatoid arthritis. The bioavailability of MTX has also been shown to be greater in the fasting state in children with JIA [45].

MTX should be taken on an empty stomach with water or clear beverages. Oral bioavailability generally is about 15% less than after intramuscular administration. The bioavailability of intramuscular and subcutaneous administration is similar, with the latter being generally more acceptable for children who require parenteral MTX [46, 47].

Several studies have reported the successful use of parenteral treatment in non-responders to oral MTX treatment, but there are no controlled comparative studies (only open-label studies are available). Alsufyani et al. found that patients switching from oral to subcutaneous administration of MTX had a 70% improvement in response [48].

Klein et al. in a retrospective study showed no differences in effectiveness between oral and parenteral administration of MTX, even if more patients on parenteral therapy discontinued it [21]. In clinical practice, MTX is preferentially administrated subcutaneously, and there is no sound study demonstrating greater efficacy for the oral route of MTX administration.

At doses over 15 mg/m^2/week, the parenteral route may be better because of the decreased oral bioavailability of the drug at high doses. It has been shown that subcutaneous administration of MTX has a 10–12% increased absorption compared with oral preparations [46, 49]. In discussion amongst the Panel members, it was noted that in clinical practice, treatment is usually started with MTX 15 mg/m^2/week, particularly in severe forms of JIA, where the patient is directly treated with MTX 15 mg/m^2/week. The Panel further suggested that, for the first administrations, the starting dose can be 10 mg/m^2/week, and then the dose can be increased at subsequent MTX administrations, if necessary. Ruperto et al. reported that MTX doses greater than 15 mg/m^2/week provided no additional clinical benefit, and that this dose should not be exceeded [9].

Research question 4: Tapering and discontinuation of methotrexate in juvenile idiopathic arthritis

Recommendation 5. *MTX could be discontinued after 6 months of stable remission (Evidence Grade 1A).*

PICO framework: P: children affected by JIA on treatment with MTX; I: tapering and discontinuing treatment six months after achieving remission; C: discontinuing MTX twelve months or longer after achieving remission; O: survival free of flares after stopping treatment.

MTX is a slow-acting drug, generally displaying its full therapeutic effect in 6–8 weeks (from 3 to 18 weeks among different studies), so there is general agreement to wait at least 12 weeks to assess its efficacy. On the contrary, there is a wide variability on the tapering and discontinuation of MTX doses in everyday clinical practice. There have been many studies in children treated with variable doses of MTX for variable periods in whom discontinuation of MTX was attempted after clinical "remission" of variable length was achieved [50].

The criteria for "remission" or "relapse" have usually not been well defined or standardized among various studies, and the assessment of outcomes has been nonblinded.

Only Foell et al. in a randomized clinical trial proved the safety of withdrawing MTX therapy after 6 months of stable remission versus 12 months. The results of this study that included 364 patients showed that a 12-month versus 6-month withdrawal of MTX did not reduce the relapse rate [51].

MTX withdrawal may result in disease flare in more than 50% of patients, and even more in younger children. A longer period on MTX treatment after remission may not prolong the duration of improvement after stopping treatment, but the duration of clinical remission may be predicted by the degree of subclinical synovial inflammation (using myeloid related proteins 8 and 14 [MRP8/MRP14]) at the time of stopping MTX [52].

Research question 5: Folic acid supplementation for the prevention of methotrexate toxicity in patients with juvenile idiopathic arthritis

Recommendation 6. *Folic or folinic acid supplementation is recommended to prevent MTX side effects (Evidence Grade 1A). The advised dose is approximately one third of the MTX dose, at least 24 h after the weekly dose of MTX for folinic acid; for folic acid 1 mg/day skipping the day when MTX is administered (Evidence Grade 4C).*

PICO framework: P: children affected by JIA on treatment with MTX; I: MTX and folic acid supplementation; C: MTX alone; O: frequency (prevalence/incidence) of nausea and dyspepsia.

MTX toxicity, such as hepatotoxicity, hematologic changes, gastrointestinal and mucocutaneous intolerance, has been hypothesized to be a result of an induced state of folate depletion. The addition of folate, therefore, can counteract the signs of toxicity, either as folic or folinic acid (a reduced form of folic acid), since they can function in biosynthetic pathways independent of dihydrofolate reductase.

In a double-blind placebo-controlled study in RA, 1–5 mg of folic acid led to a significant reduction of side effects whilst preserving the efficacy of MTX therapy, even if, in order to preserve the anti-inflammatory effect, a slightly higher dosage of MTX was necessary [53]. Several clinical studies showed also that folic acid supplementation is associated with a reduced MTX discontinuation rate [53–55]. According to available data, folic acid supplementation does not appear to interfere with the therapeutic efficacy of MTX [55–57]. Indeed, there is increasing evidence that the anti-inflammatory effect of MTX is mediated by adenosine and is unrelated to folic or folinic acid [58]. A randomized controlled study, which directly compared folic acid to folinic acid in rheumatoid arthritis, showed no difference between the two forms of supplementation [53].

Studies in children are limited. A 13-week, randomized, double-blind, placebo-controlled, crossover trial of folic acid (1 mg/day) or placebo combined with a stable dose of MTX in 19 children with juvenile rheumatoid arthritis reported no effect on the clinical efficacy of oral weekly MTX. No liver function tests abnormalities were observed, but no data about other toxicities were available [59]. According to the findings of the studies conducted in adults, the frequency of increased transaminases is reduced by 60% by folinic acid supplementation [57]. Furthermore, in a retrospective non-controlled study [60] the efficacy of folinic acid supplementation was investigated in a cohort of 43 children on an intermediate dose of MTX. A significant reduction in hepatotoxicity and gastrointestinal toxicity was shown, without compromising MTX efficacy.

Administration of folic or folinic acid 24 h apart from the administration of MTX, in a dose of approximately one-third of the MTX dose, has been used to prevent MTX toxicity manifestations [61].

However, in limited cases, it is reported that at high doses folic acid supplementation seems to be associated with disease flares [62].

According to available data, it is not possible to make firm recommendations about routine folate supplementation in children receiving MTX treatment. However, data from adult studies and limited pediatric data can provide helpful information. Low-dose (1 mg/day) folic acid supplementation does not affect the anti-inflammatory efficacy of MTX and counteracts the signs of gastrointestinal and mucosal toxicities associated with it. The advisable dose is approximately one-third of the MTX dose, at least 24 h after the weekly dose of MTX, or 1 mg/day skipping the day when MTX is administered (Grade 4C). Folic acid supplementation does not appear to interfere with the therapeutic efficacy of MTX and seems to be associated with a reduced MTX discontinuation rate.

Research question 6: Efficacy of methotrexate in uveitis associated with juvenile idiopathic arthritis

Recommendation 7. *MTX is recommended for the treatment of JIA-related uveitis refractory to topical treatment (Evidence Grade 4C).*

PICO framework: P: children affected by JIA and uveitis; I: administration of MTX; C: placebo or other therapies (e.g., oral steroids); O: efficacy and safety.

Although there is a lack of randomized controlled studies on the subject, the available data suggest that MTX is useful for preventing the onset of uveitis and improving disease activity in cases of JIA. In particular, a systematic review and meta-analysis of prospective studies carried out by Simonini et al. found that there was a 73% (95% confidence interval 66–81%) likelihood of improving intraocular inflammation in patients treated with MTX [63]. The systematic review was based on data from nine retrospective chart reviews [63–72]. The number of children in studies varied from 3 to 25, and the dose of MTX ranged from 7.5 to 30 mg/m^2, with 15 mg/m^2 the most commonly used. Ninety-five of 135 children were responders to MTX. The outcome measures to assess the effectiveness of MTX were collected according to the Standardization of Uveitis Nomenclature working group criteria [73]. It was reported that additional topical steroids or systemic immunosuppressive drugs were often required. However, the lack of randomized controlled trials means that treatment with immunosuppressive drugs is supported only at evidence level III: expert opinion, clinical experience or descriptive studies [74].

Additionally, Charuvanij and colleagues [75] reviewed the medication history in 43 children with JIA and anterior uveitis. Topical corticosteroids alone permitted satisfactory disease control in few patients (16%). The addition of MTX controlled the uveitis in three-quarters of patients, but additional systemic immunosuppressive drug (infliximab) was required in 6 children, with disease control in 4 patients.

The lack of evidence from randomized controlled trials limits our understanding of MTX effectiveness in the indication and of the best time to start therapy, even though MTX is largely used in chronic uveitis, mostly when associated with JIA.

Heiligenhaus et al. [76] suggest adding an immunosoppressive drug (i.e. MTX) to steroids when the inflammation in the eyes has not resolved within 12 weeks under treatment with topical corticosteroids maximally 3 times daily or, in cases of recurring uveitis, under a systemic corticosteroid dosage of more than 0.15 mg/kg body weight or if new uveitis complications develop. The preferred dose is 15 mg/m^2/week (maximum 25 mg/m^2/week) [77]. Evidence from several sources suggested that if MTX is effective in controlling inflammation, treatment should be maintained for 12 months from when inactive uveitis has been confirmed. In patients with poor visual prognosis, MTX treatment should be maintained over 24 months [77].

In terms of preventing the onset of uveitis in children during early treatment with MTX Papadopoulou et al. [78] performed a retrospective study of 254 patients with JIA. Eighty-six patients (33.9%) were treated with MTX and 168 patients (66.1%) did not receive MTX. Over the 2-year follow-up, the frequency of uveitis was lower in patients who had received MTX than in untreated patients (10.5% vs 20.2%, respectively, $p = 0.049$). The majority of patients in the study had persistent and extended oligoarthritis (61.8 and 22.4%, respectively); 14.2% of patients had RF-negative polyarthritis. As expected, patients treated with MTX had a greater frequency of polyarticular disease, which is well known to have a lower incidence of uveitis. However, the distribution of the main risk factors for uveitis (proportion of female and antinuclear antibodies- positive subjects) and the median age at disease onset were comparable between the two groups. In a longitudinal analysis from a nationwide pediatric rheumatology database [79] the influence of MTX, TNF-α inhibitors, and a combination of the 2 medications on uveitis occurrence in JIA patients was analyzed. In a total of 3512 patients the use of any of these drugs in the year before uveitis onset significantly reduced the risk for uveitis, and the use of MTX within the first year of disease and of the combination of MTX with a TNF-α inhibitor had the highest protective effect.

In a recent systematic review [63], MTX seems an effective therapy for uveitis associated with JIA.

Research question 7: Add-on therapy with biologic drugs in patients with juvenile idiopathic arthritis not responding to methotrexate

Recommendation 8. *The combination of MTX with a TNF-α inhibitor is recommended in patients who had an inadequate clinical response to MTX alone (Evidence Grade 3B). Combination therapy is safe and may reduce the development of anti-drug antibodies (Evidence Grade 2B).*

PICO framework: P: children affected by JIA on treatment with MTX who did not achieve remission; I: MTX plus TNF-α inhibitors (etanercept and adalimumab); C: MTX alone; O: efficacy and safety.

The ACR recommendations [11] propose the addition of a TNF-α inhibitor (etanercept or adalimumab) for patients who had a partial previous clinical response to MTX with persistent disease activity, recommending, after starting combination therapy, that treatment with MTX be continued or not depending on the patient's previous response to it.

Two retrospective cohort studies recommended completion of a maximal response timeframe and to achieve the maximum effective dose by the parenteral route before considering combination therapy [48, 80].

Studies in adult patients with RA revealed a superiority of combining MTX and etanercept versus MTX only [81, 82]. This combination has also been successfully used in children and adolescents, despite a lack of double-blind, randomized controlled trials [83].

A 3-year, open-label, prospective multicenter study of children and adolescents (aged 2–18 years) with polyarticular, systemic, or extended oligoarticular JIA receiving MTX ($n = 197$), etanercept ($n = 103$), or both ($n = 294$) showed good safety and efficacy in all three groups. The results of this study indicated that patients with polyarticular (RF-positive or negative) or systemic JIA benefit from etanercept or etanercept plus MTX treatment [84]. Improvements in joint counts and physician's global assessment scores were similar across three different arms, and improvements were maintained for three years in those continuing to receive medication.

In a randomized, double-blind, stratified, placebo-controlled, multicenter, medication-withdrawal study with a 16-week open-label lead-in phase, a 32-week double-blind withdrawal phase, and an open-label extension phase, 171 children with active juvenile rheumatoid arthritis underwent stratification according to MTX use (85 patients receiving MTX, 86 not receiving MTX) and received adalimumab every other week for 16 weeks. Subsequently, those that had an ACR Pediatric 30% (ACR Pedi 30) response at week 16 (74% of patients not receiving MTX and 94% of those receiving MTX) were randomly assigned to receive adalimumab or placebo in a double-blind fashion every other week for up to 32 weeks. At 48 weeks, the percentages of patients treated with MTX who had ACR Pedi 30, 50, 70, or 90 responses were significantly greater for those receiving adalimumab than for those receiving placebo; the differences between patients not treated with MTX who received adalimumab and those who received placebo were not significant. The study was not statistically powered to detect differences between patients receiving and those not receiving MTX; however, the proportions of patients with ACR Pedi 30, 50, 70, or 90 responses were somewhat higher among those receiving adalimumab in combination with MTX than among those receiving adalimumab without MTX [85].

A diminished response to treatment with certain TNF-α inhibitors may be associated with the development of anti-drug antibodies [86], and concomitant use of MTX reduces the immunogenicity of these drugs [85, 87].

Concerning safety, several studies reported that MTX combined with anti-TNF-α does not increase its toxicity [83, 88–90].

MTX in combination with biologic therapy is safe and may reduce the development of anti-drug antibodies in addition to improving response.

Research question 8: Molecular elements and genetic markers of response to methotrexate in juvenile idiopathic arthritis – Biomarkers

Recommendation 9. *No recommendation is made regarding the use of biomarkers in current clinical practice.*

PICO framework: P: children affected by JIA undergoing treatment with MTX; I: evaluating the concentration of MTX polyglutamates and genetics variants in MTX responders; C: polyglutamate levels and genetic variants in patients with JIA non-responders to MTX; O: response to MTX in children with JIA.

Although MTX is the first choice in JIA, it is known that about one-third of patients fail to respond. Given the time lag between MTX treatment initiation and the patient response (about 3 months), it would be particularly useful to determine a priori the probability of beneficial therapeutic response [91, 92].

In fact, the delay in identifying the optimal treatment at an early stage of disease can influence long-term joint damage. Several biomarkers have been investigated so far. Recent studies found that the effect of MTX in JIA is associated with MTX polyglutamate intracellular concentrations: elevated long chain MTX polyglutamate levels are associated with lower disease activity indexes (JADAS) during 1 year of MTX treatment in JIA [93–95].

Other studies have evaluated the effects of genetic variants in the complex pathway of candidate genes involved in MTX pharmacokinetics and pharmacodynamics on the response to the medication in children with JIA. These studies found that genetic variants that predict MTX response in JIA are those in 5-aminoimidazole-4-carboxamide ribonucleotide-transformylase (ATIC), inosine triphosphate-pyrophosphatase (ITPA) and SLC19A1 genes [96–99].

Pastore et al. showed that reduced activity of ITPA, an enzyme involved in nucleotides' homeostasis, is related to reduced MTX efficacy in patients with JIA [100]. The same group also found that a common functional variant in ATIC gene is associated with good response to MTX, while a variant in ITPA is associated with reduced response to MTX. However, there are suggestions that genetic variability, specifically single-nucleotide polymorphisms (SNP), in MTX metabolic pathways may be a better marker for MTX toxicity than for efficacy [99].

The conclusions of these studies may suggest that patients with variants associated with lack of efficacy for MTX should be switched more rapidly to a more aggressive treatment, but studies specifically addressing this issue are still lacking. In the future, therapy personalization in JIA may be achieved by a pharmacological approach integrating pharmacokinetic and pharmacogenomic evaluations. However, the supporting evidence is not yet sufficiently robust to form the basis of a recommendation.

Therefore, it was determined that the place of pharmacokinetic and pharmacogenomic analysis performed before MTX treatment in patients with JIA to identify those predisposed to better responses currently undefined and, furthermore, in current clinical practice no assessment of the biomarkers predictive of treatment response is carried out. Therefore, it was decided that no recommendation regarding the use of biomarkers in the treatment of patients with JIA should be made.

Research question 9: Use of vaccination in patients with juvenile idiopathic arthritis treated with methotrexate

Recommendation 10. *Vaccination with non-live vaccines is not contraindicated during MTX treatment (Evidence Grade 2B).*

No recommendation can be formulated for live-attenuated vaccines, but the available data for measles, mumps, rubella (MMR) booster indicate that it is safe and adequately immunogenic.

PICO framework: P: children affected by JIA on treatment with MTX; I: vaccinations during treatment with MTX; C: no vaccinations during treatment with MTX; O: safety and efficacy of vaccinations, safety of drugs.

Considering that children with JIA have an increased risk of infection, which contributes to the morbidity of their disease, non-live vaccines, and live-attenuated vaccines can be recommended in these patients. However, the presence of immunosuppressive drugs can interfere with effectiveness and safety of vaccinations.

In 2011, the European League Against Rheumatism (EULAR) published recommendations regarding the vaccination of children with rheumatic diseases [101], based on a systematic literature review published in that same year [102]. The EULAR guidelines recommend adherence to the national vaccination guidelines for live-attenuated vaccines in pediatric patients unless the patients are on high-dose immunosuppressants, high-dose cortisone or biological agents. Booster vaccinations against varicella, yellow fever, and measles, mumps, rubella (MMR) can be considered in patients receiving MTX less than15mg/m^2 or low-dose corticosteroids. However, it should be noted that the MTX summary of product characteristics states that live vaccines are contraindicated in patients taking MTX.

Recently Groot et colleagues provided an update to July 2014 of the systematic literature study of 2011 [103]. Eight studies on MTX and vaccinations, counting in total 420 patients, were available in the Groot review concerning the most common vaccines, i.e., seasonal influenza virus and H1N1, hepatitis B virus (HBV), meningococcus C, pneumococcus, measles, mumps and rubella (MMR), varicella zoster virus (VZV), bacillus Calmette-Guérin (BCG) [104–111]. Further we found five more articles about the above-mentioned vaccines including subgroups of patients on MTX [112–116], and one more concerning the bivalent human papillomavirus (HPV) vaccine [117].

In a prospective controlled observational cohort study, the immunogenicity of the bivalent HPV 16/18 vaccine in 68 patients with JIA was compared to 55 healthy controls, showing that all participants were seropositive up to 12 months after vaccination. No deleterious effect of MTX on antibodies was detected in the subgroup of 24 patients on MTX. No relevant differences in adverse events were found, and HPV vaccination did not aggravate JIA disease activity [117].

In two prospective open-label studies, influenza vaccine response and safety among patients treated with MTX were compared with a control group. Both studies showed that influenza vaccination in JIA induces a lower but effective protective antibody response with an adequate disease safety profile [109, 111].

Kasapcopur et al. compared responsiveness and safety of hepatitis B vaccination in 39 children affected by JIA and 41 healthy children. No effect of MTX on antibody concentration or response rate and no increase in disease activity were observed. A vaccination schedule at 0, 1, 6 months appeared to be the most effective [105].

The Neisseria meningitidis C (NeisVac-C) vaccine, is also safe and immunogenic in patients with JIA [115]. A retrospective cohort study showed that persistence of MenC-specific immunoglobulin (Ig)G antibodies in patients with JIA is similar to healthy controls and there is no effect of MTX on the decline of antibody levels over time, unlike biologicals [107].

Farmaki and colleagues observed that patients with JIA, when using MTX, had a similar response and seroprotection rate to the 7-valent pneumococcal vaccine (PCV7) as in healthy controls [114]. The only study evaluating the 23-valent polysaccharide pneumococcal vaccine in patients with JIA also demonstrated vaccine safety and effectiveness [116].

In a randomized, multicenter, open-label clinical equivalence trial, 137 patients with JIA aged 4 to 9 years (60 using MTX and 15 using biologics) were randomly assigned to receive MMR booster vaccination ($n = 68$) or no vaccination (control group; $n = 69$). Disease activity during complete follow-up did not differ between revaccinated patients and controls and seroprotection rates at 12 months after vaccination were higher in revaccinated patients. It seems that MTX and biologics did not affect humoral responses, but low patient numbers precluded definite conclusions. Moreover, no disease due to infections with attenuated viruses occurred in patients treated with immunosuppressive drugs [113]. A retrospective cross-sectional study [104], a retrospective observational multicenter cohort study [108] and a prospective case-control study [110] confirm these results.

In a prospective study [112], safety and immunogenicity of the VZV vaccine among 25 patients with pediatric rheumatic diseases treated with MTX and corticosteroids were compared to 18 healthy children. The vaccine proved to be safe in MTX treated patients, and no severe treatment-related adverse effects were observed during the one year follow up period. Both patients and controls had a low seroconversion rate one year after vaccination. However, a recent study [118] showed a low seroconversion rate in susceptible healthy children after one dose of vaccine, and indeed the US Centers for Disease Control and Prevention (CDC) guidelines advocate the use of 2 doses [119]. In clinical practice, a booster dose of VZV vaccine is normally administered to patients who fail to exhibit an immunological response after the first dose.

Kiray et al. demonstrated that there is no effect of MTX on purified protein derivative (PPD) induration size several years after BCG vaccination [106]. The PPD positivity rate was similar in MTX users and nonusers, even if the response to PPD was significantly lower in BCG-vaccinated children with JIA compared to healthy children. However, because of the lack of safety data, BCG vaccinations should not be administered to patients on immunosuppressive drugs (including MTX) or biologicals.

According to available data, no detrimental effect of MTX on the short-term immunogenicity or on the persistence of antibodies over time and no relevant increase in vaccine-associated adverse events were found in patients treated with MTX. Non-live vaccines are generally adequately immunogenic and safe. It appears that live-attenuated vaccines can be safely and effectively administered to patients with JIA on MTX, unless they are also on additional immunosuppressive drugs or biologicals. In these cases, evidence on safety is scarce. Live-attenuated booster vaccinations can be considered on an individual basis, although the data do not currently support the formulation of a specific recommendation for live-attenuated vaccines. There is no evidence in pediatric patients about the safe time intervals for the administration of live vaccines after cessation of immunosuppressive/immunomodulatory drugs such as MTX.

Discussion

Although MTX is accepted as the most effective non-biologic agent for the treatment of patients with JIA, there is a wide variability in everyday practice in the use of MTX in the management of JIA. Therefore, the adoption of a consensus approach by a group of practitioners expert in the use of the drug in treating patients with JIA has the potential to guide clinicians and improve the understanding and management of this condition.

The recommendations presented in these consensus guidelines developed by the panel of experts participating in the MARAJIA Expert Consensus Meeting are based on a high level of evidence provided in large measure by robust data from randomized controlled clinical trials. Based on a set of key clinical issues developed using the PICO system and a rigorous approach to evidence review and the formulation of the research questions adopted to reduce the introduction of biases and to ensure balanced and evidence-based recommendations, we identified sound scientific support to guide the use of MTX in patients with JIA. Our consensus-based analysis integrated the scientific evidence from the literature with clinical experience to provide a set of recommendations we believe are of value in helping clinicians optimize the treatment of their patients with a diagnosis of JIA.

Conclusions

These consensus recommendations relating to the efficacy, optimal dosing and route of administration and duration of treatment with MTX in JIA, and to the important issues of folic acid supplementation to prevent MTX side effects, use of MTX in the treatment of chronic JIA-associated uveitis, combination treatment with biologic agents, and the use of vaccinations in patients with JIA provide balanced and evidence-based recommendations designed to have broad value for physicians and healthcare clinicians. We did not at this time find sufficient evidence to justify pharmacokinetic and pharmacogenomic analysis prior to MTX treatment in current clinical practice, as insufficient evidence is available on biomarkers able to predict treatment response.

Abbreviations

ACR: American College of Rheumatology; BCG: Bacillus Calmette- Guérin; DMARD: Disease-modifying antirheumatic drugs; EULAR: European League Against Rheumatism; HBV: Hepatitis B virus; HPV: Human papillomavirus; IAS: Intraarticular steroid; Ig: Immunoglobulin; ILAR: International League of Associations for Rheumatology; JIA: Juvenile idiopathic arthritis; MARAJIA: **M**ethotrexate **A**dvice and **R**ecommend**A**tions on **J**uvenile **I**diopathic **A**rthritis; MISS: MTX Intolerance Severity Score; MMR: Measles, mumps, rubella; MTX: Methotrexate; NSAIDs: Nonsteroidal anti-inflammatory drugs; PICO: Population – Intervention – Comparator – Outcome; PPD: Purified protein derivative; RF: Rheumatoid factor; TNF-α: Tumor necrosis factor-α; VZV: Varicella zoster virus

Acknowledgements

The MARAJIA project was developed with the unconditional support of Alfasigma.
The authors thank Ray Hill, an independent medical writer acting on behalf of Springer Healthcare Communications, who provided medical writing support funded by Alfasigma.

Funding

The project received no direct funding.

Authors' contributions

Project conception: RC. Formulation of PICO and the first draft of the manuscript: RC, GF, GM. Analysis and critical review of recommendations: all authors. All authors read and approved the final manuscript.

Competing interests

The authors declare they have no competing interests.

Author details

[1]University of Trieste, Trieste, Italy. [2]Rheumatology Unit, Anna Meyer Children Hospital and University of Florence, University of Florence, Florence, Italy. [3]Department of Pediatrics, University of Catania, Catania, Italy. [4]Pediatric Rheumatology Section, Pediatric Onco-Hematology Unit, Vito Fazzi Hospital, Lecce, Italy. [5]Clinica Pediatrica Università di Torino, Day-Hospital Immunoreumatologia, Turin, Italy. [6]Epidemiology & Clinical Trials Office, General Hospital, Mirano VE, Italy. [7]Pediatria II – Reumatologia, Istituto Giannina Gaslini, and Università degli Studi di Genova, Genoa, Italy. [8]Institute for Maternal and Child Health - IRCCS "Burlo Garofolo", Trieste, and University of Trieste, Trieste, Italy. [9]Department of Pediatrics, Rheumatology Unit, University of Padua, Padua, Italy.

References

1. Petty RE, Southwood TR, Manners P, Baum J, Glass DN, Goldenberg J, et al. International league of associations for rheumatology classification of juvenile idiopathic arthritis: second revision, Edmonton, 2001. J Rheumatol. 2004;31:390–2.
2. Blazina S, Markelj G, Avramovic MZ, Toplak N, Avčin T. Management of juvenile idiopathic arthritis: a clinical guide. Paediatr Drugs. 2016;18:397–412.
3. Calvo I, Anton J, Lopez Robledillo JC, de Inocencio J, Gamir ML, Merino R, et al. Recommendations for the use of methotrexate in patients with juvenile idiopathic arthritis. An Pediatr (Barc). 2016;84(177):e1–8.
4. Niehues T, Lankisch P. Recommendations for the use of methotrexate in juvenile idiopathic arthritis. Paediatr Drugs. 2006;8:347–56.
5. Higgins JPT, Green S (editors). Cochrane Handbook for Systematic Reviews of Interventions Version 5.1.0 [updated March 2011]. The Cochrane Collaboration, 2011. Available from https://handbook.cochrane.org..
6. OCEBM Levels of Evidence Working Group. The Oxford levels of evidence 2. Oxford, UK: Oxford Centre for Evidence-Based Medicine; 2011.
7. Giannini EH, Brewer EJ, Kuzmina N, Shaikov A, Maximov A, Vorontsov I, et al. Methotrexate in resistant juvenile rheumatoid arthritis. Results of the U.S.a.-U.S.S.R. double-blind, placebo-controlled trial. The pediatric rheumatology collaborative study group and the cooperative Children's study group. N Engl J Med. 1992;326:1043–9.
8. Woo P, Southwood TR, Prieur AM, Dore CJ, Grainger J, David J, et al. Randomized, placebo-controlled, crossover trial of low-dose oral methotrexate in children with extended oligoarticular or systemic arthritis. Arthritis Rheum. 2000;43:1849–57.
9. Ruperto N, Murray KJ, Gerloni V, Wulffraat N, de Oliveira SK, Falcini F, et al. A randomized trial of parenteral methotrexate comparing an intermediate dose with a higher dose in children with juvenile idiopathic arthritis who failed to respond to standard doses of methotrexate. Arthritis Rheum. 2004;50:2191–201.
10. Bader-Meunier B, Wouters C, Job-Deslandre C, Cimaz R, Hofer M, Pillet P, et al. Guidelines for diagnosis and treatment of oligoarticular and polyarticular juvenile idiopathic arthritis. Arch Pediatr. 2010;17:1085–9.
11. Beukelman T, Patkar NM, Saag KG, Tolleson-Rinehart S, Cron RQ, DeWitt EM, et al. 2011 American College of Rheumatology recommendations for the treatment of juvenile idiopathic arthritis: initiation and safety monitoring of therapeutic agents for the treatment of arthritis and systemic features. Arthritis Care Res (Hoboken). 2011;63:465–82.
12. Guellac N, Niehues T. Interdisciplinary and evidence-based treatment guideline for juvenile idiopathic arthritis. Klin Padiatr. 2008;220:392–402.
13. Niehues T, Horneff G, Michels H, Hock MS, Schuchmann L, Working Groups Pediatric Rheumatology G, et al. Evidence-based use of methotrexate in children with rheumatic diseases: a consensus statement of the working groups pediatric rheumatology Germany (AGKJR) and pediatric rheumatology Austria. Rheumatol Int. 2005;25:169–78.
14. Ravelli A, Davi S, Bracciolini G, Pistorio A, Consolaro A, van Dijkhuizen EH, et al. Intra-articular corticosteroids versus intra-articular corticosteroids plus methotrexate in oligoarticular juvenile idiopathic arthritis: a multicentre, prospective, randomised, open-label trial. Lancet. 2017;389:909–16.
15. Ringold S, Weiss PF, Beukelman T, EM DW, Ilowite NT, Kimura Y, et al. 2013 update of the 2011 American College of Rheumatology recommendations for the treatment of juvenile idiopathic arthritis: recommendations for the medical therapy of children with systemic juvenile idiopathic arthritis and tuberculosis screening among children receiving biologic medications. Arthritis Rheum. 2013;65:2499–512.
16. Otten MH, Prince FH, Twilt M, Ten Cate R, Armbrust W, Hoppenreijs EP, et al. Tumor necrosis factor-blocking agents for children with enthesitis-related arthritis–data from the dutch arthritis and biologicals in children register, 1999-2010. J Rheumatol. 2011;38:2258–63.
17. Horneff G, Burgos-Vargas R, Constantin T, Foeldvari I, Vojinovic J, Chasnyk VG, et al. Efficacy and safety of open-label etanercept on extended oligoarticular juvenile idiopathic arthritis, enthesitis-related arthritis and psoriatic arthritis: part 1 (week 12) of the CLIPPER study. Ann Rheum Dis. 2014;73:1114–22.
18. Horneff G, Fitter S, Foeldvari I, Minden K, Kuemmerle-Deschner J, Tzaribacev N, et al. Double-blind, placebo-controlled randomized trial with adalimumab for treatment of juvenile onset ankylosing spondylitis (JoAS): significant short term improvement. Arthritis Res Ther. 2012;14:R230.
19. Burgos-Vargas R, Tse SM, Horneff G, Pangan AL, Kalabic J, Goss S, et al. A randomized, double-blind, placebo-controlled multicenter study of adalimumab in pediatric patients with enthesitis-related arthritis. Arthritis Care Res (Hoboken). 2015;67:1503–12.
20. Fráňová J, Fingerhutová Š, Kobrová K, Srp R, Němcová D, Hoza J, et al. Methotrexate efficacy, but not its intolerance, is associated with the dose and route of administration. Pediatr Rheumatol. 2016;14:36.
21. Klein A, Kaul I, Foeldvari I, Ganser G, Urban A, Horneff G. Efficacy and safety of oral and parenteral methotrexate therapy in children with juvenile idiopathic arthritis: an observational study with patients from the German methotrexate registry. Arthritis Care Res (Hoboken). 2012;64:1349–56.
22. Silverman E, Mouy R, Spiegel L, Jung LK, Saurenmann RK, Lahdenne P, et al. Leflunomide or methotrexate for juvenile rheumatoid arthritis. N Engl J Med. 2005;352:1655–66.
23. Cespedes-Cruz A, Gutierrez-Suarez R, Pistorio A, Ravelli A, Loy A, Murray KJ, et al. Methotrexate improves the health-related quality of life of children with juvenile idiopathic arthritis. Ann Rheum Dis. 2008;67:309–14.
24. Ravelli A, Viola S, Ramenghi B, Beluffi G, Zonta LA, Martini A. Radiologic progression in patients with juvenile chronic arthritis treated with methotrexate. J Pediatr. 1998;133:262–5.
25. Harel L, Wagner-Weiner L, Poznanski AK, Spencer CH, Ekwo E, Magilavy DB. Effects of methotrexate on radiologic progression in juvenile rheumatoid arthritis. Arthritis Rheum. 1993;36:1370–4.
26. Graham LD, Myones BL, Rivas-Chacon RF, Pachman LM. Morbidity associated with long-term methotrexate therapy in juvenile rheumatoid arthritis. J Pediatr. 1992;120:468–73.
27. Bulatović M, Heijstek MW, Verkaaik M, van Dijkhuizen EH, Armbrust W, Hoppenreijs EP, et al. High prevalence of methotrexate intolerance in juvenile idiopathic arthritis: development and validation of a methotrexate intolerance severity score. Arthritis Rheum. 2011;63:2007–13.
28. Mulligan K, Wedderburn LR, Newman S. The experience of taking methotrexate for juvenile idiopathic arthritis: results of a cross-sectional survey with children and young people. Pediatr Rheumatol Online J. 2015;13:58.
29. Braun J, Rau R. An update on methotrexate. Curr Opin Rheumatol. 2009;21:216–23.
30. Hashkes PJ, Laxer RM. Update on the medical treatment of juvenile idiopathic arthritis. Curr Rheumatol Rep. 2006;8:450–8.
31. Hashkes PJ, Balistreri WF, Bove KE, Ballard ET, Passo MH. The long-term effect of methotrexate therapy on the liver in patients with juvenile rheumatoid arthritis. Arthritis Rheum. 1997;40:2226–34.
32. Kugathasan S, Newman AJ, Dahms BB, Boyle JT. Liver biopsy findings in patients with juvenile rheumatoid arthritis receiving long-term, weekly methotrexate therapy. J Pediatr. 1996;128:149–51.
33. Salliot C, van der Heijde D. Long-term safety of methotrexate monotherapy in patients with rheumatoid arthritis: a systematic literature research. Ann Rheum Dis. 2009;68:1100–4.
34. Cleary AG, McDowell H, Sills JA. Polyarticular juvenile idiopathic arthritis treated with methotrexate complicated by the development of non-Hodgkin's lymphoma. Arch Dis Child. 2002;86:47–9.
35. Krugmann J, Sailer-Hock M, Muller T, Gruber J, Allerberger F, Offner FA. Epstein-Barr virus-associated Hodgkin's lymphoma and legionella pneumophila infection complicating treatment of juvenile rheumatoid arthritis with methotrexate and cyclosporine a. Hum Pathol. 2000;31:253–5.
36. Munro R, Porter DR, Sturrock RD. Lymphadenopathy in a patient with systemic onset juvenile chronic arthritis. Ann Rheum Dis. 1998;57:513–7.
37. Falcini F, Taccetti G, Ermini M, Trapani S, Calzolari A, Franchi A, et al. Methotrexate-associated appearance and rapid progression of rheumatoid nodules in systemic-onset juvenile rheumatoid arthritis. Arthritis Rheum. 1997;40:175–8.
38. Muzaffer MA, Schneider R, Cameron BJ, Silverman ED, Laxer RM. Accelerated nodulosis during methotrexate therapy for juvenile rheumatoid arthritis. J Pediatr. 1996;128:698–700.
39. Merrill J, Cronstein B, Shen C, Goodman S, Paget S, Mitnick H, et al. Reversal of new but not old rheumatoid nodules by colchicine: evidence from an in vitro model and case reports of 14 patients [abstract]. Arthritis Rheum. 1996;39:1272.
40. Ortiz-Alvarez O, Morishita K, Avery G, Green J, Petty RE, Tucker LB, et al. Guidelines for blood test monitoring of methotrexate toxicity in juvenile idiopathic arthritis. J Rheumatol. 2004;31:2501–6.

41. van Dijkhuizen EH, Pouw JN, Scheuern A, Hugle B, Hardt S, Ganser G, et al. Methotrexate intolerance in oral and subcutaneous administration in patients with juvenile idiopathic arthritis: a cross-sectional, observational study. Clin Exp Rheumatol. 2016;34:148–54.
42. Reiff A, Shaham B, Wood BP, Bernstein BH, Stanley P, Szer IS. High dose methotrexate in the treatment of refractory juvenile rheumatoid arthritis. Clin Exp Rheumatol. 1995;13:113–8.
43. Petty RE, Laxer RM, Lindsley C, Wedderburn LR. Textbook of pediatric rheumatology 7th edition. Philadelphia. USA: Saunders; 2016.
44. Ravelli A, Di Fuccia G, Molinaro M, Ramenghi B, Zonta L, Regazzi MB, et al. Plasma levels after oral methotrexate in children with juvenile rheumatoid arthritis. J Rheumatol. 1993;20:1573–7.
45. Dupuis LL, Koren G, Silverman ED, Laxer RM. Influence of food on the bioavailability of oral methotrexate in children. J Rheumatol. 1995;22:1570–3.
46. Jundt JW, Browne BA, Fiocco GP, Steele AD, Mock D. A comparison of low dose methotrexate bioavailability: oral solution, oral tablet, subcutaneous and intramuscular dosing. J Rheumatol. 1993;20:1845–9.
47. Pinkerton CR, Welshman SG, Glasgow JF, Bridges JM. Can food influence the absorption of methotrexate in children with acute lymphoblastic leukaemia? Lancet. 1980;2:944–6.
48. Alsufyani K, Ortiz-Alvarez O, Cabral DA, Tucker LB, Petty RE, Malleson PN. The role of subcutaneous administration of methotrexate in children with juvenile idiopathic arthritis who have failed oral methotrexate. J Rheumatol. 2004;31:179–82.
49. Tuková J, Chládek J, Němcová D, Chládková J, Doležalová P. Methotrexate bioavailability after oral and subcutaneous dministration in children with juvenile idiopathic arthritis. Clin Exp Rheumatol. 2009;27:1047–53.
50. Gottlieb BS, Keenan GF, Lu T, Ilowite NT. Discontinuation of methotrexate treatment in juvenile rheumatoid arthritis. Pediatrics. 1997;100:994–7.
51. Foell D, Wulffraat N, Wedderburn LR, Wittkowski H, Frosch M, Gerss J, et al. Methotrexate withdrawal at 6 vs 12 months in juvenile idiopathic arthritis in remission: a randomized clinical trial. JAMA. 2010;303:1266–73.
52. Foell D, Frosch M, Schulze zur Wiesch A, Vogl T, Sorg C, Roth J. Methotrexate treatment in juvenile idiopathic arthritis: when is the right time to stop? Ann Rheum Dis. 2004;63:206–8.
53. van Ede AE, Laan RF, Rood MJ, Huizinga TW, van de Laar MA, van Denderen CJ, et al. Effect of folic or folinic acid supplementation on the toxicity and efficacy of methotrexate in rheumatoid arthritis: a forty-eight week, multicenter, randomized, double-blind, placebo-controlled study. Arthritis Rheum. 2001;44:1515–24.
54. Pavy S, Constantin A, Pham T, Gossec L, Maillefert JF, Cantagrel A, et al. Methotrexate therapy for rheumatoid arthritis: clinical practice guidelines based on published evidence and expert opinion. Joint Bone Spine. 2006;73:388–95.
55. Shiroky JB, Neville C, Esdaile JM, Choquette D, Zummer M, Hazeltine M, et al. Low-dose methotrexate with leucovorin (folinic acid) in the management of rheumatoid arthritis. Results of a multicenter randomized, double-blind, placebo-controlled trial. Arthritis Rheum. 1993;36:795–803.
56. Prey S, Paul C. Effect of folic or folinic acid supplementation on methotrexate-associated safety and efficacy in inflammatory disease: a systematic review. Br J Dermatol. 2009;160:622–8.
57. Shea B, Swinden MV, Ghogomu ET, Ortiz Z, Katchamart W, Rader T, et al. Folic acid and folinic acid for reducing side effects in patients receiving methotrexate for rheumatoid arthritis. J Rheumatol. 2014;41:1049–60.
58. Dervieux T, Furst D, Lein DO, Capps R, Smith K, Walsh M, et al. Polyglutamation of methotrexate with common polymorphisms in reduced folate carrier, aminoimidazole carboxamide ribonucleotide transformylase, and thymidylate synthase are associated with methotrexate effects in rheumatoid arthritis. Arthritis Rheum. 2004;50:2766–74.
59. Hunt PG, Rose CD, McIlvain-Simpson G, Tejani S. The effects of daily intake of folic acid on the efficacy of methotrexate therapy in children with juvenile rheumatoid arthritis. A controlled study. J Rheumatol. 1997;24:2230–2.
60. Ravelli A, Migliavacca D, Viola S, Ruperto N, Pistorio A, Martini A. Efficacy of folinic acid in reducing methotrexate toxicity in juvenile idiopathic arthritis. Clin Exp Rheumatol. 1999;17:625–7.
61. West SG. Methotrexate hepatotoxicity. Rheum Dis Clin N Am. 1997;23:883–915.
62. Modesto C, Castro L. Folinic acid supplementation in patients with juvenile rheumatoid arthritis treated with methotrexate. J Rheumatol. 1996;23:403–4.
63. Simonini G, Paudyal P, Jones GT, Cimaz R, Macfarlane GJ. Current evidence of methotrexate efficacy in childhood chronic uveitis: a systematic review and meta-analysis approach. Rheumatology (Oxford). 2013;52:825–31.
64. Foeldvari I, Wierk A. Methotrexate is an effective treatment for chronic uveitis associated with juvenile idiopathic arthritis. J Rheumatol. 2005;32:362–5.
65. Gion N, Stavrou P, Foster CS. Immunomodulatory therapy for chronic tubulointerstitial nephritis-associated uveitis. Am J Ophthalmol. 2000;129:764–8.
66. Heiligenhaus A, Mingels A, Heinz C, Ganser G. Methotrexate for uveitis associated with juvenile idiopathic arthritis: value and requirement for additional anti-inflammatory medication. Eur J Ophthalmol. 2007;17:743–8.
67. Kalinina Ayuso V, van de Winkel EL, Rothova A, de Boer JH. Relapse rate of uveitis post-methotrexate treatment in juvenile idiopathic arthritis. Am J Ophthalmol. 2011;151:217–22.
68. Kaplan-Messas A, Barkana Y, Avni I, Neumann R. Methotrexate as a first-line corticosteroid-sparing therapy in a cohort of uveitis and scleritis. Ocul Immunol Inflamm. 2003;11:131–9.
69. Malik AR, Pavesio C. The use of low dose methotrexate in children with chronic anterior and intermediate uveitis. Br J Ophthalmol. 2005;89:806–8.
70. Samson CM, Waheed N, Baltatzis S, Foster CS. Methotrexate therapy for chronic noninfectious uveitis: analysis of a case series of 160 patients. Ophthalmology. 2001;108:1134–9.
71. Shetty AK, Zganjar BE, Ellis GS Jr, Ludwig IH, Gedalia A. Low-dose methotrexate in the treatment of severe juvenile rheumatoid arthritis and sarcoid iritis. J Pediatr Ophthalmol Strabismus. 1999;36:125–8.
72. Weiss AH, Wallace CA, Sherry DD. Methotrexate for resistant chronic uveitis in children with juvenile rheumatoid arthritis. J Pediatr. 1998;133:266–8.
73. Jabs DA, Nussenblatt RB, Rosenbaum JT. Standardization of uveitis nomenclature working group. Standardization of uveitis nomenclature for reporting clinical data. Results of the first international workshop. Am J Ophthalmol. 2005;140:509–16.
74. Simonini G, Cantarini L, Bresci C, Lorusso M, Galeazzi M, Cimaz R. Current therapeutic approaches to autoimmune chronic uveitis in children. Autoimmun Rev. 2010;9:674–83.
75. Charuvanij S, Guzman J, Lyons C, Petty R. Determination of response to treatment of anterior uveitis with juvenile idiopathic arthritis and isolated chronic idiopathic uveitis [abstract]. Arthritis Rheum. 2009;60:258.
76. Heiligenhaus A, Michels H, Schumacher C, Kopp I, Neudorf U, Niehues T, et al. Evidence-based, interdisciplinary guidelines for anti-inflammatory treatment of uveitis associated with juvenile idiopathic arthritis. Rheumatol Int. 2012;32:1121–33.
77. Bou R, Adan A, Borras F, Bravo B, Calvo I, De Inocencio J, et al. Clinical management algorithm of uveitis associated with juvenile idiopathic arthritis: interdisciplinary panel consensus. Rheumatol Int. 2015;35:777–85.
78. Papadopoulou C, Kostik M, Böhm M, Nieto-Gonzalez JC, Gonzalez-Fernandez MI, Pistorio A, et al. Methotrexate therapy may prevent the onset of uveitis in juvenile idiopathic arthritis. J Pediatr. 2013;163:879–84.
79. Tappeiner C, Schenck S, Niewerth M, Heiligenhaus A, Minden K, Klotsche J. Impact of antiinflammatory treatment on the onset of uveitis in juvenile idiopathic arthritis: longitudinal analysis from a nationwide pediatric rheumatology database. Arthritis Care Res (Hoboken). 2016;68:46–54.
80. Albers HM, Wessels JA, van der Straaten RJ, Brinkman DM, Suijlekom-Smit LW, Kamphuis SS, et al. Time to treatment as an important factor for the response to methotrexate in juvenile idiopathic arthritis. Arthritis Rheum. 2009;61:46–51.
81. Weinblatt ME, Kremer JM, Bankhurst AD, Bulpitt KJ, Fleischmann RM, Fox RI, et al. A trial of etanercept, a recombinant tumor necrosis factor receptor:fc fusion protein, in patients with rheumatoid arthritis receiving methotrexate. N Engl J Med. 1999;340:253–9.
82. Klareskog L, van der Heijde D, de Jager JP, Gough A, Kalden J, Malaise M, et al. Therapeutic effect of the combination of etanercept and methotrexate compared with each treatment alone in patients with rheumatoid arthritis: double-blind randomised controlled trial. Lancet. 2004;363:675–81.
83. Schmeling H, Mathony K, John V, Keysser G, Burdach S, Horneff G. A combination of etanercept and methotrexate for the treatment of refractory juvenile idiopathic arthritis: a pilot study. Ann Rheum Dis. 2001;60:410–2.
84. Giannini EH, Ilowite NT, Lovell DJ, Wallace CA, Rabinovich CE, Reiff A, et al. Long-term safety and effectiveness of etanercept in children with selected categories of juvenile idiopathic arthritis. Arthritis Rheum. 2009;60:2794–804.
85. Lovell DJ, Ruperto N, Goodman S, Reiff A, Jung L, Jarosova K, et al. Adalimumab with or without methotrexate in juvenile rheumatoid arthritis. N Engl J Med. 2008;359:810–20.

86. Murias S, Alcobendas R, Pascual-Salcedo D, Remesal A, Peralta J, Merino R. Anti-adalimumab antibodies in paediatric rheumatology patients: a pilot experience. Rheumatology (Oxford). 2014;53:2124–6.
87. Krieckaert CL, Nurmohamed MT, Wolbink GJ. Methotrexate reduces immunogenicity in adalimumab treated rheumatoid arthritis patients in a dose dependent manner. Ann Rheum Dis. 2012;71:1914–5.
88. Russo RA, Katsicas MM, Zelazko M. Etanercept in systemic juvenile idiopathic arthritis. Clin Exp Rheumatol. 2002;20:723–6.
89. Quartier P, Taupin P, Bourdeaut F, Lemelle I, Pillet P, Bost M, et al. Efficacy of etanercept for the treatment of juvenile idiopathic arthritis according to the onset type. Arthritis Rheum. 2003;48:1093–101.
90. Lahdenne P, Vahasalo P, Honkanen V. Infliximab or etanercept in the treatment of children with refractory juvenile idiopathic arthritis: an open label study. Ann Rheum Dis. 2003;62:245–7.
91. Schmeling H, Horneff G, Benseler SM, Fritzler MJ. Pharmacogenetics: can genes determine treatment efficacy and safety in JIA? Nat Rev Rheumatol. 2014;10:682–90.
92. Pastore S, Stocco G, Favretto D, De Iudicibus S, Taddio A, d'Adamo P, et al. Genetic determinants for methotrexate response in juvenile idiopathic arthritis. Front Pharmacol. 2015;6:52.
93. Calasan MB, den Boer E, de Rotte MC, Vastert SJ, Kamphuis S, de Jonge R, et al. Methotrexate polyglutamates in erythrocytes are associated with lower disease activity in juvenile idiopathic arthritis patients. Ann Rheum Dis. 2015;74:402–7.
94. Chabner BA, Allegra CJ, Curt GA, Clendeninn NJ, Baram J, Koizumi S, et al. Polyglutamation of methotrexate. Is methotrexate a prodrug? J Clin Invest. 1985;76:907–12.
95. Vilca I, Munitis PG, Pistorio A, Ravelli A, Buoncompagni A, Bica B, et al. Predictors of poor response to methotrexate in polyarticular-course juvenile idiopathic arthritis: analysis of the PRINTO methotrexate trial. Ann Rheum Dis. 2010;69:1479–83.
96. Cobb J, Cule E, Moncrieffe H, Hinks A, Ursu S, Patrick F, et al. Genome-wide data reveal novel genes for methotrexate response in a large cohort of juvenile idiopathic arthritis cases. Pharmacogenomics J. 2014;14:356–64.
97. Hinks A, Moncrieffe H, Martin P, Ursu S, Lal S, Kassoumeri L, et al. Association of the 5-aminoimidazole-4-carboxamide ribonucleotide transformylase gene with response to methotrexate in juvenile idiopathic arthritis. Ann Rheum Dis. 2011;70:1395–400.
98. de Rotte MC, Bulatović M, Heijstek MW, Jansen G, Heil SG, van Schaik RH, et al. ABCB1 and ABCC3 gene polymorphisms are associated with first-year response to methotrexate in juvenile idiopathic arthritis. J Rheumatol. 2012;39:2032–40.
99. Avramovič MZ, Dolžan V, Toplak N, Accetto M, Lusa L, Avčin T. Relationship between polymorphisms in methotrexate pathway genes and outcome of methotrexate treatment in a cohort of 119 patients with juvenile idiopathic arthritis. J Rheumatol. 2017;44:1216–23.
100. Pastore S, Stocco G, Moressa V, Zandona L, Favretto D, Malusa N, et al. 5-Aminoimidazole-4-carboxamide ribonucleotide-transformylase and inosine-triphosphate-pyrophosphatase genes variants predict remission rate during methotrexate therapy in patients with juvenile idiopathic arthritis. Rheumatol Int. 2015;35:619–27.
101. Heijstek MW, Ott de Bruin LM, Bijl M, Borrow R, van der Klis F, Kone-Paut I, et al. EULAR recommendations for vaccination in paediatric patients with rheumatic diseases. Ann Rheum Dis. 2011;70:1704–12.
102. Heijstek MW, Ott de Bruin LM, Borrow R, van der Klis F, Kone-Paut I, Fasth A, et al. Vaccination in paediatric patients with auto-immune rheumatic diseases: a systemic literature review for the European league against rheumatism evidence-based recommendations. Autoimmun Rev. 2011;11:112–22.
103. Groot N, Heijstek MW, Wulffraat NM. Vaccinations in paediatric rheumatology: an update on current developments. Curr Rheumatol Rep. 2015;17:46.
104. Heijstek MW, van Gageldonk PG, Berbers GA, Wulffraat NM. Differences in persistence of measles, mumps, rubella, diphtheria and tetanus antibodies between children with rheumatic disease and healthy controls: a retrospective cross-sectional study. Ann Rheum Dis. 2012;71:948–54.
105. Kasapcopur O, Cullu F, Kamburoglu-Goksel A, Cam H, Akdenizli E, Calykan S, et al. Hepatitis B vaccination in children with juvenile idiopathic arthritis. Ann Rheum Dis. 2004;63:1128–30.
106. Kiray E, Kasapcopur O, Bas V, Kamburoglu-Goksel A, Midilli K, Arisoy N, et al. Purified protein derivative response in juvenile idiopathic arthritis. J Rheumatol. 2009;36:2029–32.
107. Stoof SP, Heijstek MW, Sijssens KM, van der Klis F, Sanders EA, Teunis PF, et al. Kinetics of the long-term antibody response after meningococcal C vaccination in patients with juvenile idiopathic arthritis: a retrospective cohort study. Ann Rheum Dis. 2014;73:728–34.
108. Heijstek MW, Pileggi GC, Zonneveld-Huijssoon E, Armbrust W, Hoppenreijs EP, Uiterwaal CS, et al. Safety of measles, mumps and rubella vaccination in juvenile idiopathic arthritis. Ann Rheum Dis. 2007;66:1384–7.
109. Woerner A, Sauvain MJ, Aebi C, Otth M, Bolt IB. Immune response to influenza vaccination in children treated with methotrexate or/and tumor necrosis factor-alpha inhibitors. Hum Vaccin. 2011;7:1293–8.
110. Borte S, Liebert UG, Borte M, Sack U. Efficacy of measles, mumps and rubella revaccination in children with juvenile idiopathic arthritis treated with methotrexate and etanercept. Rheumatology (Oxford). 2009;48:144–8.
111. Aikawa NE, Campos LM, Goldenstein-Schainberg C, Saad CG, Ribeiro AC, Bueno C, et al. Effective seroconversion and safety following the pandemic influenza vaccination (anti-H1N1) in patients with juvenile idiopathic arthritis. Scand J Rheumatol. 2013;42:34–40.
112. Pileggi GS, de Souza CB, Ferriani VP. Safety and immunogenicity of varicella vaccine in patients with juvenile rheumatic diseases receiving methotrexate and corticosteroids. Arthritis Care Res (Hoboken). 2010;62:1034–9.
113. Heijstek MW, Kamphuis S, Armbrust W, Swart J, Gorter S, de Vries LD, et al. Effects of the live attenuated measles-mumps-rubella booster vaccination on disease activity in patients with juvenile idiopathic arthritis: a randomized trial. JAMA. 2013;309:2449–56.
114. Farmaki E, Kanakoudi-Tsakalidou F, Spoulou V, Trachana M, Pratsidou-Gertsi P, Tritsoni M, et al. The effect of anti-TNF treatment on the immunogenicity and safety of the 7-valent conjugate pneumococcal vaccine in children with juvenile idiopathic arthritis. Vaccine. 2010;28:5109–13.
115. Zonneveld-Huijssoon E, Ronaghy A, Van Rossum MA, Rijkers GT, van der Klis FR, Sanders EA, et al. Safety and efficacy of meningococcal c vaccination in juvenile idiopathic arthritis. Arthritis Rheum. 2007;56:639–46.
116. Aikawa NE, Franca IL, Ribeiro AC, Sallum AM, Bonfa E, Silva CA. Short and long-term immunogenicity and safety following the 23-valent polysaccharide pneumococcal vaccine in juvenile idiopathic arthritis patients under conventional DMARDs with or without anti-TNF therapy. Vaccine. 2015;33:604–9.
117. Heijstek MW, Scherpenisse M, Groot N, Tacke C, Schepp RM, Buisman AM, et al. Immunogenicity and safety of the bivalent HPV vaccine in female patients with juvenile idiopathic arthritis: a prospective controlled observational cohort study. Ann Rheum Dis. 2014;73:1500–7.
118. Michalik DE, Steinberg SP, Larussa PS, Edwards KM, Wright PF, Arvin AM, et al. Primary vaccine failure after 1 dose of varicella vaccine in healthy children. J Infect Dis. 2008;197:944–9.
119. Marin M, Guris D, Chaves SS, Schmid S, Seward JF. Advisory committee on immunization practices of the Centers for Disease Control and Prevention (CDC). Prevention of varicella: recommendations of the advisory committee on immunization practices (ACIP). MMWR Recomm Rep. 2007;56:1–40.

Comparing the importance of quality measurement themes in juvenile idiopathic inflammatory myositis between patients and families and healthcare professionals

Heather O. Tory[1,2*], Ruy Carrasco[3], Thomas Griffin[4], Adam M. Huber[5], Philip Kahn[6], Angela Byun Robinson[7], David Zurakowski[8], Susan Kim[9] and the CARRA Juvenile Dermatomyositis Quality Measures Workgroup

Abstract

Background: A standardized set of quality measures for juvenile idiopathic inflammatory myopathies (JIIM) is not in use. Discordance has been shown between the importance ascribed to quality measures between patients and families and physicians. The objective of this study was to assess and compare the importance of various aspects of high quality care to patients with JIIM and their families with healthcare providers, to aid in future development of comprehensive quality measures.

Methods: Surveys were developed by members of the Childhood Arthritis and Rheumatology Research Alliance (CARRA) Juvenile Dermatomyositis Workgroup through a consensus process and administered to patients and families through the CureJM Foundation and to healthcare professionals through CARRA. The survey asked respondents to rate the importance of 19 items related to aspects of high quality care, using a Likert scale.

Results: Patients and families gave generally higher scores for importance to most of the quality measurement themes compared with healthcare professionals, with ratings of 13 of the 19 measures reaching statistical significance ($p < 0.05$). Of particular importance, however, was consensus between the groups on the top five most important items: quality of life, timely diagnosis, access to rheumatology, normalization of functioning/strength, and ability for self care.

Conclusions: Despite overall differences in the rating of importance of quality indicators between patients and families and healthcare professionals, the groups agreed on the most important aspects of care. Recognizing areas of particular importance to patients and families, and overlapping in importance with providers, will promote the development of standardized quality measures with the greatest potential for improving care and outcomes for children with JIIM.

Keywords: Juvenile dermatomyositis, Quality measures, Physician perspective, Patient perspective, Patient reported outcomes

Background

The juvenile idiopathic inflammatory myopathies (JIIM) represent a group of rare conditions with the common feature of muscle weakness, the most frequent of which is juvenile dermatomyositis (JDM). These are chronic conditions, often associated with long-term morbidity due to the disease itself and medication toxicities, which can lead to significant functional impairment. While there are well documented clinical and laboratory criteria for assessment and ongoing monitoring of disease activity in patients with JIIM, and published core sets of outcome measures including disease activity and damage assessment [1, 2], there is currently no standardized, comprehensive set of quality measures for monitoring disease activity, disease chronicity, response to therapy and functional impact in patients with JIIM in clinical practice.

* Correspondence: htory@connecticutchildrens.org
[1]Pediatric Rheumatology, Connecticut Children's Medical Center, 282 Washington Street, Hartford, CT 06106, USA
[2]Department of Pediatrics, University of Connecticut School of Medicine, 263 Farmington Avenue, Farmington 06032, CT, USA
Full list of author information is available at the end of the article

Quality measures have been developed and adopted largely to enable the evaluation of the quality and performance of healthcare delivery by a healthcare provider or entity. They facilitate standardized comparisons of clinical care across care providers and are becoming increasingly important in assessing healthcare delivery processes and outcomes [3]. At the level of the individual clinician, they should serve as a roadmap to delivering the highest quality care for patients and represent the standard to achieve for every patient.

The Patient-Reported Outcomes Measurement Information System (PROMIS) measures are quickly becoming standards in evaluation of clinical practice monitoring for a multitude of disease processes, including the rheumatic diseases [4]. Involving patients in their own care significantly improves healthcare outcomes, healthcare utilization and patient satisfaction [5]; however, most patient reported outcomes (PROs) have been developed without significant patient input. Standard sets of quality measures to guide clinical care have been established for some pediatric rheumatic diseases, but have not been widely used or well defined for JIIM [6, 7].

The development of quality measures in JIIM, with a focus on PROs, is critical for giving medical providers the tools to monitor and treat patients with the disease in a manner that reflects the desired health outcomes of patients. This is also important for providing patients, parents, and caregivers the tools and information they need to make informed decisions about their healthcare. At the same time, the correlation between patient-reported and physician-reported outcome measures is not clearly established, with some studies suggesting significant discordance [8–10].

In this study, we sought to assess the importance of various aspects of high quality care to patients with JIIM and their families and assess the concordance with the importance ascribed by physicians and other clinical care providers. The ultimate goal of this work is to develop a standardized set of quality measures for use by pediatric rheumatologists and health professionals to aid in the assessment and long-term monitoring of patients with this disease.

Methods

Patient and family survey

A survey was developed by members of the Childhood Arthritis and Rheumatology Research Alliance (CARRA) JDM Quality Measures Workgroup through a consensus process. First, a list of candidate themes important in the clinical care of patients with JIIM was generated in round robin fashion, based on discussion among the ten workgroup members (including pediatric rheumatology attending physicians and trainees as well as allied health professionals) at an annual CARRA meeting. This was followed by selection of a draft list to include on the survey, using nominal group technique. Following the workgroup session, the survey underwent review and editing for additional input, suggestions regarding missing items, and evaluation of comprehensibility/readability by three parent members of the CureJM Foundation, a nonprofit organization dedicated to enhancing awareness and raising research funds for juvenile myositis. The final included list of variables then underwent an additional review online by the workgroup members for final approval.

The survey questions gathered information on patient demographics, myositis characteristics, functional disability, and asked respondents to rate the importance of 19 aspects of high quality care: timely diagnosis, access to rheumatology (ease of getting an appointment), access to dermatology, access to physical therapy, medication counseling, monitoring of medication toxicity, medication tolerance, discontinuation of steroids/prednisone, discontinuation of medications, normalization of labs, overall quality of life, ability for self-care/activities of daily living, resolution of pain, resolution of fatigue, resolution of rash, normalization of functioning/strength, school attendance, work attendance, and minimizing hospital/clinic visits. For these questions, respondents were asked to rank each measure independently on a 5-point scale, with "1" indicating very low importance and "5" indicating the greatest importance.

In June 2014, the survey was distributed electronically via e-mail to patients and family members of patients with JIIM through the CureJM Foundation patient and family database (https://www.surveymonkey.com/r/JM_QI). This database included contact information for approximately 1500 families of patients with JIIM. Responses were collated and data were abstracted in a standardized database for analysis. IRB approval was obtained at one institution and participants were informed that consent to participate was implied by completion of the questionnaire.

Healthcare professional survey

The survey sent to patients and families of patients with JIIM was adapted for use with healthcare professionals. The survey questions assessed characteristics of the responding healthcare professionals and asked respondents to rate the importance of the same 19 quality of care themes. The survey was electronically distributed via e-mail to all registered CARRA healthcare professionals in the CARRA database (approximate $n = 400$, including physicians, nurses and other allied health professionals) in June 2015, with an additional reminder in July 2015 (https://www.surveymonkey.com/r/9WG3WWB). These responses were collated and data were abstracted in the same standardized database for analysis. IRB approval was obtained at one institution and participants were informed that consent to participate was implied by completion of the questionnaire.

Statistical analysis

Student t-test comparisons were used to assess difference in the ranking of quality themes between parents and families and healthcare professionals. We used 2-tailed Student t-tests with p-values based on equal or unequal variances, as assessed by Levine's test. Two-tailed values of $p < 0.05$ were considered statistically significant. Analysis was performed using IBM SPSS Statistics version 23.0 (IBM Corporation, Armonk, NY).

Results

Patient and family survey

Overall, there were 194 respondents (approximate response rate of 13%) to the survey, the majority of whom were parents of children with JIIM and the remainder of whom were mainly other relatives acting as caregivers. Most respondents described significant functional impact when the disease was at its worst, but currently had well-controlled disease, with minimal or no impact within the preceding two weeks (Table 1).

Families of patients with JIIM rated overall quality of life as the variable with the highest average importance. Timely diagnosis and access to rheumatology were the next most important, followed by patient reported outcomes of normalization of functioning and strength, resolution of pain, and resolution of fatigue. Conversely, access to a dermatologist and concerns related to work attendance and number of hospital and clinic visits, were rated as least important (Fig. 1); however, all of the items were highly rated, with the lowest ranked (access to dermatology) receiving an average score of 3.8 out of five.

In subgroup analysis, there was no significant difference in rating of quality themes when comparing patients diagnosed in the past two years, compared to patients diagnosed more than 2 years ago, except for normalization of labs (mean rating 4.6 +/− 0.755 vs. 4.3 +/− 1.136, respectively, $p = 0.01$). There were also no significant differences found in the ratings between patients reporting high and low levels of current functional limitations.

Healthcare professional survey

There were 86 responses (approximate response rate of 22%) to the healthcare professional survey: 82 (95%) pediatric rheumatologists, 2 (2.5%) pediatric nurse practitioners, and 2 (2.5%) adult rheumatologists, all practicing in the United States (89.5%) and Canada (10.5%). Respondents were evenly divided among clinicians with 1–5 years of experience (25%), 6–10 years (22.6%), 11–20 years (23.8%) and more than 20 years (28.6%). Most respondents reported following less than 15 patients (80.7%), with only seven respondents (8.4%) reporting following more than 30 patients with JIIM.

Healthcare professionals rated timely diagnosis as the most important aspect of high quality care, followed by normalization of functioning/strength and access to rheumatology (Fig. 1).

Table 1 Demographic information of patients represented by respondents to the patient and family survey

Characteristic	All patients ($N = 194$)
Diagnosis	
Juvenile dermatomyositis, N (%)	189 (97)
Juvenile polymyositis, N (%)	5 (3)
Respondent[a]	
Parent, N (%)	168 (87)
Grandparent, N (%)	10 (5)
Aunt/Uncle, N (%)	2 (1)
Female, N (%)	140 (72)
Ethnicity, N (%)	
Caucasian/White	150 (77)
Hispanic/Latino	10 (5)
African American/Black	11 (6)
Asian/Pacific Islander	2 (1)
American Indian/Alaskan Native	1 (0.5)
Multiple Ethnicity	18 (9)
Prefer not to answer	1 (1)
Time to diagnosis (months): mean (range)	6.7 (1–40)
Functional disability when disease at worst	
Significant impact, N (%)	145 (75%)
Intermediate impact, N (%)	24 (12%)
Functional disability in prior two weeks	
Minimal or no impact, N (%)	131 (69%)
Significant impact, N (%)	19 (10%)

[a]Total less than 100%: 14 (7%) of respondents skipped question

Patient and family and healthcare professional survey comparison

While there were differences observed in the relative ratings of the importance of various quality indicators between patients and families and healthcare professionals (Fig. 1), the groups agreed on the top five most important themes (Table 2). Overall, patients and families gave higher rankings than healthcare professionals to all of the variables except school attendance and medication counseling, although this difference was not statistically significant. There were 13 quality themes that parents rated as statistically significantly more important than healthcare providers. These areas were

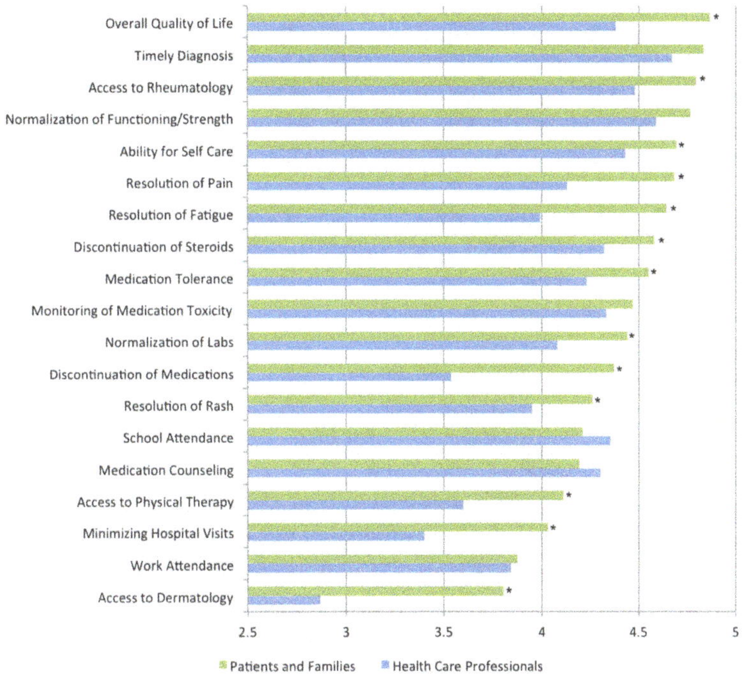

Fig. 1 Relative rating of quality measurement themes to patients and families of patients with JIIM and healthcare professionals caring for patients with JIIM. *Denotes statistical significance of $p < 0.05$ using Student t-test

overall quality of life, access to a rheumatologist, ability for self care, resolution of pain and fatigue, discontinuation of steroids, medication tolerance, normalization of labs, discontinuation of medications, resolution of rash, access to physical therapy, minimization of hospital visits, and access to dermatology (all $p < 0.05$) (Fig. 1).

Discussion

Healthcare providers and systems are increasingly focused on patient centered care, with the ultimate goal of improving care in a manner most relevant to patients. This study was performed to identify and compare the importance of various aspects of high quality care to patients and families with JIIM and their healthcare providers, to help guide the future development of a standardized set of clearly defined quality measures that are relevant to both clinical care providers and patients and their families. This is an area of great need in JIIM, as standardized quality measures are important for improving the assessment and long-term monitoring of patients with chronic diseases [11]. While collecting an exhaustive list of measures would be comprehensive, it is impractical. With limitations in economic resources and time, identifying areas for development of quality measures with overlapping importance to patients and healthcare providers will highlight the best areas for initial focus.

Previous work completed by the Outcome Measures in Rheumatology (OMERACT) myositis working group, and others, has also shown the importance of patient input in the development of PROs in myositis [12]. Using qualitative studies with focused interview and cognitive debriefing methodologies to inform their work, this group found that currently used PROs do not measure the outcomes that are most important to patients. Similarly, our work also revealed differences between patient and provider perspectives in the ratings of importance of different variables, such as minimizing hospital visits and access to other health care professionals.

Table 2 Top five quality measurement themes rated as being most important by both patients and families with JIIM and healthcare professionals

Patients and Families	Healthcare Professionals	Top Five Quality Measurement Themes
1	5	Overall Quality of Life
2	1	Timely Diagnosis
3	3	Access to Rheumatology
4	2	Normalization of Functioning/Strength
5	4	Ability for Self Care

Importantly, however, our study found that both groups mutually agreed upon the top five aspects of high quality care. This suggests that creating a standardized set of quality measures with relevance and meaning to patients and families and healthcare professionals is feasible and appropriate. These items are important to pursue in further quality measurement development, and may be the cornerstone in defining a standardized set of quality measures in JIIM.

There are limitations to consider in our work. The patient and family and healthcare professional surveys did not undergo formal reliability or validity testing, as they were exploratory in nature. The healthcare provider survey was sent to the entire CARRA membership, with a response rate of approximately 22%. While this rate can be considered low, it is similar to the response rates in other recent CARRA surveys [13] and is comparable to currently reported online survey response rates [14]. This rate is lower than that reported in some earlier surveys of CARRA work [15, 16]. The current survey was sent to the entire CARRA membership, not a specific membership subset as with some of these prior surveys (such as only to the JDM disease subcommittee), so it may be that clinicians with more exposure and expertise in JIIM were more likely to respond. With the limited response rate, it is possible that these findings are not representative of all CARRA members; however, there was broad representation of healthcare professionals, with a similar proportion of responses across all years of experience.

The patient and family survey was sent to members of the CureJM Foundation, which may represent a specific demographic population rather than the entire population of patients and families with JIIM. For example, the majority of patients appeared to be in remission, with relatively low disease impact at the time of the survey. The survey was also administered solely in English, which likely excluded a subset of patients. Furthermore, the majority of respondents were parents, not patients, which may alter the perspective and responses as well, although this is common in pediatrics. This was likely due to greater parent membership in the CureJM Foundation, compared with patients. Finally, the quality measurement themes that were presented for ranking of importance were selected and incorporated into the survey by healthcare providers and three parent reviewers, but there may be other measures that are important to patients and families that they were not given the opportunity to rank. This would benefit from additional input from a broader patient and family audience through focus groups and other methods of communication.

In general, the overall rankings of importance of all the variables were scored higher by patients and families compared to healthcare providers. Although this could be an accurate measurement, it may reflect the differences in perspective when comparing patients' and providers' experiences and goals. It is also likely that healthcare professionals are more accustomed to scales/rankings, leading to a larger range of rankings when compared to patients and families. This may have been minimized if the ratings were measured in an ordinal scale, which should be applied to future work. In addition, these differences may be related to the finding that patients and families are more likely to use temporal comparisons (considering these measures based on their personal condition), while clinicians appear to use social comparisons (considering measures based on the full range of disease in the population) [17].

We had hypothesized that there might be differences in the ranking of importance of all of the themes based on duration of disease or current level of functional impairment from disease among patients and families, but this was not shown in statistical analysis. This may have been due to the relatively low percentage of patients with any current functional impact, as nearly 70% of respondents reported minimal or no current functional impact from JIIM at the time of their response to the survey. Access to dermatology was rated lowest by patients and families compared to other items and may have been influenced by the fact that the survey was administered by a group of rheumatologists through CARRA.

Healthcare professionals must be thoughtful in aligning standardized quality measures with those that are considered important by patients and their families, to ensure that the patient voice and perspective is being incorporated into decision making for disease assessment, monitoring and treatment. Attention to quality measures that are important to patients and their families will also promote partnership in care and alignment of goals between patients and care providers which may, in turn, help to improve adherence to therapy, satisfaction, and outcomes. Understanding and appreciating differences in the perceptions of relative importance of the aspects of quality care between these groups should be considered in future plans to design and implement a standardized set of quality measures for this disease, with particular attention paid to those areas that showed overlapping highest importance (quality of life, timely diagnosis, access to rheumatology, normalization of functioning/strength, and ability for self care). With limited resources, the integration of measures that are considered important by both patients and families and clinicians may allow for future pragmatic collection of high-yield outcome measures, and maximize the opportunities to measure and improve outcomes for children with JIIM. To move this work forward and reach that goal, the themes discussed here will need to be explored and transformed into clearly developed quality measures with robust measurement specifications. This will require discussion of the measurement domains and methods, as well as the tools and methodology that are required to assess the variables. Some of the quality of care themes explored here will more readily translate into specific quality measures for use by individual pediatric rheumatologists. For example, quality of life can be assessed with the use of validated tools [18], while timely diagnosis is influenced by a variety of factors other than the care of the treating pediatric rheumatologist, as many delays in care are experienced prior to referral to rheumatology. This will need to be taken into account when designing specific, measurable parameters for quality measurement.

Conclusions

The results of this study support prior work showing differences in the relative importance that patients and families ascribed to various quality measures, compared with healthcare providers. This highlights the importance of obtaining input and feedback from patients and families when designing and implementing quality measures for use in monitoring disease activity, progress and response to treatment. This study found that the top five themes for quality care ranked by patients and families and healthcare professionals were overlapping, suggesting that these domains should be given special attention and incorporated into future quality measure development for JIIM.

Abbreviations

CARRA: Childhood Arthritis and Rheumatology Research Alliance; JDM: Juvenile Dermatomyositis; JIIM: Juvenile idiopathic inflammatory myopathies; OMERACT: Outcome Measures in Rheumatology; PROMIS: Patient-Reported Outcomes Measurement Information System

Acknowledgements

The authors wish to acknowledge CARRA and the ongoing Arthritis Foundation financial support of CARRA. In addition, we would like to acknowledge CureJM Foundation Members, who helped to review and distribute our survey, and participate in the survey.

Funding

The work of the corresponding author of this study was supported, in part, by a small grant from the Childhood Arthritis and Rheumatology Research Alliance and the Arthritis Foundation. The funding body had no impact on the study design, collection, analysis or interpretation of data, or in the writing of this manuscript.

Authors' contributions

SK, HT and DZ made substantial contributions to conception and design, acquisition of data, analysis and interpretation of data, and drafting the manuscript. AH, ABR, PK, RC and TG made substantial contributions to conception and design and critical revision of the manuscript. All authors read and approved the final manuscript.

Competing interests

The authors declare that they have no competing interests.

Author details

[1]Pediatric Rheumatology, Connecticut Children's Medical Center, 282 Washington Street, Hartford, CT 06106, USA. [2]Department of Pediatrics, University of Connecticut School of Medicine, 263 Farmington Avenue, Farmington 06032, CT, USA. [3]Pediatric Rheumatology, Dell Children's Medical Center of Central Texas, 4900 Mueller Boulevard, Austin, TX 78723, USA. [4]Pediatric Rheumatology, Carolinas HealthCare System, Levine Children's Hospital Specialty Center, 1781 Tate Boulevard, SE, Suite 206, Hickory, NC 28054, USA. [5]Pediatric Rheumatology, IWK Health Centre and Dalhousie University, 5980 University Avenue, Halifax, NS B3K 6R8, Canada. [6]Pediatric Rheumatology, New York University Medical Center, 160 E 32nd Street, New York, NY 10016, USA. [7]Pediatric Rheumatology, Rainbow Babies & Children's Hospital, 11100 Euclid Avenue, Cleveland, OH 44106, USA. [8]Departments of Anesthesia and Surgery, Boston Children's Hospital and Harvard Medical School, 300 Longwood Avenue, Boston, MA 02115, USA. [9]Pediatric Rheumatology, Benioff Children's Hospital and University of San Francisco Medical Center, 1975 4th Street, San Francisco, CA 94158, USA.

References

1. Ruperto N, Ravelli A, Murray KJ, Lovell DJ, Andersson-Gare B, Feldman BM, et al. Preliminary core sets of measures for disease activity and damage assessment in juvenile systemic lupus erythematosus and juvenile dermatomyositis. Rheumatology. 2003;42:1452–9.
2. Rider LG, Werth VP, Huber AM. Measures for adult and juvenile dermatomyositis, polymyositis, and inclusion body myositis. Arthritis Care Res. 2011;63:S118–57.
3. Suter L, Barber CE, Herrin J, Leong A, Losina E, Miller A, et al. American College of Rheumatology White Paper on performance outcome measures in rheumatology. Arthritis Care Res. 2016;68(10):1390–401.
4. Orbai AM, Bingham CO. Patient reported outcomes in rheumatoid arthritis clinical trials. Curr Rheumatol Rep. 2015;17(4):501.
5. Michaud K, Vera-Llonch M, Oster G. Mortality risk by functional status and health-related quality of life in patients with rheumatoid arthritis. J Rheumatol. 2012;39(1):54–9.
6. Lovell DJ, Passo MH, Beukelman T, Bowyer SL, Gottlieb BS, Henrickson M, et al. Measuring process of arthritis care: a proposed set of quality measures for the process of care in juvenile idiopathic arthritis. Arthritis Care Res. 2011;63:10–6.
7. Harris JG, Maletta KI, Kuhn EM, Olson JC. Evaluation of quality indicators and disease damage in childhood-onset systemic lupus erythematosus. Clin Rheumatol. 2017;36:351–9.
8. Desthieux C, Hermet A, Granger B, Fautrel B, Gossec L. Patient-physician discordance in global assessment in rheumatoid arthritis: a systematic literature review with meta-analysis. Arthritis Care Res. 2016;68:1767–73.
9. Barton JL, Imboden J, Graf J, Glidden D, Yelin EH, Schillinger D. Patient-physician discordance in assessments of global disease severity in rheumatoid arthritis. Arthritis Care Res. 2010;62:857–64.
10. Desthieux C, Granger B, Balanescu AR, Balint P, Braun J, Canete JD, et al. Determinants of patient-physician discordance in global assessment in psoriatic arthritis: a multicenter European study. Arthritis Care Res. 2017;69:1606–11.
11. Adirim T, Meade K, Mistry K. American Academy of Pediatrics Council on quality improvement and patient safety. A new era in quality measurement: the development and application of quality measures. Pediatrics. 2017; 139(1):e20163442.
12. Regardt M, Basharat P, Christopher-Stine L, Sarver C, Bjorn A, Lundberg IE, et al. Patients' experience of myositis and further validation of a myositis-specific patient reported outcome measure – establishing core domains and expanding patient input on clinical assessment in myositis. Report from OMERACT 12. J Rheumatol. 2015;42(12):2492–5.

13. Kim S, Kahn P, Robinson AB, Lang B, Shulman A, Oberle EJ, et al. Childhood arthritis and rheumatology research alliance consensus clinical treatment plans for juvenile dermatomyositis with skin predominant disease. Pediatr Rheumatol. 2017;15(1):1.
14. Cunningham CT, Quan H, Hemmelgarn B, Noseworthy T, Beck CA, Dixon E, et al. Exploring physician specialist response rates to web-based surveys. BMC Med Res Methodol. 2015;15:32.
15. Huber AM, Giannini EH, Bowyer SL, Kim S, Lang B, Lindsley CB, et al. Protocols for the initial treatment of moderately severe juvenile dermatomyositis: results of a children's arthritis and rheumatology research alliance consensus conference. Arthritis Care Res. 2010;62:219–25.
16. DeWitt EM, Kimura Y, Beukelman T, Nigrovic PA, Onel K, Prahalad S, et al. Consensus treatment plans for new-onset systemic juvenile idiopathic arthritis. Arthritis Care Res. 2012;64:1001–10.
17. Ward MM, Guthrie LC, Alba MI. Standards of comparison and discordance in rheumatoid arthritis global assessments between patients and clinicians. Arthritis Care Res. 2016;69(8):1260–5.
18. Varni JW, Seid M, Rode CA. The PedsQL: measurement model for the pediatric quality of life inventory. Med Care. 1999;37(2):126–39.

28

Reliability of ultrasonography to detect inflammatory lesions and structural damage in juvenile idiopathic arthritis

Lucio Ventura-Ríos[1*], Enrique Faugier[2], Laura Barzola[3], L. B. De la Cruz-Becerra[4], Guadalupe Sánchez-Bringas[5], Andrés Rodríguez García[2], Rocío Maldonado[2], Johannes Roth[6] and Cristina Hernández-Díaz[1]

Abstract

Background: Musculoskeletal Ultrasonography (MSUS) is an important tool for the clinical assessment in Juvenile Idiopathic Arthritis (JIA). The objective of this study was to evaluate the reliability of MSUS to detect elementary lesions: synovitis, tenosynovitis, cartilage damage and bone erosions in the wrist and metacarpal (MCP) joints of patients with JIA.

Methods: Thirty children in various subgroups of JIA according to ILAR criteria, were included in this cross-sectional study. Clinical data including painful, swollen and limited joints were recorded. Five rheumatologist ultrasonographers, blinded to the clinical evaluation, evaluated the presence of elementary lesions in the wrist and MCP 2 and 3 joints bilaterally. The synovitis was graded in B-Mode and Power Doppler (PD). In addition to descriptive statistics intra- and inter-observer reliability was calculated using Cohen's kappa according to Landis and Koch.

Results: US detected more synovitis than the clinical examination (62% vs 28%, 30% vs 23% and 22% vs 17% in the wrist, second and third MCP joints respectively). The intra-observer concordance for synovitis in all joints was excellent in B-Mode (k 0.84 .63–1.0 $p = 0.001$), except for MCP 2, where it was good (0.61, IC 95% .34–89, $p = 0.001$). For both modalities (PD, B-Mode) tenosynovitis, cartilage damage and bone erosions it was also excellent. Regarding synovitis grading the concordance was excellent for all grades (0.83–1.0, IC 95% 0.51.1.0, $p = 0.001$), except for grade 1 where it was good (0.61, IC 95% 0.43–.83, $p = 0.001$). Reliability inter-observer for grayscale synovitis (0.67–0.95, IC 95% 0.67–1.0, $p = 0.001$), tenosynovitis grayscale (0.89, IC 95% 0.78–0.99, p.001), damage cartilage (0.89, IC 95% 0.78–0.99, $p = 0.001$), PD (0.66, IC 95% 0.39–1.0, $p = 0.001$). The concordance for grading synovitis was excellent, but for grayscale grade 1 and 2 (.66, IC 95% .53–.74, $p = 0.007$) and PD grade 1 and 2 (0.63, IC 95% .58–.91, $p = 004$) was good.

Conclusions: The intra- and inter-observer reliability of MSUS for inflammatory and structural lesions is good to excellent for the wrist and MCP in patients with JIA.

Keywords: Reliability, Musculoskeletal ultrasound, Juvenile idiopathic arthritis

Background

In recent years, musculoskeletal ultrasound has been recommended for the evaluation of treatment response and the detection of subclinical synovitis in rheumatoid arthritis [1]. MSUS may be equally important in children [2]. It has many advantages over other imaging techniques being easily accessible, fast, dynamic, not exposure to radiation and not requiring sedation [3]. It is being used increasingly for patients with juvenile idiopathic arthritis (JIA) to confirm suspected clinical findings, subclinical synovitis, define specific anatomic structures and guide interventional procedures like joint injections [4–6]. MSUS has been shown to be superior to the clinical exam in the detection of synovitis in JIA [7, 8]. Despite the increasing use in daily clinical practice, there is still a lack of data on the reliability of MSUS in the evaluation of joint inflammation and

* Correspondence: venturarioslucio@gmail.com
[1]Laboratorio de ultrasonido musculoesquelético y articular, Instituto Nacional de Rehabilitación, Luis Guillermo Ibarra Ibarra, Calzada México-Xochimilco 289, Arenal de Guadalupe, Tlalpan, 14389 Mexico city, Mexico
Full list of author information is available at the end of the article

structural damage [9]. Magni-Manzoni S et al. evaluated 52 joints demonstrating excellent intra- and inter-observer reliability in the assessment of synovitis by B-Mode and Power Doppler (PD) [7]. Two other studies reported good and excellent intra- and inter-observer reliability specifically in MCP joints [8, 9]. However, these studies were done before pediatric-specific definitions of synovitis have been established.

The pediatric joint does display unique features on MSUS and the lack of a MSUS definition of synovitis in JIA may have contributed to the lack of data on the reliability of MSUS assessments. Recently, the OMERACT-US Pediatric subtask force has provided the basis for the standardized assessment by defining MSUS features of synovitis [10]. This group also proposed a synovitis scoring system and showed good reliability of it in four joints including the wrist and second MCP [11]. No pediatric specific MSUS definitions exist yet for tenosynovitis, cartilage damage and bone erosions but these lesions have been defined for adults [12, 13].

The objective of this study was to evaluate the reliability of MSUS to detect synovitis, tenosynovitis, bone erosions and cartilage damage in the wrist and MCP joints of patients with JIA.

Methods

This research was conducted in compliance with the declaration of Helsinki and the study was approved by the research ethics committee at the National Institute of Rehabilitation under protocol number 52/16.

Thirty children were recruited for this study from the Pediatric rheumatology service at the Hospital Infantil de México, all diagnosed with JIA according to the ILAR criteria independently of clinical status [14]. One pediatric rheumatologist performed the clinical exam to detect painful, swollen and limited joints on 2 consecutive days (fifteen children every day). The MSUS was done in two rounds on each child by five rheumatologists with variable experience in pediatric MSUS who were blind to the clinical evaluation (fifteen children every day). After clinical examination, the child was evaluated by the ultrasonographers. The wrist (radio-carpal and mid-carpal joint recesses), 2nd and 3rd metacarpophalangeal (MCP) joints were evaluated bilaterally. Prior to the intra and interobserver exercise, the rheumatology sonographers completed a session to review definitions of synovitis, tenosynovitis, cartilage damage, and erosions. Before to the assessments, written informed consent was taken from all the study participants and their parents/guardians.

Clinical characteristics such as age, gender, time since disease diagnosis, painful and swollen joint count, number of joints with limited range of motion, erythrosedimentation rate (ESR) and C-reactive protein (CRP) were recorded.

MSUS definition of pathology, scanning protocol and equipment

According to the OMERACT pediatric MSUS definitions for synovitis, synovial effusion was defined as abnormal intra-articular fluid that is anechoic or hypoechoic and displaceable. Synovial hypertrophy as intra-articular and hypoechoic material that is non-displaceable. For pathologic Doppler signals, the term abnormal Doppler signals was used to differentiate to normal Doppler signal in normal tissue as suggested by OMERACT-US Pediatric subtask force [10]. The abnormal Doppler signals have to be shown within an area of synovial hypertrophy [11]. The primary goal of the study was a dichotomous assessment of synovitis being present or absent but in addition grading was done as well to demonstrate the degree of synovitis present in our patients. This was also done in light of the fact that there is currently no agreement on the significance of low grade Doppler signals. We used a scoring system developed by the OMERACT pediatric ultrasound task force to graduate B-mode findings as follows: Grade 1: synovial effusion and/or synovial hypertrophy that leads to a mild change of the joint recess appearance, Grade 2: synovial effusion and/or synovial hypertrophy that leads to a moderate change of the joint recess appearance (Fig. 1a) and Grade 3: synovial effusion and/or synovial hypertrophy that leads to a severe change of the joint

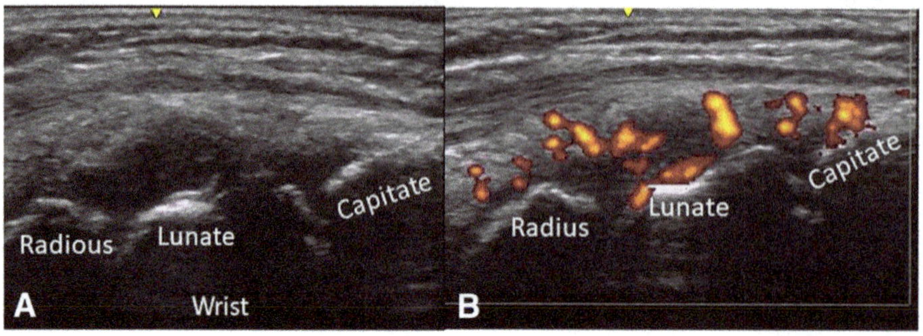

Fig. 1 **a** Synovitis (grayscale) grade 2 in wrist. **b** Power Doppler grade 2. Both in longitudinal view

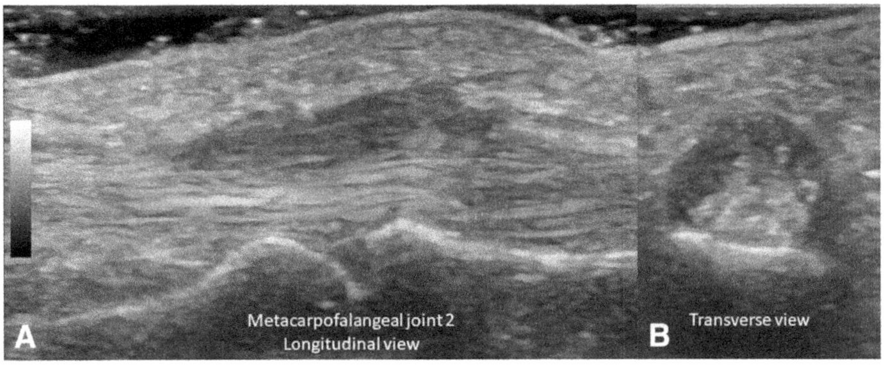

Fig. 2 a and **b** Tenosynovitis of flexor tendon in longitudinal and transverse view, respectively

recess appearance. For PD Grade 1 was defined as a detection of up to 3 single Doppler signals within the area synovial hypertrophy with or without normal physiological Doppler signals, Grade 2 as the detection of more than 3 Doppler signals but less than 30% of the area of synovial hypertrophy with or without normal physiological Doppler signals (Fig. 1b) and Grade 3 as the detection of Doppler signals within more than 30% of the area of synovial hypertrophy with or without normal physiological Doppler signals [10]. For tenosynovitis, the OMERACT definition for rheumatoid arthritis was used. It is defined as an abnormal, hypoechoic or anechoic (relative to tendon fibers) tendon sheath widening [12] (Fig. 2a, b). Similarly bone erosions were defined according to OMERACT as an intra-articular discontinuity of the bone surface visible in 2 perpendicular planes [12] (Fig. 3a, b). To evaluate cartilage thickness, the child were placed in supine position with both hands palm-side down on the examination table, then measurements of the cartilage thickness of the second and third MCP was obtained from a longitudinal dorsal scan with the MCP joints in a 90-degree flexion [15] (Fig. 4a, b). In this position, the delineation of cartilage of the epiphyses of the metacarpal head and proximal phalange is better [9]. Tenosynovitis, cartilage damage and bone erosions were evaluated dichotomously as absent/present.

The views to assess the wrist and MCP on MSUS were chosen according to the recommendations for standardized scanning by the OMERACT pediatric ultrasound group [16]. With the palm facing downwards, the wrist was assessed in neutral position with the transducer placed longitudinally in sagittal midline of the wrist, the proximal end of transducer positioned just distal to the radius diaphysis. The 2nd MCP joint was assessed with the palm facing downwards, laterally, or upwards and the finger was positioned flat in neutral position with the transducer placed longitudinally to evaluate the dorsal, lateral and volar aspect of the MCP joint. For the 3rd MCP joint, only the dorsal and volar aspects were evaluated [16].

Two GE NEXTGEN LOGIQ e R6 ultrasound machines with L8-18i-RS wide band linear were used for the assessments. Low flow settings were used for Power Doppler with a PRF 500 and low wall filter and gain was increased until a signal appeared below the cortical bone surface [17].

Statistical analysis

Qualitative data were expressed as frequencies and proportions. The mean and standard deviation (SD) was

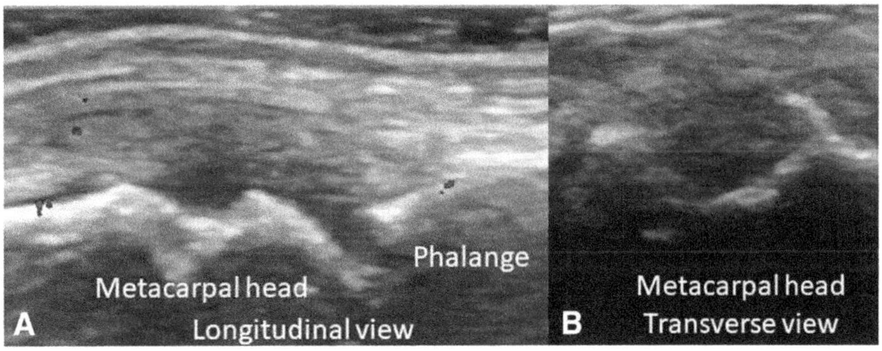

Fig. 3 a and **b** Bone erosion of metacarpal head in longitudinal and transverse view

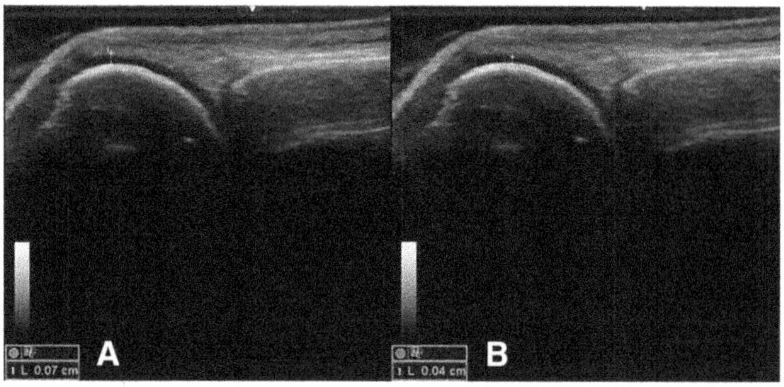

Fig. 4 **a** Bone cartilage with a well-defined border. **b** Bone cartilage with irregular border and reduced thickness

calculated for quantitative data. Intra and inter-reader concordance was determined by Cohen's kappa for qualitative variables. The following cut offs were used for Kappa values: below 0.20 poor, 0.21–0.40 fair, 0.41–0.60 moderate, 0.61–0.80 good, and 0.81–1 excellent [18]. Statistics analysis was using SPSS 15.0 (SPSS, Inc., Chicago, IL, USA).

Results

Table 1 shows demographic and clinical characteristics of the study participants. The majority was female with 60% being of the polyarticular subtype and a relatively high prevalence of rheumatoid factor at 43%. Low prevalence of synovitis in wrist, second and third MCP was detected clinically. Most of the patients were also on Disease Modifying Antirheumatic Drugs (DMARD) and/or biologic therapies suggesting more severe phenotypes of synovitis in the study.

Table 1 Demographic and Clinical characteristics

Age (years) mean ± SD	10.6 ± 5.1
Gender: # female/male	23/7
JIA Subtype n(%)	Polyarticular 18 (60%)
	Oligoarticular 12 (40%)
Disease duration (years) mean ± SD	5.4 + 1.9
Painful joint count mean ± SD	4.9 ± 1.7
Swollen joint count mean ± SD	3.5 ± 1.8
Limited joint count mean ± SD	1.9 ± 0.9
Joints clinically affected n (%)	
Wrist	17 (28)
MCP 2	14 (23)
MCP 3	10 (17)
ESR mm/hr mean ± SD	17.5 ± 14.2
CRP mg/L mean ± SD	15 ± 0.7
Positive Rheumatoid factor number (%)	14 (43%)
Positive Antinuclear antibodies number (%)	19 (57%)
Treatment n (%)	Methotrexate 28 (86%) Sulfasalazine 10 (30%) Biologic therapy 6 (20%) Prednisone 5 (16%)

Table 2 shows the number and percentages of synovitis detected by US in B-Mode and Power Doppler per joint. We observed more synovitis by US than clinical examination as expected (62% vs 28%, 30% vs 23% and 22% vs 17% in the wrist, second and third MCP respectively). The wrist was the most affected joint and MCP 3 the least. Regarding the grade of synovitis we found a higher percentage of grade 1 in the wrist and grade 2 in the MCP joints. Less than 10% of joints evaluated had grade 3 in B-Mode. The PD was present in 60% (18 joints), in one patient the PD was present in bilateral wrist. The grade I was most frequent in all joints and the wrist had more prevalence of PD. Almost all patients had one joint with this abnormal signal.

The intra-observer concordance for synovitis in all joints was excellent in B-Mode, except for MCP 2, where it was good. For Power Doppler, B-Mode tenosynovitis, cartilage damage and bone erosions it was also excellent. Regarding synovitis grading the concordance was excellent for all grades, except for grade 1 where it was good as observed in Table 3.

Table 4 shows the inter-observer reliability. The concordance was excellent for all lesions except for presence of abnormal power Doppler signal in tenosynovitis. Synovitis grading has good concordance for grade 1 and 2 in either B-Mode and Power Doppler. For grade 3 it was excellent.

The association between joint pain, motion limitation and synovitis detected clinically and synovitis by US was moderate (k = 0.46, CI 95% 0.08–.09).

Although the thickness of the articular cartilage of the MCP was measured and compared with the contralateral joint, it was considered only in a dichotomous

Table 2 Prevalence of synovitis grading in recesses by US grayscale and abnormal PD signal

Joint	Presence of synovitis n (%)	Grayscale grade 1 n (%)	PD grade 1 n (%)	Grayscale grade 2 n (%)	PD grade 2 n (%)	Grayscale grade 3 n (%)	PD grade 3 n (%)
Wrist	37 (62)	15 (30)	6 (10)	17 (28)	0 (0)	5 (8)	2 (3)
MCP 2	18 (30)	5 (8)	3 (5)	8 (13)	1 (2)	5 (8)	3 (5)
MCP 3	13 (22)	2 (3)	3 (5)	8 (13)	0 (0)	3 (5)	0 (0)

manner when there was a decrease in thickness, there was no standard mean, due to the variation in the age of the patients.

Cartilage thinning was seen in 34 (28%) and bone erosion in 12/60 (10%) MCP evaluated respectively, while tenosynovitis, most in flexors tendons, presented in 7/30 (23%) patients,.

Discussion

To our knowledge, this is the first study that evaluated MSUS reliability for both inflammatory changes and structural damage in wrists and MCPs joints in patients with JIA.

Karmazyn et al. assessed synovitis, tenosynovitis, bone erosions and cartilage thinning in MCP joints by MSUS, finding abnormalities in 32% of 200 joints, however, no data on the reliability of this technique is provided [9]. Other studies have evaluated the concordance of clinical abnormalities and synovitis detected by MSUS and in one study clinical swelling, pain on motion and limitation in the range of motion were significantly associated with MSUS findings at the MCP [8]. Two other studies have

Table 3 Intra-observer concordance in wrist and MCP joints

Elementary lesions by US	Overall agreement (%) Presence/absence	Kappa Cohen	95% CI	P value
Synovitis				
Wrist	95	.87	.71–1.0	.001
MCP 2	84	.61	.34–89	.001
MCP 3	95	.84	.63–1.0	.001
Abnormal power Doppler signal				
Wrist	95	.87	.71–1.0	.001
MCP 2	100	1.0	1.0–1.0	.001
MCP 3	100	1.0	1.0–1.0	.001
Tenosinovitis flexor tendon				
Grayscale	95	.88	.74–1.0	.001
Power Doppler	100	1.0	1.0–1.0	.001
Cartilage Damage				
MCP 2	94	.82	.59–1.0	.001
MCP 3	97	.94	.84–1.0	.001
Bone erosion	100	1.0	1.0–1.0	.001
Synovitis grading	Agreement (%)	Weighted kappa	95% CI	P value
Synovitis in all joints by US grayscale				
Grade 0	100	1.0	1.0–1.0	.001
Grade 1	73	.61	.43–.83	.004
Grade 2	83	.71	.51–87	.003
Grade 3	87	.84	.63–.91	.001
Abnormal power Doppler signal				
Grade 0	100	1.0	1.0–10	.001
Grade 1	95	.88	.71–1.0	.001
Grade 2	87	.83	.69–.96	.001
Grade 3	100	1.0	1.0–1.0	.001

Table 4 Inter-observer concordance in wrist and MCP joints

Elementary lesions by US	Overall agreement (%) Presence/absence	Kappa Cohen	95% CI	P value
Synovitis				
Wrist	96	.90	.80–1.0	.001
MCP 2	92	.81	.67–95	.001
MCP 3	97	.92	.82–1.0	.001
Abnormal power Doppler signal				
Wrist	97	.93	.85–1.0	.001
MCP 2	100	1.0	1.0–1.0	.001
MCP 3	97	.87	.74–1.0	.001
Tenosinovitis flexor tendon				
Grayscale	94	.89	.78–.99	.001
Power Doppler	98	.66	.39–1.0	.001
Cartilage Damage				
MCP 2	94	.89	.78–.99	.001
MCP 3	94	.89	.78–.99	.001
Bone erosion	100	1.0	1.0–1.0	.001
Synovitis grading	Agreement (%)	Weighted kappa	95% CI	P value
Synovitis in all joints by US grayscale				
Grade 0	100	1.0	1.0–1.0	.001
Grade 1	66	.61	.53–.74	.007
Grade 2	69	.64	.57–.86	.004
Grade 3	91	.81	.63–.97	.001
Abnormal power Doppler signal				
Grade 0	100	1.0	1.0–10	.001
Grade 1	67	.63	.58–.91	.004
Grade 2	72	.67	.60–.93	.002
Grade 3	88	.85	.67–.96	.001

shown poor agreement between MSUS and clinical abnormalities [7]. In one study intra-observer reproducibility was excellent, with high kappa values for both B-Mode and PD as in our study [9]. Magni-Manzoni S et al., had observed excellent intra- and inter-reliability for joint effusion, synovial hypertrophy, and PD signal, but had not explored this for specific grades of these lesions [7]. In relation to the synovitis grading, intra and inter-observer concordance was similar to the one observed by the OMERACT-US pediatric task force [10], suggesting that US is a reliable technique. On the other hand, concordance between clinical assessments and US findings was moderate, in line with other studies [7, 8].

Cartilage damage

One study has demonstrated an acceptable coefficient of variation (16%) between US and MRI for all joints except the wrist, suggesting the US as valid method for measurement of cartilage thickness [19]. The intra and inter-observer concordance relating to cartilage thickness on MCPs were excellent in our sample, similar to reported by Spannow [20]. The importance to detect cartilage loss in children with JIA is due because it represents an early indicator of joint damage and raises the need to intensify therapy before irreversible structural damage development [21].

Tenosynovitis

In one study, tenosynovitis in wrist was observed in 20% (40) of 200 MCPs evaluated in a longitudinal assessment [9]; this is similar to our study, where we had seen 23% of 30 patients evaluated. Even though, tenosynovitis is commonly seen in the extensor tendons of the wrist [22], we saw more changes in the flexor tendons. Tenosynovitis may be a very relevant finding with some studies in rheumatoid arthritis demonstrating that the presence of tenosynovitis predicts structural damage [23, 24] although it is not known whether the situation in JIA will be similar. The intra observer concordance was excellent for grayscale and PD, while inter-observer concordance was excellent for grayscale and good for PD. As far as we know, there is no study in children in which the reliability of ultrasonography to detect tenosynovitis has been evaluated to compare our results.

Bone erosions

We evaluated bone erosions only in the MCP joints and not in the wrist, as one study has found wrist changes on MRI, namely carpal depressions, in a large proportion of healthy children [25]. The interpretation of bone irregularities/erosions of the wrist is therefore challenging. [26]. We observed a low prevalence of bone erosions in MCPs in our patients (10%), little less than Karmazyn et al. had found (18% in 36/200 MCPs) [9]. The reliability of the US to detect bone erosions was excellent in our population. However assessing for bony erosive changes in children is difficult because some irregularities in recently ossified bones can be misinterpreted as cortical erosions, highlighting the need for further knowledge of normal bone anatomy throughout the pediatric age groups and for a reference standard like MRI for comparison [27]. Further validation and large-scale studies are required to determine the potential role of US in the detection of bone erosions in children [28].

We consider that including the assessment of tenosynovitis, cartilage damage and bone erosion to the exploration of synovitis in children by ultrasonography, could help the clinician to make a more appropriate therapeutic decision for patients with JIA. Cartilage damage and bone erosions are indicators of joint damage and suggests the need for intensify therapy to prevent major irreversible structural changes [21]. A larger population and long-term follow-up are required to assess the impact this might have.

Abnormal power Doppler signals

The intra and inter-observer concordance of abnormal power Doppler signals for synovitis was excellent in all regions and good for tenosynovitis. The clear definition of pathologic Doppler signals within an area of synovial hypertrophy [11] helps to improve reliability, given the significant presence of physiologic intraarticular blood flow in children. Doppler signal detection had better reliability than the detection of B-mode changes in other studies [29].

Limitations

There are some limitations in our study, such as the absence of patients with other disorders like finger pain or hypermobility joint syndrome. In addition, we do not include patients without treatment. Furthermore, we did not use a gold standard examination such as MRI to evaluate the accuracy of the US.

Conclusions

The intra- and inter-observer reliability of MSUS for inflammatory and structural lesions is good to excellent for the wrist and MCP in patients with JIA.

Abbreviations

CRP: C-reactive protein; DMARD: Disease Modifying Antirheumatic Drugs; ESR: Erythrosedimentation rate; JIA: Juvenile Idiopathic Arthritis; MCP: Metacarpophallangeal joint; MSUS: Musculoskeletal ultrasound; PD: Power Doppler; SD: Standard deviation

Authors' contributions

V-R L, H-D C, RJ and FE had made substantial contributions to conception, design, and acquisition, analysis and interpretation of data. BL, DC-B L, SB G, RG A and MR had been involved in acquisition of data, analysis and interpretation of data. All authors had been involved in drafting the manuscript or revising it critically for intellectual content. All authors read and approved the final manuscript.

Competing interests

The authors declare that they have no competing interests.

Author details

[1]Laboratorio de ultrasonido musculoesquelético y articular, Instituto Nacional de Rehabilitación, Luis Guillermo Ibarra Ibarra, Calzada México-Xochimilco 289, Arenal de Guadalupe, Tlalpan, 14389 Mexico city, Mexico. [2]Reumatología Pediátrica, Hospital Infantil de México, Mexico city, Mexico. [3]Reumatología, Hospital de Niños Dr. Ricardo Gutiérrez, Buenos Aires, Argentina. [4]Hospital Universitario "Dr. José E. González", UANL, Monterrey, Nuevo León, Mexico. [5]Embriology Department, Medicine School, Universidad Nacional Autónoma de Mexico, Mexico City, Mexico. [6]Division of Pediatric Dermatology & Rheumatology, Children's Hospital of Eastern Ontario, Ottawa, Canada.

References

1. Colebatch AN, Edwards CJ, Østergaard M, et al. EULAR recommendations for the use of imaging of the joints in the clinical management of rheumatoid arthritis. Ann Rheum Dis. 2013;72:804–14.
2. Colebatch-Bourn AN, Edwards CJ, Collado P, D'Agostino MA, Hemke R, Jousse-Joulin S, et al. EULAR-PReS points to consider for the use of imaging in the diagnosis and management of juvenile idiopathic arthritis in clinical practice. Ann Rheum Dis. 2015;74:1946–57.
3. HAS B, Humphries PD. Juvenile idiopathic arthritis: what is the utility of ultrasound? Br J Radiol. 2017;90:201609204.
4. Filippou G, Cantarini L, Bertoli I, Picerno V, Frediani B, Galeazzi M. Ultrasonography vs. clinical examination in children with suspected arthritis. Does it make sense to use poliarticular ultrasonographic screening? Clin Exp Rheumatol. 2011;29:345–50.

5. Laurell L, Court-Payen M, Nielsen S, Zak M, Boesen M, Fasth A. Ultrasonography and color Doppler in juvenile idiopathic arthritis: diagnosis and follow-up of ultrasound-guided steroid injection in the ankle region. A descriptive interventional study. Pediatr Rheumatol Online. 2011;9:4.
6. Haslam K, Mc Cann L, Wyat S, Wakefield RJ. The detection of subclinical synovitis by ultrasound in oligoarticular juvenile idiopathic arthritis: a pilot study. Rheumatology. 2010;49:123–7.
7. Magni-Manzoni S, Epis O, Ravelli A, Klersy C, Ch V, Lanni S, et al. Comparison of clinical versus ultrasound-determined synovitis in juvenile idiopathic arthritis. Arthritis Rheum. 2009;61:1497–504.
8. Breton S, Jousse-Joulin S, Cangemi C, de Parscau L, Colin D, Bressolette L, et al. Comparison of clinical and ultrasonographic evaluations for peripheral synovitis in juvenile idiopathic arthritis. Semin Arthritis Rheum. 2011;41:272–8.
9. Karmazyn B, Bowyer SL, Schmidt KM, Ballinger SH, Buckwalter K, Beam TT, et al. US findings of metacarpophalangeal joints in children with idiopathic juvenile arthritis. Pediatr Radiol. 2007;37:475–82.
10. Roth J, Ravagnani V, Backhaus M, Balint P, Bruns A, Bruyn GA, et al. Preliminary definitions for the sonographic features of synovitis in children. Arthritis Care Res. https://doi.org/10.1002/acr.23130.
11. Vojinovic J, Magni-Manzoni S, Collado P, Windschall D, Ravagnani V, Hernandez-Diaz C, et al. Ultrasonography definitions for synovitis grading in children: the Omeract pediatric ultrasound task force. Ann Rheum Dis. 2016; 76(Suppl 2):SAT0636.
12. Wakefield R, Balint P, Skudlarek M, Filippuci E, Backhaus M, D'Agostino MA, et al. Musculoskeletal ultrasound including definitions for Ultrasonographic pathology. J Rheumatol. 2005;32:2485–7.
13. Naredo E, DAgostino MA, Wakefield RJ, Möller I, Balint PV, Filippucci E, et al. Reliability of a consensus-based ultrasound score for tenosynovitis in rheumatoid arthritis. Ann Rheum Dis. 2013;72:1328–34.
14. Fink CW. Proposal for the development of classification criteria for idiopathic arthritides of childhood. J Rheumatol. 1995;22:1566–9.
15. Spannow AH, Pfeiffer-Jensen M, Andersen NT, Stenbog E, Herlin T. Inter-and intraobserver variation of ultrasonographic cartilage thickness assessments in small and large joints in healthy children. Pediatric Rheumatol. 2009;7:12.
16. Collado P, Vojinovic J, Nieto JC, Windschall D, Magni-Manozni S, Bryun GAW, et al. Toward standardized musculoskeletal ultrasound in pediatric rheumatology: Normal age-related ultrasound findings. Arthritis Car Res. 2016;68:348–56.
17. Torp-Pedersen ST, Terslev L. Settings and artefacts relevant in colour/power Doppler ultrasound in rheumatology. Ann Rheum Dis. 2008;67:143–9.
18. Landis JR, Koch GG. The measurement of observer agreement for categorical data. Biometrics. 1997;33:159–74.
19. Spannow AH, Stenboeg E, Pfeiffer-Jensen M, Fiirgaard B, Haislund M, Ostergaard M, et al. Ultrasound and MRI measurements of joint cartilage in healthy children: a validation study. Ultraschall Med. 2011;32:S110–6.
20. Spannow AH, Stenboeg E, Pfeiffer-Jensen M, Herlin T. Ultrasound measurement of joint cartilage thickness in large and small joints in healthy children: a clinical pilot study assessing observer variability. Pediatr Rheumatol Online J. 2007;5:3.
21. Magni-Manzoni S. Ultrasound Measurement of Cartilage Thickness in Childhood Arthritis- Target the Tissue, Tailor the technique. J Rheumatol. 2015;42:360–2.
22. Sheybani EF, Khanna G, White AJ, et al. Imaging of juvenile idiopathic arthritis: a multimodality approach. Radiographics. 2013;33:1253–73.
23. Javadi S, Kan JH, Orth RC, DeGuzman M. Wrist and ankle MRI of patients with juvenile idiopathic arthritis: identification of unsuspected multicompartmental tenosynovitis and arthritis. Am J Roentgenol. 2014; 202:413–7.
24. Janta I, Stanciu D, Hinojosa M, Nieto-González JC, Valor L, Bello N, et al. Structural damage in rheumatoid arthritis: comparison between tendon damage evaluated by ultrasound and radiographic damage. Rheumatol. 2016;55:1042–6.
25. Avenarius DM, Ording Müller LS, Eldevik P, Owens CM, Rosendahl K. The paediatric wrist revisited—findings of bony depressions in healthy children on radiographs compared to MRI. Pediatr Radiol. 2012;42:791–8.
26. DFM A, Ording Müller LS, Rosendahl K. Erosion or normal variant? 4-year MRI follow-up of the wrists in healthy children. Pediatr Radiol. 2016;46:322–30.
27. Chauvin NA, Doria AS. Ultrasound imaging of synovial inflammation in juvenile idiopathic arthritis. Pediatr Radiol. 2017;47:1160–70.
28. Dimitriou C, Boitsios G, Badot V, Le PQ GL, Simoni P. Imaging of juvenile idiopathic arthritis. Radiol Clin N Am. 2017;55(5):1071–108.
29. Cheung PP, Dougados M, Gossec L. Reliability of ultrasonography to detect synovitis in rheumatoid arthritis: a systematic literature review of 35 studies (1,415 patients). Arthritis Care Res. 2010;62:323–34.

Permissions

All chapters in this book were first published in PR, by BioMed Central; hereby published with permission under the Creative Commons Attribution License or equivalent. Every chapter published in this book has been scrutinized by our experts. Their significance has been extensively debated. The topics covered herein carry significant findings which will fuel the growth of the discipline. They may even be implemented as practical applications or may be referred to as a beginning point for another development.

The contributors of this book come from diverse backgrounds, making this book a truly international effort. This book will bring forth new frontiers with its revolutionizing research information and detailed analysis of the nascent developments around the world.

We would like to thank all the contributing authors for lending their expertise to make the book truly unique. They have played a crucial role in the development of this book. Without their invaluable contributions this book wouldn't have been possible. They have made vital efforts to compile up to date information on the varied aspects of this subject to make this book a valuable addition to the collection of many professionals and students.

This book was conceptualized with the vision of imparting up-to-date information and advanced data in this field. To ensure the same, a matchless editorial board was set up. Every individual on the board went through rigorous rounds of assessment to prove their worth. After which they invested a large part of their time researching and compiling the most relevant data for our readers.

The editorial board has been involved in producing this book since its inception. They have spent rigorous hours researching and exploring the diverse topics which have resulted in the successful publishing of this book. They have passed on their knowledge of decades through this book. To expedite this challenging task, the publisher supported the team at every step. A small team of assistant editors was also appointed to further simplify the editing procedure and attain best results for the readers.

Apart from the editorial board, the designing team has also invested a significant amount of their time in understanding the subject and creating the most relevant covers. They scrutinized every image to scout for the most suitable representation of the subject and create an appropriate cover for the book.

The publishing team has been an ardent support to the editorial, designing and production team. Their endless efforts to recruit the best for this project, has resulted in the accomplishment of this book. They are a veteran in the field of academics and their pool of knowledge is as vast as their experience in printing. Their expertise and guidance has proved useful at every step. Their uncompromising quality standards have made this book an exceptional effort. Their encouragement from time to time has been an inspiration for everyone.

The publisher and the editorial board hope that this book will prove to be a valuable piece of knowledge for researchers, students, practitioners and scholars across the globe.

List of Contributors

Megan Cann and Catherine M. Guly
University Hospitals Bristol NHS Foundation Trust, Bristol, UK

Athimalaipet V. Ramanan
University Hospitals Bristol NHS Foundation Trust, Bristol, UK
Translational Health Sciences, Bristol Medical School, Faculty of Health sciences, Bristol, UK

Sarah L. N. Clarke
University Hospitals Bristol NHS Foundation Trust, Bristol, UK
MRC Integrative Epidemiology Unit, Population Health Sciences, University of Bristol, Bristol, UK

Andrew D. Dick
University Hospitals Bristol NHS Foundation Trust, Bristol, UK
Translational Health Sciences, Bristol Medical School, Faculty of Health sciences, Bristol, UK
National Institute for Health Research (NIHR) Biomedical Research Centre at Moorfield
Eye Hospital, London, UK
University College London Institute of Ophthalmology, London, UK

Fatima Rashed
Translational Health Sciences, Bristol Medical School, Faculty of Health sciences, Bristol, UK

Andrew Crawford
BHF Centre for Cardiovascular Science, Queen's Medical Research Institute,
University of Edinburgh, Edinburgh, UK
MRC Integrative Epidemiology Unit, Population Health Sciences, University of Bristol, Bristol, UK

P. Collado
Hospital Universitario Severo Ochoa., Madrid, Spain

D. Windschall
Department of Pediatrics, Asklepios Hospital Weissenfels, Weissenfels, Germany

J. Vojinovic
Department of Pediatrics, Clinical Center, Faculty of Medicine, University of Nis, Nis, Serbia

S. Magni-Manzoni
Rheumatology Division, IRCCS Ospedale Pediatrico Bambino Gesù, Rome, Italy

P. Balint
3rd Department of Rheumatology, National Institute of Rheumatology and Physiotherapy, Budapest, Hungary

G. A. W. Bruyn
Department of Rheumatology, MC Groep, Lelystad, the Netherlands

C. Hernandez-Diaz
Instituto Nacional de Rehabilitación, Mexico City, Mexico

J. C. Nieto
Department of Rheumatology, Hospital Universitario Gregorio Marañon, Madrid, Spain

V. Ravagnani
Department of Internal Medicine, ASST Mantova, C. Poma Hospital, Mantova, Italy

N. Tzaribachev
Pediatric Rheumatology Research Institute, Bad Bramstedt, Germany

A. Iagnocco
Rheumatology Unit, Sapienza Università di Roma, Rome, Italy

M. A. D'Agostino
Rheumatology Department, Hôspital Ambroise Paré, Boulogne Billancourt; INSERM U1173, Laboratoire d'Excellence INFLAMEX, UFR Simone Veil, Versailles-Saint-Quentin University, Yvelines, France

E. Naredo
Department of Rheumatology, Hospital Universitario Fundación Jimenez Díaz and Autonoma University, Madrid, Spain

Massimo Gregori, Serena Pastore and Alberto Tommasini
Institute for Maternal and Child Health, IRCCS "Burlo Garofolo", Trieste, Italy

Andrea Taddio and Alessandro Ventura
Institute for Maternal and Child Health, IRCCS "Burlo Garofolo", Trieste, Italy
University of Trieste, Via dell'Istria 65/1, 34100 Trieste, Italy

Giovanna Ferrara
University of Trieste, Via dell'Istria 65/1, 34100 Trieste, Italy

Antonella Insalaco and Manuela Pardeo
Division of Rheumatology, Department of Paediatric Medicine, Bambino Gesù Children's
Hospital, IRCCS, Piazza di Sant'Onofrio, 4, 00165 Rome, Italy

Martina Finetti and Marco Gattorno
Pediatria 2, Istituto Gaslini, Via Gerolamo Gaslini, 5, 16148 Genoa, Italy

Eve M. D. Smith
Department of Women's and Children's Health, University of Liverpool, Institute In The Park, Alder Hey Children's Hospital, East Prescott Road, Liverpool L14 5AB, UK
Department of Paediatric Rheumatology, Alder Hey Children's NHS Foundation Trust, Liverpool, UK

Michael W. Beresford
Department of Women's and Children's Health, University of Liverpool, Institute In The Park, Alder Hey Children's Hospital, East Prescott Road, Liverpool L14 5AB, UK
Department of Paediatric Rheumatology, Alder Hey Children's NHS Foundation Trust, Liverpool, UK

Peng Yin
Research Center for Biomedical Information Technology, Shenzhen Institutes of Advanced Technology, Chinese Academy of Sciences, Shenzhen, China

Andrea L. Jorgensen
Department of Biostatistics, Block F, Waterhouse Building, University of Liverpool, Liverpool, UK

Jerold Jeyaratnam and Joost Frenkel
Department of General Pediatrics, University Medical Center Utrecht, Room
KE 04 133 1, PO-Box 85090, 3508, AB Utrecht, The Netherlands

Nienke M. ter Haar
Laboratory for Translational Immunology, University Medical Center Utrecht, Utrecht, the
Netherlands

Helen J. Lachmann
University College Medical School, National Amyloidosis Center, Royal Free Campus, London, UK

Ozgur Kasapcopur
Department of Pediatric Rheumatology, Cerrahpasa Medical School-Istanbul University, Istanbul, Turkey

Amanda K. Ombrello
Inflammatory Disease section, National Human Genome Research Institute, Bethesda, MA, USA

Donato Rigante
Institute of Pediatrics, Università Cattolica Sacro Cuore, Rome, Italy

Fatma Dedeoglu and Ezgi H. Baris
Division of Immunology, Boston Children's Hospital, Boston, MA, USA

Sebastiaan J. Vastert and Nico M. Wulffraat
Department of Pediatric Rheumatology, University Medical Center Utrecht, Utrecht, the Netherlands

Hanna Rahimi and Troels Herlin
Department of Pediatrics, Aarhus University Hospital, Palle Juul-Jensens
Boulevard 121, 8200 Aarhus N, Denmark

Marinka Twilt
Department of Pediatrics, Division of Rheumatology, Alberta Children's Hospital, 2888 Shaganappi Trail NW, Calgary, AB, Canada

Lynn Spiegel
Division of Rheumatology, The Hospital for Sick Children, 555 University Avenue, Toronto, ON, Canada

Thomas Klit Pedersen and Annelise Küseler
Department of Oral and Maxillofacial Surgery, Aarhus University Hospital, Nørrebrogade 44, 8000 Aarhus C, Denmark
Section of Orthodontics, Department of Dentistry and Oral Health, Aarhus University, Vennelyst Boulevard 9-11, 8000 Aarhus C, Denmark

Peter Stoustrup
Section of Orthodontics, Department of Dentistry and Oral Health, Aarhus University, Vennelyst Boulevard 9-11, 8000 Aarhus C, Denmark

Xin-yan Zhang, Ting-ting Yang, Xiu-fen Hu, Yu Wen and Feng Fang
Tongji Hospital, Tongji Medical College, Huazhong University of Science and Technology, Wuhan 430000, Hubei, China

Hui-ling Lu
Tongji Hospital, Tongji Medical College, Huazhong University of Science and Technology, Wuhan 430000, Hubei, China
Department of Pediatrics, Tongji Hospital, No.1095. Jiefang Road, Qiaokou District, Wuhan City 430000, Hubei Province, China

Surabhi S. Vinod
Department of Pediatrics, University of Alabama School of Medicine, Birmingham, AL, USA

Randy Q. Cron and Matthew L. Stoll
Department of Pediatrics, University of Alabama School of Medicine, Birmingham, AL, USA
Division of Pediatric Rheumatology, Children's of Alabama, Birmingham, AL 35233-1711, USA

Annelle B. Reed and Jamelle Maxwell
Division of Pediatric Rheumatology, Children's of Alabama, Birmingham, AL 35233-1711, USA

Matthew L. Stoll and Randy Q. Cron
Department of Pediatrics, University of Alabama at Birmingham (UAB), 1600 7th Avenue South, Children's Park Place North Suite G10, Birmingham 35233, AL, USA

Chung H. Kau
Department of Orthodontics, UAB, 1720 2nd Avenue South, School of Dentistry Building 305, Birmingham 35294, AL, USA

Peter D. Waite
Department of Oral and Maxillofacial Surgery, UAB, 1720 2nd Avenue South, School of Dentistry Building 419, Birmingham 35294, AL, USA

Valerie Li-Thiao-Te
Onco-Hématologie Pédiatrique, Centre Hospitalier Universitaire Amiens,
Amiens, France

Florence Uettwiller
Unité d'Immunologie-Hématologie et Rhumatologie Pédiatrique, Centre de référence pour la Rhumatologie et les maladies Auto-immunes Systémiques de l'Enfant, Hôpital Necker-Enfants Malades, Assistance Publique Hôpitaux de Paris, Paris, France

Pierre Quartier and Brigitte Bader-Meunier
Unité d'Immunologie-Hématologie et Rhumatologie Pédiatrique, Centre de référence pour la Rhumatologie et les maladies Auto-immunes Systémiques de l'Enfant, Hôpital Necker-Enfants Malades, Assistance Publique Hôpitaux de Paris, Paris, France
Université Paris-Descartes, Paris, France
IMAGINE Institute, Paris, France

Florence Lacaille
Hépatologie-Gastroentérologie-Nutrition Pédiatrique, Hôpital Necker-Enfants Malades, Assistance Publique Hôpitaux de Paris, Paris, France

Valentine Brousse and Mariane de Montalembert
Pédiatrie Générale, Centre de Référence des Hémoglobinopathies, Hôpital Necker-Enfants Malades, Assistance Publique Hôpitaux de Paris Labex-GR-Ex, Paris, France

Kim Ohl, Helge Nickel, Patricia Klemm, Anja Scheufen, Angela Schippers, Norbert Wagner and Klaus Tenbrock
Department of Pediatrics, Medical Faculty, RWTH Aachen, Pauwelsstr. 30, D-52074 Aachen, Germany

Halima Moncrieffe
Center for Autoimmune Genomics and Etiology, Cincinnati Children's Hospital Medical Center, Cincinnati, OH, USA
Department of Pediatrics, University of Cincinnati, College of Medicine, Cincinnati, OH, USA

Dirk Föll
Department of Pediatric Rheumatology and Immunology, University Hospital Muenster, Muenster, Germany

Viktor Wixler
Institute of Virology, Westfaelische Wilhelms University, 48149 Muenster, Germany

Lucy R. Wedderburn
Arthritis Research UK Centre for Adolescent Rheumatology at UCL UCLH and GOSH, London, UK
UCL GOS Institute of Child Health, University College London, London, UK
NIHR- Great Ormond Street Hospital Biomedical Research Centre (BRC), London, UK

Maher Hassan Gomaa, Shawkey Sadik Ali and Mohamed Mohamed Badr
Biochemistry Department-Faculty of Pharmacy (Boys), Al-Azhar University, Almokhayam Aldaem Street, 6th Province - 13465 Nasr City, Cairo, Egypt

Aya Mohamed Fattouh and Hala Salah Hamza
Department of Pediatrics, Kasr Al-Aini School of Medicine, Cairo University, Manial El-Roda, Cairo 11553, Egypt

Matthew L. Stoll, Melissa L. Mannion and Randy Q. Cron
Department of Pediatrics, University of Alabama at Birmingham, CPP N G10 / 1600 7th Avenue South, Birmingham, AL 35233, USA

Daniel W. Young, Stuart A. Royal and Yoginder N. Vaid
Department of Radiology at Children's of Alabama, CH 2 FL / 1600 7th Avenue South,
Birmingham, AL 35233, USA

Saurabh Guleria
Department of Radiology at Children's of Alabama, CH 2 FL / 1600 7th Avenue South Birmingham, AL 35233, USA

Present affiliation: Austin Radiological Associates, Austin, TX, USA

Anna Zejden
Department of Radiology, Aarhus University Hospital, Noerrebrogade 44, 8000 Aarhus C, Denmark

Anne Grethe Jurik
Department of Clinical Medicine, Aarhus University, Nordre Ringgade 1, 8000 Aarhus C, Denmark

Merav Heshin-Bekenstein, Emily von Scheven and Erica F. Lawson
Division of Pediatric Rheumatology, University of California San Francisco, Benioff Children's Hospital, 550 16th Street, 5th Floor, San Francisco, CA 94143-0632, USA

Liat Perl
Division of Pediatric Endocrinology, University of California San Francisco, San Francisco, CA, USA

Aimee O. Hersh
Division of Pediatric Rheumatology, University of Utah, Salt Lake City, UT, USA

Laura Trupin and Jinoos Yazdany
Division of Rheumatology, University of California San Francisco, San Francisco, CA, USA

Ed Yelin
Division of Rheumatology, University of California San Francisco, San Francisco, CA, USA
Philip R Lee Institute for Health Policy Studies, University of California, San Francisco, CA, USA

Alaina M. Davis
Division of Pediatric Rheumatology, Vanderbilt University Medical Center, Monroe Carell Junior Children's Hospital at Vanderbilt, 2200 Children's Way, Doctor's Office Tower 11240, Nashville, TN 37232, USA

Tamar B. Rubinstein
Division of Pediatric Rheumatology, Albert Einstein College of Medicine, Children's Hospital at Montefiore/ Albert Einstein College of Medicine, 3415 Bainbridge Avenue, Bronx, NY 10467, USA

Martha Rodriguez
Section of Pediatric Rheumatology, Riley Hospital for Children at Indiana University Health, 705 Riley Hospital Dr, Indianapolis, IN 46202, USA

Andrea M. Knight
Division of Rheumatology, The Children's Hospital of Philadelphia, Roberts Center for Pediatric Research, 2716 South St, Ste 10253, Philadelphia, PA 19146, USA
The Children's Hospital of Philadelphia, Roberts Center for Pediatric Research, Center for Pediatric Clinical Effectiveness, 2716 South St, Ste 10253, Philadelphia, PA 19146, USA
The Children's Hospital of Philadelphia, Roberts Center for Pediatric Research, PolicyLab, 2716 South St, Ste 10253, Philadelphia, PA 19146, USA

Wei-Te Lei, Szu-Hung Chu, Yu-Hsuan Kao, Li-Ching Fang and Shyh-Dar Shyur
Division of Allergy, Immunology, Rheumatology Disease, Department of Pediatrics, Mackay Memorial Hospital, Hsinchu, Taiwan

Po-Li Tsai
Division of Colorectal Surgery, Department of Surgery, Mackey Memorial Hospital, Taipei, Taiwan

Chien-Yu Lin
Department of Pediatrics, Mackay Memorial Hospital, Hsinchu, Taiwan

Yu-Wen Lin
Department of Medical Research, Mackay Memorial Hospital, Taipei, Taiwan

Shu-I Wu
Department of Medicine, Mackay Medical College, No.45, Minsheng Rd., Tamsui Dist., New Taipei City 25160, Taiwan
Audiology and Speech Language Pathology, Mackay Medical College, No.45, Minsheng Rd., Tamsui Dist., New Taipei City 25160, Taiwan
Department of Psychiatry, Mackay Memorial Hospital, No.45, Minsheng Rd., Tamsui Dist., New Taipei City 25160, Taiwan

Georgina Tiller, Roger Allen, Peter Gowdie and Angela Cox
Department of Rheumatology, The Royal Children's Hospital, 50 Flemington Rd, Parkville, Melbourne, VIC 3052, Australia

Joanne Buckle, Jane Munro and Jonathan Akikusa
Department of Rheumatology, The Royal Children's Hospital, 50 Flemington Rd, Parkville, Melbourne, VIC 3052, Australia
Murdoch Childrens Research Institute, Melbourne, Australia

Suzanne Parsons and Katharine Cresswell
Public Programmes Team, Manchester University NHS Foundation Trust, Manchester, UK
NIHR Manchester Biomedical Research Centre, Manchester University NHS Foundation Trust, Manchester, UK
Manchester Academic Health Science Centre, Manchester, UK

Bella Starling
NIHR Manchester Biomedical Research Centre, Manchester University NHS Foundation Trust, Manchester, UK
Research and Innovation Division, Manchester University NHS Foundation Trust, Manchester, UK

Wendy Thomson
NIHR Manchester Biomedical Research Centre, Manchester University NHS Foundation Trust, Manchester, UK
Manchester Academic Health Science Centre, Manchester, UK
Arthritis Research UK Centre for Genetics and Genomics, Centre for Musculoskeletal Research, Division of Musculoskeletal and Dermatological Sciences, Manchester, UK
School of Biological Sciences, Faculty of Biology, Medicine and Health, The University of Manchester, Manchester, UK

Janet E. McDonagh
School of Biological Sciences, Faculty of Biology, Medicine and Health, The University of Manchester, Manchester, UK
Arthritis Research UK Centre for Epidemiology, Centre for Musculoskeletal Research, Division of Musculoskeletal and Dermatological Sciences, Manchester, UK
Centre for MSK Research, University of Manchester, Stopford Building 2nd floor, Oxford Rd, Manchester M13 9PT, UK

Qianzi Zhao and Lawrence K. Jung
Division of Rheumatology, Children's National Medical Center, 111 Michigan Ave, NW, Washington, DC 20010, USA

Michael C. Kwa
Department of Dermatology, Northwestern University Feinberg School of Medicine, Chicago, IL 60611, USA

Jonathan I. Silverberg
Departments of Dermatology, Preventive Medicine and Medical Social Sciences, Northwestern University Feinberg School of Medicine, Chicago, IL 60611, USA

Kaveh Ardalan
Division of Rheumatology, Departments of Pediatrics and Medical Social Sciences, Ann and Robert H. Lurie Children's Hospital of Chicago/Northwestern University Feinberg School of Medicine, 225 E Chicago Ave Box 50, Chicago, IL 60611, USA

Hsiao-Feng Chou
Song Zhan Clinics, No.88, Songlong Rd, Taipei City 110, Taiwan

Yu-Hung Wu
Department of Dermatology, Mackay Memorial Hospital, No. 92, Sec. 2, Zhong-shan N. Rd, Taipei City 10449, Taiwan

Che-Sheng Ho
Section of Neurology, Department of Pediatrics, Mackay Memorial Hospital, No. 92, Sec. 2, Zhong-shan N. Rd, Taipei City 10449, Taiwan

Yu-Hsuan Kao
Section of Immunology, Rheumatology and Allergy, Department of Pediatrics, Mackay Memorial Hospital, No. 92, Sec. 2, Zhong-shan N. Rd, Taipei City 10449, Taiwan

Elina Liu
Rheumatology, Department of Pediatrics, Alberta Children's Hospital, 2888 Shaganappi Trail NW, Calgary, AB T3B 6A8, Canada
School of Medicine, Queen's University, Kingston, ON, Canada

Marinka Twilt, Anastasia Dropol and Susanne M. Benseler
Rheumatology, Department of Pediatrics, Alberta Children's Hospital, 2888 Shaganappi Trail NW, Calgary, AB T3B 6A8, Canada
Cumming School of Medicine, University of Calgary, Calgary, AB, Canada
Alberta Children's Hospital Research Institute, Calgary, AB, Canada

Pascal N. Tyrrell
Department of Medical Imaging and Department of Statistical Sciences, University of Toronto, Toronto, ON, Canada

Shehla Sheikh
Department of Rheumatology, Hospital for Sick Children, Toronto, ON, Canada

Mark Gorman
Boston's Children Hospital, Boston, MA, USA

Susan Kim
Boston's Children Hospital, Boston, MA, USA
Benioff Children's Hospital, University of California, San Francisco, California, USA

David A. Cabral
BC Children's Hospital, Vancouver, BC, Canada

Rob Forsyth
Institute of Neuroscience, Newcastle University, Newcastle upon Tyne, UK

Heather Van Mater
Duke Children's Hospital and Health Centre, Durham, North Carolina, USA

Suzanne Li
Joseph M. Sanzari Children's Hospital, Hackensack, NJ, USA

Adam M. Huber and Elizabeth Stringer
IWK Health Centre and Dalhousie University, Halifax, NS, Canada

Eyal Muscal
Texas Children's Hospital, Houston, TX, USA

Dawn Wahezi
Children's Hospital at Montefiore, Bronx, New York, USA

Mary Toth
Akron Children's Hospital, Akron, OH, USA

Pavla Dolezalova and Katerina Kobrova
Charles University in Prague, Prague, Czech Republic

Goran Ristic
Mother and Child Health Care Institute of Serbia, Belgrade, Serbia

Jia Zhu, Gaixiu Su, Jianming Lai, Boya Dong, Min Kang, Shengnan Li, Zhixuan Zhou and Fengqi Wu
Division of Rheumatology and Immunology, The Affiliated Children's Hospital, Capital Institute of Pediatrics, Beijing 100020, China

Rens van Vliet and Marlous J. Fernhout
Pediatric Rheumatology and Immunology, Wilhelmina Children's Hospital, University Medical Center Utrecht, Utrecht, Netherlands
Netherlands JIA Patient and Parent Organisation, member of ENCA, Amsterdam, The Netherlands

Sebastiaan J. Vastert, Jorg van Loosdregt, Anouk Verwoerd and Nico M. Wulffraat
Pediatric Rheumatology and Immunology, Wilhelmina Children's Hospital, University Medical Center Utrecht, Utrecht, Netherlands
Faculty of Medicine, Utrecht University, Utrecht, The Netherlands

Joost F. Swart
Pediatric Rheumatology and Immunology, Wilhelmina Children's Hospital, University Medical Center Utrecht, Utrecht, Netherlands
Dutch Association for Pediatric Rheumatology, Amsterdam, The Netherlands
Faculty of Medicine, Utrecht University, Utrecht, The Netherlands

Casper G. Schoemaker
Pediatric Rheumatology and Immunology, Wilhelmina Children's Hospital, University Medical Center Utrecht, Utrecht, Netherlands
Netherlands JIA Patient and Parent Organisation, member of ENCA, Amsterdam, The Netherlands
National Institute for Public Health and the Environment (RIVM), Bilthoven, The Netherlands
Department of Paediatric Rheumatology, University Medical Centre Utrecht, Wilhelmina Children's Hospital, Room KC.03.063.0, 3508 AB Utrecht, The Netherlands

Els Versluis and Sanne L. Bookelman
Netherlands JIA Patient and Parent Organisation, member of ENCA, Amsterdam, The Netherlands

Wineke Armbrust
University Medical Center Groningen (UMCG), Beatrix Childrens Hospital, Dept Pediatric Rheumatology and Immunology, University of Groningen, Groningen, The Netherlands
Dutch Association for Pediatric Rheumatology, Amsterdam, The Netherlands

Caroline Whiting and Katherine Cowan
James Lind Alliance, National Institute for Health Research Evaluation, Trials and Studies Coordinating Centre (NETSCC), based at the University of Southampton, Southampton, UK

Wendy Olsder
Youth-R-Well.com, Young Patient Organisation, The Netherlands, member of EULAR PARE, Amsterdam, The Netherlands

Jeannette Cappon
Reade, Centre for Rehabilitation and Rheumatology, Department Rehabilitation, Amsterdam, The Netherlands
Dutch Health Professionals in Pediatric Rheumatology (DHPPR), Amsterdam, The Netherlands

J. Merlijn van den Berg
Paediatric rheumatology, Emma Children's Hospital, University Medical Centre Amsterdam, Amsterdam, The Netherlands
Dutch Association for Pediatric Rheumatology, Amsterdam, The Netherlands

Ellen Schatorjé
Paediatric Rheumatology, Amalia Children's Hospital, Radboudumc, Nijmegen, The Netherlands

Paediatric Rheumatology, St. Maartenskliniek, Nijmegen, The Netherlands
Dutch Association for Pediatric Rheumatology, Amsterdam, The Netherlands

Petra C. E. Hissink Muller
Paediatric Rheumatology, Leiden University Medical Centre, Leiden, The Netherlands
Paediatric Rheumatology, Sophia Children's Hospital, Erasmus University Medical Centre, Rotterdam, The Netherlands
Dutch Association for Pediatric Rheumatology, Amsterdam, The Netherlands

Sylvia Kamphuis
Paediatric Rheumatology, Sophia Children's Hospital, Erasmus University Medical Centre, Rotterdam, The Netherlands
Dutch Association for Pediatric Rheumatology, Amsterdam, The Netherlands

Joke de Boer
Department of Ophthalmology, University Medical Centre Utrecht, Utrecht, The Netherlands
Faculty of Medicine, Utrecht University, Utrecht, The Netherlands

Otto T. H. M. Lelieveld
University Medical Center Groningen, Center for Rehabilitation, University of Groningen, Groningen, The Netherlands
Dutch Health Professionals in Pediatric Rheumatology (DHPPR), Amsterdam, The Netherlands

Janjaap van der Net
Child Development and Exercise Center, Division of Pediatrics. Wilhelmina Children's Hospital, University Medical Centre Utrecht, Utrecht, The Netherlands
Dutch Health Professionals in Pediatric Rheumatology (DHPPR), Amsterdam, The Netherlands
Faculty of Medicine, Utrecht University, Utrecht, The Netherlands

Karin R. Jongsma
Julius Center for Health Sciences and Primary Care Utrecht, University Medical Center Utrecht, Utrecht, The Netherlands

Annemiek van Rensen
PGOsupport, Dutch Networking Organisation for Patient Organisations, Utrecht, The Netherlands

Christine Dedding
Department of Medical Humanities, Amsterdam UMC, Amsterdam, The Netherlands

Giovanna Ferrara
University of Trieste, Trieste, Italy

Greta Mastrangelo and Rolando Cimaz
Rheumatology Unit, Anna Meyer Children Hospital and University of Florence, University of Florence, Florence, Italy

Patrizia Barone
Department of Pediatrics, University of Catania, Catania, Italy

Francesco La Torre
Pediatric Rheumatology Section, Pediatric Onco-Hematology Unit, Vito Fazzi Hospital, Lecce, Italy

Silvana Martino
Clinica Pediatrica Università di Torino, Day-Hospital Immunoreumatologia, Turin, Italy

Giovanni Pappagallo
Epidemiology and Clinical Trials Office, General Hospital, Mirano VE, Italy

Angelo Ravelli
Pediatria II - Reumatologia, Istituto Giannina Gaslini, and Università degli Studi di Genova, Genoa, Italy

Andrea Taddio
Institute for Maternal and Child Health - IRCCS "Burlo Garofolo", Trieste, and University of Trieste, Trieste, Italy

Francesco Zulian
Department of Pediatrics, Rheumatology Unit, University of Padua, Padua, Italy

Heather O. Tory
1Pediatric Rheumatology, Connecticut Children's Medical Center, 282 Washington Street, Hartford, CT 06106, USA
Department of Pediatrics, University of Connecticut School of Medicine, 263 Farmington Avenue, Farmington 06032, CT, USA

Ruy Carrasco
Pediatric Rheumatology, Dell Children's Medical Center of Central Texas, 4900 Mueller Boulevard, Austin, TX 78723, USA

Thomas Griffin
Pediatric Rheumatology, Carolinas HealthCare System, Levine Children's Hospital Specialty Center, 1781 Tate Boulevard, SE, Suite 206, Hickory, NC 28054, USA

Adam M. Huber
Pediatric Rheumatology, IWK Health Centre and Dalhousie University, 5980 University Avenue, Halifax, NS B3K 6R8, Canada

Philip Kahn
Pediatric Rheumatology, New York University Medical Center, 160 E 32nd Street, New York, NY 10016, USA

Angela Byun Robinson
Pediatric Rheumatology, Rainbow Babies and Children's Hospital, 11100 Euclid Avenue, Cleveland, OH 44106, USA

David Zurakowski
Departments of Anesthesia and Surgery, Boston Children's Hospital and Harvard Medical School, 300 Longwood Avenue, Boston, MA 02115, USA

Susan Kim
Pediatric Rheumatology, Benioff Children's Hospital and University of San Francisco Medical Center, 1975 4th Street, San Francisco, CA 94158, USA

Lucio Ventura-Ríos and Cristina Hernández-Díaz
Laboratorio de ultrasonido musculoesquelético y articular, Instituto Nacional de Rehabilitación, Luis Guillermo Ibarra Ibarra, Calzada México-Xochimilco 289, Arenal de Guadalupe, Tlalpan, 14389 Mexico city, Mexico

Enrique Faugier, Andrés Rodríguez García and Rocío Maldonado
Reumatología Pediátrica, Hospital Infantil de México, Mexico city, Mexico

Laura Barzola
Reumatología, Hospital de Niños Dr. Ricardo Gutiérrez, Buenos Aires, Argentina

L. B. De la Cruz-Becerra
Hospital Universitario "Dr. José E. González", UANL, Monterrey, Nuevo León, Mexico

Guadalupe Sánchez-Bringas
Embriology Department, Medicine School, Universidad Nacional Autónoma de Mexico, Mexico City, Mexico

Johannes Roth
Division of Pediatric Dermatology and Rheumatology, Children's Hospital of Eastern Ontario, Ottawa, Canada

Index